HORMONE REPLACEMENT THERAPY

CONTEMPORARY ENDOCRINOLOGY

P. Michael Conn, SERIES EDITOR

HORMONE
REPLACEMENT
THERAPY

Edited by

A. WAYNE MEIKLE, MD

University of Utah School of Medicine,
Salt Lake City, UT

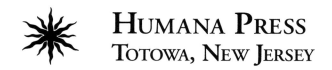

HUMANA PRESS
TOTOWA, NEW JERSEY

© 1999 Humana Press Inc.
999 Riverview Drive, Suite 208
Totowa, New Jersey 07512

For additional copies, pricing for bulk purchases, and/or information about other Humana titles,
contact Humana at the above address or at any of the following numbers: Tel: 973-256-1699;
Fax: 973-256-8341; E-mail: humana@humanapr.com or visit our website at http://humanapress.com

This publication is printed on acid-free paper. ∞
ANSI Z39.48-1984 (American National Standards Institute)
Permanence of Paper for Printed Library Materials.

Cover design by Patricia F. Cleary.

Printed in the United States of America.   10 9 8 7 6 5 4 3 2 1

Hormone replacement therapy / edited by A. Wayne Meikle
      p. cm. — (Contemporary endocrinology ; 13)
   Includes index.
   ISBN 0-89603-601-4 (alk. paper)
   1. Hormone therapy. I. Meikle, A. Wayne. II. Series:
Contemporary endocrinology (Totowa, NJ) ; 13.
   [DNLM: 1. Endocrine Diseases—drug therapy. 2. Hormone
Replacement Therapy. WK 190 H812 1999]
RM288.H67 1999
616.4' 061—dc21
DNLM/DLC
for Library of Congress   99-13398
                                            CIP

PREFACE

Replacement therapy for disorders of endocrine function is a highly specialized area of medicine and is discussed in comprehensive textbooks of endocrinology. These textbooks have reviewed current physiology, pathophysiology, differential diagnosis, and therapy. *Hormone Replacement Therapy* will focus on current replacement therapy for endocrine diseases and can assist the endocrinologist, gynecologist, pediatrician, urologist, general surgeon, neurologist, neurosurgery, psychiatrist, generalist, and trainee in the management of their patients. Endocrine testing used to monitor replacement therapy will be reviewed, but the reader is referred to appropriate diagnostic testing as covered in other textbooks of endocrinology. The authors have extensive knowledge and experience in the management of patients with specific endocrine disorders requiring replacement treatment. It is recognized that none is considered an expert in all areas of endocrine therapy, but the experts are sharing their knowledge and experience to facilitate use of the best approach available.

Differences of opinion exist in replacement therapy and each endocrinologist has a favorite regimen. Each review will attempt to be balanced without bias. If equivalent regimens exist, the authors will make this apparent to the reader, who can then choose which is best for the patient. Considerations of cost for similar regimens are important and must be discussed with the patient; thus, various options will make selection of replacement therapy an individual process.

Hormone Replacement Therapy is divided into six sections that cover hormone replacement therapy of the pituitary (I), parathyroid and vitamin D (II), thyroid (III), diabetes (IV), adrenal (V), and gonads of men and women (VI). In the pituitary section the management of diabetes insipidus and polydipsia in children is presented by Donald Zimmerman and Greg Uramoto and in adults by Andjela T. Drincic and Gary L. Robertson. Catherine K. Lum and Darrell M. Wilson review growth hormone therapy, with emphasis on growth disorders of children, whereas David E. Cummings and George R. Merriam focus on growth hormone and growth hormone secretagogues in adults.

In Part II, issues related to treatment of disorders of calcium metabolism caused by diseases affecting parathyroid hormone and vitamin D are presented by Robert F. Klein, Michael Bliziotes, and Eric S. Orwoll. In the thyroid section (III), current guidelines for thyroid hormone replacement therapy in patients with primary and secondary hypothyroidism are reviewed by David S. Cooper and special issues related to thyroid hormone replacement therapy during pregnancy are discussed by Jorge H. Mestman.

Part IV has four chapters discussing hormone replacement therapy of diabetes. R. Philip Eaton and Martin Conway focus on insulin management of the insulin-dependent diabetic, and David G. Johnson and Rubin Bressler provide guidelines for management of the type 2 diabetic. The special issues associated with the management of diabetes during pregnancy are highlighted by Kay F. McFarland and Laura S. Irwin, and Susan S. Braithwaite, Walter G. Barr, Amer Rahman, and Shaista Quddusi have developed an algorithm for diabetic therapy during glucocorticoid treatment of nonendocrine disease. The unique problems of treatment of the diabetic during exercise are summarized by Robert E. Jones.

v

There are three chapters in the adrenal section (V). One is by Lynnette K. Nieman and Kristina I. Rother, and covers glucocorticoid therapy for postnatal adrenal cortical insufficiency and for congenital adrenal hyperplasia. Therapy of mineralocorticoid deficiency disorders is summarized by W. Reid Litchfield and Robert G. Dluhy, and the pros and cons for dehydroepiandrosterone and pregnenolone therapy are carefully analyzed by Rakhmawati Sih, Hosam Kamel, Mohamad Horani, and John E. Morley.

Part VI covers sex hormone replacement issues in both men and women. Wayne Meikle details issues related to androgen replacement therapy in children and men with androgen deficiency, and the influence of androgen replacement therapy on sexual behavior, affect, and cognition is presented by Max Hirshkowitz, Claudia Orengo, and Glenn Cunningham. The merits and safety issues associated with testosterone therapy in older men are summarized by J. Lisa Tenover. Shalender Bhasin and Marjan Javanbakht present the rationale and recommendations for androgen therapy in men with muscle wasting disorders and particularly as related to AIDS. Hormonal contraception, which is becoming more commonly used in men and requires hormonal therapy to suppress spermatogenesis while maintaining normal testosterone concentrations, is discussed by Christina Wang and Ronald S. Swerdloff.

C. Matthew Peterson and Lawrence C. Udoff make recommendations for hormone replacement therapy in women with primary and secondary hypogonadism. Androgen replacement therapy in women is still somewhat controversial, but is becoming more accepted. A rationale basis for androgen therapy in women is made by Susan R. Davis and Henry G. Burger.

This work will serve as a great reference source to students, fellows, residents, and clinicians in many disciplines. Ultimately, the patient will benefit by receiving the best regimen to correct their hormonal deficit.

I express thanks to the distinguished authors who are recognized internationally and who accepted the invitation to contribute to the project and share their expertise. Sarah Fletcher provided invaluable assistance in correspondence and in compilation of the manuscripts. My sincere thanks to Dr. P. Michael Conn for his trust and encouragement in making the project a reality, and to Paul Dolgert and Debra Koch of Humana Press for their helpful suggestions.

A. Wayne Meikle, MD

CONTENTS

CONTRIBUTORS

WALTER G. BARR, MD, *Department of Rheumatology, Loyola University Medical Center, Maywood, IL*

SHALENDER BHASIN, MD, *Department of Medicine, UCLA School of Medicine; Divison of Endocrinology, Metabolism, and Molecular Medicine, Charles R. Drew University of Medicine and Science, Los Angeles, CA*

MICHAEL BLIZIOTES, MD, *Division of Endocrinology, Diabetes and Clinical Nutrition, Oregon Health Sciences University; Portland VA Medical Center, Portland, OR*

SUSAN S. BRAITHWAITE, MD, *Section of Endocrinology, Rush-Presbyterian St. Lukes, Chicago, IL*

RUBIN BRESSLER, MD, PHD, *Departments of Medicine and Pharmacology, University of Arizona, Tucson, AZ*

HENRY G. BURGER, MBBS, FRACP, *Prince Henry's Institute of Medical Research, Monash Medical Center, Clayton, Australia*

MARTIN CONWAY, MD, *Division of Endocrinology and Metabolism, Department of Medicine, School of Medicine, University of New Mexico; Lovelace Scientific Resources, Albuquerque, NM*

DAVID S. COOPER, MD, *Division of Endocrinology, Sinai Hospital of Baltimore; Thyroid Clinic, The Johns Hopkins Hospital, The Johns Hopkins University School of Medicine, Baltimore, MD*

DAVID E. CUMMINGS, MD, *Division of Metabolism, Endocrinology, and Nutrition, Department of Medicine, University of Washington School of Medicine, Veteran's Administration Puget Sound Health Care System, Seattle, WA*

GLENN R. CUNNINGHAM, MD, *Department of Research and Development, Veteran's Affairs Medical Center, Houston, TX*

SUSAN R. DAVIS, MBBS, FRACP, PHD, *The Jean Hailes Foundation; Department of Epidemiology and Preventive Medicine, Monash University, Clayton, Victoria, Australia*

ANDJELA T. DRINCIC, MD, *Clinical Research Center, Northwestern University Medical School, Chicago, IL*

ROBERT G. DLUHY, MD, *Endocrine-Hypertension Division, Brigham and Women's Hospital, Harvard Medical School, Boston, MA*

R. PHILIP EATON, MD, *Division of Endocrinology and Metabolism, Department of Medicine, School of Medicine, University of New Mexico, Albuquerque, NM*

MAX HIRSHKOWITZ, PHD, *Department of Psychiatry, Baylor College of Medicine; Sleep Research Center, Houston Veterans Affairs Medical Center, Houston, TX*

MOHAMAD HORANI, MD, *Division of Geriatric Medicine, St. Louis University Health Sciences Center; Geriatric Research Education and Clinical Center, St. Louis Veteran's Administration Medical Center, St. Louis, MO*

LAURA S. IRWIN, MD, *Department of Obstetrics and Gynecology, University Specialty Clinics, School of Medicine, University of South Carolina, Columbia, SC*

MARJAN JAVANBAKHT, MPH, *Divison of Endocrinology, Metabolism, and Molecular Medicine, Charles R. Drew University of Medicine and Science, Los Angeles, CA*

ROBERT E. JONES, MD, *Division of Endocrinology, Metabolism and Diabetes, University of Utah School of Medicine, Salt Lake City, UT*

DAVID G. JOHNSON, MD, *Section of Endocrinology, Departments of Medicine and Pharmacology, University of Arizona, Tucson, AZ*

HOSAM KAMEL, MD, *Division of Geriatric Medicine, St. Louis University School of Medicine, St. Louis, MO*

ROBERT F. KLEIN, MD, *Division of Endocrinology, Diabetes and Clinical Nutrition, Oregon Health Sciences University; Portland VA Medical Center, Portland, OR*

W. REID LITCHFIELD, MD, *Endocrine-Hypertension Division, Brigham and Women's Hospital, Harvard Medical School, Boston, MA*

CATHERINE K. LUM, MD, MPH, *Department of Pediatric Endocrinology and Diabetes, Stanford University, Stanford, CA*

KAY F. MCFARLAND, MD, *Department of Medicine, University of South Carolina School of Medicine, Columbia, SC*

A. WAYNE MEIKLE, MD, *Division of Endocrinology and Medicine, Department of Internal Medicine, University of Utah School of Medicine, Salt Lake City, UT*

GEORGE R. MERRIAM, MD, *Division of Metabolism, Endocrinology, and Nutrition, Department of Medicine, University of Washington School of Medicine, Veteran's Administration Puget Sound Health Care System, Seattle, WA*

JORGE H. MESTMAN, MD, *Department of Medicine, USC Ambulatory Health Center, University of Southern California, Los Angeles, CA*

JOHN E. MORELY, MB, BCH, *Division of Geriatric Medicine, St. Louis University Health Sciences Center; Geriatric Research Education and Clinical Center, St. Louis Veteran's Administration Medical Center, St. Louis, MO*

LYNNETTE K. NIEMAN, MD, *Developmental Endocrinology Branch, National Institute of Child Health and Human Development, National Institutes of Health, Bethesda, MD*

CLAUDIA ORENGO, MD, PHD, *Department of Medicine, Veteran's Affairs Medical Center, Houston, TX*

ERIC S. ORWOLL, MD, *Division of Endocrinology, Diabetes and Clinical Nutrition, Oregon Health Sciences University; Department of Endocrinology and Metabolism, Portland VA Medical Center, Portland, OR*

C. MATTHEW PETERSON, MD, FACOG, *Division of Reproductive Endocrinology and Infertility, Department of Obstetrics/Gynecology, University of Utah School of Medicine, University of Utah, Salt Lake City, UT*

SHAISTA QUDDUSI, MD, *Department of Medicine, University of Washington, Seattle, WA*

AMER RAHMAN, MD, *Section of Endocrinology, Rush-Presbyterian St. Lukes, Chicago, IL*

GARY L. ROBERTSON, MD, *Clinical Research Center, Northwestern University Medical School, Chicago, IL*

KRISTINA I. ROTHER, MD, *Developmental Endocrinology Branch, National Institute of Child Health and Human Development, National Institutes of Health, Bethesda, MD*

RAKHMAWATI SIH, MD, *Department of Internal Medicine and Geriatrics, Loyola Family Health Center at North Riverside, North Riverside, IL*

RONALD S. SWERDLOFF, MD, *Department of Medicine, UCLA School of Medicine; Division of Endocrinology, Department of Medicine, Harbor-UCLA Medical Center, Torrance, CA*

J. LISA TENOVER, MD, PHD, *Division of Geriatric Medicine and Gerontology, Emory University School of Medicine; Department of Medicine, Wesley Woods Geriatric Hospital, Atlanta, GA*

LAWRENCE C. UDOFF, MD, FACOG, *Division of Reproductive Endocrinology and Infertility, Department of Obstetrics/Gynecology, University of Utah School of Medicine, University of Utah, Salt Lake City, UT*

GREG URAMOTO, MD, *Department of Pediatrics, Mayo Clinic, Rochester, MN*

CHRISTINA WANG, MD, *Department of Medicine, UCLA School of Medicine; Clinical Research Center, Harbor-UCLA Medical Center, Torrance, CA*

DARRELL M. WILSON, MD, *Department of Pediatric Endocrinology and Diabetes, Stanford University, Stanford, CA*

DONALD ZIMMERMAN, MD, *Department of Adolescence and Pediatric Medicine, Mayo Clinic, Mayo Medical School, Rochester, MN*

I

PITUITARY

1

Diabetes Insipidus in Pediatrics

Donald Zimmerman, MD,
and Greg Uramoto, MD

INTRODUCTION

Separate mechanisms supply and eliminate water to maintain fluid homeostasis. A variety of sensors modulate thirst to drive water-seeking behavior and water intake. The elimination of water is achieved via hormonal control of the kidney. To insure that a healthy fluid balance is maintained, the mechanisms that accrue water can compensate for defects in the mechanisms that eliminate water and vice versa. Clinical problems arise when the capacity for this compensation is exceeded or when such compensation becomes unduly demanding.

When water losses increase for any reason, adults and children will drink more water in response to thirst if access to water is not limited. In this way, increased water intake can balance obligatory water outputs such as sweating or even mild diabetes. Infants, however, face unique problems with their inability to control their own water intake and their reliance on fluids to meet both water and caloric needs. Compounding this problem, infants cannot differentially communicate thirst, hunger, pain, and other messages. Because of the inability of infants to precisely control their water intake, the mechanisms of water elimination primarily maintain their water balance. Problems with their elimination systems, therefore, rapidly lead to clinical problems. As infants mature into ambulatory and communicative children, their control over their water intake improves and problems with water balance resemble those found in adults.

In this chapter, we will discuss the hormonal aspects of water balance and the problems that arise in this balance with emphasis on the pediatric population.

From: *Contemporary Endocrinology: Hormone Replacement Therapy*
Edited by: A. W. Meikle © Humana Press Inc., Totowa, NJ

ANATOMY AND PHYSIOLOGY

Water Consumption

THIRST INDUCTION

The driving force behind water intake is the sensation of thirst. Consumed water replaces fluid losses to maintain the osmolality of body fluids and to increase the vascular volume. No receptors found to date directly sense the absolute volume of the vascular space. This critical parameter is inferred from several indicators including the tonicity of the blood *(1)* and the blood pressure *(2)*. Inputs that influence thirst include baroreceptors of the cardiovascular system, osmoreceptors of the hypothalamus, and possibly osmoreceptors of the viscera.

The sensation of thirst is mediated at least in part by angiotensin II or by a molecule that is similar to this peptide. Receptors that bind angiotensin can be found in the lamina terminalis and in other areas of the brain that are associated with fluid homeostasis and with hemodynamic control *(3)*. Stimulation of these receptors is associated with increased thirst. Closely tied to the sensation of thirst is the appetite for salt (sodium). This is the most active osmotic ion in the extracellular space and greatly influences the fluid shifts between the intra- and extracellular spaces *(4)*.

Several conditions contribute to the induction and suppression of this sensation. Increasing the serum osmolality by 1 to 2% or decreasing the plasma volume by 10% increases thirst. Plasma osmolalities above 290 mOsmol/kg have also been strongly associated with the desire to drink *(5)*. The systemic infusion of solutes that do not easily traverse cell membranes like sodium chloride and sucrose will influence thirst more than permeable solutes like urea and glycerol. This probably reflects cellular fluid shifts between the intra- and extracellular fluid spaces.

THIRST SUPPRESSION

Thirst is suppressed by decreasing plasma osmolality by 1 to 2% or by increasing plasma volume by 10%. Drinking water will suppresses thirst before the serum osmolality decreases. Gastrointestinal (GI) stretch receptors convey a sense of fullness that inhibits thirst. In addition, temperature receptors in the oropharynx will inhibit thirst and vasopressin release when they are cooled *(6)*.

The stimuli for water seeking behavior are related to the vascular fullness and to the osmolality of the plasma. Inhibitors of thirst, however, cannot be exclusively tied to these parameters because of the lag time between drinking water, absorbing water, and the desired effects on vascular volume and osmolality. If the drive to drink water were inhibited only when the vascular space was affected, an excessively large amount of water may be consumed. To prevent this, other mechanisms including oropharyngeal temperature receptors and GI stretch receptors help to inhibit thirst more promptly. The subject of thirst and sodium hunger is complex. For a more thorough review, *see* refs. *(3)* and *(4)*.

Water Excretion

OVERVIEW

As organisms took to the land and as access to water became more restricted, opportunities to drink became more periodic. The intermittent acquisition of water necessitated a system that could dispose of water at controlled rates to keep the serum osmolality within a narrow window. The kidneys, under endocrine control, can excrete very dilute

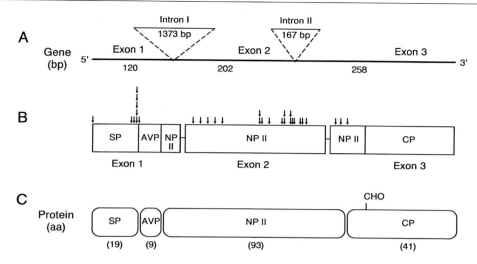

Fig. 1. Arginine vasopressin-neurophysin II-copeptin gene on chromosome 20. (**A**) Introns and exons. Exon 1 codes for a signal peptide (SP), arginine vasopressin (AVP), and the N-terminus of neurophysin II (NPII). Exon 2 codes for most of NPII. Exon 3 codes for the C-terminus of NPII and copeptin (CP). (**B**) The positions of known mutations in the gene. (**C**) Gene product. The signal peptide, AVP, neurophysin, and the glycopeptide (copeptin) are cleaved from this precurser.

or very concentrated urine to accomplish this vital task. The hormone in large part responsible for this endocrine control is arginine vasopressin (AVP). To conserve water by concentrating the urine, AVP increases the permeability of the collecting duct and thus allows the osmotic gradient in the renal medulla to draw free water out of the filtrate flowing through these ducts. Drawing free water from these ducts concentrates the urine and saves this water for physiologic needs.

Under physiological conditions, AVP adjusts the water output of the kidney and helps to preserve both plasma osmolality and vascular volume. Conserving water in the vascular space by limiting the kidney excretion of water is important, but not sufficient to maintain the vascular volume; osmotic pressure may draw free water out of the vascular space and into the tissues. The most important solute in maintaining the osmolality of the serum, sodium, is conserved via the renin-angiotensin-aldosterone pathways. Working together, AVP and aldosterone help to maintain the serum volume and osmolality. The interaction between these pathways provides physiologic flexibility and allows for fine control of the system.

AVP PRODUCTION AND RELEASE

The gene for vasopressin has been localized to chromosome region 20p13 *(7,8)* (*see* Fig. 1). Expression of this 2.5-kb prepro-AVP-NPII gene occurs in the magnocellular neurons of the hypothalamic and paraventricular nuclei in the hypothalamus. The gene consists of three exons and two introns that code for a macromolecular protein that contains vasopressin. This macromolecular protein is cleaved at dibasic amino acid sites by trypsin-like cleavage as the molecule travels down the pituitary stalk in secretory granules. Along with vasopressin, this macromolecular protein contains a signal peptide, neurophysin II binding protein, and a glycoprotein of uncertain function called copeptin. Upon reaching the posterior pituitary, the AVP nonapeptide is ready for release (*see* Fig. 2).

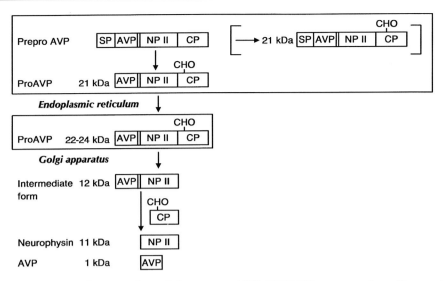

Fig. 2. Compartmental processing of the prepro-AVP-NPII-CP gene product. Prepro-AVP is converted to pro-AVP by removal of the signal peptide and the addition of carbohydrate side chains in the endoplasmic reticulum. Pro-AVP, which is partially glycosylated in the endoplasmic reticulum, is further glycosylated in the golgi apparatus. The glycosylated portion, copeptin, is cleaved in the process of axonal transport in secretory vesicles. Upon reaching the posterior pituitary, vasopressin is available for release into the blood stream.

Arginine vasopressin is comprised of a 6-amino acid disulfide ring plus a 3-amino acid tail that has an amide group attached to the carboxy terminus. This molecule is evolutionarily related to oxytocin, differing in two amino acids, but retaining the disulfide ring. Vasopressin is bound to neurophysin II while stored in the neurohypophysis. The function of this combination is still under investigation, but it has been hypothesized that the binding of neurophysin to vasopressin conveys some protection against degredation.

Vasopressin release is mediated by a stimulus-release coupling mechanism commonly found in many types of neurons. The action potential stimulus for the release of vasopressin permits the influx of extracellular calcium. This influx, in turn, stimulates the movement of the stored granules to the cell membrane and subsequent exocytosis.

STIMULI OF AVP RELEASE

AVP allows for the reabsorption of water at the level of the kidney. The need for more or less water reabsorption is estimated by the blood tonicity, the blood pressure, and the blood volume. These parameters, then, influence AVP release.

The tonicity of the blood is sensed by osmoreceptors of the anterolateral hypothalamus near the supraoptic nuclei in the anterolateral hypothalamus *(9)* (*see* Fig. 3). These osmoreceptors are functionally outside of the blood brain barrier, as evidenced by the measurement of similar serum levels of AVP in response to changing the serum tonicity with urea and with sodium. These receptors synapse with both the paraventricular (PVN) and supraoptic (SON) nuclei to influence the release of AVP from the magnocellular neurons in these nuclei. The amount of AVP released in response to the osmolality of the serum is precisely controlled. Under physiologic conditions, vasopressin blood levels rise linearly in response to rising serum osmolalities after a minimum set point of serum

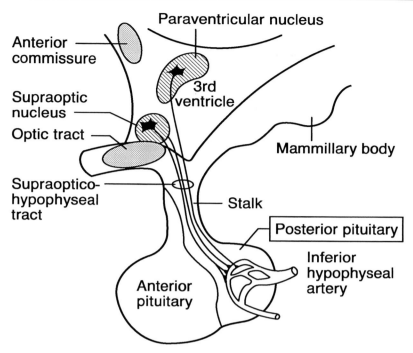

Fig. 3. Anatomy of the hypothalamus and the pituitary. Magnocellular neurons of the supraoptic (SON) and paraventricular nuclei (PVN) extend down the supraopticohypophyseal tract and synapse with capillaries of the posterior pituitary.

osmolality is reached. This set point of AVP release has been shown to be approximately 275 mOsm/kg *(10)*. Studies have shown that AVP rises approximately 1pg/mL for every 3 mOsm/kg above this threshold for vasopressin release. The levels of vasopressin are also influenced by diurnal variations in older children with night-time vasopressin levels that are approx two to three times higher than daytime levels *(11)*. Released in response to increasing serum tonicity, AVP will induce more water conservation through the kidney and thus counteract the rising serum tonicity.

Blood pressure changes contribute to the release of AVP via the high-pressure baroreceptors of aortic arch and the carotid sinuses. The baroreceptors of the aortic arch and the carotid sinuses send projections to the SON and the PVN via cranial nerves IX and X *(12)*. Signals from these pressure receptors are first routed through the nucleus tractus solitarious in the brainstem. Neurons from this nucleus then synapse with the supraoptic and paraventricular nuclei and tonically inhibit vasopressin release. Under normal physiologic conditions, these neurons tonically inhibit AVP release. Blood pressure decreases of 5 to 15% will lead to an exponential increase in vasopressin levels due to baroreceptor stimulation *(13)*. This is unlike the linear increase in vasopressin levels in response changes in osmolality as described above (*see* Fig. 4). The levels of AVP found in hypotensive states will far exceed the 5 pg/mL needed for maximal antidiuresis. AVP concentrations in this range will induce vasoconstriction via the V1 receptor on the vascular smooth muscle and will help to support the falling blood pressure. The true physiologic importance of this effect is not yet clear *(14)*.

Stretch receptors of the left atrium respond to changes in atrial blood volume. Like the baroreceptors of the aortic arch and the carotid sinuses, these stretch receptors induce

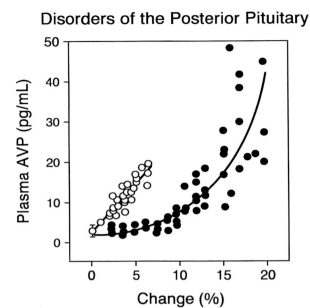

Fig. 4. Relationship between osmotic and nonosmotic stimuli for vasopressin release. Relationship of plasma AVP concentration to the percent increase in blood osmolality (open circles) or decrease in blood volume (closed circles).

vasopressin release during hypovolemic states. The influence of these neurons, however, is thought to be less important than that of the baroreceptors of the carotid sinuses and the aortic arch.

Nausea increases vasopressin levels above those needed for maximum antidiuresis. Nausea due to motion sickness, drugs, or illness can increase vasopressin levels 100-fold. The mechanism for this vasopressin release in these settings seems to be unrelated to the mechanisms that mediate vasopressin release due to changes in blood pressure and blood osmolality. Blockade of nausea with antiemetics will not suppress the vasopressin response to hypovolemia and hypernatremia.

Vasopressin release is inhibited by glucocorticoids. This modulating effect is illustrated by patients with glucocorticoid deficiency where vasopressin is inappropriately released *(15)*. The mechanism for this tonic inhibition of vasoressin by glucocorticoids remains elusive. Studies in transgenic mice implicate the involvement of a proximal *cis*-acting element that is suppressed by glucocorticoid action *(16)*.

RESPONSE TO AVP

The kidneys respond to serum vasopressin via the V_2 receptor. The binding of vasopressin to this receptor induces incorporation of aquaporin-2 molecules into the luminal membrane of the collecting ducts. This incorporation creates water channels through the walls of the collecting duct that allow water to flow down the concentration gradient in the renal medulla *(17,18)* *(see* Fig. 5). This flow draws free water out of the filtrate in the collecting ducts and thus concentrates the urine. These aquaporin-2 molecules are a part of a family of membrane proteins that are responsible for channel-mediated water transport. They are stored in the membranes of intracytoplasmic vesicles until these

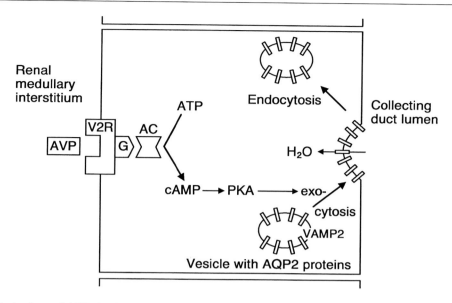

Fig. 5. Action of AVP in the collecting duct cell. AVP binds to the V_2 receptor, causing the G-protein to activate adenylate cyclase (AC), resulting in an increase in cAMP and activation of protein kinase A (PKA). The catalytic subunit of PKA, via an undetermined phosphorylation step, causes fusion of membrane bodies bearing aquaporin-2 (AQP2) water channel and VAMP2 with the collecting duct luminal membrane, resulting in an increase in water flow from the urine into the renal medullary interstium. Demeclocycline, lithium, high calcium, and low potassium interfere with these processes, possibly at the level of cAMP generation and AQP2 synthesis or action.

vesicles are incorporated into the cellular membranes by an exocytotic process. Without the stimulation of AVP, membrane endocytosis pulls these transmembrane proteins back into intracytoplasmic vesicles. The incorporation and removal of aquaporins from the luminal surface via exocytosis and endocytosis comprises a membrane shuttle mechanism.

DIABETES INSIPIDUS

The term diabetes insipidus is applied to conditions in which patients produce high volumes of dilute and glucose-free urine. Diabetes insipidus (DI) may arise from different underlying causes. A lack of AVP secretion is usually termed neurogenic, cranial, central, or hypothalamic DI. A failure to respond to circulating AVP is termed nephrogenic DI. Excessive water intake due to a lesion in the thirst centers is termed dipsogenic DI. Excessive water intake due to psychosis or other mental illnesses is termed psychogenic DI. And finally, symptoms of DI associated with a pregnancy-associated physiologically higher metabolism of AVP is termed gestational DI. Moreover, patients may have only a partial defect in either their production of or response to AVP. Each of the above categories can be further subdivided (*see* Table 1).

Pathology of DI

Problems with either vasopressin production or vasopressin response can lead to DI. The pathologies are divided at an anatomic level according to the site of the defect.

Table 1
Causes of Diabetes Insipidus

Neurogenic:	Idiopathic
	Hypothalamic or pituitary lesion
	Head trauma/surgical trauma
	CNS infection
	Lymphocytic infundibulohypophysitis
	Ischemia
	Mass lesion
	Germinoma
	Craniopharyngioma
	Hematoma
	Infiltrative lesion
	Langerhans cell histiocytosis
	Neurosarcoid
	Familial
	Autosomal dominant
	X-linked recessive
	Part of other syndrome
	DIDMOAD
Nephrogenic:	Idiopathic
	Kidney lesion
	Nephrocalcinosis
	Obstructive uropathy
	Medullary cystic disease
	Sickle cell disease
	Drugs
	Lithium
	Rifampin
	Aminoglycosides
	Acetohexamide
	Vinblastine
	Cisplatin
	Methoxyflurane
	Electrolyte Abnormalities
	Hypokalemia
	Hypercalcemia
	Familial
	X-linked recessive: V_2 receptor
	Autosomal recessive: aquaporin II
	Unknown: DIDMOAD
Dipsogenic:	Idiopathic
	Hypothalamic lesion
	Head trauma
	Drugs
	Lithium
	Carbamazepine
	Infection
	Tuberculosis
	Mass lesion
	Germinoma
	Infiltrative lesion
	Neurosarcoidosis
	Langerhans cell histiocytosis
Psychogenic:	Compulsive water drinking
	Schizophrenia

NEUROGENIC DIABETES INSIPIDUS

The pathologies involved in neurogenic DI are quite varied. Any lesion, which damages the neurons that produce and release vasopressin, will lead to DI. In broad cateories, these lesions include trauma, surgical damage, mass lesions, and infiltrative lesions. Of particular interest are the genetically transmitted forms of the disease. In patients with this pathology, vasopressin-producing neurons selectively degenerate, leaving the rest of the brain intact *(19)*. The genetic defects are in the AVP-neurophysin II gene on chromosome 20. The mutations isolated to date mainly cluster within the coding sequences of either the signal peptide of the precursor or within the coding sequence for neurophysin II *(20,21)*. At the time of this writing, only one mutation in the vasopressin sequence has been described. Accumulation of the improperly cleaved molecule most likely leads to the destruction of AVP-producing cells. Idiopathic DI is usually sporadic, although autosomal-dominant and X-linked recessive forms have been described. The prevalence of this condition in the two sexes is approximately equal. Antibodies may be found against AVP-secreting cells in approximately 30% of cases *(22)*.

NEPHROGENIC DIABETES INSIPIDUS

In nephrogenic diabetes insipidus, the kidneys fail to respond to AVP. This failure can result from an inability to establish and maintain a hyperosmotic medullary interstitium or from an inability to sense the AVP signal. The osmotic gradient in the kidney is necessary to pull water from the collecting ducts in order to concentrate the urine. The collecting ducts must also be able to allow this gradient to draw water from the collecting ducts. The permeability of the collecting duct membrane is under vasopressin control.

The concentration gradient in the kidneys is generated by sodium-potassium pumps in the ascending loops of Henle. In renal failure, the kidneys may not be able to generate an effective concentration gradient. Several primary kidney diseases, including obstructive pathologies, medullary cystic disease, and infarctions, may impair the kidneys' ability to establish a concentration gradient. Similarly, systemic diseases such as sarcoidosis, amyloidosis, and Sjogren syndrome, lead at times to DI. The loops of Henle, and the concentration gradients that they produce, are also affected in hypercalcemia and hypokalemia *(23)*. Studies in animals have shown that hypokalemia interferes with sodium transport in the thick ascending limb of the loop of Henle *(24,25)*. Recent work has suggested that a particular calcium receptor, the Ca (2+)-sensing receptor, may play a role in water metabolism and may explain hypercalcemia-mediated DI *(26)*. In addition to influencing the concentration gradient in the kidney, hypercalcemia may also play a role in the response of the kidney to AVP *(27,28)*.

A defect in the receptor for AVP can also lead to an inability to respond to AVP *(29,30)*. Familial transmission of the disorder has been reported, and it most commonly manifests an X-linked dominant pattern of inheritance *(31,32)*. The females in these families manifest some degree of DI but do not have as many clinical problems as do the males. The gene involved has been localized using linkage analysis to the long arm of the X chromosome at band 28 *(33,34)*. It codes for the V_2 receptor, which activates the membrane shuttle mechanism via cyclic AMP production, in response to arginine vasopressin.

Specific mutations in the V_2 receptor have been elucidated in patients with nephrogenic DI *(35,36)*. These can be classified into at least three distinct phenotypes *(37)* (*see* Fig. 6). In the first phenotype, the mutant receptor can be transported to the surface of the cell, but is unable to combine with vasopressin. In the second phenotype, the mutant receptor may

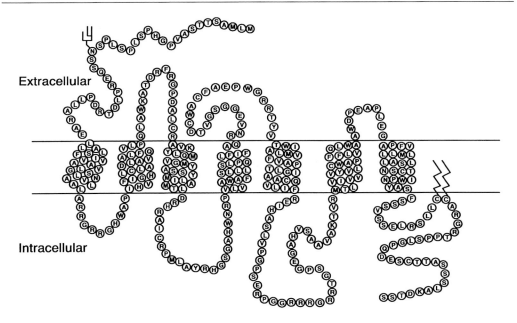

Fig. 6. Schematic representation of the V$_2$ receptor.

accumulate in intracellular compartments, but is unable to reach the cell surface. In the third phenotype, the mutant gene is ineffectively translated, or the protein is rapidly degraded.

Mutations in the gene for aquaporin-2 can also lead to nephrogenic DI (*see* Fig. 7). The family history is consistent with autosomal recessive inheritance *(38)*. Defects in the aquaporin-2 gene have included a missense mutation *(39)* that probably result in an inability to properly transport the protein to the plasma membrane and a nonsense mutation *(40)* that results in an early stop codon for the aquaporin-2 molecule.

Evaluation of Children

The most common presenting symptoms of post-infancy DI include polyuria and polydipsia with a preference for consuming ice-cold water. In a patient with this history, the differential diagnosis includes diabetes insipidus, diabetes mellitus, hypercalcemia, hypokalemia, renal failure, and psychogenic polydipsia. An initial screen for serum osmolality, serum electrolytes, BUN, serum glucose, serum calcium, and urine osmolality will aid in establishing the diagnosis of the patient. The hallmark of DI is a urine osmolality that is inappropriately low compared to the serum osmolality. In normal subjects, serum osmolalities above 295 mOsm/L will induce urine concentrations above 700 mOsm/L. In patients with partial DI, serum sodium levels greater than 143 mmol/L and serum osmolality of above 295 mOsm/L induce urine concentrations of approx 500–700 mOsm/L. Patients with complete DI will concentrate their urine to approx 250 mOsm/L or less under these conditions. To definitively establish an inability to concentrate the urine owing to a defect in the release of vasopressin or in the response to vasopressin, a water deprivation test can be used.

WATER DEPRIVATION TEST IN CHILDREN

The purpose of this test is to evaluate the urine osmolality in response to a slightly hyperosmolal and volume-contracted state. Under these conditions, the urine concentra-

Extracellular

Intracellular

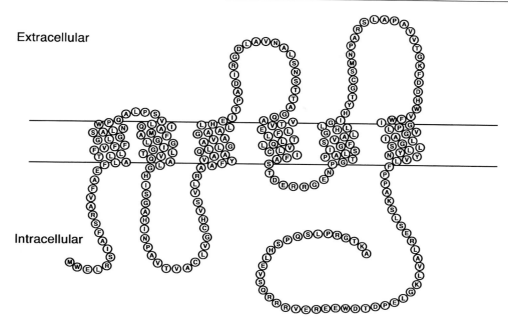

Fig. 7. Schematic representation of aquaporin-2 protein based on the proposed topology of the rat homolog and of aquaporin-1.

tion should rise as free water is conserved. Before starting the test, children should be taken off of any desmopressin acetate or diuretics for at least one day. Children should be endocrinologically normal besides the suspected deficit in vasopressin or should be well replaced with appropriate hormone treatment before starting the test.

The test would optimally begin with the child's first void in the morning after awakening. Serum should be drawn at this time and both the serum and the urine should be analyzed for osmolality. The initial blood pressure and weight should be recorded. From this time to the end of the study, the child must be prevented from consuming any food or fluids and watched carefully for compliance. The volume and timing of all urine samples should be recorded. With each void, serum is collected and the osmolality of both the serum and the urine should be determined. Weights should be determined every 1–2 h and an early termination of the test should be considered if the weight falls by > 3%. Patients with psychogenic polydipsia may be overhydrated by more than 3% of the body weight. Thus, if this diagnosis is strongly suspected, body weight may be allowed to fall more markedly. If symptoms of hypoglycemia develop, a serum glucose or a reflectance meter glucose level should be obtained.

If the urine osmolalities exceed 1000 mOsm/L at any time, a diagnosis of DI can be ruled out. If the urine osmolality is <250 mOsm/L with a concurrent serum osmolality of >295 mOsm/L, a diagnosis of DI is confirmed. If neither of these conditions is met, the test could continue for 12 h in children and 9 h in toddlers.

When a diagnosis of DI is confirmed, a distinction between nephrogenic and neurogenic DI can be made by injecting aqueous vasopressin subcutaneously at a dose of 1 U/m^2 *(41)*. Patients with neurogenic DI will respond by doubling the concentration of their urine within appropriately 3 h. If available, measuring the AVP levels at the time of maximal dehydration, is also helpful in differentiating between nephrogenic and neurogenic DI.

In psychogenic DI, the initial polyuric state is an appropriate response to the increased water intake. The urine concentrating ability, as demonstrated by a water deprivation test, is therefore, usually normal. With a long standing problem, the high turnover of water may compromise the kidney's ability to concentrate urine. Under these circumstances, they may be resistant to AVP and may transiently resemble other forms of nephrogenic DI.

RADIOLOGY

Patients with DI often have characteristic magnetic resonance imaging (MRI) findings of the posterior pituitary. In normal subjects, the T-1 weighted MR image shows a distinctly bright signal that is thought to represent intracellular storage granules of processed vasopressin and neurophysin (42,43). This bright signal is lost in patients with DI owing to a wide range of pathologies associated with injury to the magnocellular neurons including trauma, mass lesions, and infiltrative lesions. In patients with nephrogenic DI, the magnocellular neurons are intact, but much of the stored vasopressin has been released, giving a similar loss of the bright signal. In some instances, the development of this MRI finding may lag behind clinical signs of DI (44). For this reason, the initial MRI may be normal in patients with polyuria and polydipsia who eventually are found to have a central nervous system (CNS) lesion. Because MRI findings will change over time, serial scans may be useful (45).

FUTURE DIAGNOSTIC APPROACHES

Given the time and cost needed to establish a diagnosis of neurogenic DI in some patients, new ways to test for the condition are being sought. One promising avenue of exploration is the measurement of urinary aquaporins. Saito et al. found that patients with neurogenic DI secrete much less aquaporin-2 per mg of creatinine in the urine compared to normal patients under ad libitum water intake (46).

Evaluation of Infants

In the infant age range, the most common clinical presentation of DI is failure to thrive. The differential diagnosis, then, is very broad and includes both organic and inorganic pathologies. The major endocrine disorders, which could present as failure to thrive, include hypothyroidism, adrenal insufficiency, hyperparathyroidism, diabetes mellitus, and diabetes insipidus. Infants with DI may not be satisfied with feedings, but are quieted by water. Vomiting and constipation may be present. Parents may report that the infant's diaper is always wet. In decompensated states, the infant will lose enough water to develop dehydration, hypernatremia, and hyperthermia. Repeated episodes of hypernatremia and seizures may lead to brain damage and mental impairment.

WATER DEPRIVATION TEST IN INFANTS

In infants with frank polyuria, a dilute urine, and a classic serum profile (high sodium and osmolality with normal potassium, glucose calcium, and creatinine) a diagnosis of DI may be made without a water deprivation test. In cases when the diagnosis is not clear, a water deprivation test may be helpful. The purpose of this test is still to evaluate the ability of the kidney to concentrate urine appropriately. Serum samples should be obtained with each void after starting the test in the morning. Both of these samples should be sent to the laboratory for determinations of osmolalities. This test should be done in a hospital

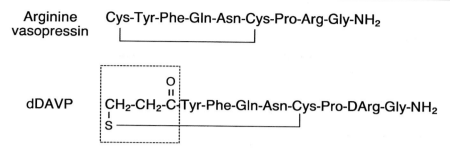

Fig. 8. Structural sequence of arginine vasopressin and desmopressin acetate (dDAVP).

setting, especially since infants may easily develop hypoglycemia with prolonged fasting. For this reason, testing should include a serum glucose with the serum osmolalities and should stop after 6–7 h if no definitive results are obtained. The period of time between determinations of the serum glucose should not exceed 1 h during the test. If the infant does not void for over an hour, a glucose level should be obtained without waiting for the void. Interpreting the results of the serum and urine osmolalities resembles that for children.

THERAPUTIC COMPOUNDS AND TREATMENT STRATEGIES

Desmopressin Acetate

Desmopressin acetate is a clinically valuable tool for treating DI (*see* Fig. 8). In children with neurogenic diabetes insipdus who have free access to water, desmopressin acetate is used widely. Treatment with desmopressin acetate in infants and any other patient who cannot directly control their own fluid intake can be difficult and requires extremely close monitoring.

Desmopressin acetate (1-deamino-8-D-arginine vasopressin) is an arginine vasopressin analog that has approximately twice the antidiuretic potency of the parent molecule in addition to a greatly decreased pressor effect *(47,48)*. Tablets, nasal solutions, and injectable forms are available. Orally administered desmopressin acetate doses are 20-fold larger than the usual nasal doses. For the oral route, antidiuretic effects may be seen approx 1 h after administration of the medication with a peak effect seen approx 4–7 h after administration. The peak effects of nasally administered desmopressin acetate can be seen at approx 1–5 h with a duration of 5–20 h. The exact mechanism of the metabolism of the drug are unknown, but the duration of the effect has been shown clincally to depend on the size of the dose. Owing probably to more predictable absorption, the clinical effects following nasal administration of desmopressin acetate usually varies less than that following the oral route. The timing, duration and magnitude of the antidiuresis of a single dose can be quite variable between different patients.

The optimum route of administration and the dosage will be influenced most strongly by the patient's ability to swallow pills, by the absorption rate of desmopressin acetate from the GI track and the nasal mucosa in the individual patient, and by the presence of nasal congestion. The convenience of the tablet forms of desmopressin acetate, which do not have to be refrigerated, may be preferred by teenagers.

A low starting dose and titration of this dose for effect is recommended. A nasal dose of desmopressin acetate at 1 µg/kg daily divided into two doses has been used successfully in premature infants *(49)*. Term infants can be started on 1 μg nasally every 12 h. In children less than 12 years old, a reasonable initial dose of nasally administered desmopressin acetate is approximately 5 μg/d divided qd or bid. In children able to swallow tablets, the initial dosage can be 0.1 mg–0.2 mg/d divided qd or bid. The dosages of both of these routes should be adjusted to allow for periods of diuresis between doses. Controlling nocturia is usually a priority for toilet-trained patients and may be the only goal of treatment. In patients with only mild symptoms, a single dose at night without a morning dose, can be enough to sufficiently control their problem.

Diuretics

This pharmacologic strategy is used in patients with nephrogenic DI, in infants, and as an adjunct to desmopressin acetate therapy. Thiazide and furosemide diuretics have been found to help conserve water by inducing a mildly hypovolemic state. By doing this, these diuretics promote better sodium resorption in the proximal tubules of the kidney with a resulting reabsorption of more water at this level of the nephron. Thus, the volume of the filtrate that reaches the collecting ducts, the site of AVP action, will be modestly reduced. A failure to concentrate the urine at the level of the collecting ducts will then have a smaller clinical impact.

Treatment with hydrochlorothiazide in combination with mild salt depletion would be a reasonable first choice in the management of DI in infants. Doses can range from 1–3 mg/kg/d divided into three doses. If this treatment is unsuccessful in ameliorating the infant's failure to thrive, then treatment with vasopressin or a vasopressin analogue can be considered. The use of desmopressin acetate in an infant is difficult because fluid intake is regulated by both hunger and thirst. With this dual control of fluid intake, infants may drink when they are already fluid overloaded.

In children, a reasonable starting dose of hydrochlorothiazide is 1–3 mg/kg/d divided bid or tid. The addition of ameloride at 0.2–0.7 mg/kg/d may improve the potassium status in patients receiving diuretic therapy *(50)*. A salt-restricted diet is usually necessary to induce the slight degree of hypovolemia and to prevent hypokalemia.

Inhibitors of Prostaglandin Synthesis

When used alone, these drugs have little effect on water conservation. When used with a thiazide diuretic, however, water conservation improves markedly in patients with nephrogenic DI *(51)*. This property has been attributed to the elimination of the prostaglandin inhibition of sodium absorption at the renal tubules. As a result, sodium reabsorption improves, and the osmolality of the renal interstitium is more efficiently increased. Following the solute reabsorption, water reabsorption is also augmented. This effect has been shown with indomethacin, tolmetin and acetylsalicylic acid *(52,53)*.

SPECIAL CONDITIONS

Primary Polydipsia and Psychogenic Polydipsia

Mimicking DI, these disorders can present with polydipsia and polyuria. In primary polydipsia, the patient has an increased desire to drink. With our incomplete knowledge of mechanisms of thirst, the exact etiology of this disorder remains unexplained. Patients with this disorder may consume excessive amounts of water in belief of specific health benefits or other reasons. Excessive water intake leads to chronic volume expansion and impairment of AVP release *(54)*. The differentiation of primary polydipsia and DI can be aided by the use of MRI. A hyperintense signal in the neurohypophysis on a T_1 weighted scan has been demonstrated in one series of patients with primary polydipsia, but not in patients with diabetes insipidus *(55)*.

Hypodipsia

Lesions due to trauma, hydrocephalus, granulomatous disease, tumor, histiocytosis, surgery, or congenital malformation can involve the thirst centers of the brain and can lead to hypodipsic states. Patients who lack thirst to control water intake rely heavily on varying urine concentrations to maintain water homeostasis. In patients with DI in addition to hypodipsia, the mechanisms, which control both fluid intake and fluid conservation, are lost. The combination of DI and hypodipsia, then, is very clinically challenging. In children with this combination of problems, the treatment regimen must be tailored to meet the needs of the patient and the family. A careful account of the water intake is necessary. Weights should be obtained once or twice each day and should be checked more often with illnesses. Desmopressin acetate may be used to reduce urine output. Serum sodium levels should be monitored frequently when starting or changing regimens. In growing children, target weights must be changed to take appropriate weight gain into account.

Chemotherapy

Children receiving chemotherapy need adequate fluid management for optimal care. Saline diuresis is often employed to reduce the renal toxicity of the chemotherapy agents. Children with DI in addition to their oncologic problem require special attention. Longer acting preparations of AVP such as desmopressin acetate are difficult to use in this setting since the effects are difficult to turn off quickly. Aqueous vasopressin is available and has been used successfully to manage DI in patients receiving chemotherapy *(56)*. This agent has a short half-life and can be administered intravenously via a continuous infusion. By adjusting the rate of infusion, the patient's urine output can be varied to achieve the goals of the chemotherapy protocol. As an initial dose, a continuous infusion of aqueous AVP at a rate of between 0.08–0.1 mU/kg/h during the hydration phase is recommended. This rate is much lower than the 1.0–3.0 mU/kg/h necessary to maintain homeostasis in a patient receiving maintenance fluids *(57)*. Frequent monitoring of urine output, urine specific gravity, weight, and serum sodium levels are needed to allow appropriate hydration. Blood pressure and pulse must also be monitored closely as well in view of the pressor effects of AVP.

Surgery

Fluid management during surgery of DI patients may follow one of two general strategies. The first strategy comprises administration of the long-acting vasopressin analog desmopressin acetate. Fluids should be given to replace insensible fluid losses and urine output. Alternatively, an intravenous infusion of aqueous vasopressin may be given and titrated to allow for fine control of the urine output. Aqueous vasopressin doses of 1–3 mU/kg/h has been used in this setting. Monitoring the urine output, urine specific gravity, and the serum sodium levels is necessary during and after the procedure. Fluids should be administered to replace insensible fluid losses in addition to urine output. This method allows minute-to-minute control of both the intake and output of fluids. The first strategy allows close regulation of fluid intake whereas output is changeable only when the activity of medications used to treat the DI begins to wane.

SUMMARY

DI may arise from abnormalities of vasopressin secretion or from aberrations of renal responsiveness to vasopressin. It presents with polyuria and polydipsia in childhood, but it may present as failure to thrive in infancy. Treatment is predicated of adequate understanding of the etiology.

Chronic treatment of children with desmopressin is usually straightforward. Other strategies may be needed for special circumstances. Infants may be effectively treated with thiazide diuretics. Adipsic patients may be treated with desmopressin acetate, but must be given maintenance fluids with appropriate supplements as directed by frequent body weight determinations and by less frequent measurements of serum sodium. Intravenous fluid administration should comprise insensible losses in addition to urine output. Urine output may be controlled with desmopressin or with aqueous vasopressin.

REFERENCES

1. Robertson GL. Physiology of ADH secretion. Kidney Int 1987;21:S20–S26.
2. McKinley MJ. Common aspects of the cerebral regulation of thirst and renal sodium excretion. Kidney Int 1992;37:S102–S106.
3. Denton DA, McKinley MJ, Weisinger RS. Hypothalmic integration of body fluid regulation. Proc Natl Acad Sci USA 1996;93(14):7397–7404.
4. Johnson AK, Thunhorst RL. The neuroendocrinology of thirst and salt appetite: visceral sensory signals and mechanisms of central integration. Frontiers Neuroendocrinol 1997;18(3):292–353.
5. Coggins CH, Leaf A. Diabetes insipidus. Am J Med 1967;42(5):807–813.
6. Salata RA, Verbalis JG, Robinson AG. Cold water stimulation of oropharyngeal receptors in man inhibits release of vasopressin. J Clin Endocrinol Metab 1987;65(3):561–567.
7. Rao VV, Loffler C, Battey J, Hansmann I. The human gene for oxytocin-neurophysin I (OXT) is physically mapped to chromosome 20p13 by in situ hybridization. Cell Genet 1992;61:271–273.
8. Riddell DC, Mallonnee R, Phillips JA. Chromosomal assignment of human sequences encoding arginine vasopressin-neurophysin II and growth hormone releasing factor. Somat Cell Molec Genet 1985;11(2): 189–195.
9. Robertson GL, Shelton RL, Athar S. The osmoregulation of the vasopressin. Kidney Int 1976;10: 25–37.
10. Zerbe, RL, Robertson GL. Osmoregulation of thirst and vasopressin secretion in human subjects: effects of various solutes. Am J Physiol 1983;224(6):E607–E614.
11. Rittig S, Knudsen UB, Norgaard JP, Abnormal diurnal rhythm of plasma vasopressin and urinary output in patients with enuresis. Am J Physiol 1989;256:F664–F671.
12. Robertson GL. Thirst and vasopressin function in normal and disordered states of water balance. J Lab Clin Med 1983;101(3):351–371.
13. Wiggins RC, Basar I, Slater JD, et al. Vasovagal hypotension and vasopressin release. Clin Endocrinol 1977;6(5):387–393.
14. Hirsch AT, Majzoub JA, Ren CJ, et al. Contribution of vasopressin to blood pressure regulation during hypovolemic hypotension in humans. J Appl Physiol 1993;75(5):1984–1988.
15. Green HH, Harrington AR, Valtin H. On the role of antidiuretic hormone in the inhibition of acute water diuresis in adrenal insufficiency and the effects of gluco- and mineralocorticoids in reversing the inhibition. J Clin Invest 1970;49(9):1724–1736.
16. Burke ZD, Ho MY, Morgan H, Smith M, Murphy D, Carter D. Repression of vasopressin gene expression by glucocorticoids in transgenic mice: evidence of a direct mechanism mediated by proximal 5' flanking sequence. Neuroscience 1997;78(4):1177–1185.
17. Deen PM, Verdijk MA, Knoers NV, et al. Requirement of human renal water channel aquaporin-2 for vasopressin-dependent concentration of urine. Science 1994;264:92–95.

18. Saito T, Ishikawa SE, Sasaki S, et al. Urinary excretion of aquaporin-2 in the diagnosis of central diabetes insipidus. J Clin Endocrinol Metab 1997;82(6):1823–1827.
19. Ito M, Oiso Y, Murase T, et al. Possible involvement of inefficient cleavage of preprovasopressin by signal peptidase as a cause for familial central diabetes insipidus. J Clin Invest 1993;91(6):2565–2571.
20. Rittig S, Robertson GL, Siggaard C, et al. Identification of 13 new mutations in the vasopressin-neurophysin II gene in 17 kindreds with familial autosomal dominant neurohypophyseal diabetes insipidus. Am J Hum Genet 1996;58(1):107–117.
21. Rauch F, Lenzner C, Nurnberg P, Frommel C, Vetter U. A novel mutation in the coding region of neurophysin II is associated with autosomal dominant neurohypophyseal diabetes insipidus. Clin Endocrinol 1996;44(1):45–51.
22. Scherbaum WA, Wass JA, Besser GM, Bottazzo GF, Doniach D. Autoimmune cranial diabetes insipidus: its association with other endocrine diseases and with histiocytosis X. Clin Endocrinol 1986;25(4):411–420.
23. Schwartz WB, Relman AS. Effects of electrolyte disorders on renal structure and function. N Engl J Med 1967;276(8):452–458.
24. Bennett CM. Urine concentration and dilution in hypokalemic and hypercalcemic dogs. J Clin Invest 1970;49(7):1447–1457.
25. Galla JH, Booker BB, Luke RG. Role of loop segment in the concentrating defect of hypercalcemia. Kidney Intl 1986;29(5):977–982.
26. Hebert SC, Brown EM, Harris HW. Role of the Ca(2+)- sensing receptor in divalent mineral ion homeostasis. J Exp Biol 1997;200:295–302.
27. Berl T. The cAMP system in vasopressin-sensitive nephron segments of the vitamin D-treated rat. Kidney Intl 1987;31(5):1065–1071.
28. Beck N, Singh H Reed SW, et al. Pathogenic role of cyclic AMP in the impairment of urinary concentrating ability in acute hypercalcemia. J Clin Invest 1974;54(5):1049–1055.
29. Bichet DG, Razi M, Lonergan M, et al. Hemodynanic and coagulation responses to 1-desamino (8-D-arginine) vasopressin in patients with congenital nephrogenic diabetes insipidus. N Engl J Med 1988;318(14):881–887.
30. Moses AM, Miller JL, Levine MA. Two distinct pathophysiological mechanisms in congenital nephrogenic diabetes insipidus. J Clin Endocrinol Metab 1988;66(6):1259–1264.
31. Knoers N, van der Heyden H, van Oost BA, et al. Three-point linkage analysis using multiple DNA polymorphic markers in families with X-linked nephrogenic diabetes insipidus. Genomics 1989;4(3):434–437.
32. Oksche A, Schulein R, Rutz C, Liebenhoff U, Dickson J, Muller H, Birnbaumer M, Rosenthal W. Vasopressin V2 receptor mutants that cause X-linked nephrogenic diabetes insipidus: analysis of expression, processing, and function. Molec Pharmacol 1996;50(4):820–828.
33. Kambouris M, Dlouhy SR, Trofatter JA, et al. Localization of the gene for X-linked nephrogenic diabetes insipidus to Xq28. Am J Med Genet 1988;29(1):239–246.
34. Rosenthal W, Seibold A, Antaramian A, et al. Molecular identification of the gene responsible for congenital nephrogenic diabetes insipidus. Nature 1992;359:233–235.
35. Merendino JJ Jr, Speigel AM, Crawford JD, et al. Brief report: A mutation in the vasopressin V2-receptor gene in a kindred with X-linked nephrogenic diabetes insipidus. N Engl J Med 1993;328:1538.
36. Holtzman EJ, Harris HW Jr, Kolakowski LF, et al. Brief report: A molecular defect in the vasopressin V2-receptor gene causing nephrogenic diabetes insipidus. N Engl J Med 1993;328(21):1562,1563.
37. Tsukaguchi H, Matsubara H, Taketani S, Mori Y, Seido T, Inada M. Binding-, intracellular transport-, and biosynthesis-defective mutations of vasopressin type-2 receptor in patients with X-linked nephrogenic diabetes insipidus. J Clin Invest 1995;96(4):2043–2050.
38. Langley JM, Balfe JW, Selander T, Ray PN, Clarke JT. Autosomal recessive inheritance of vasopressin-resistant diabetes insipidus. Am J Med Genet 1991;38(1):90–94.
39. Deen PMT, Croes H, van Aubel RA, Ginsel LA, van Os CH. Water channels encoded by mutant aquaporin-2 genes in nephrogenic diabetes insipidus are impaired in their cellular routing. J Clin Invest 1995;95(5):2291–2296.
40. Hochberg Z, Van Lieburg A, Even L, Brenner B, Lanir N, van Oost BA, Knoers NV. Autosomal recessive nephrogenic diabetes insipidus caused by an aquaporin-2 mutation. J Clin Endocrinol Metab 1997;82(2):686–689.
41. Muglia LJ, Majzoub JA. Pediatric endocrinology. In: Sperling MA, ed. Disorders of the Posterior Pituitary. WB Saunders Co, Philadelphia, 1996, p. 206.

42. Abernethy LJ, Qunibi MA, Smith CS. Normal MR appearances of the posterior pituitary in central diabetes insipidus associated with septo-optic dysplasia. Pediatr Radiol 1997;27(1):45–47.
43. Colombo N, Berry I, Kucharczyk J, Kucharczyk W, de Groot J, Larson T, Norman D, Newton TH. Posterior pituitary gland: appearance on MR images in normal and pathologic states. Radiology 1987;165(2):481–485.
44. Weimann E, Molenkemp G, Bohles HJ. Diabetes insipidus due to hypophysis. Horm Res 1997;47(2):81–84.
45. Mootha SL, Barkovich AJ, Grumbach MM, Edwards MS, Gitelman SE, Kaplan SL, Conte FA. Idiopathic hypothalamic diabetes insipidus, pituitary stalk thickening, and the occult intracranial germinoma in children and adolescents. J Clin Endocrinol Metab 1997;82(5):1362–1367.
46. Saito T, Ishikawa S, Sasaki S, Nakamura T, Rokkaku K, Kawakami A, Honda K, Marumo F, Saito T. Urinary excretion of aquaporin-2 in the diagnosis of central diabetes insipidus. J Clin Endocrinol Metab 1997;82(6):1823–1827.
47. Kimbrough RD, Cash WD, Branden LA, et al. Synthesis and biologic properties of 1-desamino-8-lysine vasopressin. J Biol Chem 1963;238:1411.
48. Sawyer WH, Grzonka Z, Manning M. Neurohypophysial peptides: design of tissue specific agonists and antagonists. Molec Cell Endocrinol 1981;22(2):117–134.
49. Giacoia GP, Watson S, Karathanos A. Treatment of neonatal diabetes insipidus with desmopressin. Southern Med J 1984;77(1):75–77.
50. Knoers N, Monnens LA. Amiloride-hydrochlorothiazide versus indomethacin-hydrochlorothiazide in the treatment of nephrogenic diabetes insipidus. J Pediatr 1990;117(3):499–502.
51. Fichman MP, Speckhart P, Zia P, Lee A. Antidiuretic response to prostaglandin inhibition by indomethacin in nephrogenic diabetes insipidus. Clin Res 1976;24:161A.
52. Chevalier RL, Rogol AD. Tolmetin sodium in the management of nephrogenic diabetes insipidus. J Pediatr 1982;101(5):787–789.
53. Monn E. Prostaglandin synthetase inhibitors in the treatment of nephrogenic diabetes insipidus. Acta Pediatr Scand 1981;70(1):39–42.
54. Moses AM, Clayton B. Impairment of osmotically stimulated AVP release in patients with primary polydipsia. Am J Physiol 1993;265:R1247–R1252.
55. Moses AM, Clayton B, Hochhauser L. The use of T1-weighted MR imaging to differentiate between primary polydipsia and central diabetes insipidus. AM J Neuroradiol 1992;13(5):1273–1277.
56. Bryant WP, O'Marcaigh AS, Ledger GA, Zimmerman D. Aqueous vasopressin infusion during chemotherapy in patients with DI. Cancer 1994;74(9):2589–2592.
57. McDonald JA, Martha PM, Kerrigan J, Clarke WL, Rogol AD, Blizzard RM. Treatment of the young child with postoperative central diabetes insipidus. Am J Dis Child 1989;143(2):201–204.

2

Treatment of Diabetes Insipidus in Adults

Andjela T. Drincic, MD,
and Gary L. Robertson, MD

Contents

INTRODUCTION

Diabetes insipidus (DI) is a syndrome characterized by the excretion of abnormally large volumes of dilute urine. The polyuria causes symptoms of urinary frequency and nocturia and sometimes, incontinence and enuresis. It is also associated with thirst and/or a commensurate increase in fluid intake (polydipsia).

DI is divisible into 3 types, each of which has a different pathogenesis and must be managed in a different way *(1)*. The most common type of DI is that owing to a deficiency of the antidiuretic hormone, arginine–vasopressin (AVP). It is usually if not always caused by destruction of the neurohypophysis and is variously referred to as pituitary, neurohypophyseal, cranial, or central DI. This destruction can be caused by various acquired *(1)* or genetic causes *(2)*. It can also be caused or uncovered by the increased metabolism of AVP that occurs during pregnancy, in which case it is known as gestational DI *(3)*. A second type of DI is owing to renal insensitivity to the antidiuretic effect of AVP. It is caused by defects in the AVP receptor or postreceptor elements that mediate antidiuresis and is usually referred to as nephrogenic DI. It too can be caused by acquired diseases *(1)* or genetic mutations *(4)*. The third type of DI is owing to excessive intake of water. It is generally referred to as primary polydipsia and is divisible into two subtypes: one is caused by an

From: *Contemporary Endocrinology: Hormone Replacement Therapy*
Edited by: A. W. Meikle © Humana Press Inc., Totowa, NJ

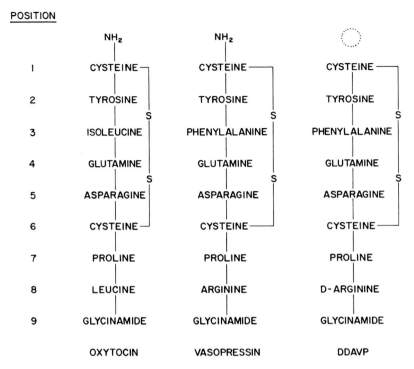

Fig. 1. The amino-acid sequence of oxytocin, vasopressin, and DDAVP.

abnormality in the thirst mechanism and may be referred to as dipsogenic DI *(5)*; the other is owing to a more generalized cognitive defect and is usually called psychogenic polydipsia *(6,7)*. Because it is important, but not always easy, to distinguish between the three types of DI, a brief review of the basic anatomy, biochemistry, physiology, and diagnostic methodology of antidiuretic function is in order before discussing management.

VASOPRESSIN

AVP is a nonapeptide hormone (Fig. 1) synthesized and secreted by magnocellular neurohypophyseal neurons that originate in the supraoptic and paraventricaular nuclei and terminate on capillaries in the median eminence and posterior lobe of the pituitary gland *(8)*. The gene encoding AVP is located on chromosome 20 near the gene for a closely related neurosecretory hormone, oxytocin *(9)*. It has three exons and directs the production of a preprohormone that contains 166 amino acids and comprises a signal peptide, AVP, an AVP binding protein known as neurophysin II (NP) and a glycosylated peptide known as copeptin (CP). Like other preprohormones, the AVP precursor is formed by cleavage of signal peptide in the endoplasmatic reticulum, transported through the Golgi to neurosecretory vesicles, where it is further processed to AVP, NPII, and CP and stored until release into the systemic circulation.

The main if not the only important physiological action of AVP in humans is to regulate urinary concentration and flow by altering the hydro-osmotic readsorption of solute free water in the distal and collecting tubules of the kidney. This effect is mediated by special receptors (V2) that activate adenyl cyclase and cause preformed water channels composed of a protein known as aquaporin II to be inserted in the luminal membrane of tubular cells *(10,11)*. The insertion of these water channels permits solute free water to be readsorbed osmotically down the gradient that exists between the hypertonic medulla and the hypotonic tubular fluid. This results in a reduction in urine volume and a rise in urine concentration to levels 3 to 4 times that of plasma (osmolality = 1200–1500 mosmoles/kg). When AVP is low or absent, relatively little solute free water is reabsorbed and the urine that remains is increased in volume and unconcentrated (osmolality < 100 mosmoles/ kg), a condition known as water diuresis.

Supraphysiologic amounts of AVP or a synthetic analog desmopressin (DDAVP) also act via V2 receptors to stimulate the release of Factor VIII and von Willebrand factor from endothelium *(12)*. This effect is probably of no physiologic importance but has important implications for treatment of certain bleeding disorders *(see below,* DDAVP). AVP can also act via a different type of receptor (V1) to stimulate contraction of vascular and gastrointestinal smooth muscle, urinary excretion of potassium and prostaglandin production by the kidney. However, it is not yet clear if these effects are of any physiologic or pharmacologic importance.

The secretion of AVP and, presumably, NPII and CP are regulated primarily by the effective osmotic pressure of extracellular fluid *(13)*. This effect is mediated via osmoreceptors that are located in the anterior hypothalamus near the supraoptic nucleus. These osmoreceptors appear to operate like a discontinuous or "set -point" receptor and are extremely sensitive to changes in the plasma concentration of sodium and certain other solutes. Among healthy adults, the "set" and sensitivity of the osmoregulatory system shows relatively large, genetically determined differences. On average, however, plasma AVP begins to rise at a plasma osmolality or sodium concentration around 280 mosmoles/kg or 135 meq/L and it reaches levels sufficient to produce maximum antidiuresis at a plasma osmolality and sodium of only about 295 mosmoles/kg and 143 meq/L. AVP secretion can also be stimulated by hypotension, hypovolemia, nausea, and certain other nonosmotic factors but these influences probably are important only under certain pathological conditions.

DIFFERENTIAL DIAGNOSIS OF DI

Once the diagnosis of DI has been established by determining that a 24-h urine volume has an increased volume (> 50 mL/kg), subnormal concentration (< 300 mOsm/kg) and no excessive glucose or other solutes, it is necessary to determine which type of DI is present *(14)*.

Measurements of basal plasma osmolality and/or sodium are of limited value in the differential diagnosis of DI. Although one would expect them to be high in pituitary or nephrogenic DI and low in primary polydipsia, the values in the three groups vary widely and overlap extensively probably as a consequence of inherent individual differences in the "set" of their osmoregulatory systems. In patients with uncomplicated pituitary and nephrogenic DI, basal plasma osmolality and sodium are usually within normal limits because an increase in plasma osmolality of as little as 1–2 % induces thirst and a compensatory increase in fluid intake. Conversely, in patients with primary polydipsia, a decrease in plasma osmolality and sodium of the same magnitude suppresses AVP secretion and induces a maximum water diuresis that serves to prevent overhydration. Thus, unless basal plasma osmolality and sodium are elevated, a fluid deprivation test is indicated to determine if mild hypertonic dehydration causes concentration of the urine (maximum Uosm > 300 mOsm/kg). If not, primary polydipsia is excluded and an injection of AVP (1 IU Pitressin) or its synthetic analog, desmopressin (4 μg DDAVP) will suffice to differentiate between severe pituitary and nephrogenic DI. However, if dehydration results in concentration of the urine, partial pituitary or nephrogenic DI are not excluded and the subsequent urinary response to AVP or DDAVP is of no diagnostic value. In this case, other approaches to the differential diagnosis are required.

In patients who concentrate their urine during the dehydration test, the simplest, least expensive and most accurate way to differentiate between primary polydipsia, partial pituitary and partial nephrogenic DI is to measure the plasma AVP level before and during a standard fluid deprivation test and then plot the results as a function of concurrent plasma and urine osmolalities. The sample collected before the start of the fluid deprivation test is the most useful for diagnosing nephrogenic DI. If plasma AVP is normal or high (> 1.0 pg/mL) when urine osmolality is low (< 300 mOsm/kg), the patient has nephrogenic DI. The most informative value for differentiating partial pituitary DI from either form of primary polydipsia is obtained at the end of dehydration test. However this distinction will be clear only if the levels of plasma osmolality and sodium concentration achieved are above the normal range. This is often difficult to achieve by fluid deprivation alone in patients who concentrate their urine–i.e., in those with primary polydipsia or partial defects in AVP secretion or action. Therefore, it is also usually necessary to give them a short infusion of 3% saline (1–2 h at 0.1 mL/kg/min) to achieve the desired level of plasma hypertonicity. In pituitary DI, plasma AVP may rise slightly but its relationship to plasma osmolality is subnormal reflecting their primary deficiency in secretion of vasopressin. In dipsogenic DI, however the rise in plasma AVP is normal for the rise in plasma osmolality. Measuring AVP is not recommended as a routine approach to the diagnosis of DI in pregnancy because special protease inhibitors must be used during collection of the sample to prevent rapid degradation of AVP in vitro.

An alternate way to differentiate between the three types of DI is to give a short (24–48 h) closely monitored therapeutic trial of DDAVP (2–4 μg subcutaneously [sc] every 12 h or 20 μg intravenously [in] every 8 h). If DDAVP promptly abolishes thirst and polyuria as well as polyuria without excessive retention of water (i.e., plasma sodium concentration remains within the normal limits) the patient probably has pituitary DI. If DDAVP has no effect, the most likely diagnosis is nephrogenic DI. If DDAVP abolishes the polyuria but causes smaller reductions in thirst and polydipsia and/or results in development of water intoxication (i.e., plasma sodium concentration below the normal limits) the odds are about 20 to 1 that the patient has dipsogenic DI.

In addition to these diagnostic studies, an MRI of the brain can be obtained to determine the absence of the posterior pituitary " bright" spot that is seen in noninfused T1 weighted images of most (70–90%) normal individuals (15). This spot appears to be absent in most if not all patients with pituitary DI but is usually present in those with nephrogenic DI or primary polydipsia. Apart from expense, the problem with this approach is that it does not distinguish between primary polydipsia and nephrogenic DI. Moreover, it may be misleading because 20% of normal adults do not emit the signal where as a few patients with pituitary DI do. Nevertheless, the presence of a completely normal posterior pituitary bright spot speaks strongly against pituitary DI.

TREATMENT OF DI

In general, the goal of DI treatment is to improve the patients quality of life by restoring urinary volume to normal, or, at least reducing urinary frequency to minimize interference with daytime activities or sleep at night. Because DI *per se* usually does not cause significant morbidity (if the patient has intact thirst mechanism and unrestricted access to water), the modality of treatment chosen should not be only effective but safe as well.

TREATMENT OF PITUITARY DI

Because pituitary DI is owing to a primary deficiency of AVP that is rarely if ever reversible, it can be and should be treated by replacing the hormone or giving other drugs that mimic its antidiuretic effect. Agents currently available are as follows:

1. ARGININE VASOPRESSIN (PITRESSIN®) is a synthetic form of the natural hormone. When given as a subcutaneous injection in a dose of 1–5 U, aqueous Pitressin has a very short half-life with onset of action within 30 min and duration of action of 3–6 h. Given intravenously, it has an equally rapid onset of action, and a duration that persists for 1–2 h after stopping the infusion. Therefore, its principal use is for acute, short-term treatment of DI. Aqueous pitressin comes as a buffered solution of L-arginine vasopressin in 1 mL snap-top vials at a concentration of 20 U/mL. Because it is so highly concentrated, it must be diluted several thousand fold to achieve the desired concentration in the infusate. We recommend that it be prepared in 5% dextrose and water at a concentration of 1–2 mU/mL and infused at a rate of 0.5 mL/kg/h. Side effects of Pitressin occur only at very high doses and are primarily nausea, vomiting, and abdominal cramps.
2. VASOPRESSIN TANNATE IN OIL (PITRESSIN TANNATE®) is an extract of bovine posterior pituitary in depot preparation. When given in a dose of 5–10 U sc or im, it has an antidiuretic effect that lasts up to 72 h. The duration of action varies markedly because of variable bioavailability. For many years it was a standard of treatment for pituitary DI. However, it is no longer available in the US.
3. LYSINE VASOPRESSIN (LYPRESSIN, DIAPID®) is a synthetic vasopressin which has a lysine in place of arginine at position 8. 50 USP posterior pituitary (pressor) U/mL. When given intranasally, Diapid has a very short half life with rapid onset of action (30 min) and short duration of action (4–6 h). The recommended dose is 1–2 sprays intranasally (providing 2–4 U of vasopressin) 4–6 times/d. Side effects are essentially the same as those encountered with AVP. Diapid is currently available on a compassionate basis through Novartis Pharmaceutical.
4. DESMOPRESSIN: 1 DEAMINO 8 D ARGININE VASOPRESSINE (DDAVP®) *(16)* is a synthetic analog of L arginine vasopressin in which the amino group at position 1 has been removed and the naturally occurring levoisomer of arginine at position 8 has been replaced by its dextroisomer (Fig 1). DDAVP has no significant side effects except for a slight reduction in blood pressure and tachycardia when given iv or sc at supraphysiologic doses. Because it is less susceptible to degradation by N–terminal peptidases, it can be given by the oral as well as parenteral and intranasal routes.
   a. Oral DDAVP is provided as tablets of 0.1 or 0.2 mg *(17,18)*. It is easy to use, does not require refrigeration, and is the treatment of choice in situations where poor absorption from intranasal mucosa is expected (*see below,* intranasal DDAVVP). It may also be preferred in children. The usual dose is 100–200 µg PO two or three times daily. In

some patients, its effects can be erratic owing, presumably, to variable absorption of the peptide from the gastrointestinal (GI) tract.

b. Intranasal DDAVP is supplied as a 2.5-mL bottle containing 100 μg/mL of desmopressin. It is available for two different modes of administration; a calibrated rhinal tube applicator that can be used to deliver volumes of 50–200 μL containing 5–20 μg of DDAVP, respectively; or a nasal spray pump that delivers a fixed 100 μL vol containing 10 μg of desmopressin. The main advantage of the rhinal tube is the ability to give small, graded doses of medication. However, the technical skills required for proper use render it impractical for many patients. The nasal spray is easier to use, but provides a higher minimal dose and larger graduations of 10 μg which may be more than is necessary for some patients. The usual dose by either route is 10–20 μg intranasally two or three times a day but individual requirements vary widely. Poor or erratic responses usually result from incomplete absorption owing to inflammation of the nasal mucosa secondary to upper respiratory infections, allergic rhinitis, or sinusitis. Poor vision and severe arthritis also make intranasal DDAVP difficult to use. Allergy to DDAVP, with or without resistance to its biologic effects is rare.

c. Parenteral DDAVP is supplied as a 10-mL vial containing 4 μg/mL of desmopressin and is available for intravenous and subcutaneous use. It is the treatment of choice for patients who, because of their age or intercurrent illness, are unable to take or absorb the drug by the intranasal or oral route. The usual dose in adults is 1–4 μg once or twice daily.

After more than 20 yr of clinical experience, desmopressin has become the drug of choice for the treatment of pituitary DI. In uncomplicated patients, administration of the drug completely eliminates the polyuria and polydipsia (Fig. 2)—both acutely and during long-term therapy—without any recognized side effects. Desmopressin is equally effective in all patients with pituitary DI, irrespective of the severity or cause of their vasopressin deficiency. Because of individual differences in absorption and metabolism, the dose required to achieve complete, around-the-clock control varies from patient to patient. Increasing the dose size generally increases the duration of action rather than magnitude of antidiuresis. Thus, once-a-day dosing is possible, but it is more expensive because higher total dose must be used. Desmopressin therapy is also completely safe for patients with uncomplicated pituitary DI. At doses that are 5–10 times higher than those conventionally used to treat pituitary DI, DDAVP does stimulate the release of Factor VIII and Von Willebrand factor, (which is the basis of its hemostatic applications). However hypercoagulability is not a risk with the usual antidiuretic doses.

A major misconception in DDAVP therapy is the fear that the drug will induce hyponatremia unless the patient is allowed to "escape" frequently from the antidiuretic effect. However, even high doses of DDAVP do not induce hyponatremia in patients with uncomplicated pituitary DI because the drug induces slight retention of water which reduces plasma osmolality/sodium and promptly suppresses thirst and fluid intake. Hyponatremia develops only if the patient has an associated abnormality in thirst or drinks excessively for other reasons. Thus, patients should be instructed to drink only to satisfy their thirst and avoid excessive social drinking. In addition, patients should be advised that any increase in fluid intake, for example, to treat a cold or "flu," can lead to life-threatening water intoxication. When hospitalized for other medical or surgical reasons, even routine maintenance or "keep open" rates of iv fluids may induce water intoxication if given together with DDAVP. Therefore, whenever intravenous fluids are given to a patient on antidiuretic therapy, plasma sodium should be monitored frequently and the rate of fluid adjusted as needed to prevent overhydration (*see below*, Special Considerations, Postoperative and Posttraumatic DI).

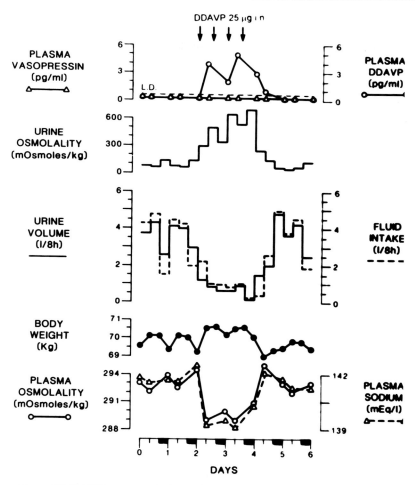

DDAVP 25 μg i n

PLASMA
VASOPRESSIN
(pg/ml)
Δ——Δ

PLASMA
DDAVP
(pg/ml)
○——

URINE
OSMOLALITY
(mOsmoles/kg)

URINE
VOLUME
(l/8h)
——

FLUID
INTAKE
(l/8h)
- - - -

BODY
WEIGHT
(Kg)

PLASMA
OSMOLALITY
(mOsmoles/kg)
○——○

PLASMA
SODIUM
(mEq/l)
Δ - - - Δ

DAYS

Fig. 2. The effect of DDAVP on water balance in pituitary DI. DDAVP was given intranasally in dose of 25 μg every 8 h. The urinary values are for successive 8 h collections. Note that the treatment produced a commensurate, contemporaneous decrease in fluid intake and urinary output with minimal retention of water as indicated by slight increase in body weight and decrease in plasma osmolality/sodium, both of which remain within normal range.

5. CHLORPROPAMIDE also increases urine concentration and reduces urine volume in patients with pituitary DI (Fig. 3) *(19,20)*. Its mechanism of action is uncertain, but may involve enhancing the secretion as well as the antidiuretic action of residual AVP *(21)*. It may also act via some independent mechanism *(20)*, because it is often most effective in patients with severe if not complete deficiencies of vasopressin (*see below*; this section) and its antidiuretic action begins sooner in patients with a prolonged deficiency of antidiuretic hormone (often in 24–48 h) than in patients recently exposed to AVP or DDAVP (in which case the maximum effect may not occur for 7–10 d). This fact as well as the lack of antidiuretic effect of chlorpropamide in normal subjects or patients with primary polydipsia suggests that the mechanism requires some change in antidiuretic function that results from prolonged deficiency of the hormone.

Contrary to long held views, chlorpropamide is equally effective in patients with severe or partial pituitary DI. For unknown reasons unrelated to the severity of the AVP

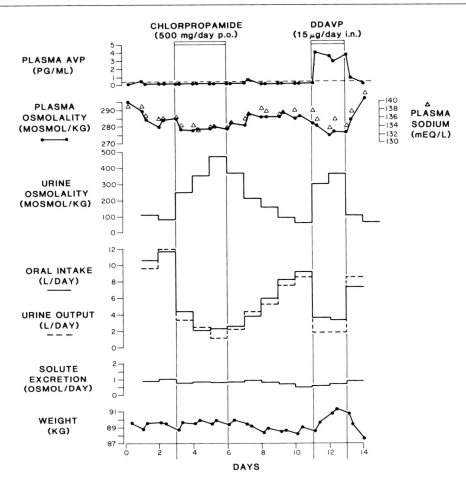

Fig. 3. The effect of chlorpropamide and DDAVP on water balance in pituitary DI. Note that the urinary volumes are for 24 h urinary collections. Given separately, both chlorpropamide and DDAVP produced a significant rise in urine osmolality and a decrease in fluid intake and urinary output with minimal water retention as indicated by the slight increase in body weight and decrease in plasma osmolality/sodium, both of which remain within the normal range. Note that the magnitude of antidiuretic effect is similar in both drugs.

deficiency, the magnitude of antidiuretic effect varies widely from patient to patient. Thus, some can be completely controlled on a dose as low as 100 mg/d, whereas others will achieve only a 50% reduction in urine output at doses as high as 500 mg/d. In these cases, the addition of chlorothiazide (250–500 mg bid) or hydrochlorothiazide (25–50 mg bid) potentiates the antidiuretic effect of chlorpropamide and usually reduces urine production to the normal range. However, chlorpropamide should not be combined with DDAVP, because this combination is no more effective than DDAVP alone. The most serious side effect of chlorpropamide is hypoglycemia but this is uncommon unless the patient engages in strenuous, prolonged physical activity or severely restricts food intake. Nevertheless, because of this risk, the drug should be used with caution (if at all) in children, the elderly and patients with chronic renal failure or concurrent hypopituitarism—mainly hypoadrenalism.

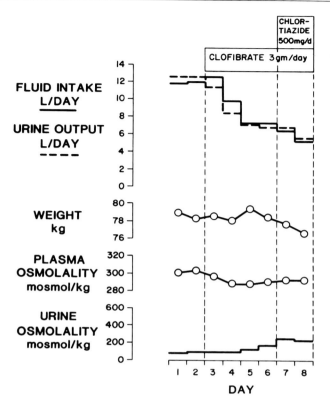

Fig. 4. The effect of clofibrate and HCTZ on water balance in pituitary DI. Note that both clofibrate given alone or with HCTZ produce an increase in urine osmolality as well as a fall in fluid intake and urine output with minimal water retention as evidenced by the slight fall in plasma osmolality and increase in body weight that remains within normal limits.

Chlorpropamide can also produce antabus-like reaction to alcohol in about 30% of patients but this effect is well tolerated if the patient is forewarned and usually attenuates or stops with repeated exposure.

6. CLOFIBRATE in divided doses of 1–3 gm/d also increases urine concentration and decreases urine volume in patients with pituitary DI (Fig. 4). Like chlorpropamide, its mechanism of action is uncertain and may involve potentiation of AVP action, enhanced secretion or an AVP independent effect *(22)*. Its antidiuretic effect is usually but not always less than that of chlorpropamide *(23)*. It is not widely used because of limited efficacy and related side effects, the most important being induction of gallstone formation and subsequent increase in risk for gallbladder cancer.

7. CARBAMAZEPINE in doses of 200–600 mg/d has a pronounced antidiuretic effect in patients with pituitary DI. Its mechanism of action is unknown *(24–26)*. Its most serious potential side effect is agranulocytosis, which necessitates periodical hematologic monitoring.

8. THIAZIDE DIURETICS also reduce urine volume and increase urine concentration in patients with pituitary DI (Fig. 4). They act via two vasopressin-independent mechanisms related to their natriuretic effect. One is interference with sodium absorption in the ascending limb of Henle's loop, which impairs urine dilution, and the other is mild volume depletion, which increases reabsorption of glomerular filtrate in proximal tubule,

thereby decreasing distal delivery *(27–29)*. When combined with dietary sodium restriction, the thiazides reduce urine volume by an average of 50%. This effect is inadequate for sole therapy of pituitary DI but is very useful as an adjunct to the other oral agents. The usual recommended dose of hydrochlorothiazide is 25–50 mg once or twice daily. Side effects are mainly related to consequences of electrolyte and metabolic disturbances, namely hypokalemia, hypercalcemia and rarely hyperglycemia with glycosuria.

Special Considerations in Therapy of Pituitary DI

POSTOPERATIVE AND POSTTRAUMATIC DI

Postsurgical and post-traumatic DI occur secondary to trauma to the median eminence, pituitary stalk or posterior pituitary *(30)*. Incidence of postsurgical DI varies from 5–25% following transsphenoidal surgery to almost 75% after suprasellar operations for craniopharyngeoma *(31)*. Post-traumatic DI usually occurs in a setting of a head trauma in a motor vehicle accident and is thought to be owing to a shearing force on a pituitary stalk or hemorrhagic ischemia of the hypothalamus or posterior pituitary. In either case, more than 80% of supraoptic nuclei need to be destroyed in order for clinically overt DI to occur. There are several special problems associated with diagnosis and treatment of DI in this clinical setting:

1. The first issue is whether the patient's polyuria is due to excessive administration of fluids, to pituitary DI, to nephrogenic DI that occasionally results from certain anesthetics used during the surgery, or to osmotic diuresis caused by administration of mannitol, contrast dyes or hyperglycemia. The first possibility can be assessed simply by slowing (or if possible stopping) the rate of parenterally administered fluids and remeasuring urinary output, urine osmolality and serum sodium. If the patient does not concentrate his or her urine before plasma sodium reaches 145 mq/l, excessive fluid intake can be eliminated as a cause and AVP or DDAVP can be injected to rule out nephrogenic DI. The last possibility of an osmotic diuresis can be evaluated by the clinical setting, tests for glucosuria, or by determining if the product of urine volume × osmolality exceeds 15 µmoles/kg/min.

2. When the presence of pituitary DI is established, the next problem is choosing the mode of therapy. Edema and inflammation after transsphenoidal surgery often preclude the use of nasal DDAVP and altered mental status and unreliability of gastrointestinal absorption are a relative contraindication to the use of oral DDAVP. Therefore, parenteral DDAVP in a dose of 1–2 µg im or iv once or twice daily is usually the initial treatment of choice. The intravenous route is sometimes preferable to im or sq administration because it provides rapid delivery and a quick "off" time if water intoxication occurs. When maintenance therapy is required, the parenteral can be changed to intranasal therapy as soon as the nasal mucosa has healed (usually 1–2 wk after transsphenoidal surgery) and the patient is capable of learning the technique.

3. The third problem is choosing optimal fluid replacement. Initially, owing to altered mental status, the patient may be dependent on administered iv fluids. During DDAVP treatment, fluids cannot be given indiscriminately but must be carefully matched to total urinary and insensible losses to prevent over or under hydration. The effectiveness of the regimen should be monitored by measuring plasma osmolality or sodium at least twice a day. A rise in either variable indicates dehydration and should be treated by administering supplemental fluid and increasing the dose of DDAVP if DI is not adequately controlled. An excessive decrease in plasma osmolality or sodium indicates overhydration and should be treated by reducing fluid intake or, as a last resort, discontinuing antidiuretic therapy.

Attempting to regulate water balance by titrating the dose of DDAVP is not recommended, because the resultant changes in urinary flow are impossible to control precisely and often lead to large and rapid fluctuations in salt and water balance. In some patients, massive head trauma and/or radical surgeries may be associated with damage to hypothalamic osmoreceptors for thirst and vasopressin secretion. Therefore, DDAVP treatment in such patient poses a risk for water intoxication when the patient attempts to regulate his or her own fluid balance. We shall deal with management of this challenging clinical scenario in a separate section.

4. A fourth problem in the management of postsurgical and post-traumatic DI results from the possible fluctuations in the course of the disease during the first 4–6 wk. This is often referred to as the triple phase response, which is characterized by initial DI followed by SIADH with or without return of permanent DI *(32,33)*. For this reason, it is advisable to stop treatment for the first month to determine if DI recurs. It should be remembered that the development of associated adrenal insufficiency will mask signs of DI. Therefore, spontaneous resolution of signs or symptoms should always prompt evaluation of adrenal function.

THIRST DISORDERS WITH DI

Hyperdipsia. As previously mentioned, water intoxication is an uncommon side effect of desmopressin therapy in uncomplicated pituitary DI. However, it may arise in patients who also have hyperdipsia owing to associated damage to the inhibitory component of the thirst mechanism *(34)*. The treatment of this combined defect is problematic because no method has been devised for abolishing abnormal thirst. Therefore, standard doses of DDAVP cannot be given to these patients, because they will invariably result in water intoxication. However, the nocturia and sleep disturbances can be prevented by a small dose of desmopressin at bedtime. This regimen will not result in water intoxication if the dose of desmopressin is titrated to permit recurrence of polyuria during the day, when most of the abnormal water intake occurs. Chlorpropamide may also be useful in treating patients with a combined defect because it allows more modulation of urine output in accordance with changes in hydration.

Hypodipsia. Patients with pituitary DI can also develop hypernatremic dehydration if they have hypodipsia due to associated damage to the stimulatory component of the thirst mechanism. This condition has been observed with head trauma, tumors such as craniopharyngioma, histiocytosis, neurosarcoidosis and congenital developmental defects. It can also occur with aging *(35)*. The dehydration results presumably from failure to sense and replenish excessive free water loss caused by untreated DI or insensible loss. However, in some cases it is also aggravated by a secondary carbohydrate intolerance that results in hyperglycemia, glucosuria and a solute diuresis. The carbohydrate intolerance is usually a temporary phenomenon caused by the dehydration, but the basic mechanism is unclear. Hypokalemia may also be present as a result of hypovolemia and secondary hyperaldosteronism.

The acute treatment of hypernatremic dehydration entails first the elimination of excessive urinary water losses and, second, replacement of the free water deficit (FWD) as well as ongoing urinary or insensible losses. If DI is present, AVP or DDAVP should be given parenterally as described in the previous section. If glucosuria is present, the patient should also be given regular insulin in doses sufficient to control blood sugar until the dehydration is corrected when the carbohydrate intolerance usually subsides. Parenteral potassium supplementation should also be given as needed to correct the hypokalemia. If hypotension and/or hyperglycemia are present, the free water deficit should be replaced initially with normal (0.9%) saline, because it is slightly hypotonic relative to body fluids, does not aggravate the hyperglycemia, and restores extracellular volume more rapidly with less effect on osmolality than comparable volumes of free water (i.e., 5% dextrose). Once the blood pressure or blood sugar are normalized, fluid can be given iv as half normal saline and 5% dextrose in water or 5% dextrose in water alone.

The amount required to replenish the FWD can be estimated from the formula:

$$FWD = 0.55 \times BW \times (p\,Na^*-140)/140 \qquad (1)$$

where BW=body weight and pNa* = effective plasma sodium. The latter should be corrected for any hyperglycemia that may be present by the formula:

$$pNa^* = pNa\text{-m} + 0.5\,(BS-100)/18 \qquad (2)$$

where BS stands for measured blood sugar in mg/dl and p Na-m stands for measured plasma sodium. This volume should be supplemented by amounts equal to ongoing urinary and estimated insensible losses and administered over a 24–48 h period. Progress should be monitored continuously by repeat measurements of plasma sodium and glucose and the rate of fluid administration adjusted accordingly.

Once the acute dehydration has been corrected, the patient should be placed on an individually tailored regimen of weight-controlled water intake in conjunction with DDAVP *(36,37)*. In some patients, chlorpropamide may be more effective than DDAVP because it allows more modulation of urine output in accordance with changes in hydration and may also stimulate thirst *(38)*.

Vasopressin Antibodies

Antibodies to vasopressin do not occur spontaneously in untreated DI *(39)*. However, they occasionally develop during treatment with antidiuretic hormone, usually lysine vasopressin, and when they do, almost always result in secondary resistance to its antidiuretic effect. Antibodies to vasopressin do not impair the response to other forms of therapy such as chlorpropamide. They may interfere with the diagnosis of DI by falsely suggesting partial nephrogenic DI probably because the hormone that is extracted and assayed is biologically inactive owing to antibody binding.

Pregnancy

Women who develop DI during pregnancy usually have a deficiency of AVP caused by the combination of a preexisting subclinical impairment in secretion and a marked increase in metabolic clearance by a vasopressinase produced by placenta *(40–42)*. DDAVP is ideal treatment for such a condition because it is not degraded by vasopressinase and because it is free of any uterotonic effect. Use of DDAVP during pregnancy does not constitute a significant risk for the fetus *(43)*. Nursing while using DDAVP is also safe since the baby is not exposed to the clinically significant amounts of hormone and it is not at risk for water intoxication.

Women with preexisting pituitary DI who are on a stable dose of DDAVP usually do not need any dose adjustment during pregnancy. The occasional reports of a need to increase the dose may reflect the misinterpretation of symptoms associated with physiological decrease in the threshold for thirst that normally occurs during pregnancy *(43)*. AVP and lysine vasopressin are much less effective for treating DI during pregnancy because they are quickly degraded by vasopressinase. Chlorpropamide and clofibrate are contraindicated because of possible teratogenic effects.

WOLFRAM SYNDROME

Wolfram's is a rare disorder characterized by diabetes insipidus, diabetes mellitus, optic atrophy and deafness (DIDMOAD syndrome) *(44,45)*. Dilatation of the urinary tract and gonadal dysfunction have also been noted. Many cases appear to be inherited in a autosomal recessive manner due to a mutation in a gene on chromosome 4 *(46)*.

The DI in DIDMOAD syndrome appears to be secondary to an AVP deficiency *(47)*. It ranges in severity from partial to complete and the vast majority of patients respond to treatment with DDAVP. The reason for poor response to DDAVP that is occasionally noted is unclear but may represent a partial nephrogenic component to the DI resulting from chronic dilatation of the collecting system.

Diabetes mellitus in DIDMOAD varies from impaired glucose tolerance to diabetic ketoacidosis. Chlorpropamide can be used to treat both DI and DM, but one should be alert to a progressive decline in insulin secretory capacity and institute insulin treatment when needed.

TREATMENT OF NEPHROGENIC DI

Because nephrogenic DI is caused by renal resistance to AVP, it cannot be treated with standard therapeutic doses of desmopressin or any of the other agents effective in pituitary DI (except thiazide diuretics). Some patients with partial nephrogenic DI do respond to high doses of DDAVP but the great expense of this approach currently makes it impractical for long term treatment. Therefore, treatment is currently limited to sodium restriction in combination with a few drugs that reduce urine output by vasopressin-independent mechanisms. They are:

1. THIAZIDE DIURETICS are the mainstay of therapy for nephrogenic DI. Their pharmacology has been described earlier in the section on pituitary DI. One should remember that thiazide induced hypokalemia may impair glucose tolerance and urinary concentrating ability, either of which could exaggerate polyuria and polydipsia in patients with nephrogenic DI.
2. AMILORIDE reduces polyuria in nephrogenic DI. In most forms, it tends to be less effective than chlorothiazide because it is a weak natriuretic. However, it can be used to augment the effect of the thiazides *(48)*. Moreover, it is the drug of choice for treatment of lithium induced nephrogenic DI *(49)* because it acts at least in part by blocking aldosterone sensitive sodium channels that are the site of lithium entry into the collecting tubule cell. Thus, it reduces lithium toxicity by minimizing lithium accumulation in the distal nephron. At the usual recommended dose of 5–10 mg bid, urinary volume is reduced by 35% but the onset of action may require several weeks *(49)*. Because blockade of sodium sensitive aldosterone channel also impairs secretion of potassium and hydrogen ions, amiloride may cause hyperkalemia and metabolic acidosis.
3. NONSTEROIDAL ANTIINFLAMMATORY AGENTS also have an antidiuretic effect in patients with nephrogenic diabetes insipidus. They appear to act by inhibiting the synthesis of prostaglandins which impair urinary concentration by increasing medullary blood flow and solute washout thereby decreasing osmolar gradient and water reabsorption *(50–52)*. When given in recommended dose of 1.5–3 mg/kg/d or 50 mg bid or tid,

indomethacin can decrease urinary volume 30–52 % both acutely (within hours of administration) and during chronic use *(52,53)*. It should be remembered that chronic use of nonsteroidal agents is associated with gastrointestinal, hematopoetic, central nervous system, and renal toxicity. Combining NSAIDS with hydrochlorothiazide diuretics may or may not give additive effects on urine output *(51,54)*.

Special Considerations in the Therapy of Nephrogenic DI (NDI)

1. Lithium is the most common cause of acquired NDI. The impairment in urinary concentrating ability correlates with duration of therapy, average serum lithium ion level, and total lithium carbonate dose *(55)*. Because lithium-induced NDI may be fully reversible if the drug is discontinued in the first year or two of treatment, the necessity of prolonged lithium use should be discussed with the prescribing physician before alternatives are considered. If discontinuation of lithium is not possible or effective, lithium-induced polyuria can be reduced by thiazide diuretics *(56)*, nonsteroidal agents *(53)*, or amiloride *(49)*. Thiazide diuretics cause volume contraction, which increases renal reabsorption of lithium and increases the risk of lithium toxicity. Therefore, it is important to closely monitor serum lithium levels after starting the treatment. Nonsteroidal agents appear to be efficacious but have not been extensively studied. Amiloride is currently considered to be the drug of choice for treatment of this form of nephrogenic DI. The major drawback is slow onset of action and relatively modest antidiuretic effect. The limited efficacy probably can be explained by the presence of lithium-induced structural tubulointerstitial damage *(55)*.
2. Demeclocycline, usually used for acne therapy, often causes a dose, and duration-dependent, reversible form of NDI. Complete restoration of renal concentration capacity usually occurs several weeks after treatment is stopped.
3. Because electrolyte imbalances such as hypokalemia (with potassium deficit greater than 200 meq) and hypercalcemia (Ca > 11 mg/dL) cause a reversible form of NDI, the mainstay of therapy in these forms remains the treatment of underlying cause.

TREATMENT OF PRIMARY POLYDIPSIA

Because patients with primary polydipsia have a physiological or psychological compulsion to drink excessive amounts of fluid, treatment with standard doses of AVP, DDAVP, thiazides, or any other drugs that reduce free water excretion is contraindicated because they invariably cause symptomatic water intoxication (Fig. 5). The only safe and effective way to treat this type of DI is to eliminate the excessive fluid intake. Unfortunately, there is currently no way to do this in either the psychogenic or the dipsogenic form of primary polydipsia. Therefore, the only treatment possible at present is to ameliorate some of the more annoying symptoms of nocturia and to educate the patient to prevent, recognize, and rapidly treat potentially serious complication of water intoxication.

1. The symptoms of nocturia can be relieved by small bedtime doses of DDAVP or lysine vasopressin. This treatment generally should be limited to patients with dipsogenic DI because the potential for misuse is much greater in patients with psychogenic polydipsia. To minimize the risk of water intoxication, the dose and/or form of treatment should be selected to permit recurrence of polyuria the following morning. Because of its shorter duration of action (only 4–6 h), Diapid may offer an advantage over DDAVP, whose effect can last 12 h or longer. Regardless of the medication used, patients should have plasma osmolality and/or sodium measured periodically to rule out excessive free water retention.

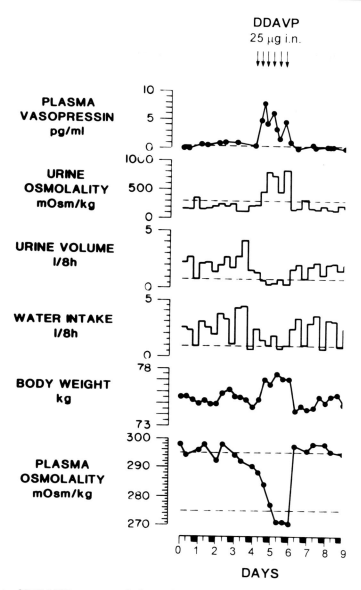

DDAVP
25 μg i.n.

Fig. 5. The effect of DDAVP on water balance in a patient with dipsogenic DI. DDAVP was administered intranasally in a dose of 25 μg every 8 h. Note that the treatment produced an increase in urine osmolality and a decrease in fluid intake but only after excessive water retention as evidenced by an abnormally large gain in weight and a fall in plasma osmolality and sodium to well below normal limits.

2. The risk of water intoxication can be minimized by instructing patients with either form of primary polydipsia to avoid the use of nicotine or drugs such as thiazide diuretics, which can impair water excretion *(27,57,58)*. In addition, they should be warned about the possibility of developing acute SIADH during influenza or other febrile illnesses. Specifically, they should be advised to obtain measurements of plasma sodium at the first suggestion of symptoms of water intoxication such as headaches, nausea, and anorexia.

CONCLUSIONS

Optimal treatment of DI requires an adequate diagnostic evaluation to determine the cause and the type of DI. A search for possible collateral damage to other organ systems is also needed. In pituitary or dipsogenic DI, the search should include computed tomography and/or magnetic resonance imaging (MRI) of the brain and tests of anterior pituitary function. In nephrogenic DI, the search should include screening for potentially reversible metabolic causes such as hypercalcemia, as well as drugs. In both forms, a search for genetic causes *(2,4)* may also be indicated, particularly if there is a family history.

ACKNOWLEDGMENTS

The authors thank the staff of Northwestern University's General Clinical Research Center for assistance in caring for the patients who have greatly contributed to the understanding of this topic. The authors also express their appreciation to Mary Beth Gaskill for help with figure preparation and to James Macchione for technical assistance in preparation of this manuscript.

REFERENCES

1. Robertson GL. Diabetes insipidus. Endocrinol Metab Clin North Am 1995;24:549–572.
2. Hansen LK, Rittig S, Robertson GL. Genetic basis of familial neurohypophyseal diabetes insipidus. TEM 1997;8:363–372.
3. Durr JA. Diabetes insipidus in pregnancy. Am J Kidney Dis 1987;9:276–283.
4. Knoers N, Monnens LAH. Nephrogenic diabetes insipidus: clinical symptoms, pathogenesis, genetics and treatment (invited review). Pediatr Nephrol 1992;6:476–482.
5. Robertson GL. Dipsogenic Diabetes insipidus: a newly recognized syndrome caused by a selective defect in the osmoregulation of thirst. Trans Assoc Physician 1987;100:241–249.
6. Illowsky BP, Kirch DG. Polydipsia and hyponatremia in psychiatric patients. Am J Psychiatry 1988;145:675–683.
7. Goldman MB, Luchins DJ, Robertson GL. Mechanisms of altered water metabolism in psychotic patients with polydipsia and hyponatremia. N Engl J Med 1988;318:397–403.
8. Zimmerman EA, Ma LY, Nilaver G. Anatomical basis of thirst and vasopressin secretion. Kidney Int 1987;32(suppl 21):S14–S19.
9. Schmale H, Fehr S, Richter D. Vasopressin biosynthesis–from gene to peptide hormone. Kidney Int 1987;32(suppl 21):S8–S13.
10. Knepper MA, Wade JB, Terris J, et al. Renal aquaporins. Kidney Int 1996;49:1712–1717.
11. Nielsen S, Marples D, Frokiaer J, et al. The aquaporin family of water channels in kidney: an update on physiology and pathophysiology of aquaporin-2. Kidney Int 1996;49:1718–1723.
12. Mannucci PM. Desmopressin: a nontransfusional form of treatment for congenital and acquired bleeding disorders. Blood 1988;72:1449–1455.
13. Zerbe RL, Robertson GL. Osmotic and nonosmotic regulation of thirst and vasopressin secretion. In: Narins RG, ed. Clinical disorders of fluid and electrolyte metabolism. McGraw Hill, New York, NY, 1994, pp. 81–100.
14. Robertson GL. Differential diagnosis of polyuria. Ann Rev Med 1988;39:425–442.
15. Elster AD. Modern imaging of the pituitary. Radiology 1993;187:1–14.
16. Richardson DW, Robinson AG. Desmopressin. Ann Intern Med 1985;103:228–239.
17. Fjellstad-Paulsen A, Paulsen O, d'Agay–Abensour L, Lundin S, Czernichow P. Central diabetes insipidus:oral treatment with dDAVP. Reg Pep 1993;45:303–307.
18. Lam KS, Wat MS, Choi KL, Ip TP, Pang RWC, Kumana CR. Pharmacokinetics, pharmacodynamics, long-term efficacy and safety of oral 1-deamino-8-D-arginie vasopressin in adult patients with central diabetes insipidus. Br J Clin Pharm 1996;42:379–385.

19. Robertson GL. Posterior pituitary. In: Felig P, Baxter JD, Frohman LA, eds. Endocrinology and Metabolism, 3rd ed. McGraw Hill, New York, 1995, pp. 385–432.

20. Byun KY, Gaskill MB, Robertson GL. The mechanism of chlorpropamide antidiuresis in diabetes insipidus. Clin Res 1984;32:483 A.

21. Moses AM, Numann P, Miller M. Mechanism of chlorpropamide-induced antidiuresis in man: evidence for release of ADH and enchancement of peripheral action. Metabolism 1973;22:59–66.

22. Moses AM, Howanitz J, van Gemert M, Miller M. Clofibrate-induced antidiuresis. J Clin Invest (1973) 52:535–542.

23. Thompson P Jr, Earll JM, Schaaf M. Comparison of clofibrate and chlorpropamide in vasopressin-responsive diabetes insipidus. Metabolism 1977;26:749–762.

24. Van Amelsvoort T, Bakshi R, Devaux CB, Schwabe S. Hyponatremia associated with carbamazepine and oxacarbazepine therapy: a review. Epilepsia 1994;35:181–188.

25. Stephens WP, Coe JY, Baylis PH. Plasma arginine vasopressin concentration and antidiuretic action of carbamazepine. Br Med J 1978;1:1445–1447.

26. Gold PW, Robertson GL, Ballenger JC, et al. Carbamazepine diminishes the sensitivity of the plasma arginine vasopressin response to osmotic stimulation. J Clin Endocrinol Metab 1983;57:952–957.

27. Friedman E, Shadel M, Halkin H, Farfel Z. Thiazide-induced hyponatremia: Reproducibility by single dose rechalenge and an analysis of pathogenesis. Ann Intern Med 1989;110:24–30.

28. Walter SJ, Skinner J, Laycock JF, et al. The antidiuretic effect of chronic hydrochlorothiazide treatment in rats with diabetes insipidus: Water and electrolyte balance. Clin Sci 1982;63:525–532.

29. Shirley DG, Walter SJ, Laycock JF. The antidiuretic effect of chronic hydrochlorothiazide treatment in rats with diabetes insipidus: renal mechanisms. Clin Sci 1982;63:533–538.

30. Seckl JR, Dunger DB. Postoperative DI. Br Med J 1989;298:2–3.

31. Ciric I, Ragin A, Baumgartner C, Pierce D. Complications of transsphenoidal surgery: results of a national survey, review of the literature and personal experience. Neurosurgery 1997;40:225–236.

32. Seckl JR, Dunger DB. Neurohypophyseal peptide function during early postoperative diabetes insipidus. Brain 1987;110:737–746.

33. Lindsay RS, Seckl JR, Padfield PL. The triple phase response-problems of water balance after pituitary surgery. Postgrad Med J 1995;71:439–441.

34. Robertson GL. Disorders of thirst in man. In: Ramsay DJ, Booth DA, eds. Thirst: Physiological and Psychological Aspects. Springer-Verlag, New York, 1991, pp. 453–475.

35. Phillips PA, Phil D, Rolls BJ, Ledingahm JGG, Forsling ML, Morton JJ, Crowe MJ, Wollner L. Reduced thirst after water deprivation in healthy elderly men. NEJM 1984;311:753–759.

36. Robertson GL. Abnormalities of thirst regulation. Kidney Internat 1984;25:460–469.

37. Perez GO, Ostre JR, Robertson GL. Severe hypernatremia with impaired thirst. Am J Nephrol 1989;9:421–434.

38. Nandi M, Harrington AR. Succesful treatment of hypernatremic thirst deficiency with chlorpropamide. Clin Nephrol 1978;10:90–95.

39. Vokes TJ, Gaskill MB, Robertson GL. Antibodies to vasopressin in patients with diabetes insipidus. Ann Inter Med 1988;108:190–195.

40. Iwasacki Y, Oiso Y, Kondo K, et al. Aggravation of subclinical diabetes insipidus during pregnancy. N Engl J Med 1991;324:522–526.

41. Durr JA, Hoggard JG, Hunt JM, Schrier RW. Diabetes insipidus in pregnancy associated with abnormally high circulating vasopressinase activity. N Engl J Med 1987;316:1070–1074.

42. Lindheimer MD, Davison JM. Osmoregulation, the secretion of arginine vasopressin and its metabolism during pregnancy. Eur J Endocrinol 1995;132:133–143.

43. Kallen BAJ, Carlsson SS, Bengtsson BKA. Diabetes insipidus and use of desmopressin (Minirin®) during pregnancy. Eur J Endocrinol 1995;132:144–146.

44. Kinsley BT, Swift M, Dumont RH, Swift RG. Morbidity and mortality in the Wolfram syndrome. Diabetes Care 1995;18:1566–1570.

45. Barett TG, Bundey SE. Wolfram (DIDMOAD) syndrome. J Med Genet 1997;34:838–841.

46. Karasik A, O'Hara C, Sriknata S, et al. Genetically Programmed Selective Islet β-cell loss in diabetic subjects with Wolfram's syndrome. Diabetes Care 1989;12:135–138.

47. Thompson CJ, Charlton SW, Walford S, et al. Vasopresson secretion in the DIDMOAD (Wolfram) syndrome. QJM 1989;71:333–345.

48. Alon U, Chan JCM. Hydrochlorothiazide-amiloride in the treatment of congenital nephrogenic diabetes insipidus. Am J Nephrol 1985;5:9–13.

49. Battle DC, von Riotte AB, Gaviria M, Grupp M. Amelioration of polyuria by amiloride in patients receiving long-term lithium therapy. N Engl J Med 1985;312:408–414.
50. Libber S, Harrison H, Spector D. Treatment of nephrogenic diabetes insipidus with prostaglandin synthesis inhibitors. J Pediatr 1986;108:305–311.
51. Jakobsson B, Berg U. Effect of hydrochlorothiazide and indomethacin treatment on ranal function in nephrogenic diabetes insipidus. Acta Pediatr 1994;83:522–525.
52. Monn E. Prostaglandin synthetase inhibitors in the treatment of nephrogenic diabetes insipidus. Acta Pediatr Scand 1981;70:39–42.
53. Allen HM, Jackson RL, Winchester MD, Deck LV, Allon M. Indomethacin in the treatment of lithium-induced nephrogenic diabetes insipidus. Arch Intern Med 1989;149:1123–1126.
54. Monnens L, Jonkman A, Thomas C. Response to indomethacin and hydrochlorothiazide in nephrogenic diabetes insipidus. Clin Sci 1984;66:709–715.
55. Boton R, Gaviria M, Battle DC. Prevalence, pathogenesis and treatment of renal dysfunction associated with chronic lithium therapy. Am J Kidney Dis 1987;10(5):329–345.
56. Himmelhoch JM, Forrest J, Neil JF, Detre TP. Thiazide-lithium synergy in refractory mood swings. Am J Psychiatry 1977;134:149–152.
57. Hariprasad MK, Eisinger RP, et al. Hyponatremia in psychogenic polydipsia. Arch Intern Med 1980;140:1639–1642.
58. Siegler El, Tamres D, Berlin JA, et al. Risk factors for the development of hyponatremia in psychiatric inpatients. Arch Intern Med 1995;155:953–957.

3

Growth Hormone Therapy in Children

Catherine K. Lum, MD, MPH,
and Darrell M. Wilson, MD

Contents

INTRODUCTION

The first documented therapeutic use of growth hormone (GH) occurred in 1958 in an effort to treat a GH-deficient adolescent *(1)*. Further studies confirmed that human GH improved the growth of children with severe GH deficiency (GHD). However, owing to the limited supply of pituitary-derived GH, treatment was limited to only a few thousand patients, and therapy was often sporadic. The use of the pituitary-derived human GH continued until 1985. At that time, a link between the pituitary derived hormone and Jakob-Creutzfeldt disease was reported, resulting in the cessation of the therapeutic use of this medication *(2,3)* in the US. Fortunately, biosynthetic forms of GH quickly became available. With improved safety and essentially limitless supplies, the therapeutic use of GH has increased dramatically.

GH therapy remains extremely expensive and quite cumbersome. Despite decades of use, substantial debate regarding appropriate therapy candidates remains. The role of GH stimulation tests, the traditional tests of GH axis in selecting patients who will benefit

From: *Contemporary Endocrinology: Hormone Replacement Therapy*
Edited by: A. W. Meikle © Humana Press Inc., Totowa, NJ

from GH therapy, is increasingly controversial. Although GH's recent approval for use in GHD adults has the potential to alter significantly the care of these patients, questions about the long-term benefits of this therapy remain. There are many potential uses for GH therapy, but because it can induce serious adverse reactions, the efficacy and benefits must be thoroughly studied in each clinical condition before it should be accepted as an appropriate therapy.

GROWTH IN CHILDREN

The primary goal of GH therapy in children and adolescents with growth abnormalities is to increase linear growth and final adult height. Essential to this process is the identification of abnormal growth patterns. The initial evaluation of growth involves accurate measurement and recording of height. Height is most consistently and accurately measured by using a calibrated, wall-mounted stadiometer for those children who can stand unassisted. The flexible arm type of measuring devices, as often attached to scales, give misleading measurements. If the child is too young or unable to stand, then a lying height, using fixed measurement devices, is the next best option. Although not necessary for screening purposes, triplicate height measurements ensure accuracy in children receiving GH therapy. Wherever possible, height should be measured by a single experienced person.

Once an accurate height is obtained, it should be recorded on a standard growth curve. There are two families of growth curves available—cross-sectional curves and longitudinal curves. The most common cross-sectional curve is based on height and weight data of normal US children, compiled by the National Center for Health Statistics *(4)*. These curves list the height values from the 5th to 95th percentile of normal children. Although these curves are useful for screening children, the limited percentile ranges make it difficult to quantify the deviation from normal of the very short or very tall child. Furthermore, these curves reflect heights for children going through puberty at various ages and can be misleading for the evaluation of growth of adolescents. The longitudinal curves, based on the expected growth during puberty, may be more helpful for an adolescent patient *(5)*. When compared to the cross-sectional curve, the longitudinal curve better reflects the transient increase in growth velocity at the time of puberty (Table 1).

In addition to noting the impact of pubertal development on growth, it is also important to assess other factors that influence growth. Chronic diseases, malnutrition, genetic abnormalities, and a history of intrauterine growth retardation (IUGR) can all play a significant role in affecting growth and final height. The genetic potential, based on parental heights, is also a strong determinant of adult height. It is helpful to adjust population-derived growth curves for genetic growth potential of the patient. Formulas can be used to calculate patient specific 5th and 95th percentile target range, based on parental heights (Table 1).

In addition to assessing stature, it is important to assess the growth velocity. The growth velocity should be at a reasonable rate, when compared to normal standards *(5)*. In the US, the minimum growth rate is approx 4–5 cm/yr in the prepubertal ages, and 8–9 cm/yr during puberty. The growth rate is calculated by re-assessing growth every 4–6 mo.

EVALUATION OF ABNORMAL GROWTH IN CHILDREN

The initial growth assessment entails a thorough history *(6)*. Birth history, including birth weight, past medical history of chronic illness, and use of chronic medications,

Table 1
Calculating a Target Height Range Based on Parental Heights

1. Calculate midparental height (cm) accounting for the mean difference between adult men and women of 13 cm.
   For a boy (Father's height + Mother's height + 13)/2
   For a girl (Father's height −13 + Mother's height)/2
2. Adjust the midparental height for the tendency of children's height to regress to the mean. The difference between the calculated midparental height and average adult height (177 cm for men, 164 cm for women) should be reduced to 80% of original difference.
3. Calculated the 95% confidence interval for the target range by adding and subtracting 10 cm for boys and 9 cm for girls.
   Example:
   For a boy:
       Father's height is 165 cm
       Mother's height is 154 cm
           Midparental height (165 + 154 + 13)/2 = 166 cm
           Regression to the mean (177–166) = 11
               $11 \times 0.8 = 8.8$
           Corrected midparental height: 177–8.8 = 168.2 cm
           Target range 158.2–178.2 cm
   For a girl:
       Father's height is 165 cm
       Mother's height is 154 cm
           Midparental height (165 − 13 + 154)/2 = 153 cm
           Regression to the mean (164–153) = 11
               $11 \times 0.8 = 8.8$
           Corrected midparental height: 164–8.8 = 155.2 cm
           Target range 146.2–164.2 cm

should be detailed. The pregnancy history and birth weight are especially important, because approx one-third of patients with IUGR will continue to have poor growth velocity beyond infancy and will have a subnormal adult height (7), despite normal pituitary function. Family history should include parental heights, any endocrine abnormalities, and age of onset of puberty of the parents as an indication of a family history of constitutional delay.

A complete physical exam should include height, measured with a stadiometer, and complete pubertal staging. It is important to assess the weight and weight gain in relation to the height and growth velocity. If the weight gain has been inadequate then malnutrition, which negatively impacts growth velocity, must be initially addressed. Follow-up measurements, using the same equipment, should be performed at 4–6 mo intervals to assess the growth velocity.

Many factors, both endocrine and nonendocrine, play important roles in growth. Hypothyroidism is one of the more common endocrine disorders that causes growth failure in children. Thyroid stimulating hormone (TSH) and thyroxine levels are essential to determine if hypothyroidism is present. Other endocrine disorders that can present as poor growth velocity include cortisol excess, delayed puberty, and poorly controlled diabetes mellitus. These endocrine maladies can be assessed with a thorough history, physical exam, and specific blood tests.

If the growth rate is subnormal, based on historical data or follow-up data, and there are no confounding factors, GHD should be considered. However, as discussed later, the interpretation of GH testing has become increasingly controversial.

GH SECRETION

GH is one of the primary hormones influencing linear growth. Produced by the anterior pituitary gland, it is regulated by GH releasing hormone and somatostatin, both hypothalamic hormones. GH secretion is pulsatile, with peak secretion occurring during sleep in the early morning hours *(8)*. GH values are initially high in the newborn and decline by 1 mo of age towards the prepuberty GH levels *(9)*. GH values increase in puberty with an increase primarily in the amplitude of the GH pulses. The mean GH secretion peaks during early puberty in girls and late puberty in boys *(10,11)*. The daily GH secretion plateaus in adulthood, followed by a decline by the fourth decade of life *(8)*. By the eighth decade of life in men, the mean GH values are less than one-third of the values found in men in their 20s to 30s *(12)*.

Severe stress, exercise, and hypoglycemia also increase the secretion of GH. Severe psychosocial deprivation reduces the GH secretion and obesity is associated with a decrease in the frequency and intensity of the peaks of GH secretion, primarily during the day *(13)*.

GH mediates its growth effects primarily through insulin-like growth factor-I (IGF-I). The production of IGF-I, stimulated by GH, occurs mainly in the liver, but also takes place in many other tissues in the body *(14)*. IGF-I stimulates tissue proliferation and thus directly affects growth. Most of the circulating IGF-I is bound to specific binding proteins, with the majority bound to IGF-binding protein-3 (IGFBP-3). Both IGF-I and IGFBP-3 concentrations are stable in the serum and lack the pulsatile variation as observed in serum GH measurements. Similar to GH, IGF-I and IGFBP-3 vary with age, gender and the degree of pubertal development. Serum IGF-I levels increase from infancy to puberty *(11)*, with pubertal IGF-I peaks occurring later in boys than girls (14.4 yr of age form males, compared to 12.6 yr for females) *(15)*. The IGF-I levels tend to decrease after the 30th year of life and by the seventh decade of life, the values are approx 60% of the young adult level and by the 90th year, at 30% of the 20–30-yr-old level (15). These two proteins also correlate with the peak stimulated GH levels *(16,17)* and may be good indicators of GH production.

EVALUATION OF GH AXIS

Clinical Signs in Children

GHD in children should be suspected when a patient's height is less than three standard deviations below the mean or when the growth velocity declines with the growth curve crossing percentile lines *(18)*. Traditionally, children have been considered GHD if they have a peak GH response of less than 10 μ/L following two stimulation tests (e.g., using clonidine, insulin-induced hypoglycemia, exercise, etc.) *(19)*. In the past, the insulin induced hypoglycemia test was considered to be the best method to assess GHD *(18)*, however, these tests are not without their inherent risks. Many children experience side effects from the tests, including vomiting, abdominal pain, and hypoglycemic symptoms *(20)*. More serious complications, such as hypotension, bradycardia, seizures, and death, have also been reported *(21,22)*.

GH Testing Problems

Serum GH has a short half-life in blood and is normally secreted in a pulsatile manner. As such, random sampling to measure GH directly rarely yields useful information. GH can be measured following a large variety of physiologic and metabolic/hormonal stimuli *(19)*. Most clinicians have used the peak GH concentration obtained during a combination of GH stimulation tests (GHST) as the gold standard of diagnosing GHD. The data regarding these GHST make this a questionable practice.

Golden Standard

Rather than validating various tests for GHD by comparing them to GHST, the utility of any diagnostic test (including GHST) should be determined in a population where the diagnosis of GHD has been made using other criteria. Patients who have had their pituitaries surgically removed demonstrate this point. Adan et al. *(23)* used clinical criteria (pituitary stalk interruption, familial GHD, and/or microphallus and hypoglycemia) as the golden standard for GHD in children. Stimulated GH, 24-h GH profiles, IGF-I, or IGFBP-3 are all dramatically low. For children and adolescents with classical GHD, all of the GH assessment procedures are quite consistent with the clinical impression. Except for these classically GHD patients, meeting all these criteria is quite difficult.

Without growth as a clinical sign, the diagnosis of GHD in adults is potentially more difficult. Moreover, many investigators report that impaired IGF-I and IGFBP-3 concentrations are not found as consistently among adults with GHD.

Reproducibility

GHST have poor reproducibility *(20)*. Carel et al. *(24)* reviewed paired GHST in over 3200 children and adolescents and concluded reliability of the estimate of the GH peak value was poor. The 95% confidence limits for the difference in GH concentration on two GH stimulation tests was –5 to +5 ng/L. These data confirm those of Tassoni et al. *(25)* who performed various GHST twice in a group of 49 short children. Repeated arginine GHST were discordant in 40% of the patients (using a GH concentration cutoff of 7 µg/L).

In severe GHD, with peak-stimulated GH values less than 4 µ/L, the stimulation tests are generally reliable. However, peak GHST are notoriously unreliable for the majority of patients with GH responses between 5–9.9 µ/L *(24,26)*. Therefore, the interpretation of GHST results must be evaluated in context with the clinical history and data.

Many of the studies involving GHD adults are using lower GH cutoffs to confirm the diagnosis of GHD. This seems to improve the reliability of GHST.

Physiological Factors

A number of factors alter both the endogenous production of GH and the GH response to various stimuli. Patients in puberty have a more robust response to GHST. Many investigators advocate priming prepubertal children with sex steroids immediately prior to GHST. Marin et al. *(27)* performed arginine-insulin and exercise GH stimulation tests in 84 children and adolescents with heights in the expected range. They demonstrated a dramatic effect of the stage of puberty on the GH response in adolescents. The mean peak GH concentration of 6.9 µg/L among the prepubertal subjects was four times lower than that found among adolescents with stage 5 puberty. In fact, only 4 out of 18 (22%) of stage 1 subjects had unprimed peak GH concentrations greater than 10 µg/L on any of the three tests. Eleven prepubertal subjects had a second set of tests following 2 d of pretreatment with estrogen. The lower limit of the 95% confidence interval for stimulated GH concentrations increased from 1.7 to 7.2 µg/L. Of note, this value is still substantially below commonly accepted pediatric cutoff of 10 µg/L.

As previously discussed, both GH and IGF-I concentrations rise with puberty *(8,15)* and decrease with aging *(28)*, implying that age specific normal ranges be used to develop criteria for diagnosing GHD.

Finally, obese patients have reduced endogenous GH production *(29)* and decreased GH response to GHST.

GH Assays

GH assays are quite variable. Celniker et al. *(30)* compared two different RIAs and two immunoradiometric assays for GH and found a threefold difference in GH concentrations. Granada et al. *(31)* compared 11 commercially available GH assays, and found 3.3-fold variation in mean GH concentration done on the same samples. Many investigators have found that polyclonal RIAs generally gave higher serum GH values than two-site immunoradiometric assays employing monoclonal antibodies. Factors found to contribute to these discrepancies included variable standards, different buffers, and the ability of the different antibodies to recognize the 20 K GH variant. The variable nature of these assays make the common practice of using a fixed cutoff value untenable.

24-H GH Profiles

The most consistent period of GH secretion occurs approximately one hour after the onset of deep sleep. Spontaneous GH secretory patterns are generally obtained by obtaining serum at 20- to 30-min intervals. However, GH secretion can be affected by many factors, and it is not clear what GH secretory patterns reflect. The reproducibility of such patterns is poor *(32)*.

Spiliotis et al. *(33)* measured serum GH levels in samples obtained at 20-min intervals from indwelling catheters and found minimal overlap between GHD children and controls. The correlation of pharmacologic provocative tests and measures of physiologic GH secretion (measured at 30-min intervals) in short children was assessed by Plotnick et al. *(34)*. They found a significant correlation between the 24-h integrated serum GH concentration and the peak stimulatory GH levels ($r = 0.67$). Despite this correlation, 25% of the children who were considered GHD (peak GH of less than 10 µ/L following a stimulation test) had 24-h GH concentrations that were within the normal range. Furthermore, Bercu et al. *(35)* and Rose et al. *(36)* have reported that measurements of spontaneous GH secretion correlated poorly with provocative testing or with any gold standard for the diagnosis of GHD.

IGF-I and IGFBP-3

The diagnostic significance of low serum levels of radioimmunoassayable IGF-I was first reported in the mid 1970s. It was quickly discovered that normal concentrations are influenced by chronological age, degree of sexual maturation, and nutritional status. Thus, clinical information is essential to properly interpret IGF-I or IGFBP-3 concentrations.

Rosenfeld et al. *(37)* subsequently measured plasma IGF-I levels in 197 patients with normal heights, compared with 68 children with GHD (provocative GH levels < 7 µ/L) and 44 normal short children (provocative GH levels > 7 µ/L). Eighteen percent of the

GHD children had IGF-I levels within the normal range for age. Furthermore, 32% of normal short children had low IGF-I levels, although all children in this group had provocative GH levels >7 µ/L. Many other investigators have shown similar overlaps. Measurement of IGF-II levels provided limited discrimination between GHD and GH replete patients.

Among children, the general lack of good concordance between measurements of GH secretion (either provocative or spontaneous) and plasma IGF-I or IGFBP-3 levels appears to primarily reflect the failure of standard GH tests to adequately measure GH secretion *(38)*.

Among adult patients, a different picture may be emerging. Hoffman et al. *(39)* compared 23 subjects with organic pituitary disease (age range 17–77 yr) with 35 normal subjects. The subjects were defined as having GHD if they had a structural lesion of the pituitary or hypothalamus that was treated with surgery and/or radiotherapy (n = 20), or if they required replacement therapy of at least two other pituitary hormones (n = 3). The investigators found complete separation of the two groups when they used insulin-induced hypoglycemia as a GH stimulus and a GH cutoff of 4 µg/L. However, integrated 24-h GH, IGF-I, and IGFBP-3 concentrations all showed substantial overlap between the two groups. Despite the dangers and inconvenience of insulin-induced hypoglycemia, these authors conclude that it is the test of choice.

In contrast, Baum et al. *(40)* compared the GH secretion of 23 adult men (aged 32–62 yr) with adult-onset GHD with 17 normal adult men. All of the GHD subjects had undetectable GH concentrations (less than 0.5 µg/L) following two GHST. Of note, these investigators did not use insulin-induced hypoglycemia in any subjects older than 50 yr because of concerns of cardiovascular complications of hypoglycemia. Each GHD subject had additional pituitary hormone deficiencies. Because the diagnosis of GHD was based on GHST, these data cannot be used to evaluate the role of stimulation tests in the diagnosing GHD among adults. These subjects, however, met clinically reasonable criteria for GHD and can be used to evaluate other biochemical measures that might be useful to diagnose GHD. Of note, the mean peak GH response following arginine stimulation among the normal subjects was only 5.8 µg/L (range 0.8–16.6). Thirty-five percent of the normal subjects had no GH response at all to clonidine (0.15 mg). Twenty four-hour GH sampling revealed mean GH concentrations that were clearly lower in the GHD group. The overlap seen with the normal subjects resulted from the very low GH concentrations seen in about 30% of normal subjects, a phenomenon also seen among children.

IGF-I concentrations demonstrated good separation between the groups with only three of the GHD subjects overlapping with the concentrations seen in normal subject. Unfortunately, the investigators did not normalize the IGF-I concentrations for age. Of note, the mean IGF-I concentration falls by approx 30% over the age range of the GHD subjects *(28)*. IGFBP-3 fared less well, with substantial overlap between the two groups.

As part of the baseline evaluation for a trial of GH therapy, Attanasio et al. *(41)* reported on 173 subjects with GHD as diagnosed by a peak GH follow a single GHST of less than 5 µg/L. Seventy-four of these subjects had the onset of their GHD in childhood, whereas 99 had adult onset. Of note, the mean concentrations of both IGF-I and IGFBP-3 among those with adult onset GHD were nearly twice as high as the mean concentrations among the child onset group.

Among adults, IGF-I remains an effective indicator of GH secretion. However, IGFBP-3, a useful indicator of GHD in children, is frequently normal among adults with GHD.

Table 2
Uses for Recombinant Human Growth Hormone

FDA approved uses
  Growth failure as a result of lack of adequate endogenous GH secretion
  Short stature associated with Turner's syndrome
  Growth failure associated with chronic renal insufficiency
    (up to time of renal transplantation)
  Replacement therapy in adults with somatotropin deficiency syndrome
  AIDS wasting (cachexia)
Possible uses
  Idiopathic short stature in children
  Short stature due to syndromes or bone dysplasias in children
  Short stature due to intrauterine growth retardation in children
  Severe malnutrition in children and adults
Speculative uses
  Fertility
  Elderly subjects without GHD

Paradoxically, one possible explanation for this may be the generally lower IGF-I concentrations seen in older adults. The molar concentration of serum IGFBP-3 approximates the sum of IGF-I and IGF-II in most clinical settings. Among pediatric subjects, normal IGF-I concentrations are high and fall with GHD ,whereas IGF-II concentrations remain more constant. The lower normal IGF-I concentrations found in adults implies that IGFBP-3 concentration mainly reflect serum IGF-II, a hormone that is not as GH dependent as IGF-I.

Auxiologic Assessment

Among children, poor growth is the most important sign of GHD. Thus, auxiologic data are essential in the diagnosis of GHD. In Australia, auxiologic data and close clinical follow-up alone (rather than biochemical testing) have been used to select patients for GH therapy and dictate the duration of treatment *(42)*. Although concerns exist about over-prescribing GH by using auxiologic data alone, the preliminary study indicates that the percentage of children treated with GH in Australia is comparable to many other countries and less than the US, Sweden, and Japan *(42)*. The rate of adverse side effects is low and the authors assert that this method is effective in selecting appropriate candidates for GH therapy. However, final height data are not yet available on children selected by auxiologic criteria alone.

APPROVED USES OF RECOMBINANT GH

Currently, GH has been approved by the US Food and Drug Administration (FDA) for children and adults with GHD, girls with Turner's syndrome, and children with chronic renal insufficiency (Table 2). GH therapy has been effectively used clinically for other problems such as hypoglycemia in infants and children owing to secondary panhypopituitarism. GH therapy trials, assessing the effectiveness of therapy among short non-GH deficient children *(43)* and short IUGR children *(44)*, have yielded variable results. GH therapy for severely malnourished patients has shown short term improvement in the nitrogen balance, although long-term effectiveness is unknown *(45)*. Furthermore, extensive studies are underway to determine if GH therapy is beneficial for elderly patients.

GH THERAPY

Historically, patients were treated with GH purified from human pituitaries obtained at autopsy. Following the reports of Jakob-Creutzfeldt disease in 1985, the use of human-derived GH stopped in the US. Since that time, all US GH preparations have been biosynthetically produced.

GH Preparations

GH is supplied as either a premixed solution or a powder. The premixed solution is dispensed in vials or cartridges, which can be used in a pen injection system. The pen device, in which one can "dial" the appropriate volume, is beneficial to those patients who have difficulties in drawing up medication and for some children who seek independence when administering their GH. However, the dosing quantity can be more accurately administered with the needle and syringe method.

Although the premixed solution is convenient and reduces the risk of dilution error, there are some reports that the injection site is more painful with this solution, especially among patients who were previously on another GH product *(46)*. Many patients still use the powder, which requires the addition of a diluent to create the injectable solution. The concentration can be adjusted so that the smallest volume can be administered by diluting the GH solution. Most preparations of GH require refrigeration, although some are stable at room temperature.

GH Dose for Children

In children, GH therapy, given as subcutaneous injection, is most effective if given daily or six times/wk *(47)*. Dosing is usually in the range of 25–50 µg/kg/d, with most children receiving approx 50 µg/kg/d.

Children are generally followed every 3–4 mo in the first year, then at a minimum of every 6 mo thereafter to assess growth rate and to monitor for complications. Most children, regardless of their diagnosis, have an increase in their growth velocity in the first 1–3 yr of treatment. Whenever the growth velocity on GH is lower than expected, the patient should be re-evaluated with particular attention to compliance.

GH Dose for Adults

Early studies of GH therapy among adults generally used dosing regimens similar to those used in pediatric patients. These doses of GH resulted in a high incidence of complications *(40)*. De Boer et al. *(48)* compared three doses of GH (approx 5, 10, and 15 µg/kg/d) in 46 GHD adult males. The dose of GH was reduced in 67% of the subjects receiving the highest dose because of side effects. Dose reductions were required in 35% and 18% of subjects in the middle and lowest dose groups. Using normalization of IGF-I concentrations as a goal, these authors recommend a maintenance dose of about 7 µg/kg/d, roughly sevenfold lower than the pediatric dose. The current suggested starting dose in the FDA approved package insert is 6 µg/kg/d, rising to a maximum of 12.5 µg/kg/d.

Table 3
Complications Associated with Growth Hormone Therapy

Complications in children
    Site hypertrophy
    Pain/bruising at injection site
    Glucose intolerance/hyperglycemia
    Benign idiopathic intracranial hypertension/pseudotumor cerebri
    GH antibody production
    Slipped capital femoral epiphysis
    Leukemia (?)
    Gynecomastia (?)
    Worsening of scoliosis (?)
    Allergic reaction (?)
Complications in adults
    Site hypertrophy
    Pain/bruising at injection site
    Glucose intolerance/hyperglycemia
    Benign idiopathic intracranial hypertension/pseudotumor cerebri
    GH antibody production
    Fluid retention/edema
    Carpel tunnel syndrom
    Arthralgia
    Psycologic effects/depression

Psychosocial Aspects of GH Therapy

Effective GH therapy in children requires intense parental involvement and commitment. If there is concern about poor compliance with therapy, this can be assessed through the pharmacy records and biochemically. If GH is not requested in a timely fashion, or if a given supply lasts for an inappropriately long time, then noncompliance is very likely. IGF-I and IGF-BP3 levels increase with GH therapy *(16)*, so these tests can be used to monitor compliance. Not all children will have an improved growth velocity in response to GH, despite good compliance. If the growth response is poor, continuation of GH therapy must be re-evaluated.

Complications of GH Therapy in Children and Adults

Therapy with GH is not only costly, but is also associated with some significant side effects (Table 3). GH is a parenteral drug and small bruises or pain can occur at the injection sites. Furthermore, hypertrophy at injection sites can occur if the injection sites are not rotated. This hypertrophy may interfere with GH drug absorption.

Development of antibodies to the GH preparation occurs in some patients. Antibody production was more notable in the patients receiving earlier human-derived GH preparations and methionyl-recombinant human growth hormone *(49)*. A high percentage of patients (65–95%) who received methionyl-GH developed anitbodies, although the titers were low and there was no effect in the growth velocity in these patient *(49–51)*. A more recent study *(52)* showed that the GH preparations derived from *Escherichia coli* DNA recombinant techniques induced very little immunogenicity (1.4–2.8%), and the GH produced by mammalian cell lines resulted in 8.5%

antibody rate. The antibody presence was transitory and at low titers and did not influence the growth velocity.

Benign increased intracranial hypertension (pseudotumor cerebri) is a rare complication. Twenty-three cases (22 children and 1 adult) were reported between 1986 and 1993 *(53)*. It usually occurs within the first 8 wk of therapy; however, some patients reported symptoms up to 5 yr after the initiation of therapy *(53)*. Over one-third of the reported cases involved children with chronic renal insufficiency. Symptoms include headache, nausea, vomiting, and vision changes. Signs include papilledema, which may only be evident with a thorough ophthalmology examination. If pseudotumor cerebri is suspected, GH treatment should be suspended, and an ophthalmology referral and brain-imaging study considered. Of the reported cases, all patients had papilledema, the majority had increased cerebral spinal fluid (CSF) pressure, and most had normal brain-imaging studies *(53)*. The increased pressure, and associated symptoms resolves after discontinuation of GH therapy.

Hyperglycemia and glucose intolerance can also occur with GH therapy in children and adults, although it is very rare. Among 19,000 patients on GH therapy followed by the National Cooperative Growth Study, fewer than 30 cases of hyperglycemia were reported *(54)*. Furthermore, most of these cases occurred among individuals who had an increased risk of glucose intolerance, such as patients with Turner's syndrome or children with syndromes with a known increased risk for glucose intolerance. In the majority of the reported cases, the hyperglycemia resolved once GH therapy was discontinued. However, any signs of hyperglycemia, such as polyuria, polydypsia, and polyphagia, must be immediately investigated. Long-term studies do not indicate any increased risk for the future development of diabetes among GH-treated patients *(45)*.

A slight increased risk of slipped capital femoral epiphysis (SCFE) has also been reported among children receiving GH. The incidence of SCFE among treated children is 21:7719 *(45)*, whereas the incidence of SCFE observed in adolescents is 1–8:100,000 *(55)*. Furthermore, animal models suggest that GH may weaken growth plates *(45)*, which may play a role in the development of SCFE. Any complaints of knee or hip pain when on GH therapy should be assessed with a complete examination and radiologic studies, as indicated.

Fifty to seventy-five percent of normal boys experience some transient increase in the breast glandular tissue during puberty, and spontaneous resolution occurs in the majority of these males *(56)*. The occurrence of prepubertal gynecosmastia is much less frequent, although incidence rates are unknown. Among boys treated with GH therapy through 1995, there were 28 reported cases of gynecomastia, with over half of them occurring in pubertal boys. Of the prepubertal boys, about half had some resolution of the gynecomastia when continuing GH therapy, and the remaining had resolution with GH therapy cessation *(57)*. The etiology of the breast enlargement among these patients is not clear. Whether it was a normal physiologic occurrence or related to the GH therapy is unknown and, why only a limited number of treated boys experienced it remains a mystery. GH may have played a causal role in the development of gynecomastia in some of these males.

Scoliosis is also a fairly prevalent complaint in the general pediatric population, with mild scoliosis (10–20° curvature) occurring in up to 3% of the population *(57)*. It is more commonly seen in girls and tends to progress during childhood and worsen during peak growth periods. Among children treated with GH and followed by the National Cooperative Growth Study, less than 1% of the patients reported a new diagnosis of scoliosis *(57)*.

Table 4
Etiology of Growth Hormone Deficiency in Children

Congenital
    Pituitary dysplasia or absence
        Septo-optic dysplasia, midline defects
    Hypothalamus dysplasia
    Neurosecretory disorders
    Biochemically inactive GH
Acquired
    Chemotherapy/irradiation
    Trauma
    Infection/Inflammation
    Hypoxia
    Central nervous system tumor/mass
        Hamartoma, craniopharyngioma
    Histiocytosis
    Vascular lesion or infarction
    Idiopathic

Therefore, there does not seem to be an increased risk of the development of scoliosis among GH-treated individuals. However, because GH therapy does result in increased growth velocity, it is important to monitor existing cases of scoliosis for progression so appropriate intervention can be provided.

There was initial concern that GH therapy increased a child's risk for malignancy, however recent data casts doubt on that assertion. Watanabe et al. *(58)* reported an increase risk of leukemia in pediatric GHD patients following GH therapy. To date, these results have not been duplicated *(59)*. Among over 24,000 children followed by the National Cooperative Growth Study, no increased risk of leukemia was detected. Eleven cases of new leukemia were found among 24,417 GH treated individuals; however eight of these children had known risk factors for leukemia, such as previous CNS tumor or aplastic anemia. Therefore, when compared to the incidence rate of leukemia in the general pediatric population (approx 1:2,000 persons under 15 yr of age *[59]*), there was not an increased cancer risk among GH-treated children. However, reports imply a greater risk of cancer among children who have risk factors *(57)*, such as previous cancer or radiation therapy. Therefore, caution should be taken when treating recovered cancer patients with GH.

Among adults, GH therapy has been associated with increased fluid retention and edema. In a small study, 18% of the adult patients experienced edema with therapy, although the majority had resolution of symptoms when the GH dose was decreased *(60)*. Other reported side effects included carpel tunnel syndrome and arthralgias, which also resolved when dosing was reduced *(61)*. One study *(60)* reported emotional lability and depression when on GH therapy.

GHD

GHD in Children

GHD can be congenital or acquired (Table 4). Patients with structural brain defects, such as with septo-optic dysplasia, or genetic defects may present in the neonatal period with hypoglycemia. Poor growth issues tend to present later in life, frequently around 6 mo of age.

The acquired forms of GHD can present at any age and are clinically detected by an acute decline in the growth velocity with the growth rate at less than that expected for age. The reported incidence of GHD varies widely from 1:1,500 to 1:30,000. A recent US survey of school children reported GHD in 1:3,500 children, with a slight male:female predominance of 2.7:1 *(62)*.

If GHD is suspected, an magnetic resonance imaging (MRI) of the brain, with specific attention to the hypothalamus and pituitary, should be considered to detect tumors or other structural abnormalities. Furthermore, other pituitary hormone deficiencies, such as TSH, adrenocorticotropic hormone (ACTH), and in pubertal-aged children, gonadotropins, should be sought.

Most studies indicate that children with classic GHD dramatically improve their growth rate in the first few years of GH therapy. Growth velocity in one study increased from a mean of 4 cm/yr to 10 cm/yr *(18)*. One can expect at least a doubling in the pretreatment growth velocity in the first year of treatment (63). Children also experience an improvement in their final adult height; however, historically, many children do not reach their predicted genetic height based on their parental heights *(63)*. This long-term deficit in adult height may be due to the late diagnoses or the limited supply of GH at the time of these earlier studies.

A recent study *(64)* evaluated GH therapy in children with GHD and suggested that the normal genetic growth pattern was not restored, despite therapy. This study initially enrolled over 3000 patients, however, approx 35% did not complete the study (as a result of insufficient response or "tiredness"). The mean age at the start of treatment was 10.5 yr, and most were diagnosed with GHD, based on stimulation tests with a mean peak GH level of 6.7 μg/L. The treatment ended when the growth velocity was less than 2 cm in 6 mo, and the bone age was greater or equal to 13 yr for girls and 14.5 yr for boys.

The average treatment time was 4.3 yr, and most children did have a gain in their growth velocity in the first year of treatment. The pubertal children in the study had a change in their final height standard deviation (SD) score ranging from 0.5–0.8. Among the prepubertal children, their final height was at −1.9 SD curve and lower than the genetic target, but their height SD score increased by 1.2 SD over the treatment years.

This study reports smaller gains in height SD scores compared to previous studies; however, many of these children were pubertal and the injection doses and frequencies were 30–50% lower than doses recommended and routinely used in other countries (13 μg/kg/wk vs 35 μg/kg/wk). The diagnosis of GHD was based on stimulation tests that are difficult to interpret, especially the range in which most of the study children were detected. It is quite possible that many of these children were not truly GHD. These children were also treated for only a relatively short period, and it is unclear from this study if the final height may have improved if the children began treatment earlier. It is generally believed that the earlier that GH therapy is started, the better the final height outcome. Furthermore, the study only reports near final adult height. Therefore, this study does not provide definitive information about treatment of GHD.

GHD in Adults

Meling and Nylen *(65)* and Juul et al. *(66)* recently reviewed GH therapy in GHD adults. Possible benefits of GH therapy for adults are listed in Table 5. Although a

Table 5
Possible Benefits of GH Therapy in GHD Adults

Body composition
    Increased muscle mass
    Improved muscle strength and exercise capacity
    Decreased fat mass
Increased bone mineral density
Increased cardiac output
Improved sleep patterns
Improved perceived health status

multitude of studies has addressed the benefits of GH therapy in this group, most studies are small and uncontrolled. A few of the larger, controlled trials are reviewed in the following section.

GHD in adults can be of childhood or adult onset. Attanasia et al. (41) found significant baseline differences when comparing 74 childhood onset GHD subjects (mean age 28.8 yr) with 99 adult onset GHD (mean age 43.5 yr). Men with childhood onset GHD were 12 cm shorter (~50% shorter than –2 SD) and 22 kg lighter. Similar differences were seen among the women. Of note, the IGF-I and IGFBP-3 concentrations were nearly twice as high among the subjects with adult onset GHD. Clearly, there are substantial differences in the baseline characteristics between these two groups and it is reasonable to expect differences in the response to GH therapy.

GHD–CHILDHOOD ONSET

The primary outcome of GH treatment during childhood and adolescence is increased adult height. As such, most clinicians stopped GH therapy as linear growth waned. As the supply of GH increased, many investigators suggested that GH therapy be continued because of GHs other salutary metabolic effects. Toogood and Shalet (67) repeated GHST in 88 adults who had been treated with GH for GHD as children. Originally, these children were diagnosed as GHD if they failed to achieve a peak GH 20 mU/L (~7–10 mcg/L) following one (29 subjects) or two (59 subjects) tests. Reevaluating the initial data, the proposed peak GH cutoff for adult GHD of <9 mU/L resulted in only 65% being classified as GHD. The 88 subjects were retested as adults with either one (33 subjects) or two (55 subjects) GHSTs. Sixty percent had peak GH concentrations of <9 mU/L as adults. Of note, 26 of the 55 of the adults (47%) undergoing two GHST had discordant results using this more conservative cutoff. Fifteen of the 55 subjects who had two GHST with a GH concentration of <9 mU/L had additional pituitary hormone deficiencies.

Clearly, not all children who receive GH during adolescence should continue to receive it as adults. On the other hand, repeat GHST is not necessary in the setting of clear GHD (e.g., surgical removal of the pituitary, multiple pituitary hormone deficiencies). Which GH-treated adolescents should continue GH as adults remains unclear.

In a randomized placebo-controlled trial of 74 subjects with childhood onset GHD, Attanasia et al. (41) studied GH therapy at a dose of 12.5 µg/kg/d (half this dose for the first month) for 6 mo. The GH treated subjects had an 8.5% increase in lean body mass and a 17% decrease in body fat (measured by bioelectrical impedance). IGF-I concentrations tripled, and IGFBP-3 concentrations increased by 70%. No treatment effect was seen on quality-of-life measures (Nottingham Health Profile). Of note, these subjects reported substantially fewer adverse effects than those subjects with adult onset GHD.

GHD–Adult Onset

In a randomized placebo controlled trial of 99 subjects with adult-onset GHD, Attanasia et al. *(41)* studied GH therapy at a dose of 12.5 µg/kg/d (half this dose for the first month) for 6 mo. The GH treated subjects had an 6% increase in lean body mass and a 17% decrease in body fat. As with subjects with childhood onset GHD, IGF-I concentrations tripled. IGFBP-3 concentrations, however, increased only by 40%. Only the social isolation and physical mobility subscales of the Nottingham Health Profile were improved ($p < 0.01$).

Nass et al. *(68)* examined the effect of GH on exercise performance in 20 adults with adult onset GHD. Those randomly assigned to receive 12.5 µg/kg/d of GH for 6 mo increased their IGF-1 concentrations nearly fivefold to a mean of 303 µg/L. Their maximum oxygen consumption increased by 37% in the GH-treated group. Multiple measures of exercise performance increased in the treated group but remained constant in the placebo group.

An ever-increasing number of studies are examining the hypothesis that GH replacement in GHD adults can significantly improve their lives. Most of the published studies demonstrate some clinically significant improvement. Many questions about risk vs benefit, ideal doses, and appropriate duration of therapy remain incompletely answered at this time.

NON-GHD IDIOPATHIC SHORT STATURE (ISS)

Most short children do not have any endocrinologic abnormality; the short stature most often is explained by constitutional delay, genetic components (based on predicted midparental heights), or a combination of both *(6)*.

Some children with severe short stature and a height below the –2 standard deviation curve or a growth velocity that is slightly decreased are not GHD by standard stimulation tests. This may be a reflection of the unreliability of the provocative GH tests or, alternatively, these children may have a neurosecretory defect in GH production and delivery. The issue of whether GH therapy is effective in this group of children is controversial, because the data are inconclusive.

Studies on the final height achieved among these children with non-GHD ISS have had varied results (Table 6). Most reports indicate that these children have an initial increase in growth velocity in the first few years of treatment *(69)*, although the response is not as great as that seen in GHD patients. There were no reported side effects with treatment, and puberty was initiated at a comparable time, compared to controls. However, there is an indication that the bone age advances at a slightly greater rate during puberty among the GH-treated individuals *(70)*. Ultimately, this may affect final adult height, and whether the final adult height outcome is improved remains to seen.

There have been at least six studies that compare final height or near final height to the pretreatment predicted adult height in GH-treated non-GHD children. Although some children showed no increase in final adult height *(70–72)*, other children had an increase ranging between 2.5 and 7.5 cm *(73–76)*. When the GH treated groups were compared to untreated non-GHD controls, the results varied from no difference in height change *(72)*, improved height change *(73)*, and decreased height change *(71)*. The varied results

Table 6
Growth Response to GH Therapy Among Short Non-GHD Individuals

Study/year	Years of treatment	Change in final height
Loche (70)	4–10 yr	no increase
Kawa (71)	4.2 yr (mean)	no increase
Wi (72)	6–7 yr	0.4 cm
Hindmarsh (73)	7.5 yr (median)	2.5–2.8 cm
Guyda (74)	Minimum of 3 yr	2.6–3.0 yr
Hintz (75)	Approx 7 yr	4.6–7.5 cm[a]
Zadik (76)	4 yr	5.4 cm[b]

Change in final adult height with GH treatment, compared to pretreatment predicted adult height.
[a]Near final height.
[b]Predicted adult height change, not final height.

in final height comparisons likely reflect the age of diagnosis and length of treatment in the different studies. However, all of the final heights were less than the predicted target heights, based on parental heights.

Because the data are so varied, and the cost and potential side effects of GH therapy are quite significant, careful pre-treatment evaluation of ISS children is required. If the child's height is below the –2 standard deviation curve, but he/she is growing with a normal growth velocity, close observation–instead of medical therapy–is warranted. However, if the growth velocity declines, consideration could be made for GH therapy. It is still unclear if GH therapy improves adult height, and parents and patients should be aware of the variable outcomes with therapy, in addition to the cost and possible side effects.

TURNER'S SYNDROME

Turner's syndrome is classically associated with significant short stature. If untreated, then US women with Turner's syndrome are expected to reach a mean adult height of 142 cm (18). Although the etiology of the short stature is unknown, it is suspected that both skeletal dysplasia and GH neurosecretory defects both play roles. Often, girls with Turner's syndrome tend to have normal GH responses to stimulation tests and normal IGF1 levels (77), although the IGF-I levels tend to decrease after 10 yr of age (78). Whether the decrease in IGF-I levels is related to the delayed puberty, owing to gonadal dysgenesis is unknown. However, clinically the growth velocity tend to dramatically decrease at this time.

One study indicated that girls with Turner's syndrome with isochromosomes had a greater incidence of an abnormal GH response to a stimulation test, compared to the Turner girls with an XO or mosaic karyotype (79). However, the short- and long-term responses to GH therapy could not be predicted by the results of the GH stimulation tests (79). The short-term response to GH therapy was significantly better among the girls with mosaic karyotype, although the final height was significantly greater among the girls with isochromosomes. As discussed by Schmitt, et al. (79), this greater adult height could be explained by the greater delay in bone age at the start of GH therapy among this subgroup.

GH therapy was recently approved by the FDA for girls with Turner's syndrome. The degree of improved final height depends on treatment duration although the exact increase in final height varies according to different studies. Recent European studies indicate a mean increase in final height of 5–8 cm among Turner's syndrome girls treated with GH compared to untreated Turner's syndrome girls *(80,81)*. A recent Japanese study revealed a mean improvement of final height of 4–6 cm among GH-treated Turner's syndrome girls, with a mean treatment period of 10 yr, compared to untreated Japanese Turner's syndrome girls *(82)*. The US study showed that treatment with GH improved Turner's syndrome adult height by approx 8–9 cm, after an average of 6 years of therapy *(83)*. The optimal time to start GH therapy in Turner's syndrome is unknown but earlier treatment results in further improvement of adult height. GH therapy is often initiated when the height is less than the fifth percentile on the normal female curve, which usually occurs at 4–5 yr of age. Because the classic GH stimulation testing yields little diagnostic information, GH testing should not be routinely performed in girls diagnosed with Turner's syndrome.

In some early studies, the use of oxandrolone, in combination with GH, induced a greater growth velocity than treatment with GH alone, at least during the first few years of treatment *(18)*. However, the combination regimen causes a greater advancement of the skeletal age, when compared to GH therapy alone, so the long-term benefit appeared questionable *(18)*. Furthermore, treatment with oxandrolone, alone or in combination with GH, negatively affects glucose control and carbohydrate metabolism among Turner's syndrome girls *(84)*, whereas GH therapy alone does not. Therefore, most clinicians use GH therapy alone in girls with Turner's syndrome.

The optimal duration of GH therapy is unknown. Many physicians continue GH therapy until the growth velocity slows to less than 2.5 cm/yr and the bone age is greater than 14 yr. Although the complications with GH therapy do not differ with Turner's syndrome girls, Turner's syndrome itself is associated with glucose intolerance, so one must be vigilant about assessing possible signs of hyperglycemia when treating these patients *(84)*.

CHRONIC RENAL INSUFFICIENCY (CRI)

Severe short stature and impaired growth velocity are common complications of CRI. Many children with CRI prior to puberty will have adult heights less than 2.0 standard deviations below the mean *(85)*. GH therapy is FDA approved for children with short stature and CRI, prior to transplant. In order to optimize the response to GH therapy, these patients should be managed by an experienced pediatric nephrologist and should have good metabolic and nutritional status with minimal renal osteodystrophy.

Placebo-controlled studies indicate that GH therapy will significantly improve growth velocity–at least in the short term–among patients with CRI *(85)*. In a study of long-term treatment (5 yr) *(86)* of children with CRI, the mean increase in height was 40 cm with a 1.9 SD height improvement. Furthermore, these children did not have excessive increase in their bone age or any adverse effects. They also did not experience any significant worsening of renal function. However, it is yet unclear if the final adult height will be improved with GH therapy.

Criteria for initiation of GH in CRI does not require GHST. GH responses to GHST, IGF-I, and IGFBP-3 levels can be variable among CRI patients *(87)* and are of little diagnostic value. GH therapy should be initiated for those patients whose height is more than 2 standard deviations below the mean or whose growth velocity is subnormal such that the height falls off the curve and approaches the –2 SD level *(85)*. Patients should be followed on a quarterly basis in order to assess the responsiveness to therapy and possible complications. GH therapy is discontinued in most CRI patients at the time of renal transplant.

GH therapy following renal transplant has been shown to be effective for children with short stature. In one study *(88)*, GH therapy improved growth velocity following transplant. Furthermore, there was no relationship between therapy and rejection or graft survival. Although this study duration was only for 3 yr, further studies may indicate if GH therapy will ultimately improve adult height among these patients without any change in renal function.

GH has not been indicated in adults with CRI, although other growth factors have been studied to determine if they will improve renal function in acute renal failure. Initial trials indicated that IGF-I may improve the renal function (as measured by the glomerular filtration rate), but later controlled studies failed to show any relationship between IGF-I therapy and recovery from renal failure *(89)*.

CONCLUSIONS

The therapeutic use of GH for short stature has greatly expanded since the emergence of a biosynthetic product in 1985. In the US, recombinant GH is currently approved for children with GH deficiency, Turner's syndrome, or chronic renal insufficiency and adults with GHD. There continues to be speculative uses for GH in children for other causes of short stature, such as genetic syndromes and IUGR. GH therapy has also been used for severe malnutrition in children and adults with limited success. Furthermore, the therapeutic effectiveness of GH therapy to improve body composition and cardiac status among GHD adults continues to be investigated. Furthermore, studies on the use of GH therapy among elderly non-GHD adults are currently being researched to determine if there are any long-term benefits.

There continues to be controversy regarding GH testing issues, identification of appropriate patients for GH, and efficacy of therapy among children and adults. As the patient population for GH therapy expands, the benefits of therapy for each group need to be thoroughly explored to yield the best outcome with the least risks.

REFERENCES

1. Raben MS. Treatment of pituitary dwarf with human growth hormone. J Clin Endocrinol Metabol 1958;18:901–903.
2. Hintz RL. The prismatic case of Creutzfeldt-Jakob disease associated with pituitary growth hormone treatment. J Clin Endocrinol Metabol 1995;80:2298–2301.
3. Fradkin JE, Schonberger LB, Mills JL, Gunn WJ, Piper JM, Wysowski DK, Thomson R, Durako S, Brown P. Creutzfeldt-Jakob disease in pituitary growth hormone recipients in the United States. J Am Med Assoc 1991;265:880–884.
4. National Center for Health Statistics:NCHS Growth Curves for Children 0–18 years, United States, Vital and Health Statistics, Series 11, no. 165, Washington, D.C. Health Resources Administration, U.S. Government Printing Office, 1977.
5. Tanner JM, Davies PSW. Clinical longitudinal standards for height and height velocity for North American children. J Pediatr 1985;107:317–329.
6. Tanner J. Auxology. In: Kappy MS, Blizzard RM, Migeon CJ, eds. The Diagnosis and Treatment of Endocrine Disorders in Childhood and Adolescence, 4th ed. Charles C. Thomas, Springfield, IL, pp. 137–192.
7. Fitzhardinge PM, Inwood S. Long-term growth in small-for-date children. Acta Paediatr Scandin 1989:349:27–33.
8. Van Cauter E, Plat L. Physiology of growth hormone secretion during sleep. J Pediatr 1996:128:S32–37.
9. Radetti G, Bozzola M, Paganini C, Valentini R, Gentili L, Tettoni K, Tato L. Growth hormone bioactivity and levels of growth hormone, growth hormone-binding protein, insulinlike growth factor I, and

insulinlike growth factor-binding proteins in premature and full-term newborns during the first month of life. Arch Pediatr Adoles Med 1997:151:170–175.

10. Rose SR, Municchi G, Barnes KM, Kamp GA, Uriarte MM, Ross JL, Cassorla F, Cutler GB. Spontaneous growth hormone secretion increases during puberty in normal girls and boys. J Clin Endocrinol Metabol 1991;73:428–435.

11. Costin G, Kaufman FR, Brasel JA. Growth hormone secretory dynamics in subjects with normal stature. J Pediatr 1989;115:537–544.

12. Van Coevorden A, Mockel J, Laurent E, Kerkhofs M, L'Hermite-Baleriaux M, Decoster C, Neve P, Van Cauter E. Neuroendocrine rhythms and sleep in aging men. Am J Physiol 1991;260:E651–661.

13. Martin-Hernandez T, Galvez MD, Cuadro AT Herrera-Justiniano E. Growth hormone secretion in normal prepubertal children: importance of relations between endogenous secretion, pusatility and body mass. Clin Endocrinol 1996;44:327–344.

14. Humbel RE. Insulin-like growth factors I and II. Euro J Biochem 1990;190:445–462.

15. Hesse, V, Jahreis G, Schambach H, Vogel H, Vilser C, Seewald HJ, Borner A, Deichl A. Insulin-like growth factor I correlations to changes of the hormonal status in puberty and age. Exp Clin Endocrinol 1994;102, 289–298.

16. Attie KM, Julius JR, Stoppani C, Rundle AC. National Cooperative Growth Study substudy VI:The clinical utility of growth-hormone-binding protein, insulin-like growth factor I, and insulin-like growth factor-binding protein 3 measurements. J Pediatr 1997;131:S56–60.

17. Nunez SB, Municchi G, Barnes KM, Rose SR. Insulin-like growth factor I (IGF-I) and IGF-Binding protein-3 concentrations compared to stimulated and night growth hormone in the evaluation of short children - A clinical research center study. J Clin Endocrinol Metabol 1996;81:1927–1931.

18. Neely EK, Rosenfeld RG. Use and abuse of human growth hormone. Ann Rev Med 1994;45:407–420.

19. Frasier SD. A review of growth hormone stimulation tests in children. Pediatrics 1974;53:929–936.

20. Ghigo E, Bellone J, Aimaretti G, Bellone S, Loche S, Cappa M, Bartolotta E, Dammacco F, Camanni F. Reliability of provocative tests to assess growth hormone secretory status. Study in 472 normally growing children. J Clin Endocrinol Metabol 1996;81:3323–3327.

21. Rowe DW, Sare Z, Kelley VC. Possible complications of the levodopa-propranolol test. Pediatrics 1977;60:132,133.

22. Shah A, Stanhope R, Matthew D. Hazards of pharmacological tests of growth hormone secretion in childhood. Brit Med J 1992;304:173,174.

23. Adan L, Souberbielle JC, Brauner R. Diagnostic markers of permanent idiopathic growth hormone deficiency. J Clin Endocrinol Metabol 1994;78:353–358.

24. Carel JC, Tresca JP, Letrait M, Chaussain JL, Lebouc Y, Job JC, Coste J. Growth hormone testing for the diagnosis of growth hormone deficiency in childhood:A population register-based study. J Clin Endocrinol Metabol 1997;82:2117–2121.

25. Tassoni P, Cacciari E, Cau M, et al. Variability of growth hormone response to pharmacological and sleep test performed twice in short children. J Clin Endocrinol Metabol 1990;71:230–234.

26. Rosenfeld RG, Albertsson-Wikland K, Cassorla F, Frasier SG, Hasegawa Y, Hintz RL, LaFranchi S, Lippe B, Loriaux L, Melmed S, Preece MA, Ranke MB, Reiter EO, Rogol AD, Underwood LE, Werther GA. Diagnostic controversy: the diagnosis of childhood growth hormone deficiency revisited. J Clin Endocrinol Metabol 1995;80:1532–1540.

27. Marin G, Domene HM, Barnes KM, Blackwell BJ, Cassorla FG, Cutler Jr GB. The effects of estrogen priming and puberty on the growth hormone response to standardized treadmill exercise and arginine-insulin in normal girls and boys. J Clin Endocrinol Metabol 1994;79:537–541.

28. Florini JR, Prinz, PN, Vitiello MV, Hintz RL. Somatomedin-C levels in healthy young and old men:relationship to peak and 24-hour integrated levels of growth hormone. J Gerontol 1985;40:2–7.

29. Veldhuis JD, Iranmanesh A Physiological regulation of the human growth hormone (GH)-insulin-like growth factor type I (IGF-I) axis:predominant impact of age, obesity, gonadal function, and sleep. Sleep 1996;19(10 Suppl):S221–S224

30. Celniker AC, Chen AB, Wert RM Jr, et al. Variability in the quantitation of circulating growth hormone using commercial immunoassays. J Clin Endocrinol Metabol 1989;68:469–476.

31. Granada ML, Sanmarti A, Lucas A, Salinas I, Carrascosa A, Foz M, Audi L. Assay dependent results of immunoassayable spontaneous 24-hour growth hormone secretion in short children. Acta Paediatr Scandin 1990;370:63–70.

32. Donaldson DL, Hollowell JG, Pan F, Gifford RA, Moore WV. Growth hormone secretory profiles: variation on consecutive nights. J Pediat 1989;115:51–56.

33. Spiliotis BE, August GP, Hung W, et al. Growth hormone neurosecretory dysfunction. A treatable cause of short stature. J Am Med Assoc 1984;251:2223–2230.
34. Plotnick LP, Lee PA, Migeon CJ, et al. Comparison of physiological and pharmacological tests of growth hormone function in children with short stature. J Clin Endocrinol Metabol 1979;48:811–815.
35. Bercu BB, Shulman D, Root AW, et al. Growth hormone (GH) provocative testing frequently does not reflect endogenous GH secretion. J Clin Endocrinol Metabol 1986;63:709–716.
36. Rose SR, Ross JL, Uriarte M, et al. The advantage of measuring stimulated as compared with spontaneous growth hormone levels in the diagnosis of growth hormone deficiency. N Engl J Med 1988;319:201–207.
37. Rosenfeld RG, Wilson DM, Lee PDK, et al. Insulin-like growth factors I and II in the evaluation of growth retardation. J Pediat 1986;109:428–433.
38. Rosenfeld RG. Editorial. Is growth hormone deficiency a viable diagnosis? J Clin Endocrinol Metabol 1997;82:349–351.
39. Hoffman DM, O'Sullivan AJ, Baxter RC, Ho KKY. Diagnosis of growth-hormone deficiency in adults. Lancet 1994;343:1064–1068.
40. Baum HBA, Biller BMK, Katznelson L, et al. Assessment of growth hormone (GH) secretion in men with adult-onset GH deficiency compared with that in normal men: a Clinical Research Center Study. J Clin Endocrinol Metabol 1996;81:84–92.
41. Attanasio AF, Lamberts SWJ, Matranga AMC et al. Adult Growth Hormone (GH)-deficient patients demonstrate heterogeneity between childhood onset and adult onset before and during human GH treatment. J Clin Endocrinol Metabol 1997;82:82–88.
42. Werther GA. Growth hormone measurements versus auxiology in treatment decisions: the Australian experience. J Pediat 1996;128:S47–51.
43. Hintz RL. Current and potential therapeutic uses of growth hormone and insulin-like growth factor I. Endocrinol Metabol Clin N Am 1996;25:759–773.
44. Chernausek SD, Breen TJ, Frank GR. Linear growth in response to growth hormone treatment in children with short stature associated with intrauterine growth retardation: the National Cooperative Growth Study experience. J Pediat 1996;128:S22–27.
45. Wilson DM. Clinical actions of growth hormone. Endocrinol Metabol Clin N Am 1992:21(3):519–537.
46. Arky R, ed. Physicians' Desk Reference, 52nd ed. Medical Economics, Inc., Montvale, NJ, 1998, 990–992.
47. MacGillivray MH, Baptista J, Johanson A. Outcome of a four-year randomized study of daily versus three times weekly somatotropin treatment in prepubertal naive growth hormone-deficient children. J Clin Endocrinol Metabol 1996;81:1806–809.
48. de Boer H, Blok GJ, Popp-Snijders C, Stuurman L, Baxter RC, van der Veen E. Monitoring of growth hormone replacement therapy in adults, based on measurement of serum markers. J Clin Endocrinol Metabol 1996;81:1371–1377.
49. Massa G, Vanderschueren-Lodeweyckx M, Bouillon R. Five-year follow-up of growth hormone antibodies in growth hormone deficient children treated with recombinant human growth hormone. Clin Endocrinol 1993;38:137–142.
50. Kaplan SL, August GP, Blethen SL, Brown DR, Hintz RL, Johansen A, Plotnick LP, Underwood LE, Bell JJ, Blizzard RM, Foley TP, Hopwood NJ, Kirkland RT, Rosenfeld RG, Van Wyk JJ. Clinical studies with recombinant-DNA-derived methionyl human growth hormone in growth hormone deficient children. Lancet 1986;I:697–700.
51. Milner RDG, Barnes ND, Buckler JMH, Carson DJ, Hadden DR, Hughes IA, Johnston DI, Parkin JM, Price DA, Rayner PH, Savage DCL, Savage MO, Smith CS, Swift PG. United Kingdom multicentre clinical trial of somatrem. Arch Dis Childhood 1987;62:776–779.
52. Pirazzoli P, Cacciari E, Mandini M, Cicognani A, Zucchini S, Sganga T, Capelli M. Follow-up antibodies to growth hormone in 210 growth hormone-deficient children treated with different commercial products. Acta Paediatr 1995;84:1233–236.
53. Malozowski S, Tanner LA, Wysowski D, Fleming GA. Growth hormone, insulin-like growth factor I, and benign intracranial hypertension. N Engl J Med 1993;329:665,666.
54. Blethen SL, Allen DB, Graves D, August G, Moshang T, Rosenfeld R. Safety of recombinant deoxyribonucleic acid-derived growth hormone: The National Cooperative Growth Study experience. J Clin Endocrinol Metab 1996;81:17041710.
55. Sponseller PD, Tolo VT. Bone, joint and muscle problems. In: Oski FA, ed. Principles and Practice of Pediatrics. Lippincott, Philadelphia, pp. 943,944.
56. Styne DM. The testes: disorders of sexual differentiation and puberty. In: Sperling MA, ed. Pediatric Endocrinology. W.B. Saunders, Philadelphia, p. 467.

57. Allen DB. Safety of human growth hormone therapy: current topics. J Pediatr 1996;28:S8–13.
58. Watanabe S, Tsunematsu Y, Fujimoto J, et al. Leukaemia in patients treated with growth hormone (letter). Lancet 1988;331:1159,1160.
59. Allen DB, Rundle AC, Graves DA, Blethen SL. Risk of leukemia in children treated with human growth hormone:Review and reanalysis. J Pediatr 1997;131:S32–36.
60. Beshyah SA, Freemantle C, Shah M, Anyaoku V, Merson S, Lynch S, Skinner E, Sharp P, Foale R, Johnston DG. Replacement treatment with biosynthetic human growth hormone in growth hormone-deficient hypopituitary adults. Clin Endocrinol 1995;42:73–84.
61. Baum HBA, Biller BMK, Finkelstein JS, Cannistraro KB, Oppenheim DS, Schoenfeld DA, Michel TH, Wittink H, Klibanski A. Effects of physiologic growth hormone therapy on bone density and body composition in patients with adult-onset growth hormone deficiency. Ann Intern Med 1996; 125:883–890.
62. Lindsay R, Feldkamp M, Harris D, Robertson J, Rallison M. Utah Growth Study:Growth standards and the prevalence of growth hormone deficiency. J Pediatr 1994;125:29–35.
63. Furlanetto RW and the members of the Drug and Therapeutics Committee of the Lawson Wilkins Pediatric Endocrine Society. Guidelines for the use of growth hormone in children with short stature. J Pediatr 1995;127:857–867.
64. Coste J, Letrait M, Carel JC, Tresca JP, Chatelain P, Rochiccioli P, Chaussain JL, Job JC. Long term results of growth hormone treatment in France in children of short stature:population, register based study. Brit Med J 1997;315:708–713.
65. Meling TR, Nylen ES. Growth hormone deficiency in adults: a review. Am J Med Sci 1996;311:153–166.
66. Juul A, Jorgensen JO, Christiansen JS, Muller J, Skakkeboek NE Metabolic effects of GH: a rationale for continued GH treatment of GH-deficient adults after cessation of linear growth. Hormone Res 1995;44 Suppl 3:64–72
67. Toogood AN, Shalet SM. The prevalence of severe growth hormone deficiency in adults who received growth replacement in childhood. Clin Endocrinol 1996;44:311–316.
68. Nass R, Huber RM, Klauss V, Muller OA, Schopohl J, Strasburger CJ Effect of growth hormone (hGH) replacement therapy on physical work capacity and cardiac and pulmonary function in patients with hGH deficiency acquired in adulthood. J Clin Endocrinol Metabol 1995;80(2):552–557.
69. Allen BD, Brook CGD, Bridges NA, Hindmarsh PC, Guyda, HJ, Frazier D. Therapeutic controversies: growth hormone (GH) treatment of non-GH deficient subjects. J Clin Endocrinol Metabol 1994; 79:1239–1241.
70. Loche S, Cambiaso P, Setzu S, Carta D, Marini R, Borrelli P, Cappa M. Final height after growth hormone therapy in non-growth-hormone-deficient children with short stature. J Pediatr 1994;125:196–200.
71. Kawai m, Momoi T, Yorifuji T, Yamanaka C, Sasaki H, Furusho K. Unfavorable effects of growth hormone therapy on the final height of boys with short stature not caused by growth hormone deficiency. J Pediatr 1997;130:205–-209.
72. Wit JM, Boersma B, de Muinck Keizer-Schrama SMPF, Nienhuist HE, Oostdijk W, Otten BJ, Delemarre-Van de Waal HA, Reeser M, Waelkens JJJ, Rikken B, Massa GG. Long-term results of growth hormone therapy in children with short stature, subnormal growth rate and normal growth response to secretagogues. Clin Endocrinol 1995;42:365–372.
73. Hindmarsh PC, Brook CGD. Final height of short normal children treated with growth hormone. Lancet 1996;348:13–16.
74. Guyda HJ. Use of growth hormone in children with short stature and normal growth hormone secretion. Trends Endocrinol Metabol 1994;5:334–340.
75. Hintz RL, Attie KM, Johanson AJ, Baptista J, Roche AF and the Genentech Study Group. Near final height in GH-treated short children without classical GH deficiency (abstract). Pediatr Res 1995;37:91A.
76. Zadik A, Chalew S, Zung A, Landau H, Leiberman E, Koren R, Voet H, Hochberg Z, Kowarski AA. Effect of long-term growth hormone therapy on bone age and pubertal maturation in boys with and without classic growth hormone deficiency. J Pediatr 1994;125:189–195.
77. Wit JM, Massarano AA, Kamp GA, Hindmarsh PC, Es AV, Brook CGD, Preece MA, Matthews DR. Growth hormone secretion in patients with Turner's syndrome as determined by time series analysis. Acta Endocrinol 1992;127:7–12.
78. Ranke MB, Blum WF, Haug F, Rosendahl W, Attanasio A, Enders H, Gupta D, Bierich JR. Growth hormone, somatomedin levels and growth regulation in Turner's syndrome. Acta Endocrinol 1987; 116:305–313.

79. Schmitt K, Haeusler G, Blumel P, Plochl E, Frisch H. Short- and long-term (final height) growth responses to growth hormone (GH) therapy in patients with Turner's Syndrome: correlation of growth response to stimulated GH levels, spontaneous GH secretion, and kayotype. Hormone Res 1997;47:67–72.
80. Pasquino AM, Passeri F, Municchi G, Segni M, Pucarelli I, Larizza D, Bossi G, Severi F, Galasso C. Final height in Turner's Syndrome patients treated with growth hormone. Hormone Res 1996;46:269–272.
81. Attanasio A, James D, Reinhardt R, Rekers-Mombarg L. Final height and long-term outcome after growth hormone therapy in Turner's Syndrome: results of a German multicentre trial. Hormone Res 1995;43:147–149.
82. Takano K, Ogawa M, Tanaka T, Tachibana K, Fujita K, Hizuka N, Members of the Committee for the Treatment of Turner's Syndrome. Clinical trials of GH treatment in patients with Turner's Syndrome in Japan: a consideration of final height. Euro J Endocrinol 1997;137:138–145.
83. Rosenfeld RG, and the Genentech National Cooperative Study Group. Growth hormone therapy in Turner's syndrome: an update on final height. Acta Paediatr Suppl 1992;383:3–6.
84. Wilson DM, Frane JW, Sherman B, Johanson AJ, Hintz RL, Rosenfeld RG, and the Genentech Turner's Collaborative Group. Carbohydrate and lipid metabolism in Turner's syndrome: effect on therapy with growth hormone, oxandrolone, and a combination of both. J Pediatr 1988;112:210–217.
85. Kohaut ED, Fine RN. Testing for growth hormone release is not necessary prior to treatment of children with chronic renal insufficiency with recombinant human growth hormone. Kidney Intl 1996;49(S53): S119–122.
86. Fine RN, Kohaut E, Brown D, Kuntze J, Attie KM. Long-term treatment of growth retarded children with chronic renal insufficiency, with recombinant human growth hormone. Kidney Intl 1996;49:781–785.
87. Mehls O, Tonshoff B, Tonshoff C, Haffner D, Blum WF. Therapeutic value of recombinant human growth hormone in children with chronic renal failure. Min Electrolyte Metabol 1992;18:320–324.
88. Mentser M, Breen TJ, Sullivan D, Fine RN. Growth-hormone treatment of renal transplant recipients: the National Cooperative Growth Study experience: a report of the National Cooperative Growth Study and the North American Pediatric Renal Transplant Cooperative Study. J Pediatr 1997;131:520–524.
89. Wang R, Hirschberg R. Role of growth factors in acute renal failure. Nephrol Dialysis Transplant 1997;12:1560–1563.

4

Growth Hormone and Growth Hormone Secretagogues in Adults

David E. Cummings, MD,
and George R. Merriam, MD

CONTENTS

INTRODUCTION

The association of growth hormone (GH) with the promotion of linear growth in childhood has focused attention away from its role in adults, but GH secretion continues throughout life, reaching a maximum in adolescence and then declining progressively with age. Many age-related changes resemble those of patients with classical GH deficiency (GHD), including a reduction in muscle and bone mass, an increase in body fat, diminished exercise capacity, and adverse changes in lipoprotein profiles *(1)*. There are other changes less classically associated with GHD that may also be related to the age-related decline in GH secretion. Sleep disorders, for example, become more common with aging, and because nocturnal GH secretion is synchronized with slow-wave sleep, it has been suggested that GH, or the stimuli to GH secretion, may promote as well as respond to sleep.

These phenotypic similarities have led to the belief that GH continues to play an important metabolic role in adult life as a partitioning hormone regulating body composition and function, and that in GH-deficient patients, GH replacement should be continued even after final adult stature is attained. Studies of GH therapy in adult GH deficiency have documented changes in hormone profiles and body composition over several years of treatment. Although adults are often more sensitive to the side effects of GH and there are still no data directly demonstrating improved functional performance

From: *Contemporary Endocrinology: Hormone Replacement Therapy*
Edited by: A. W. Meikle © Humana Press Inc., Totowa, NJ

or morbidity or mortality, GH treatment of GH-deficient adults has been approved by drug regulatory agencies in the United States, Europe, and other regions.

By extension, this focus has led to speculation that GH could also be used to reverse some of the symptoms associated with normal aging in subjects without classical GH deficiency. Short-term studies of GH treatment of normal older men date to the work of Rudman and colleagues, and a number of clinics, mostly outside the U.S., have been organized specifically to promote GH treatment. However, interest in aging as a partial phenocopy of GH deficiency has also highlighted the differences between normal aging and GH deficiency syndrome in adults of similar ages. At any given age, the decrement in GH secretion remains more severe in patients with documented GH deficiency than in healthy age-matched controls (2). An indication for treatment in one group is not necessarily an indication in the other, and it remains an important goal to improve the ability to diagnose GH deficiency specifically in adult life. Nor is it clear that open-ended chronic replacement therapy is necessarily the optimum approach in so large and heterogeneous a group as the elderly; short-term treatment focused on recovery from disease or injury might better balance benefits, costs, and risks.

And these risks are not trivial. The high prevalence of side effects such as edema and carpal tunnel syndrome in studies both of GH deficiency and normal aging has forced major dose reductions below those which are well tolerated in childhood, and a recently unblinded study of high-dose GH treatment in critically ill patients found a marked increase in mortality in the GH-treated group (3). Thus, GH treatment in aging should be approached with caution and based upon appropriately focused studies of clinical outcomes, not just hormonal or body composition measurements. Few of these have yet been published.

Except in patients with hypopituitarism, pituitary somatotrophs are intrinsically normal in most cases of childhood-onset GH deficiency and in normal aging. Stimulating the

---

GH AND IGF-I: A NOTE ON UNITS

Measurements of GH and of IGF-I concentrations and the preparation of pituitary-derived GH for therapy began before their chemical identity and structure were determined. To calibrate assays and doses, reference was made to defined pools and standard preparations and expressed in somewhat arbitrary units. With defined sequences for both GH and IGF-I, calibration has shifted to mass units (ng/mL or μg/L for assays, and μg for GH dosing). However, much of the earlier literature used units, and many clinicians are still most familiar with dosing in IU.

Conversion of units to mass is fairly straightforward for GH, and more complex for IGF-I. Therefore this chapter approaches the two sets of units differently:

GH: GH levels and dosing are expressed in mass units (μg/L or ng/mL). Doses are sometimes also listed in International Units, using the conversion 1 μg = 3 IU.

IGF-I: Early studies of IGF-I reported values in U/mL. These were calibrated with reference to a standard in which the mean value for young adults was set as 1 U/mL, with a normal range of approximately 0.5–1.5 U/mL. Given the heterogeneity of antisera, there is no single conversion factor which would accurately report these values in ng/mL, and therefore we retain the original units in discussing papers which used this system. More recent studies are reported in ng/mL, but readers should be aware that the normal range varies from study to study depending upon the antisera and reference preparations used.

pituitary with GH-releasing hormone (GHRH) or with the enkephalin-derived GH-releasing peptides (GHRP's) or their non-peptide analogs can evoke a GH response, and repeated administration of these agents can chronically increase GH secretion. These agents could therefore also potentially be used as treatments for GH deficiency and normal aging, and there are both physiologic and practical reasons why their use might be attractive. Because of ongoing variability in secretion of somatostatin and perhaps other factors, GH secretion remains pulsatile even during continuous administration of GHRH or GHRP's, and there is evidence that the pattern as well as the amount of GH secreted may modulate its responses. Feedback regulation at the pituitary level is preserved during GHRH or GHRP administration, perhaps buffering somewhat against overtreatment. Of great practical importance, some GH secretagogues, particularly the GHRP's and non-peptidyl analogs, are active when administered orally, avoiding the need for GH injections. Several preliminary studies have explored the short-term effects of GHRH and GHRP's in adult GHD and aging, but their use is still investigational.

This chapter reviews replacement therapy with GH and the GH secretagogues in adult GH deficiency and aging. Of these uses, only GH for adult GH deficiency syndrome and for AIDS wasting has received full regulatory approval, but we summarize the results of clinical trials which may lead to other treatment indications in the future.

MECHANISMS OF REDUCED GH SECRETION

Physiologic Regulation of GH Secretion

GH is regulated by several hypothalamic factors. Without these signals, GH synthesis and secretion fall to low levels and pituitary somatotrophs atrophy. GHRH, a 44-amino acid peptide, is the principal stimulator of GH production. Somatostatin (SRIF), a family of 14- and 28-amino acid peptides, is a noncompetitive inhibitor of GH secretion. Since these two peptides were characterized, the prevailing consensus has until recently been that the pattern of episodic ("pulsatile") GH secretion derives from the interplay of hypothalamic GHRH and SRIF (for review see *(4)*).

In the early 1980s, a group of enkephalin derivatives were found to have GH-releasing activity which appeared to act by a different mechanism from GHRH. Successive modification of these small peptides has led to the development of GH-releasing peptides (GHRPs) rendered devoid of opioidergic activity *(5)*. High-affinity GHRP binding sites distinct from the receptors for GHRH have been demonstrated in both pituitary and hypothalamus, and recently cloned *(6)*. These findings point strongly to the existence of an endogenous ligand ("GHRP-E" of "GHS") and a separate physiologic mechanism of GH release, possibly involving further intermediate factors ("U-factors") (Fig. 1). A systematic effort to characterize the endogenous GHRP natural ligand is underway. While GHRPs can act directly and independently on the pituitary to release GH, their full GH secretagogue effect in vivo appears to involve a secondary release of endogenous GHRH and synergism with the pituitary effects of GHRH. Thus there is a potent synergism when GHRH and GHRP are given together, and administration of a GHRH antagonist markedly reduces the effect of administered GHRP *(7,8)*

GH Deficiency and Aging

Childhood-onset GH deficiency is a heterogeneous disorder, but most often results from reduced hypothalamic secretion of GHRH. Thus, the pituitary is usually intrinsically

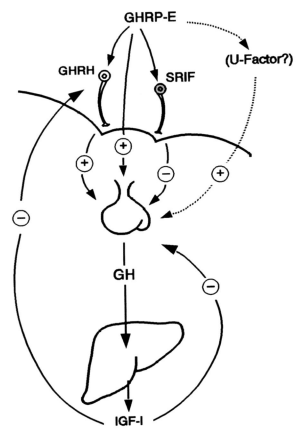

Fig. 1. Neuroendocrine regulation of growth hormone (GH) secretion. Only the most proximal hypothalamic factors and feedback regulators are shown. A large number of converging neurotransmitter and neuromodulator pathways in turn regulate the proximate loops illustrated here to provide the pattern of episodic GH secretion and the responses to factors such as sleep, stress, exercise, and meals. GHRH, GH-releasing hormone; SRIF, somatostatin; IGF-I, insulin-like growth factor-I; GHRP-E, endogenous natural ligand for the GHRP receptor; U-factor, hypothesized intermediary for some GHRP actions.

normal. Immune tolerance to GH typically develops, so that GH replacement generally does not evoke a clinically significant immune response, and the pituitary can respond to exogenous GHRH or GHRP *(9)*. The majority of adults with GH deficiency, however, acquire GHD as adults, and for most of these the deficiency results from a pituitary tumor or its treatment with radiation or surgery. In this setting patients frequently have multiple pituitary deficiencies and GH secretagogues would not be expected to be effective.

Although normal aging mimics many of the features of GH deficiency, the causes are likely to be different and the deficiency less severe. There are at least four possible mechanisms which could underlie the age-related decline in GH secretion: loss of pituitary responsivity to secretagogues, increased sensitivity to negative feedback by IGF-I, declining hypothalamic stimulation, and increased somatostatin inhibition.

Although both spontaneous and stimulated GH secretion are reduced in aging, the pituitary remains responsive to secretagogues; when some of the other factors which blunt GH responses are removed, GH responses to GHRH can remain vigorous (10). Thus, a primary loss of somatotroph responsivity is unlikely to underlie the age-related decline in GH secretion. Thorner and colleagues examined dose-response curves for the suppression of GH secretion by infusions of IGF-I, and found no age-related shift in sensitivity to IGF-I negative feedback *(11)*.

GH responses to both GHRH and to GHRPs are reduced in aging, but can be increased by agents such as arginine which are believed to suppress somatostatin secretion. The arginine effect is enhanced in older vs younger subjects *(12)*, suggesting that aging is associated with an increase in somatostatin tone, perhaps secondary to increased body fat. Although increases in GH secretion and IGF-I in response to GHRH suggest a relative deficiency of GHRH secretion in aging, it has been suggested that secretion of the endogenous GHRP may also decline. Reduced GH responses to GHRP which cannot be fully restored by antagonism of somatostatin have led Bowers and colleagues to postulate an age-related decline in a hypothesized intermediate for GHRP action, the so-called "U factor." Although several lines of evidence point to the existence of a U-factor, its identity and even its existence are not yet conclusively established.

At this stage it is reasonable to conclude that the decline in GH secretion with aging is multifactorial and arises above the pituitary level.

Differential Diagnosis: GH Deficiency vs Aging

Since the causes, severity, and consequences of adult GH deficiency and aging may differ, it is important to make the diagnosis of bona fide GH deficiency in adults. The clinical context is often highly suggestive: the presence of a pituitary macroadenoma, a history of surgical or radiation treatment, and failure of other pituitary-dependent systems should all suggest GH deficiency.

There is less information available on the best tests for GH deficiency in adults than in children. Ho and colleagues compared several potential measures in hypopituitary patients with presumed GH deficiency vs age-matched controls. GH stimulation with insulin-induced hypoglycemia (ITT) provided the clearest distinction between patients and controls, while indirect measures such as levels of IGF-I and IGFBP-3 showed substantial overlap and thus were poor discriminants *(2)*. The ITT was the only provocative test examined in this comparison, and although it is reasonable to believe that other tests such as arginine infusion, which may be preferable to insulin especially in frail or elderly patients, will provide comparable discrimination, this has not yet been directly tested. Patients with longstanding GHD and pituitary atrophy have markedly reduced responses to acute administration of GHRH or GHRP, and it has been argued that the combination of GHRH with arginine (to eliminate the variable effects of somatostatin) also discriminates well between GHD and normal aging *(12)*.

Even after many years of using GH for the treatment of childhood GHD, there is still a vigorous debate in the pediatric literature as to which (if any) provocative tests best correlate with GH deficiency as measured by 24-h GH profiles. Thus it is premature to rely too exclusively on any single test for the diagnosis of GHD in adults. FDA-approved guidelines for treatment with GH in adults in the U.S. recommend using a peak GH response to provocative testing of < 5 µg/L (polyclonal GH antibody) or <2.5 µg/L (monoclonal GH antibody) as a cutoff. The prudent clinician will weigh the results of one or two provocative tests with the clinical context. In the gray zone of possible "partial" or "mild" GH deficiency, a definite diagnosis may not be possible, and one may choose to undertake a trial of 6–12 mos of therapy to determine whether there is a beneficial response.

GH Deficiency vs GH Resistance

The somatic response to GH involves several intermediate steps, most visibly the generation of insulin-like growth factor (IGF-I); and inhibition of IGF-I can create a syndrome of relative GH resistance in which GH effects are reduced while GH secretion remains high. For example, fasting or malnutrition causes a rapid fall in IGF-I levels, often with a compenstory increase in GH secretion. In severe systemic illness, however, GH secretion can also fail. Several studies of critically ill hospitalized patients have shown reduced spontaneous GH secretion and profoundly decreased levels of IGF-I (13). These patients most likely have both GH deficiency and GH resistance. It has been suggested that in some catabolic states, such as burns and fractures, high-dose GH administration might overcome GH resistance, promote an anabolic response, and hasten recovery. Strictly speaking, this is pharmacologic rather than replacement therapy. The indications, doses, and side effects—some of which may be severe—are different in the two contexts, and the clinician should keep clearly in mind whether the intent of therapy is physiologic replacement or supraphysiologic therapy.

GH TREATMENT OF ADULT GH DEFICIENCY SYNDROME

Adult GH deficiency is commonly categorized in terms of whether the defect arose in childhood or adulthood. The former condition is usually congenital and idiopathic, and may be characterized by an isolated GH deficit. Adult-onset GH deficiency, which is far more prevalent, is most often iatrogenic, resulting from the treatment of pituitary or peripituitary tumors. Less common causes include trauma, pituitary apoplexy, Sheehan's syndrome, autoimmune or infiltrative diseases, infections, and metastases. Adult-onset GH deficiency is generally accompanied by deficits in other anterior pituitary hormones. This is because treatment of pituitary tumors usually causes panhypopituitarism, and GH is often the first hormone to be lost from most noniatrogenic causes of hypopituitarism, typically followed in sequence by gonadotropins, TSH, then ACTH. Consequently, GH deficiency is almost always a component of adult hypopituitarism, regardless of the cause. Yet traditionally GH shortfalls have not been treated in adults who have completed linear bone growth, while inadequate thyroid, adrenal, and reproductive hormonal axes are exogenously restored.

Adult GH Syndrome

In recent years, it has become widely accepted that GH and/or its downstream effector IGF-I subserve numerous important functions throughout adult life. GH-deficient adults are physically and emotionally less healthy than age-matched peers, and suffer from a distinct clinical syndrome with widespread manifestations that are evident even when other pituitary hormone deficits are adequately corrected (Table 1) (reviewed in refs. 14–19).

This syndrome includes several undesirable perturbations in body composition. GH has been shown to promote lipolysis and inhibit lipogenesis, as well as to redistribute fat from an android to a gynoid pattern. Accordingly, fat mass (LBM) in GH-deficient adults is increased by 7–10%. The excess fat is located preferentially in the visceral compartment of the abdomen, a pattern which in other contexts is associated with increased risk

Table 1
Clinical Features of the Adult GH Deficiency Syndrome

↑ Fat mass (especially abdominal fat)
↓ Lean body mass
↓ Muscle strength
↓ Cardiac capacity
↓ RBC volume
↓ Exercise performance
↓ Bone mineral density
Atherogenic lipid profile
Thin, dry skin; poor venous access
Impaired sweating
Psychosocial problems:
  low self-esteem
  depression
  anxiety
  fatigue/listlessness
  sleep disturbances
  emotional lability and impaired self-control
  social isolation
  poor marital and socioeconomic performance

of cardiovascular disease and diabetes. Conversely, lean body mass is decreased 7–8% in GH-deficient adults, and skeletal muscle volume at various sites has been shown to be diminished by up to 15%. GH exerts anti-natriuretic effects, both directly by stimulating renal tubular sodium-potassium pumps, and indirectly by facilitating the renin/aldosterone system. The net effect is that GH increases total body water. Consequently, at least some of the loss of lean body mass (LBM) seen in GH-deficient adults arises from deficits in total body sodium and fluid, especially in the extracellular compartment. However, GH is also anabolic towards muscle. It has been shown to increase the proliferation of muscle satellite cells, which can become myofibers. In mature muscle cells GH stimulates glucose and amino acid uptake, as well as amino acid and protein synthesis. This suggests that the reduced LBM found in GH-deficient adults probably does not result solely from decreased total body water, but also from muscular atrophy.

GH-deficient adults lose cardiac muscle in addition to skeletal muscle. Most notably, diminished left ventricular (LV) wall thickness has been demonstrated. This is associated with impaired ventricular function and cardiac capacity, as revealed by decreases in LV ejection fraction, stroke volume, and cardiac index. Furthermore, GH deficiency generates an atherogenic lipid profile characterized by increased total cholesterol (by 20%), LDL-C (34%), and triglycerides (76%), and decreased HDL-C (34%). Thrombogenic blood components such as fibrinogen and plasminogen activator inhibitor-1 are also elevated, and hypertension may be more common. These changes conspire to cause premature atherosclerosis (20). Hypopituitary patients suffer a 2-fold increase in cardiovascular mortality, a 3.4-fold increase in cerebrovascular mortality, and decreased life expectancy overall compared with normals (21,22). Since thyroid, adrenal, and gonadal hormones are replaced in these individuals, GH deficiency has been implicated as the cause of increased mortality (23). It remains possible, however, that other factors such as the sequelae of pituitary radiotherapy are also involved, especially in the increase in cerebrovascular disease.

Exercise capacity is markedly compromised in GH-deficient adults. Maximal oxygen intake (VO$_2$ max), an indicator of overall aerobic fitness, is decreased by 20–30%. This can be explained in part by a 10–15% loss of strength in various muscle groups that accompanies the reduced muscle mass. However, exercise performance is impaired out of proportion to muscular defects alone, and is undoubtedly exacerbated by diminished cardiac capacity, as well as reduced red blood count (RBC) volume.

GH exerts important influences on bone physiology even after linear bone growth has ceased, and its absence in post-pubertal adults is unequivocally associated with osseous pathology. In general, GH is anabolic with regard to bone, as it is with muscle. It enhances all of the following: intestinal absorption of Ca^{++} and PO4^{---}, 25-hydroxy-vitamin D-1α-hydroxylase activity, renal tubular PO4^{---} reabsorption, osteoblast proliferation, and synthesis of DNA and procollagen mRNA in bone. The overall effect is a stimulation of both bone formation and resorption. Bone mineral density at various skeletal sites is decreased in GH-deficient adults by at least one standard deviation compared with age-matched controls. Consequently, these individuals have an increased incidence of osteoporotic fractures.

The skin of GH-deficient adults is cool, dry, and thin. Patients have poor venous access and are often cold intolerant. These changes are partially due to compromised cardiac capacity. However, the fact that acromegalics develop abnormally thick skin suggests that GH also stimulates skin growth directly. In addition, eccrine sweat glands express GH receptors, and acromegalics suffer from excessive sweating. Conversely, GH deficiency leads to impaired sweat formation, probably contributing to exercise intolerance.

GH-deficient adults suffer numerous psychological and social difficulties. Using a variety of validated questionnaires, investigators have described these as including diminished self-esteem, depressed mood, low energy and vitality, listlessness, fatigue, disturbed sleep, social isolation, anxiety, emotional lability, and impaired self control. Objectively, patients demonstrate poor marital and socioeconomic performance. In the studies conducted to establish these findings, controls are typically matched for age, gender, socio-economic status, and sometimes height. Nevertheless, it is difficult to determine to what degree the impaired well-being and quality of life arises directly from effects of insufficient GH vs from self- consciousness regarding a body habitus that is likely to be abnormally fatty, and possibly short if the disease originated prepubertally.

Benefits of GH Replacement in GH-Deficient Adults

In view of the manifold ailments suffered by GH-deficient adults, it is reasonable to query whether some or all of these problems would be alleviated by GH replacement. Historically, GH treatment has been reserved for children. It was first proposed in 1921 that pituitary extracts might have growth-promoting effects (24). Beginning in the 1950s such extracts were administered to GH-deficient children, and it quickly became axiomatic that GH increases linear bone growth in these patients. The severely limited availability of pituitary extracts prohibited serious research into the impact of exogenous GH on adults for another three decades. However, a case study was reported in 1962 describing improved vigor, ambition, and well-being in a 35-yr-old hypopituitary adult who received pituitary-derived GH, suggesting that the hormone might perform meaningful functions in adults (25). Purified recombinant human GH (rhGH) became available in 1984, and one year later pituitary-derived GH was removed from the market because of concerns over the transmission of Creutzfeldt-Jakob disease (26). The first placebo-controlled trials of GH repletion in GH-deficient adults were reported in 1989

(27,28). At least 45 related human trials have ensued in less than a decade since that time, each seeking to determine whether specific facets of the adult GH-deficiency syndrome are ameliorated by GH replacement (reviewed in *(14,16–17,19,29–35)*). The results of these studies were sufficient to justify approval by the FDA in late 1996 for the use of rhGH in GH-deficient adults.

Bona fide primary GH deficiency arising in adulthood is rare (roughly 10 cases/million people/yr) *(36)*. However, GH levels fall approximately 50% in the course of normal aging *(37)*, and there is considerable overlap between the geriatric and GH- deficient phenotypes. Furthermore, it has been proposed that the anabolic actions of GH on muscle and bone might benefit patients with diverse catabolic conditions such as AIDS, severe burns, extensive surgery, and malnutrition, despite the fact that GH levels are generally normal in these situations. GH has recently been approved by the FDA for use in AIDS-related wasting under the auspices of an expanded access program, despite a relative paucity of convincing evidence to justify its use in this setting. Thus, there is a potentially vast target population for GH therapy. However, before exploring this market it was necessary to prove that GH replacement is worthwhile in genuine nonaging-related GH deficiency, which is the most logical paradigm for its use.

Several hundred GH-deficient adults have now been administered rhGH in controlled trials. In order to recruit adequate study cohorts, investigators have typically combined patients with childhood-onset and adult-onset GH deficiency. In most cases where these groups were analyzed separately, the findings were qualitatively similar, although a recent direct comparison of the two suggested that there may be some important differences in the response to GH therapy. Table 2 summarizes the major effects of GH replacement in GH-deficient adults, for which there is a general consensus among published reports.

Among the two dozen reported trials which examined body composition as a principal endpoint it is uncontested that GH replacement causes a loss of fat and gain of LBM. Such consensus is impressive in view of the diverse methods of measurement employed, including bioelectrical impedance, DEXA, ^{40}K-counting, D_2O dilution, CT, MRI, skin fold thickness, and waist-to-hip ratios. GH therapy decreases fat mass and volume by 7–15%, with the greatest reductions seen in abdominal visceral adipose tissue. In contrast, both LBM and skeletal muscle volume increase by 5–10%. Total body water increases, especially that in the extracellular compartment. Although this explains at least some of the increase in LBM, total body K^+ is also elevated, suggesting that GH promotes genuine muscular growth as well. Most studies showed no major changes in overall body weight, but rather a shift from fat to lean mass. Body composition changes in response to GH treatment are greatest in men (compared with women) and in young patients with low GH-binding protein levels at baseline.

There is also no controversy regarding the finding that GH replacement improves cardiac performance, as judged by increases in LV ejection fraction, stroke volume, and cardiac output, as well as decreased peripheral vascular resistance. These favorable changes are sustained for at least three years on therapy. As the GH-induced expansion of extracellular volume includes increases in plasma volume (seen at 3 wk) and total blood volume (seen at 3 mo), at least some of the enhanced cardiac capacity may be due to preload augmentation. Studies to date are fairly evenly divided between those that report minor (~5%) increases in LV muscle mass and those that deny this. The long-term impact of GH replacement on cardiac function is unknown, but warrants caution. Acromegalics develop hypertension, LV hypertrophy, and ultimately cardiac failure, which explains their increased

Table 2
Effects of GH Replacement in GH Deficient Adults

↓ Fat mass (especially abdominal fat)
↑ Lean body mass
↑ Total body water and plasma volume
↑ Muscle mass and strength
Improved cardiac capacity
↑ RBC volume
↑ Skin thickness
Improved sweating capacity
Improved exercise performance
↑ Resting energy expenditure
↑ Bone mineral density (after 1 yr of treatment)
Altered lipid profile:
    ↓ Total cholesterol
    ↓ LDL-C
    ↓ Apo B
    ↓ Triglycerides (if initially elevated)
    ↑ HDL-C (not seen in all studies)
    ↑ Lp(a)
↑ Insulin sensitivity (after changes in body composition)

Common side effects
Fluid retention; edema
Arthralgias
Carpal tunnel syndrome
↓ Insulin sensitivity (acutely); hyperglycemia

incidence of cardiovascular mortality. It is likely that these problems can be avoided by restoring GH only to physiological levels, which may need to be adjusted for age.

Another universal finding is that GH restoration significantly improves exercise performance and capacity. Usually assessed on bicycle ergometers, subjects show increases in VO$_2$ max to nearly normal levels. Isometric and isokinetic muscle strength have been tested in various muscle groups. Although muscle volume increases shortly after initiating GH therapy (owing in part to fluid retention), at least 6 mo treatment is required to generate appreciable changes in strength. One study showed no differences in skeletal muscle fiber areas and the proportions of type I vs II fibers after 6 mo of therapy (although these parameters were also unchanged in GH–deficient patients at baseline). Limb girdle strength appears to respond to therapy by approximately 6 mo, whereas quadriceps strength may take up to 1 yr to improve. Muscle strength continues to recover for as many as 3 yr of continued GH administration. The impressive GH-mediated improvement in exercise capacity is presumably due to a combination of enhanced cardiac performance, increased muscle mass and strength, and a shift in body composition from fat to lean mass. In addition, GH replacement in this setting expands RBC volume (and hence oxygen-carrying capacity), via an IGF-I-mediated stimulation of erythropoiesis. Finally, GH replacement augments the capacity to sweat (as measured by response to pilocarpine iontophoresis), and thus dissipate heat during exercise.

More than a dozen studies have examined the effects of GH replacement on bone metabolism. All have shown GH treatment to increase markers of both bone formation (osteocalcin, bone alkaline phosphatase, procollagen I and III, and bone Gla) as well as bone resorption (urinary pyridinoline and deoxypyridinoline, cross-linked telopeptides of type I collagen, and urinary hydroxyproline and Ca^{++}). The conclusion is that GH replacement stimulates bone turnover and remodeling in general. Of the more than 20 studies that have examined bone mineral density (BMD), there is a roughly even split between those that lasted less than 1 yr and reported no change in this parameter, vs those that lasted more 1 yr and reported increases in BMD of 4–10%. Interestingly, the response of bone to GH restoration is biphasic. Initially, bone resorption is predominantly stimulated, and BMD may fall within the first year on therapy. Later this change is counterbalanced by a delayed induction of bone formation, increasing BMD (up to at least 2 yr). Effects are maximal in patients with low initial BMD, and least impressive in the elderly, where unrelated causes of osteopenia may be at work. The GH-induced increase in bone mass occurs fastest in trabecular bone, and is thus manifest in vertebrae before the appendicular (cortical) skeleton. Investigators have reported no effects of GH upon PTH or 25-hydroxy-vitamin D, whereas there are conflicting reports of either increased or unchanged 1, 25-hydroxy-vitamin D.

GH regulates hepatic lipoprotein metabolism in a complex fashion, and its absence in adults is associated with an atherogenic lipid profile. Eight placebo-controlled trials, typically lasting 6 mo, have examined the impact of GH replacement on lipids in GH-deficient adults. Most reported decreases in total cholesterol, LDL-C, and apoB, although these changes were not significant in all cases. Triglycerides tended to fall in patients who had elevated baseline values. Most investigators reported GH-mediated increases in HDL-C, although this change was only statistically significant in two trials. Four additional open-label studies conducted for more than a year demonstrated that these lipoprotein changes were sustained for up to four years on GH therapy. All of the above lipid alterations are favorable with respect to cardiovascular risk. In contrast, five of six studies found that GH replacement increased Lp(a), a lipoprotein which in other contexts poses an independent risk for premature atherogenesis and myocardial infarction. Given GH's opposing actions to decrease LDL-C and increase Lp(a), it is unclear what the net effect of GH replacement would be upon cardiovascular risk.

GH-deficient adults tend to be centrally obese, and consequently demonstrate insulin resistance and elevated basal insulin levels. It is difficult to predict the effect of GH replacement on these parameters. GH directly antagonizes insulin action, which should worsen insulin resistance; yet it also decreases central obesity, which should ameliorate the problem. In fact, trials that have specifically addressed this question using hyperinsulinemic euglycemic clamps or iv glucose tolerance tests have shown that both effects occur in sequence over time. GH replacement worsens insulin resistance during the first few weeks of therapy, presumably due to its direct counter-regulatory actions. However, these changes are reversed after 3–6 mo of therapy. While resting hyperinsulinemia persists, carbohydrate metabolism returns to baseline, presumably because of lost visceral fat. Several studies in which glycemic parameters were not primary endpoints reported mild elevations in basal insulin and/or glucose levels at some point during GH therapy, although these values generally remained within normal ranges and were never associated with significant elevations of HgA_{1c}.

GH replacement in GHD results in a rapid 12–18% elevation in resting energy expenditure (REE). While much of this effect can be accounted for by increased LBM, some studies show increases in REE even when it is corrected for LBM, suggesting an actual increase in cellular metabolism. GH has been shown to facilitate T_4 to T_3 conversion, as well as to increase both protein synthesis and fat oxidation. All of these effects could contribute to its calorigenic potency.

Skin thickness and total skin collagen are reduced in adults with GH deficiency, as well as in normal aging. Although trials of GH replacement in GH-deficient adults have not examined this endpoint, GH supplementation was shown to increase skin thickness in one study of normal elderly men who had been selected on the basis of low IGF-I levels.

Despite the plethora of trials examining GH replacement in GH-deficient adults, there is a dearth of data regarding clinically germane final outcomes, as opposed to surrogate or intermediate outcomes. For example, there is a great deal of data regarding bone mineral density but none on fractures; on muscle strength and exercise capacity but not functional status; and on body composition and lipids but not morbidity or mortality. Data does exist about parameters that are overtly manifest (i.e., things that patients notice directly) in the psychosocial arena. In all controlled trials to date, subjects receiving GH replacement reported improvements in mood, energy, subjective well-being, emotional reaction, sleep, pain perception, behavior, and overall quality of life. Similar results were obtained with standardized and nonstandardized questionnaires. Not all of these parameters were significantly altered in every study in which they were examined, and the changes that were seen were often subtle and mutable over time. Furthermore, maintaining blindedness in these studies is difficult, due to GH-related symptoms such as fluid retention and arthralgias. Nevertheless, there has been remarkable concordance among numerous diverse studies suggesting that GH replacement improves overall well-being in GH-deficient adults, although the mechanism by which this occurs is not known.

Adverse Effects of GH Replacement

Because rhGH is identical to the endogenous hormone, undesired consequences of GH administration should arise solely from the hormonal effects of over-replacement. By far the most common untoward effects of GH therapy in GH-deficient adults are consequences of fluid retention arising from the anti-natriuretic actions of GH. Roughly 40% of patients studied in experimental trials developed clinically apparent edema. About 20% complained of joint swelling (especially in the hands) and/or noninflammatory arthralgias, and ~16% developed myalgias. Joint symptoms may be caused by excessive fluid in the joint space, since neither joint inflammation nor X-ray changes are detected, although the exact mechanism is unknown. These problems are generally mild, and resolve after a few weeks on therapy. However, ~10% of subjects develop symptoms of carpal tunnel syndrome. While increased blood pressure has occasionally been reported, most studies to not demonstrate this, even after as many as 3 yr of therapy. Gynecomastia has also been reported in association with GH therapy *(38)*.

As discussed above, GH replacement may mildly impair glucose tolerance, at least transiently. Thus, patients should have glycemic markers checked periodically, especially when initiating therapy. In addition, GH influences the metabolism of certain medications, which may thus require dose adjustment after GH therapy is begun.

Some concern has been expressed over potentially mitogenic properties of GH, based on highly controversial in vitro data using cells of many lineages *(39)*, as well as the observation that acromegalics have an increased incidence of colon and breast cancer compared with matched controls *(40–42)*. However, it is inappropriate to extrapolate conclusions from acromegalics, who have greatly excessive GH levels, to GH-deficient patients in whom only physiological restitution is sought. More importantly, GH replacement has been practiced for four decades in children (at higher doses/kilo than those intended for adults), and there is no convincing data to support either an increased incidence of de novo cancer due to GH therapy in these patients, nor an increased likelihood of recurrence of pre-existing malignancies. However, rates of both are higher in GHD children than in the general pediatric population—for example, in children who are GH deficient due to cranial radiotherapy for leukemia—and a controversy which still surrounds childhood GH replacement is re-emerging in the context of adult therapy. It is true that the risk of cancer is generally higher in adults than children, especially in AIDS patients and the elderly, two populations currently being considered for GH therapy. Nevertheless, at this time adults receiving GH therapy are not recommended to require additional cancer surveillance beyond standard practices for prevention and early detection.

Two recent case-control studies have suggested an association between circulating levels of IGF-I and the risk of breast or of prostate cancer *(42a,42b)*. As with concerns extrapolated from patients with acromegaly, the groups with increased incidence had IGF-I values above those likely to be seen with carefully titrated replacement therapy, and epidemiologic studies such as these do not directly speak to the effects of GH treatment. But until these reports are supplemented by extensive experience with GH treatment, it would be prudent to adhere strictly to guidelines for prostate examinations and PSA levels in men, and for mammography in women, and to discuss these reports with high-risk patients.

There have been isolated case reports associating GH therapy with cerebral side effects such as headaches, tinnitus, encephalocele, and benign intracranial hypertension (typically with papilledema). Most of these were in children receiving high-dose GH, and were reversible with cessation of therapy. Atrial fibrillation and male gynecomastia have been rarely reported in association with GH treatment in elderly adults.

GH administration is contraindicated in the setting of active malignancy, benign intracranial hypertension, and proliferative or preproliferative diabetic retinopathy. Although early pregnancy is not a contraindication, GH therapy may be discontinued in the second trimester, as a GH variant is secreted by the placenta.

Several manufacturers of GH for adults are sponsoring post-marketing surveillance studies of adult GH deficient patients. While they are not randomized, placebo controlled protocols, these studies each aim to follow several thousand patients over several years and should provide useful information on the actual rate of complications of GH therapy. Physicians prescribing GH may wish to inform their patients about the possibility of enrolling in one of these studies.

Recommended Dosing

Since all GH-related side effects are dose-dependent, they may be avoided by titrating GH injections to the minimal effective dose. Serum IGF-I levels should be used as an indicator of GH treatment since IGF-I has virtually no diurnal variation, while serum GH levels fluctuate widely due to pulsatile release, diurnal variation, and sensitivity to numerous environmental stimuli. Early studies employed GH doses extrapolated from those used in GH-deficient children (ca. 15–50 μg/Kg/d). These proved to be too high for adults, as judged by the supraphysiological IGF-I levels and high incidence of side effects that they generated, both of which improved at lower doses. More recent trials have typically used lower doses, and have still measured salutary effects. It has been noted that patients who

Table 3
Summary Recommendations for Adult Growth Hormone Replacement Therapy

Begin treatment at a dose of 150–300 µg/d in the evening. This dose approximates 2–4 µg/Kg/d
    Older patients should begin at the low end of this range.
Titrate the dose at monthly or longer intervals based on clinical response, IGF-I levels, side
    effects, and individual considerations such as glucose tolerance.
In general, aim for an IGF-I level at or slightly below the 50th percentile for age and gender unless
    side effects are significant. Sensitivity to the side effects of GH treatment varies widely; obese
    and older patients appear to be particularly sensitive.
GH should not be used in the presence of active malignancy. Glucose intolerance is not an absolute
    contraindication to GH therapy, because although insulin resistance may be acutely worsened,
    changes in body composition often improve insulin sensitivity over time. However, these
    patients require close monitoring, as do patients with pre-existing carpal tunnel syndrome.
Adults given chronic GH therapy should receive age- and gender-appropriate periodic cancer
    screening such as colonoscopy, prostate-specific antigen (PSA) levels, and mammography.
    There is currently no consensus on whether enhanced cancer surveillance is appropriate unless
    a patient has individual risk factors.

Adapted from ref. *43* and other sources.

developed adverse side effects tend to have supraphysiologic IGF-I levels, while those
whose IGF-I levels were maintained around the 50th percentile of the normal range had the
greatest level of desired responses with few no adverse effects *(38)*.

The GH Research Society Workshop on Adult GH Deficiency recently published
consensus guidelines for the diagnosis and treatment of adult GH deficiency *(43)*. They
recommend initiating GH at a low dosage (150–300 µg/d; 0.45–0.90 IU/d), administered
subcutaneously in the evening (because~2/3 of GH release usually occurs during sleep)
(44,45). The dose should be gradually titrated upwards, monitoring clinical and
biochemical responses (no more frequently than monthly) until a maintenance level is
achieved. This can be defined as the minimal dose that normalizes serum IGF-I values
without causing unacceptable side effects; we use the 50th percentile for age and sex as a
general target (Table 3). IGFBP-3 has proven to be a less helpful indicator. The considerable
inter-individual variation in GH sensitivity dictates equally variable final doses among
different patients, although these should seldom exceed 1 mg/d (3 IU/d). The most sensitive
groups are elderly and/or obese people, as well as those with either a relatively high GH
response to provocative testing or else an unusually brisk rise in IGF-I following GH
treatment. Variability in both subcutaneous absorption and individual sensitivity preclude
using body weight or surface area to predict dosage. Pulsatile GH administration enjoys the
theoretical advantage of being more physiological, but is much more cumbersome and
has not yet been proven to have clinical advantages to justify the use of pump therapy.
GH secretagogues (*see* "GH Secretagogues") may offer a more practical way to
reconsitute pulsatile GH secretion.

Recent reports have suggested that women are less sensitive to the effects of GH than
men, and may require higher GH doses to achieve similar biological responses. Burman
and colleagues gave similar doses (adjusted for body surface area) to 21 men and to
15 women for nine months, and found greater increases in IGF-I levels and greater effects
on bone markers, lipoproteins, and body fat in the men *(45a)*. Although it is possible that
this reflects the difficulty of scaling GH dose with body size, these results are supported

by the findings of Drake and colleagues *(45b)*, who used a dose-titration treatment strategy similar to that recommended by the GH Research Society *(43)*. In their study, women required significantly higher mean GH doses than did men to achieve similar results. Median doses and ranges were 1.2 (0.8-2.0) vs 0.8 (0.4–1.6) IU/d, or 400 (range 267–667) mg/day in women vs 267 (133–533) mg/day in men. These differences may reflect an effect of estrogen upon generation of IGF-I in the liver, and so may be more marked in patients receiving oral than transdermal estrogen replacement. That is consistent with the report of Bellantoni et al., who found that oral estrogens reduced IGF-I levels but that transdermal estrogens had no effect *(45c)*. However, the appearance of relative resistance to GH in a wide variety of responses in women suggests that this may not be solely a liver effect, and that estrogens may modulate GH responses in many target tissues.

Once a maintenance dosage is achieved, follow-up visits every 6–12 mo are sufficient, at which times IGF-I levels should be used for dose adjustments. Measurements to monitor efficacy might include simple anthropometric determinations such as waist-to-hip ratio or skin-fold thickness, possibly supplemented by bioelectrical impedance or DEXA. The latter is also helpful in following BMD. Lipids should be assessed when indicated.

The cost of GH therapy is significant. At a current wholesale price of approximately $35-40/mg, the annual cost of drug for a patient weighing 70 Kg receiving 6 µg/Kg/d (420 µg/d) would be about $6000. Given that cost, some insurers and health plans still question the medical necessity for GH replacement in adults, although policies vary widely.

GH THERAPY IN AGING

In the course of normal aging there is a gradual decrease in GH secretion *(1,46)*, mediated at least in part by an age-related diminishment of endogenous GHRH release *(vide supra)* *(47)*. Consequently, serum IGF-I levels in elderly people are approximately 50% as high as those in younger adults (Fig. 2). Hyposomatomedinemia is especially marked in the frail elderly *(37)*. Many of the untoward changes associated with aging mimic those seen in the GH-deficiency syndrome, including muscle atrophy, osteopenia, obesity, cardiovascular deterioration, exercise intolerance, decreased metabolic rate, dyslipidemia, thinning of the skin, mild anemia, and depression. Aging is thus a partial phenocopy of adult GH deficiency. This has led to the speculation that pituitary somatotrope activity may be a pacemaker of aging *(34)*, and raised the possibility that GH supplementation might reverse or slow some features of geriatric deterioration *(48)*.

GH Treatment Studies in Aging

The first major trial examining the impact of GH replacement in the elderly was reported by Rudman, et al. in 1990 *(49)*. Twenty-one healthy elderly men (ages 61–81) with physiologically low serum IGF-I levels (< 0.35 U/mL) (*see* Note on Units at the begining of this chapter) were randomized to receive 30 µg/kg of GH three times per week vs placebo for 6 mo. IGF-I levels in the GH group rose to a range that would be normal for men in the third decade of life (0.5–1.5 U/mL). These subjects enjoyed an 8.8% increase in LBM, a 14.4% decrease in adipose tissue mass, and a 7.1% increase in skin thickness. LBM was assessed by ^{40}K counting, which should not be falsely elevated due to fluid retention. There was a slight (1.6%) increase in lumbar vertebral BMD in the GH group, but no change in BMD in the radius or proximal femur in either group. In a larger follow-up study using a similar cohort of healthy, GH-insufficient elderly men and the

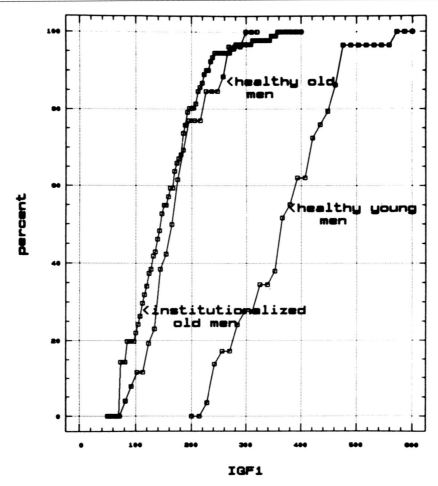

Fig. 2. Cumulative frequency distributions for circulating levels of IGF-I in young, healthy old, and institutionalized old men. There is a marked decrease in IGF-I levels with aging, regardless of functional status *(37)*.

same GH dose, Rudman and his colleagues demonstrated that increases in LBM, muscle cross-sectional area, and skin thickness persisted for as long as one year in GH-treated individuals *(50)*.

Since Rudman's landmark studies, there have been surprisingly few published investigations of GH treatment for the "somatopause" associated with normal aging. Among these, there is a consensus that GH causes similar advantageous changes in body composition among the elderly as when it is replaced in younger GH-deficient adults. For example, Thompson, et al. demonstrated significant increases in LBM and decreases in fat mass among older women (72 ± 1 yr) administered either GH or IGF-I for just 4 wk *(51)*. The treatments promoted whole-body and skeletal muscle protein synthesis and nitrogen retention. Similarly Cohn, et al. reported a 6% increase in LBM and a 16% decrease in adipose tissue mass among elderly men (69 ± 2 yr) treated with GH for 1 yr *(38)*. All of the studies of GH usage in the elderly that are described below noted changes similar to those among GH-treated subjects.

While these alterations in body composition are favorable, it would be more meaningful to demonstrate improvement in strength and functional status with GH treatment, especially since at least some of the augmentation in LBM arises from GH-mediated fluid retention rather than from actual muscle growth. Taaffe et al. reported that there was no increase in muscular response to strength training among elderly men treated with GH for 10 wk, and concluded that deficits in GH do not underlie the time-dependent leveling off of muscle strength seen with aging (52).

In a larger study, Papadakis et al. assessed whether restoration of GH to youthful physiological levels improved functional ability in older men (53). Fifty-two healthy elderly men (70–85 yr) with well preserved functional ability but low serum IGF-I levels were randomized to receive 30 μg/Kg of GH three times/wk vs placebo for 6 mo in a double-blinded fashion. Once again, LBM increased by 4.3% and fat mass decreased by 13.1% in the treatment group, while there were no significant changes in body composition seen with placebo. However, there was no difference between GH and placebo with regard to grip strength at the hand or knee, nor in systemic endurance. Several tests were employed to assess cognitive function and mood. Mean score in the Trails B Test, which measures visual and motor tracking and attention, improved by 8.5 s in the GH group and deteriorated by 5.0 s in the placebo group (p = 0.01). However, on the Mini-Mental State Examination, which assess orientation, attention, calculation, language, and memory, scores deteriorated by 0.4 in the GH group and improved by 0.2 in the placebo group (p=0.11). Neither group showed changes in results on the Digital Symbol Substitution test, which measures cognitive ability, nor in the Geriatric Depression Scale. The authors concluded that physiological GH replacement in healthy older men for 6 mo improves body composition but not functional status.

Two trials have been published examining the effects of GH administration on bone physiology in healthy, post-menopausal women. They both showed that GH increases bone turnover, but reported somewhat conflicting results regarding GH effects on BMD. Holloway, et al. randomized 27 elderly women (67 ± 3 yr) to receive either placebo or GH at an initial dose of 43 μg/kg/d for 6 mo (54). Half of the subjects receiving GH required dose reduction within the first few weeks owing to adverse side effects, most commonly related to fluid retention and carpal tunnel syndrome. GH treatment was associated with 20–80% increases in markers of both bone formation (osteocalcin) and bone resorption (urinary hydroxyproline and pyridinoline). These changes were especially marked in women not taking supplemental estrogens, and they persisted for as long as 12 mo in a subset of subjects who remained on therapy after the formal trial was completed. There was no change in BMD at the lumbar spine or hip in the GH group, whereas the placebo group showed a 1.7% decrease in BMD at the femoral trochanter and a 3.0% decrease at Ward's triangle. The authors concluded that while GH is a powerful initiator of bone remodeling in elderly women, it exerts at best a protective, not enhancing, effect on BMD. Similar increases in markers of both bone formation and resorption have been reported using GH in a mixed group of elderly men and women (55).

Since GH stimulates both bone formation and resorption, it seems logical to administer it in conjunction with a resorption inhibitor such as a bisphosphonate, in order to treat osteoporosis. Accordingly, Erdtsieck, et al. examined the effects of supplemental GH on bone turnover and mass among healthy, post-menopausal women in the presence of pamidronate (56). Twenty-one women received pamidronate for one year, either with or without concomitant GH therapy (22 μg/Kg, 3 times per week) for the first 6 mo. GH blocked the pamidronate-induced decrease in biochemical markers of bone turnover. Furthermore, while subjects receiving only pamidronate showed a 5% increase in bone mineral mass at the lumbar spine and distal forearm, these changes were not seen in individuals receiving GH as well. Thus, GH blocked the pamidronate-induced decrease in bone turnover and the accumulation of bone mineral mass.

Two groups have examined the use of GH to enhance body weight in malnourished elderly people (57,58). Subjects over 60 yr of age selected on the basis of low body weight, recent weight loss, low serum albumin, and low IGF-I levels were administered GH for 3 wk. IGF-I levels were restored to the high end of the youthful range. This was associated with significant nitrogen retention, accompanied by a 2.2–2.3 kg weight gain and increased mid-arm muscle circumference. No increase in albumin was achieved, although the duration of therapy may have been too short for this. Although these findings show that GH supplementation bolsters body weight in the malnourished elderly, the results can be attributed at least in part to fluid retention. Further studies are required to determine whether GH improves strength or functional ability in this setting.

Patient Selection, GH Dosage, and Adverse Effects in the Elderly

Two important questions must be addressed if GH supplementation is to be considered in the elderly. Who should be classified as GH deficient, and to what level should IGF-I values be normalized? The answer to both questions depends upon which healthy reference group is chosen as a standard: young adults or elderly people. As shown in Fig. 2 (37), the normal IGF-I range, as defined by 95% confidence intervals, for healthy men in their 20s is 240–460 ng/mL. Values less 240 ng/mL are below the 2.5 percentile and are classified as abnormally low if this reference group is used. More recent studies define a wider population normal range; but by this standard, 80% of men over 60 yr of age would be deemed hyposomatomedinemic. Clearly the definition of GH deficiency, and thus the prevalence of the condition, are critically dependent upon the reference range employed. The situation is similar to that encountered with the use of T vs Z scores to characterize bone density.

At present there is insufficient evidence to clarify which reference group is most sensible to use for the geriatric population, either in defining abnormal GH deficiency or in establishing target IGF-I values to dictate GH dosage. Essentially, we do not yet know whether the age-related decline in GH secretion is a pathological or an adaptive condition, nor whether it confers some still cryptic benefits in the elderly. The experimental trials cited above have generally used young adults as the standard, and corrected IGF-I levels to a range that would be normal for that population. Additional studies are required to determine whether the risk/benefit ratio for GH treatment in the elderly is optimized by this strategy or by the more conservative approach of normalizing IGF-I levels only to the middle or high end of the geriatric reference range.

Adverse effects of GH therapy are unequivocally dose-related, and several studies have shown that elderly people are considerably more susceptible to these untoward consequences than are the young. Indeed, nearly all of the trials discussed in this section reported high incidences of GH-related side effects in the geriatric population, especially fluid retention, carpal tunnel syndrome, gynecomastia, and insulin resistance. Some investigators noted that when IGF-I levels in elderly people were restored to the youthful normal range (0.5–1.5 U/mL), side effects were far more prevalent among those individuals brought to the high end of that range (1.0–1.5 U/mL) (35,38,51). Subjects with levels in the lower half of the normal range (0.5–1.0 U/mL) generally enjoyed the benefits of GH therapy with far fewer adverse consequences.

As discussed earlier, GH has mitogenic properties on a number of cell lineages in vitro *(39)*, and epidemiological evidence suggests that untreated acromegalics have an increased risk of neoplasia *(40–42)*. Although these findings do not necessarily mean that people given physiological replacement doses of GH would suffer any increased cancer risk, it will be very difficult to prove or disprove definitively whether this is the case in humans. Theoretical concerns about carcinogenic properties of GH are likely to be greatest in the elderly, where there is an increased cancer risk in general.

In summary, if GH therapy ever becomes accepted for use in aging, physicians should seek to restore IGF-I levels to no more than the lower end of the normal range for young adults because of the enhanced sensitivity of elderly people for the adverse effects of supplemental GH. These levels can often be achieved with doses much lower than those reported in the earlier studies *(59)*. It would be reasonable to adopt a strategy similar to that developed by the GH Research Society for use in adult GH deficiency, beginning with a low dose and raising it gradually. Thus, one might initiate GH therapy at 150 µg sc at bedtime (approximately 2 µg/Kg), and increase as necessary until the desired IGF-I level is achieved *(43,60)* or until limiting side effects develop. Active malignancy is considered an absolute contraindication. In principle, complications of therapy could also be minimized by excluding patients with conditions that might be exacerbated by exogenous GH, such as carpal tunnel syndrome, diabetes, arthritis, congestive heart failure, and hypertension. But as this list would exclude a large fraction of those who might benefit and sensitivity to GH side effects varies widely among individuals, these conditions are flags for caution and conservative dosing regimens rather than absolute contraindications. The effects of GH on body composition may improve glucose tolerance despite its acute insulin antagonism, and its effects on cardiac contractility may override its acute effects on fluid retention.

Both long- and short-term GH replacement strategies can be envisaged in the elderly *(48)*. Long-term therapy could theoretically reverse or slow many of the catabolic features of aging such as muscle and bone atrophy, although convincing evidence to prove this is lacking. In addition, short-term GH treatment might be indicated to maintain LBM when impaired nutrition and/or catabolic states develop, such as major surgeries, trauma such as hip fracture, or illnesses. Although no studies have been published to evaluate this possibility, it is very plausible that short-term GH therapy could facilitate the recovery of acutely debilitated elderly patients, and this is a subject of active investigation.

Summary of GH Therapy for Aging

Very little evidence exists to judge whether GH supplementation can ameliorate the physical and cognitive deterioration of aging. While there is considerable public excitement about this possibility, most of the optimistic contentions are speculations derived from the treatment of GH-deficient young adults. It is true that the handful of studies examining GH usage in healthy elderly people have all demonstrated beneficial changes in body composition: notably increased LBM and decreased adiposity. In his original paper Rudman stated that these alterations were "equivalent in magnitude to the changes incurred during 10–20 yr of aging" *(49)*— a statement which was construed by the news media to suggest that GH reverses the effects of aging. However, it has not yet been shown that these changes correlate with any more meaningful clinical outcomes. In contrast to the situation with nonelderly GH-deficient adults, investigators have tried but failed to document among healthy elderly people any improvement from GH treatment in muscle strength, functional status, cognitive ability, or overall physical or emotional well-being. Thus, scientific evidence is lacking to support the popular perception of GH as an ergogenic aid in the elderly. While GH may exert a maintenance effect on BMD in the hip among post-menopausal women, a variety of anti-resorptive agents currently perform at least as well in this regard, and it would be difficult to justify the use of GH over such agents in view of its cost and inconvenient delivery. No studies have yet been reported to assess the impact of GH in the elderly with regard to such clinically germane outcomes as fracture risk, cardiac capacity, cardiovascular risk, cost effectiveness, recovery, overall morbidity, or mortality.

In view of the fact that GH has not been clearly shown to confer important lasting benefits in the elderly, and that this population is especially susceptible to GH-related side effects, and that GH therapy remains remarkably expensive, the use of GH in otherwise healthy aging people is not yet warranted. Nevertheless, GH replacement in the elderly has many theoretical advantages, and longer studies may one day show it to have rejuvenating properties in this population. If so, it is likely that GH will be used first in frail and debilitated patients, in whom the risk/benefit ratio of treatment may be most favorable *(61)*. See ref. *61a* for a recent review of GH secretion and GH treatment in aging.

OTHER CONDITIONS: CATABOLISM, HIV, AND CRITICAL ILLNESS

GH has also been recommended as treatment for a variety of conditions in which the relationship of symptoms to reduced GH secretion is less clear—for example, fibromyalgia and chronic fatigue syndrome. It has been suggested that GH secretion may be reduced in some fibromyalgia patients. A placebo-controlled trial of GH in 50 patients with fibromyalgia and low levels of IGF-I (< 160 ng/mL) reported a reduction in symptoms over 9 mo of treatment, with most improvement occurring after 6 mo *(62)*. At this time there are no confirmatory studies, and the FDA has not approved the use of GH for this indication.

Well-controlled data supporting the use of GH are even sparser for most other non-traditional indications except for those associated with protein catabolism or wasting, such as chronic illnesses such as AIDS or renal failure, burns, fractures, or malnutrition (*vide supra* for discussion of malnutrition in aging). In these settings, GH secretion is normal or even elevated, but partial GH resistance may be present. Since the GH resistance in these conditions is relative rather than absolute, it has been suggested that pharmacologic doses of GH might overcome it and promote anabolism, often in conjunction with nutritional supplementation. For example, Horber and Haymond demonstrated that very high dose GH treatment (100 µg/Kg/d) counteracted prednisone-induced leucine and nitrogen catabolism over 1 wk of treatment *(63)*. Similar effects were shown in burn patients using even higher doses of GH (200 µg/Kg/d) (64), and the use of GH has been suggested for patients with renal failure, based upon some success in promoting growth in children (65). Because high-dose GH produces insulin resistance and often hyperglycemia, the combination of GH with recombinant IGF-I, which shares anabolic effects but reduces insulin resistance, has been advocated and evaluated in a few studies.

Early studies such as these were of brief duration and so have reported only metabolic endpoints, but a few more recent trials have reported favorable effects upon clinically relevant endpoints such as decreased hospital stays and mortality in burn patients (*see* ref. *66* for review).

Of these catabolic states, the only one that has received FDA approval for GH treatment is AIDS-associated wasting. Serono laboratories has registered a separate name for its GH for this indication, Serostin®. Published studies of GH in HIV illness are still relatively few. Mulligan and colleagues showed increased nitrogen retention and decreased protein oxidation in 6 men with HIV-associated wasting during 7 d of treatment with 100 µg/Kg/d GH *(67)*. More recently this group has reported 3 mo treatment with the same high GH dose *(68)*. There was an increase in LBM and a decrease in body fat, and an increase in treadmill work output in patients receiving GH vs placebo. Lee and colleagues administered a lower GH dose (approximately 12 µg/Kg/d) together with IGF-I (5 mg BID) for 3 mo, but found no significant anabolic effects with this regimen *(69)*. There are still no data available showing an effect of GH on meaningful functional status, quality of life, or survival in HIV; and further studies are needed to define its indications.

Hospitalized patients with critical illness appear to have a dual GH disorder. They suffer marked protein catabolism and appear to share a relative GH resistance with other catabolic states; but in severe illness GH secretion is also markedly reduced *(13)*. These patients would thus seem to be appropriate candidates for high-dose GH treatment, but recent experience also highlights the potential hazards of its use. Pharmacia and Upjohn recently halted a multicenter study of GH in several hundred ICU-hospitalized critically ill patients because of a near-doubling of the already high mortality rate, from 20 to 38% *(3)*. Although the relatively large sample size makes it unlikely that this is a statistical artifact, there does not appear to be a single or simple explanation for this adverse effect. The study has not been published and detailed information is not yet available; but this cautionary report is reminiscent of earlier studies of the use of tri-iodothyronine (T_3) in critical illness, which also showed an adverse effect.

Doses of GH proposed for use in most wasting syndromes are high, and it is not clear that GH resistance is uniform in all tissues, carrying the possibility of greater dose-related side effects in fragile patients. While protein catabolism is a serious clinical problem, the reductions in GH secretion or action may be adaptive in other ways which we override at our peril. Less acutely or seriously ill patients with catabolism report the usual gamut of GH side effects including edema and compression neuropathies but have not shown serious morbidities or the excess mortality seen in critical illness. We recommend that clinicians wishing to use GH in catabolism, even for FDA-approved indications such as AIDS, obtain informed consent after thorough discussion with their patients, use graduated doses, and monitor side effects very closely.

GH SECRETAGOGUES

Hypothalamic GH secretagogues—GHRH and the "endogenous GHRP"—stimulate physiologic GH secretion, and in patients in whom the pituitary is intact, administered GH secretagogues can replace GH by boosting endogenous secretion. GH secretagogues have several potential and practical advantages over administered GH. Even when infused continuously, GHRH and GHRPs stimulate an episodic pattern of GH pulses which resembles physiologic secretion, presumably due to the effects of intermittent endogenous somatostatin. The GH response is modulated by IGF-I negative feedback at the pituitary level, which offers a relative (but not absolute) protection against overtreatment. And as they are much smaller molecules than GH, some of the secretagogues can be administered nasally or orally. GHRH can be administered transnasally in high doses, and both the peptide and nonpeptide GHRPs are resistant to proteolysis and can be given orally.

At this writing, the only GH secretagogue approved for use as replacement therapy is GHRH(1–29)NH$_2$ (Geref ®, Serono), which has been licensed for the treatment of idiopathic GH deficiency in children. Single nightly subcutaneous injections have been given to GH-deficient children in doses of 15–30 µg/Kg/d, with restoration of normal growth velocity *(70)*. In principle, this treatment could be continued in adult patients with hypothalamic GH deficiency as well, and a few studies have examined the effects of short-term administration of GHRH in GH-deficient adults *(71)*. But since the majority of adults with GH deficiency have pituitary disorders and would be unlikely to respond, there are no published studies of long-term GHRH treatment of adult GH deficiency.

Most studies have focused instead upon the effects of GHRH in aging. Acute administration of GHRH continues to elicit an acute GH response in aging *(10)*, although the magnitude of the rise may decline. Corpas and colleagues *(72)* found that twice-daily subcutaneous administration of 1 mg GHRH (approximately 15 µg/Kg) for 2 wk to healthy older men could elevate plasma IGF-I levels to the young adult normal range *(72)*. Recently, Vittone et al. reported the effects of the same total daily GHRH given as a single 2-mg nightly injection for 6 wk *(73)*. Two measures of muscle strength improved, but IGF-I and IGFBP-3 levels did not rise, and the authors concluded that divided doses of GHRH might be more effective than single higher doses. Khorram and colleagues have described a study of 16-wk treatment with single nightly injections of a GHRH analog in healthy older men and women (74). IGF-I levels rose in both men and women, but there was a gender difference in effects on body composition, with an increase in lean body mass in men but not in women. These published studies have been of relatively brief duration, long enough to assess hormonal effects but not effects on body composition or function. We are currently conducting two studies of a 6-mo intervention with single nightly sc doses of 1–2 mg GHRH(1–29)NH$_2$. In the study examining men and estrogenized women there is an approximately 35% rise in IGF-I levels *(75)*, but functional measures are not yet available.

A small number of studies have examined the effects of GHRH upon sleep and cognition, some of which may be mediated by GH secretagogues themselves and not by GH. Sleep promotes GH secretion, but the reverse may also be true. Steiger and colleagues and Kerkhofs et al. have reported that GHRH acutely stimulates slow-wave sleep in healthy young adults *(76,77)*, and that somatostatin inhibits this effect *(76)*. Our current study will examine whether this sleep-promoting effect is also observed in older adults and persists with chronic treatment.

Short-term studies of the effects of the GHRPs and the nonpeptide GHRP mimetics in older subjects have also been conducted. Even brief 24 h infusions significantly elevated IGF-I levels. Daily oral administration of the nonpeptide GHRP agonist MK677 in two different doses (10 and 25 mg) for 14–28 d in healthy older men and women markedly elevated 24-h pulsatile GH and plasma IGF-I levels *(78)*. Effects of the GHRPs on body composition or function in adults have not yet been published. In GH-deficient children treated with GHRP for 6 mo, there was a restoration of normal growth velocity *(79)*, and thus it is reasonable to speculate that GHRPs will have effects similar to those of GHRH in adults as well.

A few studies of the effects of GHRH or GHRPs in recovery from fractures and catabolism have been conducted but are not yet published. One study of treatment of children with chronic renal failure and growth retardation using GHRH(1-29)NH$_2$ twice daily for 3–6 mo reported an acceleration of growth *(80)*, and this encourages further study of the use of GH secretagogues in adult catabolic states.

In contrast to GH administration, the effects of the GH secretagogues are affected by the same factors that modulate endogenous GHRH secretion. Increased somatostatin tone in particular can markedly reduce the GHRH response to GHRH or the GHRPs. Because obesity appears to suppress GH secretion at least in part through increased somatostatin, this inhibition can blunt the therapeutic response to repeated administration of GHRH, GHRPs, or the GHRP mimetics *(81)*. This effect has led investigators to examine the potential utility of adjuvants that could enhance the response to secretagogue treatment. Ghigo and colleagues have shown that arginine markedly potentiates the acute GH response to GHRP in aging *(12)*. Beta-adrenergic antagonists such as propranolol and atenolol also boost the acute GH response to GHRH, probably through inhibition of somatostatin secretion, and are active by oral administration. We examined the effect of atenolol co-treatment in a group of GH-deficient children treated with subcutaneous GHRH. In doses commonly used to treat hypertension, atenolol significantly increased the growth velocity acceleration during the first year of treatment, as compared to treatment with GHRH and placebo *(82)*.

Because GHRH and GHRP exert synergistic effects on GH release, in principle the combination of agents of these two categories would be more potent than either given alone. Our study of the treatment of GH children with GHRP included a final 2-mo treatment period with GHRP and GHRH given together *(79)*. Combination therapy produced a greater rise in peak nighttime GH than GHRP alone. The growth response was no greater, but the brief 2-mo treatment period limits the conclusions which can be reached from growth data. There are no comparable published studies of enhancing adjuvants to GH secretagogue therapy in adults.

In theory the moderating effects of feedback regulation should make the GH secretagogues freer from side effects than is GH. This has generally been the case in published series, but occasional patients have reported typical GH side effects such as edema and carpal tunnel syndrome, and a small number of patients have had erythema or urticarial responses consistent with allergic reactions. At this date it is not clear whether the apparently lower incidence of side effects reflects a qualitative advantage of GH secretagogues, or simply the lower potency of the doses that have been employed.

Current formulations of the GH secretagogues are quite short-acting and do not fully realize their potential for restoring physiologic pulsatile GH secretion. A preparation which provides secretagogue effect for at least 8–12 h is needed to attempt to restore the nighttime GH profile. The existing formulation of GHRH(1-29)NH$_2$ and the research formulations of the GHRPs and their mimetics appear to stimulate an acute rise in GH after administration but do not support GH secretion for the rest of the night in adults. Thus, the role for GH secretagogues in GH replacement for adults is likely to remain very limited until longer-acting drugs or formulations become available.

SUMMARY AND FUTURE PROSPECTS

Growth hormone has only recently become available for adult replacement therapy. Our evaluation of its use, effects, and side effects is current as of mid-1998, but we can expect it to change as the published experience with investigational trials is supplemented by post-marketing clinical experience in a much larger number of subjects. The recommended dosage has been reduced progressively since the first studies of GH in adult GH deficiency, and is likely to change still further or to evolve into an individualized titration as recommended by the GH Research Society and currently practiced by some endocrinologists. It is already clear that sensitivity to the side effects of GH varies widely among individuals, especially in obesity and aging, and these high-risk groups will be more fully defined in coming years. It is not yet clear whether patients receiving GH require periodic screening over and above population-based recommendations for colon, prostate, or other malignancies, or for other conditions.

Aging reduces levels of sex steroids, melatonin, and other hormones as well as growth hormone. Thus, many older people as well as hypopituitary patients are candidates for hormone replacement with more than one agent, but the interactions among these trophic factors have not been well defined. For example, many subjects given growth hormone may also receive thyroid hormone, glucocorticoids, estrogen or testosterone treatment. Their several effects may oppose, add to, or synergize with each other, and these interactions can arise from effects both on the secretion of other hormones as well as on mutual target organs. Thus, estrogen and aromatizable androgens stimulate GH secretion, and there is evidence for synergy between sex steroids and GH on some target organs *(83–85)*.

In addition to other hormones and drugs, GH may be used in conjunction with lifestyle interventions such as exercise conditioning. Exercise is also trophic, producing some of the same changes in fat, muscle, and bone as GH while improving glucose tolerance. While exercise acutely stimulates GH, most of these consequences are probably mediated through different effectors, in that even intensive exercise condition regimens do not elevate circulating levels of IGF-I *(86)*. Few data exist on the interactions between GH and exercise conditioning. Several research studies evaluating the effects of GH or GH secretagogues together with exercise are in progress, including studies of combined treatment with exercise together with GH or GHRH being conducted at the Universities of Virginia and Washington, and should yield results within the next 1–2 yr *(87)*.

Thus with new GH formulations and secretagogues under development, and new information about its beneficial and adverse effects as well as interactions with other treatment regimens, the practice of adult GH replacement therapy is in a state of rapid development. It is likely to change significantly in the coming years.

REFERENCES

1. Corpas E, Harman SM, Blackman MR. Human growth hormone and human aging. Endocr Rev 1993;14:20–39.
2. Hoffman DM, O'Sullivan AJ, Baxter RC, Ho KKY. Diagnosis of growth-hormone deficiency in adults. Lancet 1994;343:1064–1068.
3. Pharmacia and Upjohn. Letter to Physicians 1997.
4. Gelato MC, Merriam GR. Growth hormone-releasing hormone. Ann Rev Physiology 1986;48:569–591.
5. Bowers CY, Veeraragavan K, Sethumadhavan K. A typical growth hormone releasing peptides. In: Bercu BB, Walker RF, eds. Growth Hormone: Basic and Clinical Aspects. Springer-Verlag, New York, 1994, pp. 203–222.
6. Patchett AA, Nargund RP, Tata JR, Chen MH, Barakat KJ, Johnston DB, Cheng K, Chan WW, Butler B, Hickey G, Smith RG. Design and biological activites of L-163.191 (MK-0677), a potent, orally active growth hormone secretagogue. Proc Nat Acad Sci USA 1995,92:7001–7005.

7. Mericq V, Cassorla F, Garcia H, Avila A, Bowers CY, Merriam GR. Growth hormone (GH) responses to GH-releasing peptide and to GH-releasing hormone in GH-deficient children. J Clin Endocrinol Metab 1995,80:1681–1684.

8. Pandya N, DeMott-Friberg R, Bowers CY, Barkan AL, Jaffe CA. Growth hormone-releasing peptide-6 requires endogenous hypothalamic GH-releasing hormone for maximal GH stimulation. J Clin Endocrinol Metab 1998;83:1186–1189.

9. Gelato MC, Malozowski S, Caruso-Nicoletti M, Ross JL, Pescovitz OH, Rose S, Loriaux DL, Cassorla F, Merriam GR. Growth hormone (GH) responses to GH-releasing hormone during pubertal development in normal boys and girls:comparison to idiopathic short stature and GH deficiency. J Clin Endocrinol Metab 1986;63:174–179.

10. Pavlov EP, Harman SM, Merriam GR, Gelato MC, Blackman MR. Responses of growth hormone (GH) and somatomedin-C to GH-releasing hormone in healthy aging men. J Clin Endocrinol Metab 1986;62:595–600.

11. Chapman IM,. Hartman ML, Pezzoli SS,. Harrell Jr FE, Hintz RL, Alberti KG, Thorner MO. Effect of aging on the sensitivity of growth hormone secretion to insulin-like growth factor-I negative feedback. J Clin Endocrinol Metab 1997;82:2996–3004.

12. Ghigo E, Goffi S, Nicolosi M, Arvat E, Valente F, Mazza E, Ghigo MC, Camanni F. Growth hormone (GH) responsiveness to combined administration of arginine and GH-releasing hormone does not vary with age in man. J Clin Endocrinol Metab 1990;71:1481–1485.

13. VandenBerghe G, deZegher F, Veldhuis JD, et al. The somatotrophic axis in critical illness:effect of continuous growth hormone (GH)-releasing hormone and GH-releasing peptide-2 infusion. J Clin Endocrinol Metab 1997;82:590–599.

14. Christ ER, Carroll PV, Russell JDL, Sonksen PH. The consequences of growth hormone deficiency in adulthood, and the effects of growth hormone replacement. Schweiz Med Wochenschr 1997;127:1440–9.

15. Cuneo RC, Salomon F, McGauley GA, Sonksen PH. The growth hormone deficiency syndrome in adults. Clin Endocrinol Oxf 1992;37:387–397.

16. Labram EK, Wilkin TJ. Growth hormone deficiency in adults and its response to growth hormone replacement. Qjm 1995;88:391–399.

17. Ros'en T, Johannsson G, Johansson JO, Bengtsson BA. Consequences of growth hormone deficiency in adults and the benefits and risks of recombinant human growth hormone treatment. Horm Res 1995;43:93–99.

18. Jorgensen JO, Muller J, Moller J, Wolthers T, Vahl N, Juul A, Skakkebaek NE, Christiansen JS. Adult growth hormone deficiency. Horm Res 1994;42:235–241.

19. Lieberman SA, Hoffman AR. Growth hormone deficiency in adults:characteristics and response to growth hormone replacement. J Pediatr 1996;128:S58–S60.

20. Markussis V, Beshyah SA, Fisher C, Sharp P, Nicolaides AN, Johnston DG. Detection of premature atherosclerosis by high-resolution ultrasonography in symptom-free hypopituitary adults. Lancet 1992;340:1188–1192.

21. Ros'en T, Bengtsson BA. Premature mortality due to cardiovascular disease in hypopituitarism. Lancet 1990;336:285–288.

22. Bates AS, Van't HW, Jones PJ, Clayton RN. The effect of hypopituitarism on life expectancy. J Clin Endocrinol Metab 1996;81:1169–1172.

23. Shahi M, Beshyah SA, Hackett D, Sharp PS, Johnston DG, Foale RA. Myocardial dysfunction in treated adult hypopituitarism:a possible explanation for increased cardiovascular mortality. Br Heart J 1992;67:92–96.

24. Evans HM, Long JA. The effect of the anterior lobe administered intraperitoneally upon growth. Maturity and oestrous cycles of the rat. Anat Rec 1921;21:62–63.

25. Raben MS. Clinical use of human growth hormone. N Engl J Med 1962;266:82–86.

26. Buchanan CR, Preece MA, Milner RD. Mortality, neoplasia, and Creutzfeldt-Jakob disease in patients treated with human pituitary growth hormone in the United Kingdom. BMJ 1991;302:824–828.

27. Salomon F, Cuneo RC, Hesp R, Sonksen PH. The effects of treatment with recombinant human growth hormone on body composition and metabolism in adults with growth hormone deficiency. N Engl J Med 1989;321:1797–1803.

28. Jorgensen JO, Pedersen SA, Thuesen L, Jorgensen J, Ingemann HT, Skakkebaek NE, Christiansen JS. Beneficial effects of growth hormone treatment in GH-deficient adults. Lancet 1989;1:1221–1225.

29. Carroll PV, Christ ER, Bengtsson BA, Carlsson L, Christiansen JS, Clemmons D, Hintz R, Ho K, Laron Z, Sizonenko P, Sonksen PH, Tanaka T, Thorner M. Growth hormone deficiency in adulthood and the

effects of growth hormone replacement: a review. Growth Hormone Research Society Scientific Committee. J Clin Endocrinol Metab 1998;83:382–95.

30. Clark W, Kendall MJ. Growth hormone treatment for growth hormone deficient adults. J Clin Pharm Ther 1996;21:367–372.

31. Meling TR, Nylen ES. Growth hormone deficiency in adults: a review. Am J Med Sci 1996; 311:153–166.

32. MantzorosCS, Moses AC. Whither recombinant human growth hormone? Ann Intern Med 1996; 125:932–934.

33. Powrie J, Weissberger A, Sonksen P. Growth hormone replacement therapy for growth hormone-deficient adults. Drugs 1995;49:656–663.

34. Lamberts SW, Valk NK, Binnerts A. The use of growth hormone in adults:a changing scene. Clin Endocrinol Oxf 1992;37:111–115.

35. Jorgensen JO. Human growth hormone replacement therapy: pharmacological and clinical aspects. Endocr Rev 1991;12:189–207.

36. Bengtsson BA. The consequences of growth hormone deficiency in adults. Acta Endocrinol 1993;2:2–5.

37. Abbasi AA, Drinka PJ, Mattson DE, Rudman D. Low circulating levels of insulin-like growth factors and testosterone in chronically institutionalized elderly men. J Am Geriatr Soc 1993;41:975–982.

38. Cohn L, Feller AG, Draper MW, Rudman IW, Rudman D. Carpal tunnel syndrome and gynaecomastia during growth hormone treatment of elderly men with low circulating IGF-I concentrations. Clin Endocrinol Oxf 1993;39:417–425.

39. Daughaday WH. The possible autocrine/paracrine and endocrine roles of insulin–like growth factors of human tumors. Endocrinology 1990;127:1–4.

40. Ezzat S, Melmed S. Clinical review 18:Are patients with acromegaly at increased risk for neoplasia? J Clin Endocrinol Metab 1991;72:245–249.

41. Brunner JE, Johnson CC, Zafar S, Peterson EL, Brunner JF, Mellinger RC. Colon cancer and polyps in acromegaly: increased risk associated with family history of colon cancer. Clin Endocrinol Oxf 1990;32:65–71.

42. Bengtsson BA, Ed'en S, Ernest I, Od'en A, Sjogren B. Epidemiology and long-term survival in acromegaly: a study of 166 cases diagnosed between 1955 and 1984. Acta Med Scand 1988; 223:327–35.

42a. Hankinson SE, Willett WC, Colditz GA, Hunter DJ, Michaud DS, Deroo B, Rosner B, Speizer FE, Pollak M. Circulating concentrations of insulin-like growth factor-I and risk of breast cancer. Lancet 1998;351:1393–1396.

42b. Chan JM, Stampfer MJ, Giovanucci E, Gan PH, Ma J, Wilkinson P, Hennekens CH, Pollak M. Plasma insulin-like growth factor-I and prostate cancer risk: a prospective study. Science 1998;279:563–566.

43. Growth Hormone Research Society. Consensus guidelines for the diagnosis and treatment of adults with growth hormone deficiency: summary statement of the Growth Hormone Research Society Workshop on Adult Growth Hormone Deficiency. J Clin Endocrinol Metab 1998;83:379–381.

44. Zadik Z, Chalew SA, McCarter RJJ, Meistas M, Kowarski AA. The influence of age on the 24-hour integrated concentration of growth hormone in normal individuals. J Clin Endocrinol Metab 1985;60:513–516.

45. Ho KY, Evans WS, Blizzard RM, Veldhuis JD, Merriam GR, Samojlik E, Furlanetto R, Rogol AD, Kaiser DL, Thorner MO. Effects of sex and age on the 24-hour profile of growth hormone secretion in man:importance of endogenous estradiol concentrations. J Clin Endocrinol Metab 1987;64:51–58.

45a. Burman P, Johansson AG, Siegbahn A, Vessby B, Karlsson FA. Growth hormone deficient men are more responsive to GH replacement therapy than women. J Clin Endocrinol Metab 1997;82:550–555.

45b. Drake WM, Coyte D, Camacho-Hubner, Jivanji NM, Kaltsas G, Wood DF, Trainer PJ, Grossman AB, Besser GM, Monson JP. Optmizing growth hormone replacement therapy by dose titration in hypopituitary adults. J Clin Endocrinol Metab 1998;83:9313–9319.

45c. Bellantoni MF, Vittone J, Campfield AT, Bass KM, Harman SM, Blackman MR. Effects of oral vs. transermal estrogen on the growth hormone-insulin-like growth factor I axis in younger and older postmenopausal women. J Clin Endocrinol Metab 1996;81:2848–2853.

46. Harman SM, Blackman MR. Growth hormone, IGF–I, gonadal steroids, and aging. Aging Milano 1992;4:257–259.

47. Degli Uberti EC, Ambrosio MR, Cella SG, Margutti AR, Trasforini G, Rigamonti AE, Petrone E, Muller EE. Defective hypothalamic growth hormone (GH)-releasing hormone activity may contribute to declining GH secretion with age in man. J Clin Endocrinol Metab 1997;82:2885–2888.

48. Rudman D, Shetty KR. Unanswered questions concerning the treatment of hyposomatotropism and hypogonadism in elderly men. J Am Geriatr Soc 1994;42:522–527.

49. Rudman D, Feller AG, Nagraj HS, Gergans GA, Lalitha PY, Goldberg AF, Schlenker RA, Cohn L, Rudman IW, Mattson DE. Effects of human growth hormone in men over 60 years old. N Engl J Med 1990;323:1–6.

50. Rudman D, Feller AG, Cohn L, Shetty KR, Rudman IW, Draper MW. Effects of human growth hormone on body composition in elderly men. Horm Res 1991;36 (suppl):73–81.

51. Thompson JL, Butterfield GE, Marcus R, Hintz RL, Van LM, Ghiron L, Hoffman AR. The effects of recombinant human insulin-like growth factor-I and growth hormone on body composition in elderly women. J Clin Endocrinol Metab 1995;80:1845–1852.

52. Taaffe DR, Jin IH, Vu TH, Hoffman AR, Marcus R. Lack of effect of recombinant human growth hormone (GH) on muscle morphology and GH-insulin-like growth factor expression in resistance–trained elderly men. J Clin Endocrinol Metab 1996;81:421–425.

53. Papadakis MA, Grady D, Black D, Tierney MJ, Gooding GA, Schambelan M, Grunfeld C. Growth hormone replacement in healthy older men improves body composition but not functional ability. Ann Intern Med 1996;124:708–716.

54. Holloway L, Butterfield G, Hintz RL, Gesundheit N, Marcus R. Effects of recombinant human growth hormone on metabolic indices, body composition, and bone turnover in healthy elderly women. J Clin Endocrinol Metab 1994;79:470–479.

55. Marcus R, Butterfield G, Holloway L, Gilliland L, Baylink DJ, Hintz RL, Sherman BM. Effects of short term administration of recombinant human growth hormone to elderly people. J Clin Endocrinol Metab 1990;70:519–527.

56. Erdtsieck RJ, Pols HA, Valk NK, Van OBM, Lamberts SW, Mulder P, Birkenhager JC. Treatment of post-menopausal osteoporosis with a combination of growth hormone and pamidronate:a placebo controlled trial. Clin Endocrinol Oxf 1995;43:557–565.

57. Kaiser FE, Silver AJ, Morley JE. The effect of recombinant human growth hormone on malnourished older individuals. J Am Geriatr Soc 1991;39:235–240.

58. Binnerts A, Wilson JH, Lamberts SW. The effects of human growth hormone administration in elderly adults with recent weight loss. J Clin Endocrinol Metab 1988;67:1312–1316.

59. Gupta KL, Shetty KR, Agre JC, Cuisinier MC, Rudman IW, Rudman D. Human growth hormone effect on serum IGF-I and muscle function in poliomyelitis survivors. Arch Phys Med Rehabil 1994;75:889–894.

60. Weksler ME. Hormone replacement therapy for men:has the time come? Geriatrics 1995;50:52–54.

61a. Martin FC, Yeo A-L, Sonksen PH. Growth hormone secretion in the elderly: ageing and the somatopause. Balliere's Clin Endocrinol Metab 1997;11:223-250.

61. Borst SE, Millard WJ, Lowenthal DT. Growth hormone. exercise. and aging: the future of therapy for the frail elderly. J Am Geriatr Soc 1994;42:528–535.

62. Bennett RM, Clark SC, Walczyk J. A randomized. double-blind. placebo-controlled study of growth hormone in the treatment of fibromyalgia. Am J Medicine 1998;104:227–231.

63. Horber FF, Haymond MW. Human growth hormone prevents the protein catabolic side effects of prednisone in humans. J Clin Invest 1990;86:265–272.

64. Gore DC, Honeycutt D, Jahoor F, Wolfe RR, Herndon DN. Effect of exogenous growth hormone on whole-body and isolated-limb protein kinetics in burned patients. Arch Surg 1991;126:38–43.

65. Maxwell H, Rees L. Recombinant human growth hormone treatment in infants with chronic renal failure. Arch Dis Child 1996;74:40–43.

66. Jenkins RC, Ross RJ. Growth hormone therapy for protein catabolism. Quart J Med 1996;89:813–819.

67. Mulligan K, Grunfeld C, Hellerstein MK, Neese RA, Schambelan M. Anabolic effects of recombinant human growth hormone in patients with wasting associated with the human immunodeficiency virus. J Clin Endocrinol Metab 1993;77:956–962.

68. Schambelan M, Mulligan K, Grunfeld C, Daar ES, LaMarca A, Kotler DP, Wang J, Bozzette SA, Breitmeyer JB. Recombinant human growth hormone in patients with HIV-associated wasting. A randomized, placebo-controlled trial. Ann Int Med 1996;125:873–832.

69. Lee PD, Pivarnik JM, Bukar JK, et al. A randomized, placebo-controlled trial of combined insulin-like growth factor I and low dose growth hormone therapy for wasting associated with human immuno-deficiency virus. J Clin Endocrinol Metab 1996;81:2968–2975.

70. Thorner M, Rochiccioli P, Colle M, Lanes R, Grunt J, Galazka A, Landy H, Eengrand P, Shah S. Once daily subcutaneous growth hormone-releasing hormone therapy accelerates growth in growth hormone-deficient children during the first year of therapy. J Clin Endocrinol Metab 1996;81:1189–1196.

71. Borges JL, Blizzard RM, Evans WS, Furlanetto R, Rogol AD, Kaiser DL, Rivier J. Vale W, Thorner MO. Stimulation of growth hormone and somatomedin C in idiopathic GH-deficient subjects by intermittent pulsatile administration of human pancreatic tumor GH-releasing factor. J Clin Endocrinol Metab 1984;59:1–6.

72. Corpas E, Harman SM, Pineyro MA, Roberson R, Blackman MR. Growth hormone (GH)-releasing hormone-(1-29) twice daily reverses the decreased GH and insulin-like growth factor-I levels in old men. J Clin Endocrinol Metab 1992;75:530–535.

73. Vittone J, Blackman MR, Busby-Whitehead J, Tsiao C, Stewart KJ, et al. Effects of single nightly injections of growth hormone-releasing hormone GHRH 1-29) in healthy elderly men. Metabolism 1997;46:89–96.

74. Khorram O, Laughlin GA, Yen SSC. Endocrine and metabolic effects of long-term administration of [Nle27] growth hormone-releasing hormone $(1–29)NH_2$ in age-advanced men and women. J Clin Endocrinol Metab 1997;82:1472–1479.

75. Merriam GR, Barsness S, Drolet G, Galt S, Hastings R, Moe KE, Schwartz RS, Vitiello MV. IGF-I variability during GHRH treatment: effect of diet control. GH Research Society, abstract 1148, 1998.

76. Steiger A, Guldner J, Hemmeter U, Rothe B, Wiedemann K, Holsboer F. Effects of growth hormone-releasing hormone and somatostatin on sleep EEG and nocturnal hormone secretion in male controls. Neuroendocrinology 1992;56:566–573.

77. Kerkhofs M, Cauter Ev, Onderbergen Av, Caufriez A, Thorner MO, Copinschi G. Sleep-promoting effects of growth hormone-releasing hormone in normal men. Am J Physiol 1993;264:E594–E598.

78. Chapman IM, Bach MA, van Cauter E, Farmer M, Krupa D, Taylor AM, Schilling AM, Cole KY, Skiles EH, Pezzoli SS. Stimulation of the growth hormone (GH)-insulin-like growth factor I axis by daily oral administration of a GH secretagogue MK-677) in healthy elderly subjects. J Clin Endocrinol Metab 1996;81:4249–4257.

79. Mericq VG, Salazar T, Avila A, Iniguez G, Bowers CY, Cassorla FG, Merriam GR. Effects of eight months treatment with graded doses of growth hormone-releasing peptide in growth hormone-deficient children. J Clin Endocrinol Metab 1998;83:2355–2360.

80. Pasqualini T, Ferraris J, Fainstein-Day P, Eymann AA, Moyano-Caturelly S, Ruiz S, Ramirez J, Gutman R. Growth acceleration in children with chronic renal failure treated with growth hormone-releasing hormone (GHRH). Medicina (Buenos Aires) 1996;58:241–246.

81. Kelijman M, Frohman LA. Enhanced growth hormone GH) responsiveness to GH-releasing hormone after dietary manipulation in obese and nonobese subjects. J Clin Endocrinol Metab 1988;66:489–494.

82. Cassorla F, Mericq V, Garcia H, Cristiano AM, Avila A, Boric A, Iniguez G, Merriam GR. The effects of β_1-adrenergic blockade on the growth response to growth hormone (GH)-releasing hormone therapy in GH-deficient children. J Clin Endocrinol Metab 1995;80:2997–3001.

83. Liu L, Merriam GR, Sherins RJ. Chronic sex steroid exposure increases mean plasma GH concentration and pulse amplitude in men with isolated hypogonadotropic hypogonadism. J Clin Endocrinol Metab 1987;64:651–656.

84. Moe KE, Prinz PN, Larsen LH, Vitiello MV, Reed SO, Merriam GR. Growth hormone in postmenopausal women after long-term estrogen replacement therapy. J Gerontol Biol Sci 1998;53A:in press.

85. Guidice LC. Insulin-like growth factors and ovarian follicular development. Endocrine Reviews 1992;13:641–669.

86. Vitiello MV, Wilkinson CW, Merriam GR, Moe KE, Prinz PN, Ralph DD, Colasurdo EA, Schwartz RS. Successful six-month endurance training does not alter insulin-like growth factor-I in healthy older men and women. J Gerontol Med Sci 1997;52A:149–154.

87. Hodes RJ. Frailty and disability: can growth hormone or other trophic agents make a difference? J Am Geriatr Soc 1994;42:1208–1211.

II PARATHYROID AND VITAMIN D

5

Parathyroid Hormone and Vitamin D Replacement Therapy

Robert F. Klein, MD, *Michael Bliziotes,* MD, *and Eric S. Orwoll,* MD

CONTENTS

INTRODUCTION
HYPOPARATHYROIDISM
VITAMIN D DEFICIENCY
REFERENCES

INTRODUCTION

Calcium is a critically important mineral necessary for both intracellular and extracellular processes. Calcium circulates in the blood in an ionized state, bound to albumin and other serum proteins, and chelated to citrate, sulfate, and lactate. Only the free, ionized form of calcium is biologically active. Generally, total serum concentrations of calcium reflect the ionized calcium available to cells. However, there are two clinically important exceptions to this rule: 1) alkalosis will decrease ionized calcium concentration owing to an increase in the binding of calcium ions to albumin; and 2) in many chronic illnesses, substantial reductions in serum albumin concentrations occur, and this may lower total serum calcium concentrations while the ionized calcium concentration remains normal. The circulating level of ionized calcium is maintained in the physiologic range through the concerted actions of parathyroid hormone (PTH) and 1,25-dihydroxyvitamin D, which mobilize calcium stores from bone and increase the efficiency of intestinal calcium absorption and renal calcium reabsorption. Hypocalcemia, in general, is an uncommon disorder. However, defects in the production or recognition of either PTH or 1,25-dihydroxyvitamin D, or a chronic deficiency of vitamin D, can precipitate hypocalcemia. Additionally, the removal of calcium from the circulation occasionally can exceed the capacity for correction by PTH and 1,25-dihydroxyvitamin D. In this section, the clinical presentations and appropriate therapeutic approaches for disorders associated with either deficient PTH or vitamin D action will be discussed.

From: *Contemporary Endocrinology: Hormone Replacement Therapy*
Edited by: A. W. Meikle © Humana Press Inc., Totowa, NJ

HYPOPARATHYROIDISM

Differential Diagnosis

Hypoparathyroidism is a deficiency of effective parathyroid hormone (PTH) *(1)*. A pathogenetic classification of disorders that can result in hypoparathyroidism is given in Table 1. The condition can arise from a failure of the glands to secrete the hormone or a failure of the tissues to respond to it (pseudohypoparathyroidism). The most common cause of hypoparathyroidism is surgical excision of, or damage to, the parathyroid glands as a result of total thyroidectomy, radical neck dissection, or repeated operations for primary hyperparathyroidism. The frequency of impaired parathyroid function following such operations is generally related to the amount of tissue resected and the experience and skill of the surgeon. In some cases, autotransplantation of parathyroid tissue is indicated to prevent hypoparathyroidism.

The nonsurgical causes of parathyroid gland destruction are relatively uncommon. Malignant replacement of parathyroid tissue has been noted in patients with lymphoma and other neoplasms of the head and neck; however, functional impairment of the parathyroid glands is rare. Infiltrative diseases such as amyloidosis, hemochromatosis, or Wilson's disease have been associated with decreased parathyroid reserve, but clinically evident hypoparathyroidism is exceptional.

Congenital hypoplasia or agenesis of parathyroid tissue can result in a lifelong hypoparathyroid state. The parathyroid glands are derived from the third and fourth branchial pouches. Thus, hypoparathyroidism owing to branchial dysembryogenesis is frequently associated with other branchial cleft abnormalities. The most common of these is DiGeorge syndrome, which may include thymic aplasia with defective cell-mediated immunity, cleft palate, facial abnormalities, and cardiac defects. These anomalies are frequently the result of a microdeletion on the long arm of chromosome 22. The mnemonic "catch 22" has been applied to this cluster of disorders—cardiac, abnormal facies, thymic aplasia, cleft palate, hypocalcemia, and cardiac deletion. All infants with congenital hypoparathyroidism should be evaluated for other occult anomalies (e.g., subclinical heart disease) and undergo cytogenetic analysis of chromosome 22. A negative result suggests another cause of hypoparathyroidism, although the possibility of as-yet-unknown deletions cannot be excluded. More commonly, hypoparathyroidism may develop in early childhood (between 6 mo and 20 yr of age, average age 7–8 yr) and be accompanied by persistent mucocutaneous candidiasis and variable deficiencies of other endocrine glands, especially the adrenals and thyroids. This disorder may be sporadic or familial. Antibodies to endocrine tissue are a common feature of the disease, but it is uncertain as to whether these autoantibodies are of primary or secondary importance in the pathogenesis of the endocrine gland dysfunction.

Functional hypoparathyroidism can also develop as a consequence of altered regulation of parathyroid gland function. The calcium sensor in the parathyroid glands is responsible for monitoring serum ionized calcium concentrations. Hypercalcemia detected by the calcium sensor triggers an intracellular signaling cascade that results in a decrease in the synthesis and secretion of PTH. Recently, a family has been described with an inherited form of hypoparathyroidism that is the result of an activating mutation in the calcium receptor. As the calcium sensor is constitutively activated, affected subjects exhibit chronically suppressed PTH levels despite significant hypocalcemia. A much more common cause of functional hypoparathyroidism is magnesium deficiency.

Table 1
Causes of Hypoparathyroidism

Dysembryogenesis
    Isolated
    DiGeorge syndrome
    Kearns-Sayre syndrome
    Kenny-Caffey syndrome
    Barakat syndrome
Destruction
    Surgical excision
    Autoimmune
    Metal overload (Fe, Cu)
    Radiation
    Granulomatous infiltration
    Neoplastic invasion
Deficient hormone secretion
    Maternal hyperparathyroidism
    Calcium sensor mutation
    Hypomagnesemia
Deficient hormone action
    Pseudohypoparathyroidism

Hypomagnesemia both impairs PTH secretion and blunts its hypercalcemic effect. Hypomagnesemia may result from chronic alcoholism, malabsorption, excessive diuretic use, cisplatinum therapy, prolonged parenteral nutrition, hyperemesis, or as an isolated defect in intestinal magnesium absorption. Patients with hypocalcemia owing to hypomagnesemia are resistant to parenteral calcium and vitamin D therapy until magnesium concentrations are normalized and parathyroid gland function is restored. Interestingly, hypermagnesemia can also suppress PTH secretion and produce hypocalcemia. Acute alcohol intoxication has also been demonstrated to produce a reversible impairment in PTH secretion accompanied by hypocalcemia and hypercalciuria. Occasionally, functional hypoparathyroidism occurs in infants born to mothers with primary hyperparathyroidism. Hypercalcemia in the mother results in enhanced placental transport of ionized calcium to the fetus and persistent hypercalcemia in the fetus leads to suppression of its parathyroid gland function. Hypocalcemia can last for up to 6 mo after birth.

Aside from conditions that impair PTH synthesis and release, hypoparathyroidism can also result from target organ unresponsiveness. Albright initially described a syndrome of PTH resistance in 1941 and coined the term "pseudohypoparathyroidism" to describe this disorder. In these patients, exogenous administration of PTH fails to increase nephrogenous cyclic adenosine monophosphate (AMP) and/or renal phosphate excretion (biomarkers of PTH action), suggesting that there is a defect in the PTH receptor signaling pathway. The incidence of pseudohypoparathyroidism is not known. Women are affected more commonly than men and both sporadic and familial forms exist. The mode of inheritance has varied in different families with evidence for autosomal dominant, autosomal recessive, and X-linked patterns being present in different kindreds. In some families, the defect has been localized to the stimulatory guanine nucleotide regulatory protein (Gs) that couples membrane receptors to adenylyl cyclase This defect likely accounts for the variable resistance to other adenylyl cyclase-coupled hormone receptors, such as glucagon, gonadotropins, and thyrotropin, that these patients manifest. Other possible molecular mechanisms responsible for the PTH resistance may reside in the PTH receptor itself or in the intracellular signaling pathway distal to cyclic AMP generation.

Clinical Features

The clinical manifestations of hypoparathyroidism depend on the severity and chronicity of the hypocalcemia, and can range from a vague feeling of ill health to life-threatening neuromuscular and cardiovascular collapse. Neuromuscular complications are frequently seen in hypoparathyroidism, especially when serum calcium levels decrease acutely (e.g., immediately after neck surgery in the region of the parathyroid glands). Nervous tissue exposed to low calcium concentrations exhibits decreased excitation thresholds, repetitive responses to a single stimulus, reduced accommodation, and, in extreme cases, continuous activity (or tetany). The tetany may be latent or overt, and the symptoms in overt tetany can range from mild muscle cramps to frank seizures. Latent tetany may be demonstrated in otherwise asymptomatic patients by eliciting Chvostek's sign or Trousseau's sign. Chvostek's sign is performed by tapping on the facial nerve 2–3 cm anterior to the ear, evoking a contraction of the facial muscles, and a drawing up of the lip. Trousseau's sign is a carpal spasm elicited by inflation of a blood pressure cuff to 20 mm Hg above the patient's systolic blood pressure for 3–5 min. Flexion of the wrist and metacapophalangeal joints, extension of the interphalangeal joints, and adduction of the digits reflect the heightened irritability of the nerves to ischemia in the region below the cuff. Whereas upwards of 10% of normal individuals will demonstrate a slightly positive Chvestek's sign, a positive Trousseau's sign is rarely seen in the absence of significant hypocalcemia. It should be noted that significant hypocalcemia may be present in the absence of either Chvostek's or Trousseau's signs, particularly when hypocalcemia has been of gradual onset. Clinically, tetany usually begins with a prodrome of circumoral and facial paresthesias. Motor manifestations include stiffness and muscle cramps of the arms, legs, and feet that can progress to spontaneous carpopedal spasm. Other less common complications include abdominal cramps, urinary frequency, laryngeal stridor, bronchospasm, and, rarely, respiratory arrest.

Central nervous system (CNS) manifestations of hypoparathyroidism can include mental retardation, psychosis, dementia, and seizures of all types. Chronic hypocalcemia may be associated with extrapyramidal movement disorders, including classic parkinsonism. Such manifestations are presumed to be related in some way to the basal ganglia calcifications that are present in many patents. Anterior and posterior subcapsular cataracts, papilledema, dermatitis, and alopecia may also be present. The cardiovascular manifestations of hypocalcemia include arrhythmias, hypotension, and congestive heart failure. The electrocardiogram reveals a characteristic prolongation of the QT interval. The hypotension results from diminished smooth muscle tone and the congestive heart failure from inpaired myocardial contractility. The cardiovascular dysfunction is unresponsive to pharmacological interventions until the hypocalcemia is corrected. Abnormalities in tooth development are frequently observed in children with hypoparathyroidism. Depending upon the age of onset of PTH deficiency, on may find defective enamel and root formation, dental hypoplasia, or failure of adult teeth eruption. Untreated hypoparathyroidism during pregnancy has resulted in severe skeletal demineralization of the fetus and transient hypoparathyroidism in the newborn.

Patients with pseudohypoparathyroidism and deficient Gs activity exhibit a variety of phenotypic features that are not seen in other forms of hypoparathyroidism. These include short stature, obesity, round face, skeletal abnormalities (brachydactyly), and heterotopic calcifications. This constellation of somatic abnormalities has been termed Albright's hereditary osteodystrophy (AHO). The features of AHO may coexist with normal PTH responsiveness, and this is termed pseudohypoparathyroidism. Within a given family, affected individuals may show AHO with or without abnormal PTH responsiveness.

Therapy

The major goal of therapy in all hypoparathyroid states is to restore serum calcium and phosphorus to satisfactory levels so as to prevent symptoms of hypocalcemia and progression of long-term complications. The particular therapeutic approach depends on the severity of the hypocalcemia, the acuteness of onset, and the presence of symptoms. In acute, symptomatic hypocalcemia, intravenous administration of calcium salts is recommended. Available solutions include calcium chloride (272 mg elemental calcium/10 mL ampoule), calcium glucceptate (90 mg elemental calcium/5 mL ampoule), and calcium gluconate (90 mg elemental calcium/10 mL ampoule). Initial therapy should ensure the delivery of 250 mg elemental calcium. Concentrated calcium solutions are quite caustic and may cause considerable local damage if they extravasate into soft tissue. It is preferable to further dilute the calcium salts into 100 mL of a 5% dextrose solution (D5W) and administer the initial dose over 15 min by a secure intravenous route. Calcium should always be administered very cautiously in patients receiving digitalis therapy, as hypercalcemia predisposes to digitalis intoxication and arrhythmias. If the symptoms are severe or fail to resolve after the initial therapy, calcium can be administered by continuous intravenous infusion (e.g., 10–15 mg of elemental calcium/kg of body weight in 1 L of DW every 6 h). Serum calcium levels should be monitored frequently to maintain the serum calcium at 7–8.5 mg/dL. The cause of the hypocalcemia should be sought during this period and reversible causes treated. If magnesium depletion is suspected in the acute setting of hypocalcemia, a blood sample for magnesium determination should be obtained. Then, if renal function is intact, magnesium should be administered parenterally. If significant hypomagnesemia is documented, its cause should be evaluated and magnesium repletion (either parenterally or orally) should be continued until the serum value is normalized. Empiric magnesium therapy should not be considered in the presence of renal insufficiency.

The chronic hypoparathyroid states will require long-term therapy to maintain calcium levels in the normal range. Theoretically, the most appropriate therapy for hypoparathyroidism would be physiologic replacement of the absent hormone with its natural analog. Indeed, a recent study has demonstrated that once-daily subcutaneous administration of human PTH (1–34), which contains the biologically active region of intact PTH, can maintain calcium levels in the normal range throughout the day and reduce urinary calcium excretion (2). However, there are practical limitations to this approach, including the need to administer the hormone parenterally and the high cost of commercial preparations of PTH. Such treatment might become feasible in the future as an alternative for patients poorly controlled by conventional regimens. Parathyroid autotransplantation has lowered the incidence of permanent hypoparathyroidism in selected patients. Unfortunately, the immunology of parathyroid transplantation is

Table 2
Calcium Preparation for Oral Supplementation

Preparation	Common tablet size	Elemental calcium (%)	# of tabs for 1500 mg calcium
Ca gluconate	1000 mg	9	16
Ca lactate	650 mg	13	18
Ca carbonate	650 mg	40	6
	1300 mg		3
Ca citrate	950 mg	21	8

incompletely understood and the allograft success rate is too low to currently recommend this procedure on a routine basis (3,4).

Because of the absence of PTH and the consequent hyperphosphatemia, little, if any, circulating 25-hydroxyvitamin D is converted to 1,25-dihydroxyvitamin D, and there are low or undetectable serum levels of this metabolite in hypoparathyroidism. Although lowering of serum phosphate levels through low-phosphate diets (e.g., restricting dairy products and meat) and oral nonabsorbable aluminum hydroxide gels (to bind intestinal phosphate) might be expected to increase the conversion of 25-hydroxyvitamin D to 1,25-dihydroxyvitamin D, such treatment has received little attention. Rather, treatment with supplemental calcium and vitamin D has been the mainstay of therapy (5).

Generally, at least 1 g/d of elemental calcium is required in hypoparathyroid patients under 40 and 2 g/d in patients over the age of 40. The amount of supplemental calcium necessary for adequate control may vary from 1 g/d (even in the absence of vitamin D supplements) in mild, partial hypoparathyroidism to 5–10 g/d (plus supplemental vitamin D) in more severe cases. Supplements can be provided by administering calcium as the gluconate, lactate, carbonate, or citrate salt (Table 2). Calcium gluconate and lactate tablets contain relatively small quantities of elemental calcium, so that large numbers of tablets must be administered. Calcium carbonate preparations have the highest calcium content (on a weight-percent basis) and are therefore preferred by most patients. Calcium citrate may be of benefit for patients with hypercalciuria, because urinary excretion of citrate may prevent kidney stone formation. Oral calcium supplements are best absorbed in small doses and in an acidic environment (e.g., with meals).

In patients with less severe parathyroid insufficiency, oral calcium supplementation alone may be adequate. However, in most patients, therapy with vitamin D or one of its analogs is also required to prevent symptomatic hypocalcemia. As indicated in Table 3, ergocalciferol (vitamin D_2) and calcifediol are the least expensive forms of therapy. However, pharmacologic doses of these compounds are usually required (reflecting the absence of the stimulatory effect of PTH on renal synthesis of 1,25-dihydroxyvitamin D) and this, coupled with their long duration of action, can result in prolonged toxicity. For these reasons, analogs with shorter half-lives and no requirement for renal 1-α hydroxylation (such as dihydrotachysterol and calcitriol) are generally preferred. Therapy must be individualized in all cases of hypoparathyroidism (6). Because changes in calcium and vitamin D requirements may occur unpredictably during chronic treatment, routine monitoring of serum calcium levels is mandatory. Calcium should be measured weekly at the initiation of vitamin D therapy, then monthly during dosage adjustment and at least every 3 mo during long-term follow-up. A single episode of vitamin D intoxication can irreversibly impair renal function.

Table 3
Characteristics of Commonly Used Vitamin D Preparations

Preparation	Physiologic dose[a]	Pharmacologic dose[b]	Onset of action	Duration of action	Cost ($)[c]
Vitamin D$_2$ (ergocalciferol)	5–10 µg	1–10 mg	10–14 d	4–12 wk	$7.00/100 (1.25 mg)
25(OH)D[d] (calcifediol)	1–5 µg	20–200 µg	7–10 d	2–6 wk	$52.45/60 (20 µg) $119.60/60 (50 µg)
Dihydrotachysterol (DHT)	25–100 µg	375–750 µg	4–7 d	1–4 wk	$94.02/100 (125 µg)
1,25[(OH)$_2$D] (calcitriol)	0.25–0.5 µg	0.75–3.0 µg	1–2 d	2–5 d	$110.04/100 (0.25 µg) $175.98/100 (0.5 µg)

[a]Dosage for the treatment of nutritional deficiency.
[b]Dosage for the treatment of hypoparathyroidism.
[c]Average wholesale price (5a).
[d]25-hydroxyvitamin D.

The major impediment to restoration of normocalcemia with supplemental calcium and vitamin D analogs is the development of hypercalciuria with a resulting predilection for nephrolithiasis, nephrocalcinosis, and impaired renal function. Because PTH is not present to maintain normal renal tubular reabsorption of calcium, enhanced absorption of calcium from the intestines initiated by calcium and vitamin D therapy results in an increased filtered load of calcium, which is readily cleared through the kidney. Consequently, significant hypercalciuria may develop long before serum calcium is normalized. Frequently, it is necessary to accept a low–normal serum calcium concentration in order to limit the degree of hypercalciuria. Thiazide diuretics, which increase renal tubular calcium reabsorption, have been proposed as a means of reducing urine calcium in hypoparathyroidism and may have the added benefit of partially restoring eucalcemia (7,8). Although this approach is beneficial in some patients, the use of diuretics may be problematic in patients with concurrent adrenal insufficiency (owing to polyglandular failure) or impaired renal function. However, in patients with normal renal and adrenal function, thiazide diuretics, in conjunction with calcium and vitamin D supplementation, may provide a relatively inexpensive solution to the chronic hypercalciuria that is often encountered in this clinical setting.

Long-term restoration of serum calcium to normal or nearly normal ranges usually results in improvements in most manifestations of hypoparathyroidism including the ocular, neurologic, and dermatologic disorders. Improved surgical techniques and the use of parathyroid autotransplantation surgery for disorders requiring extensive removal of thyroid or parathyroid tissue may lower the incidence of permanent hypoparathyroidism. Early diagnosis of latent hypoparathyroidism with adequate long-term treatment will lead to a lower incidence of late complications.

VITAMIN D DEFICIENCY

Differential Diagnosis

Dietary vitamin D_2 (ergocalciferol) is absorbed via the intestinal lymphatic system. Absorption takes place in the proximal small intestine and requires bile acids. Vitamin D_3 (cholecalciferol) is produced in the skin by photochemical synthesis from 7-dehydrocholesterol. Vitamin D_2 and D_3 exhibit little in the way of biologic activity. Both undergo hydroxylation in the liver to form 25-hydroxyvitamin D by action of the enzyme vitamin D-25-hydroxylase. 25-hydroxyvitamin D serves as the primary storage form of vitamin D hormone. To become biologically active, 25-hydroxyvitamin D requires further hydroxylation to form 1,25-dihydroxyvitamin D by action of the enzyme 25-hydroxy-vitamin D-1α-hydroxylase. This hydroxylation step takes place primarily in the kidney and is tightly regulated by circulating PTH, phosphate, and calcium levels. Thus, vitamin D deficiency can result from nutritional deprivation, inadequate sunlight exposure, impaired gastrointestinal absorption, reduced synthesis of 25-hydroxyvitamin D, and/or 1,25-dihydroxyvitamin D or end-organ resistance to 1,25-dihydroxyvitamin D *(9)*. A pathogenetic classification of disorders that can result in vitamin D deficiency is given in Table 4.

Nutritional vitamin D deficiency is rare in the United States, because milk and cereals are commonly fortified with vitamin D_2. However, vitamin D deficiency can occur in alcoholics and the elderly because of their poor nutritional status and limited sunlight exposure. Gastrointestinal (GI) disease is now the predominant cause of vitamin D deficiency in the United States. Intestinal malabsorption syndromes that affect the small intestine (especially the duodenum and jejunum) are all associated with impaired vitamin D absorption owing to either rapid transit or enhanced fecal loss of 25-hydroxyvitamin D because of impaired enterohepatic circulation. Similarly, patients with chronic severe parenchymal and cholestatic liver disease frequently exhibit vitamin D deficiency owing to the associated malabsorption syndrome combined with a decreased hepatic capacity to convert vitamin D to 25-hydroxyvitamin D. Those patients who take phenobarbital have increased activity of microsomal hydroxylases in the liver and consequent accelerated metabolism of vitamin D can lead to functional vitamin D deficiency.

Renal disease is one of the most common causes of vitamin D deficiency. As kidney function declines, 1-α-hydroxylase activity decreases leading to reductions in circulating levels of 1,25-dihydroxyvitamin D and consequently impaired GI calcium absorption. Additionally, phosphate excretion falls as renal function declines. Hyperphosphatemia then results in further decreases in the serum calcium level by chelating ionized calcium and inhibiting any remaining 1-α-hydroxylase enzyme activity.

In rare instances, inborn errors of vitamin D metabolism can result in hypocalcemia. Patients with these disorders, generally present early in life, with hypocalcemia and skeletal abnormalities despite adequate vitamin D intake. Vitamin D-dependent rickets Type I is an autosomal recessive disorder that stems from impaired renal 1-α-hydroxylase activity. Affected patients have low concentrations of 1,25-dihydroxyvitamin D, but respond to treatment with physiological doses of 1,25-dihydroxyvitamin D. In contrast, patients with vitamin D-dependent rickets Type II have a variety of mutations in the vitamin D receptor, exhibit dramatically increased circulating concentrations of 1,25-dihydroxyvitamin D (as a consequence of their secondary hyperparathyroidism) and respond poorly even to pharmacological doses of 1,25-dihydroxyvitamin D. Patients with the more severe form of this disease frequently have alopecia.

Table 4
Causes of Vitamin D Deficiency

Decreased precursor vitamin D
    Malnutrition
    Malabsorption
    Sunscreen use
    Lack of sunlight exposure
    Antiseizure medications
Decreased conversion to active metabolites
    Liver disease
    Kidney disease
    Vitamin D-dependent rickets, type I
    Oncogenic osteomalacia
    X-linked hypophosphatemic rickets
1725-dihydroxyvitamin D resistance
    Vitamin D-dependent rickets, type II

Clinical Features

The clinical manifestations of vitamin D deficiency can include myotonia, muscle weakness, and, in severe cases, frank tetany. Additionally, skeletal abnormalities are also frequently present. The characteristic skeletal disturbance in vitamin D deficient states is osteomalacia (literally, "soft bones"). The malacic bone results from impaired mineralization and is subject to distortion in shape and to fracture. When osteomalacia develops in young, actively growing children it is referred to as "rickets." If vitamin D deficiency is present during the first year of life, the characteristic features of rachitic bone can include widened cranial sutures, frontal bossing, posterior flattening of the skull ("craniotabes"), bulging of the costochondral junctions ("rachitic rosary"), indentation of the ribs at the diaphragmatic insertions ("Harrison's groove"), and enlargement of the wrists. After the first year of life, the deformities resulting from vitamin D deficiency are most severe in the long bones because of their rapid growth and weight-bearing function. The bony shafts of the long bones can be deformed and subject to fracture. The ends of the long bones become enlarged and bowleg *("genu varum")* or knock-knee *("genu valgum")* deformities progressively worsen. In longstanding disease, there may be *coxa vara* and rachitic saber shins. Moderate deformities occurring before age 4 may resolve with adequate vitamin D treatment, but those occurring later usually result in lasting deformity, compromised adult height, or both.

The clinical features associated with osteomalacia in adults are more subtle than those with rickets in children. In the mature, fully grown skeleton, bone turnover is less than 5%/yr. Thus, a mineralization defect in adults must be present for several years to produce clinical manifestations. The characteristic symptom, if any, is pain when weight or pressure is applied to the affected bones. Low backache relieved by recumbency is one of the earlier complaints, but the pain may include other portions of the spine, ribs, and feet. Significant osteomalacia may be present without radiographic manifestations, but there is often a generalized decrease in bone mineral density. The most characteristic feature of adult osteomalacia is the pseudofracture (Looser's zone, Milkman's syndrome), a straight, transverse band localized, often symmetrically, at the concave ends of the shafts of long bones, ribs, scapulae, and pubic rami. The origin of these radiographic abnormalities is unknown, but they may arise from the pressure of overlying pulsating arteries. Skeletal fractures (sometimes superimposed upon pseudofractures) can occur and usually unite very slowly. Longstanding disease can lead to bowing of long bones and distortion of the pelvic outlet (assuming a triangular appearance on standard anteroposterior views). Loss of vertebral height can lead to kyphosis as a late manifestation. The skeletal deformities may be associated with other features of malnutrition and/or secondary hyperparathyroidism (e.g., subperiosteal resorption). Associated proximal weakness can contribute to a waddling gait or severe crippling.

Therapy

The goals of treatment in states of vitamin D deficiency are:

1. To correct hypocalcemia, alleviate related symptoms, and prevent *grand mal* seizures and cataracts;
2. To prevent the skeletal deformities of rickets and excess parathyroid hormone;
3. To prevent toxicity (hypercalcemia, hypercalciuria, and their sequelae); and
4. To promote normal growth and development in children.

The choice of the vitamin D preparation used for therapy depends on the cost of the medication and associated illnesses that may influence vitamin D metabolism. Preparations of vitamin D and its metabolites that are available for clinical use in the United States are listed in Table 3. The table also lists the onset of optimal biologic activity, duration of effect after cessation of treatment, dosage forms available, and cost. The pharmacologic advantages and disadvantages of the drugs are listed in Table 5.

The precursor molecules, ergocalciferol (vitamin D_2) and cholecalciferol (vitamin D_3), are the least expensive. These compounds and 25-hydroxyvitamin D_3 (calcifediol) have the theoretical advantage that they are precursors of the other vitamin D metabolites, so that physiologic regulation may avert toxicity. Calcifediol should be used in patients with liver disease who may have decreased activity of vitamin D-25-hydroxylase. A disadvantage of vitamin D_2 and D_3 is that they tend to be chemically unstable and to lose activity during storage. They also tend to accumulate in fat and muscle during long-term administration so that the effect becomes cumulative. With both compounds, the therapeutic dose approaches the toxic dose, a long period is required for optimal biologic effect, and activity may persist after cessation of administration, a disadvantage in the event of intoxication. The advantages of dihydrotachysterol (DHT) and calcitriol (1,25-dihydroxyvitamin D_3) are that they require only a short period for optimal biologic activity and their effects last only a short period after cessation of treatment. Both are effective when l-αhydroxylation of 25-hydroxyvitamin D is defective. However, both drugs are relatively expensive and toxicity can occur spontaneously in patients on long-term treatment. The hypercalcemia is easily managed by stopping the drug and is prevented by reducing the dose.

Optimal management of vitamin D deficiency is dependent upon the underlying cause of the disorder and treatment must be individualized with regard to pathogenesis and severity of the disorder. For cases of nutritional vitamin D deficiency, ergocalciferol or cholecalciferol are reasonable initial choices. A multivitamin that contains 400 IU of cholecalciferol will help maintain circulating levels of 25-hydroxyvitamin D above 20 ng/mL in most patients. However, in the absence of sunlight, this dose may not be sufficient. For patients who are vitamin D deficient under these conditions, the required dose may be

Table 5
Advantages and Disadvantages of Vitamin D and its Derivatives

Drug	Advantages	Disadvantages
Vitamin D2	Inexpensive; precursor of vitamin D metabolites	Therapeutic dose approaches toxic dose; long period for onset of biologic effect; may not be effective, particularly when vitamin D metabolism is defective; unstable, undergoes oxidation, photochemical decomposition, and loss of activity with storage
25-Hydroxyvitamin D$_3$	Chemically stable; precursor of vitamin D metabolites	Moderately expensive; except for stability, disadvantages are same as vitamin D$_2$
Dihydrotachysterol	Does not require 1a-hydroxylation, can be used when this step is impaired; short period for onset of biologic effect; duration of effect after cessation usually short	Therapeutic dose approaches toxic dose; moderately expensive 25-hydroxylation required for biologic effectiveness; may be ineffective in liver disease
1,25-dihydroxyvitamin D$_3$	Short period of onset for biologic effect; short duration of effect after cessation; can be highly effective when 1a-hydroxylation is impaired and may provide normal or near normal growth	Expensive; toxicity may occur spontaneously

quite variable. A regimen of 50,000 U (1.25 mg/d) of ergocalciferol is frequently used at the beginning of therapy (i.e., the first month) to more rapidly increase systemic vitamin D levels. For older patients in northern latitudes, using this regimen for several weeks may be sufficient to maintain 25-hydroxyvitamin D levels in the normal range for several months. If, however, chronic vitamin D replacement therapy is necessary, maintenance dosages should be reduced and titrated to maintain 25-hydroxyvitamin D levels between 25 and 35 ng/mL. Disorders associated with frank malabsorption may require pharmacologic amounts of ergocalciferol (10–25,000 U/d; 0.25–0.625 mg/d). In the presence of malabsorption, concurrent magnesium depletion must always be considered. Vitamin D$_2$ or D$_3$ may not be appropriate in some circumstances. If vitamin D deficiency is secondary to intestinal resection or impaired enterohepatic circulation, calcifediol (50–100 µg/d) may be absorbed more readily. In the setting of defective renal hydroxylation of 25-hydroxyvitamin D (e.g., end-stage renal disease, type I vitamin D-dependent rickets) therapy with either DHT or calcitriol is required. In general, states of vitamin D deficiency in which renal 1-α-hydroxylation is intact should not be treated with analogs such as DHT or calcitriol. These compounds bypass the renal site of feedback control of 1,25-dihydroxyvitamin D biosynthesis and thus carry a greater risk of inducing hypercalcemia.

Intoxication can be a major problem with vitamin D or any of its metabolites (10). Hypercalcemia and hypercalciuria result from increased intestinal absorption of calcium and mobilization of calcium from the skeleton and may lead to impairment in renal function, nephrocalcinosis, nephrolithiasis, urinary tract infections, renal failure, and death. Patients with intoxication are often asymptomatic, but they may have anorexia, nausea, vomiting, weight loss, polyuria, polydipsia, and alterations in mental status. Children and infants often show listlessness and hypotonia. Unfortunately, intoxication frequently occurs unexpectedly, possibly as a result of changes in diet, gastointestinal absorption of calcium, or hydration status.

The treatment of intoxication is to stop the drug and force fluids. If intoxication is profound, a short course of steroids or bisphosphonates may be required, usually only when hypercalcemia is produced by the longer acting sterols. Use of lower doses of the drugs after episodes of hypercalcemia will usually prevent recurrences. Patients who are difficult to treat with vitamin D_2 may be more easily managed with 1,25-dihydroxyvitamin D_3.

The best treatment for intoxication is prevention. Patients should be closely followed at regular intervals with measurement of serum and urinary calcium and serum creatinine. Weekly measurements of serum calcium may be needed while the treatment regimen is being established. For stable patients, quarterly measurements are probably adequate, but more frequent measurements should be done when a dosage adjustment is made. Patients should be informed of the possibility of intoxication, the symptoms to be aware of, and the potential harmful effects.

REFERENCES

1. Nusynowitz ML, Frame B, Kolb FO. The spectrum of hypoparathyroid states: A classification based on physiologic principles. Medicine 1976;55:105–119.
2. Winer KK, Yanovski JA, Cutler GB. Synthetic human parathyroid hormone 1-34 vs calcitriol and calcium in the treatment of hypoparathyroidism. JAMA 1996;276:631–636.
3. Wozniewicz B, Migaj M, Giera B, Prokurat A, Tolloczko T, Sawicki A, et al. Cell culture preparation of human parathyroid cells for allotransplantation without immunosuppression. Trans Proc 1996;28:3542–3544.
4. Tolloczko T, Wozniewicz B, Sawicki A, Gorski A, Nawrot I, Zawitkowska T, Migaj M. Clinical results of human cultured parathyroid cell allotransplantation in the treatment of surgical hypoparathyroidism. Trans Proc 1996;28:3545,3546.
5. Avioli LV. The therapeutic approach to hypoparathyroidism. Am J Med 1974;57:34–42.
5a. Cardinale V (ed.). Drug Topics Red Book. Medical Economics, Montvale, NJ, 1997.
6. Okano K, Furukawa Y, Morii H, Fujita T. Comparative efficacy of various vitamin D metabolites in the treatment of various types of hypoparathyroidism. J Clin Endocrinol Metab 1982;55:238-243.
7. Parfitt AM. The interactions of thiazide diuretics with parathyroid hormone and vitamin D. J Clin Invest 1972;51:1879–1888.
8. Porter RH, Cox BG, Heaney D, Hostetter TH, Stinebaugh BJ, Suki WN. Treatment of hypoparathyroid patients with chlorthalidone. N Engl J Med 1978;298:577–581.
9. Drezner MK. Disorders of vitamin D metabolism: rickets and osteomalacia. In: Manolagos SC, Olefsky JM, eds. Metabolic Bone and Mineral Disorders, vol. 5. Churchill Livingstone, New York, 1988, pp 103–129.

10. Davies M, Adams PH. The continuing risk of vitamin D intoxication. Lancet 1978;i:621–623.
11. Holick MF. Vitamin D: Photobiology, metabolism, mechanism of action and clinical applications. In: Favus MJ, ed. Primer in the Metabolic Bone Diseases and Disorders of Mineral Metabolism. Lippincott-Raven, Philadelphia, PA, 1996, pp. 74–81.
12. McKenna MJ, Frame B. Privational vitamin D deficiency. Comprehen Ther 1987;13:54–61.
13. Reber PM, Heath H III. Hypocalcemia emergencies. Med Clin N Am 1995;79:93–107.
14. Recker RR. Calcium absorption and achlorhydria. N Engl J Med 1985;313:70–73.
15. Dawson-Hughes B, Dallal GE, Krall EA, Harris S, Sokoll LJ, Falconer G. Effect of vitamin D supplementation on wintertime and overall bone loss in healthy postmenopausal women. Ann Int Med 1991;115:505–512.

III Thyroid

6

Thyroid Hormone Replacement Therapy for Primary and Secondary Hypothyroidism

David S. Cooper, MD

CONTENTS

INTRODUCTION

Definitions, Etiologies, and Diagnosis of Primary and Secondary Hypothyroidism

Primary hypothyroidism is defined as a deficiency of thyroid hormone owing to intrinsic failure of the thyroid gland. This leads to low levels of circulating thyroxine, insufficient levels of thyroid hormone in target tissues, and typical symptoms, signs, and laboratory abnormalities. When severe or long-standing, the clinical diagnosis is straightforward, confirmed by the finding of elevated serum levels of thyrotropin (TSH) and depressed serum concentrations of free thyroxine (fT4) or the free T4 estimate (free T4 index or FTI). Circulating serum triiodothyronine (T3) concentrations are generally low or low-normal. It is a relatively common disorder, affecting 1–3% of the population, with an annual incidence of approx 1–2 per 1000 in women and 1 per 10,000 in men *(1)*. Autoimmune (Hashimoto's) thyroiditis is the cause of spontaneous primary hypothyroidism in the vast majority of cases. Postablative hypothyroidism after therapy for hyperthyroidism or thyroid surgery is the second most common cause. Drugs may also precipitate primary hypothyroidism, especially in people with underlying autoimmune thyroid disease (i.e., positive antithyroid antibodies). Lithium and iodine-containing drugs such as the antiarrhythmic amiodarone frequently lead to hypothyroidism in such individuals. Rare congenital causes of primary hypothyroidism include thyroid agenesis

From: *Contemporary Endocrinology: Hormone Replacement Therapy*
Edited by: A. W. Meikle © Humana Press Inc., Totowa, NJ

or maldevelopment and a variety of hereditary intrathyroidal enzyme deficiencies or thyroglobulin biosynthetic abnormalities probably caused by specific genetic mutations.

The mildest form of primary hypothyroidism has been termed "subclinical hypothyroidism." Subclinical hypothyroidism is said to exist when serum fT4 levels fall but remain within the broad range of normal. Owing to the exquisite sensitivity of the pituitary to subtle changes in fT4 levels, TSH secretion increases in response to these lower–albeit "normal"–fT4 concentrations. Therefore, subclinical hypothyroidism is defined biochemically by a normal serum fT4 or fT4 estimate, a normal serum T3 concentration, and an elevated serum TSH concentration. In this situation, the serum TSH level is usually less than 20 mU/L. Obviously, the diagnosis of subclinical hypothyroidism cannot be made if only the serum fT4 or FTI is assessed. Subclinical hypothyroidism is generally associated with few symptoms or signs of hypothyroidism and minimal biochemical changes (e.g., serum lipid levels) (2). Nevertheless, many experts feel that subclinical hypothyroidism may be associated with both subtle symptoms and mild dyslipidemia that could be detrimental to the patient. Subclinical hypothyroidism is likely the precursor to overt hypothyroidism in some cases–particularly in individuals with high titers of antithyroid antibodies. Subclinical hypothyroidism is far more common than overt hypothyroidism, affecting approx 5% of people; it is particularly prevalent in women over age 60, in whom the frequency has approached 20% in some surveys (2). The same factors that are associated with the development of overt hypothyroidism (autoimmune thyroiditis and other autoimmune diseases, postablation, and certain drugs) are also associated with subclinical hypothyroidism.

Secondary hypothyroidism is defined as a deficiency of thyroid hormone caused by a lack of thyroidal stimulation by pituitary TSH. Generally, secondary hypothyroidism indicates the presence of significant underlying hypothalamic or pituitary disease. Secondary hypothyroidism is uncommon, but the actual prevalence is not known. The diagnosis may be more difficult than in the case of primary hypothyroidism, since serum TSH levels may not always be low. Thus, if the physician simply relies on the serum TSH as the sole laboratory test to screen for hypothyroidism, the diagnosis will be missed. On the other hand, if both the fT4 or FTI and the TSH are measured, the diagnosis should be entertained if either the fT4 or FTI is low, and the TSH level is either normal or low. In very rare cases, the TSH levels may be at the upper end of the normal range or slightly elevated, a situation that can masquerade as subclinical hypothyroidism. The "normal" TSH levels in secondary hypothyroidism are the result of the elaboration by the pituitary gland of a TSH molecule with normal immunoactivity but depressed bioactivity, possibly related to alterations in TSH glycosylation (3,4). It is often difficult to distinguish between hypothalamic and pituitary disease on clinical grounds. Stimulation with the hypothalamic peptide thyrotropin-releasing hormone (TRH) may be useful, since patients with pituitary disease usually do not respond or respond poorly to TRH, whereas those with hypothalamic disease respond, albeit with a delayed rise in serum TSH. However, with the almost ubiquitous use of magnetic resonance imaging (MRI) to establish the site and type of disease, TRH testing is rarely needed.

This chapter focuses on the use of thyroid hormone in the management of patients with primary and secondary hypothyroidism. There have been several recent reviews of this topic (5–7). Although thyroid hormone can be used to treat goiter and thyroid nodules (so-called "suppression" therapy), this indication is beyond the scope of this review, as are the nuances of thyroid hormone therapy in patients with differentiated thyroid cancer.

THYROID HORMONE PREPARATIONS

When one speaks of "thyroid hormone," one generally means the sodium salt of levothyroxine (L-T4). However, the US Pharmacopeia (8) lists five thyroid hormone preparations: synthetic L-T4, synthetic liothyronine (L-T3); liotrix (a fixed combination of synthetic L-T4 and L-T3 in a 4:1 ratio); desiccated thyroid manufactured from the thyroids of slaughterhouse animals, and purified animal thyroglobulin. L-T4 is the treatment of choice for the long-term management of primary and secondary hypothyroidism. L-T3 has specific, narrow, and self-limited indications, including suppression testing and in the preparation of thyroid cancer patients for radioiodine scanning or therapy. Because of its relatively short half-life of one day, its use leads to variable serum hormone levels throughout the day. Liotrix and desiccated thyroid, although still available in pharmacies, are obsolete forms of therapy; patients taking either of these two drugs should be switched to L-T4, using the guidelines presented below. Purified animal thyroglobulin (Proloid) is no longer available in the US.

Thyroxine is one of the most frequently prescribed medications in the US, with over 18 million prescriptions for the various preparations written annually (9). Another study revealed that 6.9% of an unselected cohort of older adults were taking thyroid hormone (10).

THYROXINE PHARMACOLOGY

The average daily secretion rate of thyroxine by the thyroid gland is in the range of 90 μg (Table 1), but the usual requirement for orally administered L-T4 is 100–200 μg per day (11). This indicates that the gastrointestinal absorption of L-T4 is considerably less than 100%. Studies using simultaneous oral and intravenous (IV) thyroxine have indicated that L-T4 is 60–80% absorbed, with large individual differences (50–100%) in apparently healthy people (12). There is no absorption of orally administered L-T4 from the stomach, and the main absorptive sites appear to be the proximal and midjejunum. Progressively decreasing degrees of absorption occur along the distal bowel and proximal colon, but there are no reports of L-T4 malabsorption in colectomized individuals (12). People over age 70 yr may have a slight (10%) decrease in L-T4 absorption that is probably not clinically significant (13). Thyroxine absorption is greater if the drug is given on an empty stomach (14), and food may also delay absorption (15). Hypothyroidism may lead to a slight increase in thyroxine absorption (16).

Factors Affecting L-T4 Absorption or Metabolism

A variety of intestinal diseases have been associated with increased L-T4 requirements, including sprue, Crohn's disease, and short bowel syndromes (17–19). Chronic pancreatitis and cirrhosis have also been reported to cause L-T4 malabsorption (12). A factitious form of malabsorption termed "levothyroxine pseudomalabsorption" has been reported in patients with psychiatric disease, in whom normal L-T4 absorption is found when it is directly assessed (20). Drugs that interfere with thyroxine absorption include the bile sequestrants cholestyramine (21,22), aluminum hydroxide (23), ferrous sulfate (24), and sucralfate (25). Soy-based infant formulas and diets enriched with fiber supplements (26) have also been reported to lead to higher than expected thyroxine dosing.

After ingestion, serum thyroxine levels rise 10–15%, peaking at 2–4 h (27,28). Serum T3 levels generally do not change after L-T4 administration, because of the slow

Table 1
Conditions That May Affect L-T4 Requirements

Increased requirements
    Physiologic States
        Pregnancy
        Infancy and childhood
    Gastrointestinal Disease
        Malabsorption (sprue, regional enteritis)
        Cirrhosis
        Pancreatitis
    Drugs that interfere with absorption
        Cholestyramine and colestipol
        Sucralfate
        Aluminum hydroxide
        Ferrous sulfate
        Lovastatin
    Drugs that block T4 to T3 conversion
        Amiodarone
    Drugs that accelerate L-T4 disappearance
        Phenytoin
        Carbamazepine
        Phenobarbital
        Rifampin
    Dietary factors that interfere with absorption
        Soy-based infant formula
        Fiber supplements
Decreased requirements
    Exogenous androgen use
    Aging

conversion of T4 to T3 in peripheral tissues. Thus, exogenous L-T4 provides a steady source of T3, similar to what is seen after endogenous T4 secretion and deiodination.

Certain drugs accelerate thyroxine metabolism in the liver by inducing mixed-function oxygenase enzyme systems. Patients taking phenytoin *(29)*, carbamazepine *(30)*, and rifampin *(31)* will often require an increased L-T4 dose. Patients taking amiodarone, a potent inhibitor of T4 to T3 conversion, may also require an increase in dosage because of difficulty in normalization of serum TSH levels, likely caused by blockade of intrapituitary T4 to T3 conversion *(32)*. On the other hand, patients treated with androgen for breast cancer have been reported to require a 25–50% decrease in L-T4 dose, possibly related to a decrease in serum thyroxine binding globulin concentrations, with subsequent increases in serum fT4 levels *(33)*.

REPLACEMENT THERAPY IN PRIMARY HYPOTHYROIDISM

Based on the criterion of normalization of serum TSH concentrations, the average L-T4 replacement dose is approximately 1.6 µg/kg ideal body weight *(11)*. The dose is 10–40% lower in the elderly because of decreases in thyroxine turnover with age *(34,35)*, and it is significantly higher in infants and children (10–15 µg/kg in infants and 2–3 µg/kg in children *[36]*). The reasons for these markedly increased requirements are not known. The dose to normalize the serum TSH level may differ depending on the etiology of the hypothyroidism; all else being equal, the L-T4 dose in patients with primary or postsurgical hypothyroidism may be 20% greater than the dose in patients with postablative Graves disease, presumably because of the continued presence of autonomously functioning thyroid tissue in the latter situation *(37)*.

Given the fact that the distribution of serum TSH levels is not Gaussian but is skewed to the left, it is reasonable to strive for a serum TSH level in the lower one-half of the normal range (0.5 –2.5 or 3 mU/L in an assay where the normal range is 0.5–5 mU/L). In the average otherwise healthy patient, the full replacement dose (1.6 µg/kg) can be given at the outset, without building the dosage up slowly. In extremely obese individuals, the dose should probably be based on lean body mass *(5)*. With this in mind, the average woman will require a dose in the range of 100–125 µg/d, and 125–175 µg/d will be needed for the average man. Because serum TSH levels fall at a rate of approx 50%/ wk *(38)*, it is usually recommended that serum TSH levels not be checked for 4–6 wk after therapy is initiated, especially if the serum TSH is extremely elevated to begin with. Also, L-T4 has a serum half-life of about 6 d, and 5 half-lives are required for any drug to reach steady state levels in the blood. If the serum TSH level is persistently elevated after 8–12 wk of therapy, the L-T4 dose should be increased by 25 µg, and the TSH reassessed after an additional 6–8 wk.

Clinical improvement generally begins after a few days to a few weeks, but complete recovery may take several months of therapy. Once the proper dose has been established, it should not change unless clinical circumstances change (e.g., introduction of an interfering drug, weight loss or gain, aging, pregnancy [*see* "Pregnancy" section]). In stable patients, serum TSH can be checked annually to assure compliance; it is usually not necessary to monitor the fT4 or FTI unless the TSH becomes abnormal *(39)*. If the fT4 or FTI is measured, it is often in the upper end of the normal range or may be even slightly above normal. This is likely a result of the need for a higher serum T4 and fT4 to generate adequate T3 in the absence of the thyroid gland. In normal individuals, approx 20% of circulating T3 is derived from the thyroid itself, whereas 80% comes from the conversion of T4 to T3 peripherally. In treated primary hypothyroidism, a higher T4 is required to compensate for the loss of the thyroidal component of the daily T3 production. Thus, serum T3 and TSH values are almost always normal in L-T4 treated patients with euthyroid hyperthyroxinemia.

Noncompliance always should be considered in such cases in whom the dose seems inappropriately large, assuming other factors that increase L-T4 dose requirements can be ruled out (*see* "Malabsorption" and "Pregnancy" sections). Patients with fT4 levels that are high-normal or elevated who also have elevated TSH levels most likely are taking their medications sporadically, especially in anticipation of a physician visit or laboratory testing. Because of its long half-life, thyroxine may be given once weekly to extremely noncompliant patients *(40)*.

Overreplacement with thyroxine, as judged by a suppressed serum TSH concentration, should be avoided, particularly in older patients. Some (e.g., *41,42*) but not all *(43,44)* studies have concluded that postmenopausal women on suppressive doses of L-T4 are at risk for lower bone mineral density compared to age-matched control women. Estrogen use may attenuate this effect *(45)*. In addition, a study examining the risk of atrial fibrillation, found that patients with suppressed serum TSH levels–the majority of whom were taking L-T4–had an almost threefold elevation in the risk of atrial fibrillation over a 10-yr follow-up period compared to patients with either normal, slightly elevated, or slightly low serum TSH levels *(46)*. Therefore, it behooves the clinician to carefully titrate the L-T4 dose against the serum TSH to be sure that it remains within the range of normal. Major effects on the serum TSH, and by inference, on the skeleton and heart, can be seen with changes in L-T4 dosage as small as 25 µg/d *(47)*.

Patients taking desiccated thyroid or T4/T3 combinations should be switched to L-T4. Although it has been a traditional concept that one grain of desiccated thyroid is approximately equal to 100 µg of L-T4, this conversion often leads to excessive L-T4 dosing. Practically speaking, it is better to simply stop the desiccated thyroid and start L-T4 at a dose commensurate with the patient's weight, as described above.

Brand Name or Generic Thyroxine?

There continues to be great controversy concerning the possible differences in potency and reliability of brand name (proprietary) vs generic thyroxine preparations *(48)*. With ever increasing demands for cost containment , the pressure to prescribe less expensive L-T4 preparations has increased. Since 1983, all thyroxine products have been required to contain 90–110% of the stated tablet content, measured by high-pressure liquid chromatography (HPLC). Although the proprietary products have consistently met this standard, there are troubling reports of departures from these standards with generic products *(49)*, although the prevalence of this problem is not known. In addition, differences in thyroxine bioavailability, which is related to tablet solubility and composition rather than to hormonal content, may exist. The inert ingredients (called "excipients," including lactose, corn starch, and talc) that permit a tablet to be formed into a specific shape and to have a particular consistency may be important in this regard. Neither the US Pharmacopoeia nor the Food and Drug Administration (FDA) have specific guidelines for demonstrating thyroxine bioequivalence among various products. Furthermore, FDA guidelines for bioequivalence of drugs are based on the demonstration of similar acute pharmacokinetic profiles (i.e., area under the curve and maximal concentration after dosing) rather that the more relevant physiological parameter of serum TSH. Thus, although several recent studies have claimed that some L-T4 preparations are "bioequivalent" *(50,51)*, methodological problems exist, and data on TSH levels show considerable individual variability after switching from one product to another.

One can be reasonably sure that serum levels of thyroxine and TSH will be stable if a patient consistently takes L-T4 manufactured by the same company, be it proprietary or generic. Unfortunately, if generic thyroxine is prescribed, the patient may receive thyroxine made by a different manufacturer the next time a prescription is filled. Thus, it appears that the only way to be sure of consistency is to prescribe proprietary thyroxine. There are considerable cost differences among the various proprietary products (Table 2). Switching from one brand to another is not recommended, and current guidelines published by the American Thyroid Association recommend that TSH levels should be checked if thyroxine brands are changed *(52)*.

Other Considerations

SUBCLINICAL HYPOTHYROIDISM

There continues to be controversy over whether subclinical hypothyroidism represents a disease that requires therapy or a clinically insignificant set of laboratory

Table 2
Retail Prices of Thyroxine at Four Large Baltimore Pharmacy Chains (September 1997)[a]

Pharmacy	Synthroid	Levothroid	Levoxyl	Generic
A	$28.29	N/A	$19.19	$7.39
B	$27.98	N/A	$13.49	$13.49 (Levoxyl)
C	$29.96	$10.96	$12.46	$10.96 (Levothroid)
D	$31.99	$10.99	$12.39	$10.99 (Levothroid)
Average	$29.55	$10.97	$14.38	$10.70

N/A, not available (store does not carry product).
[a]Costs of 100 0.1 mg tablets.

abnormalities. In the view of many experts, therapy is usually indicated for three reasons. First, several studies have shown that "subclinical" hypothyroidism may actually be associated with mild symptoms consistent with hypothyroidism that are reversed with L-T4 therapy (53,54). Second, when TSH values are greater than 10 mU/L, there may be improvements in serum lipids, especially low density lapoprotein (LDL)-cholesterol (55–57). Finally, patients, especially the elderly, are at risk for the development overt hypothyroidism at a rate of 5–20%/yr, especially, but not exclusively, in patients with positive antithyroid antibodies (58–60). In subclinical hypothyroidism, most patients' TSH serum levels can be normalized with modest L-T4 doses, in the range of 50–100 μg/d. Indeed, it has been shown that the final replacement dose of L-T4 correlates with the pretreatment TSH level (61).

PREGNANCY

At least 50–75% of pregnant hypothyroid women will require an increase in their L-T4 dose during pregnancy (62,63). Possible reasons include increased thyroxine binding globulin levels, transplacental passage of T4, and placental deiodination of T4. In one study, the mean daily increment to normalize the serum TSH was 37 μg/d (62); in another, it was 52 μg/d (63). Increases in L-T4 requirements may begin in the first trimester; consequently, serum TSH should be checked at the end of the first trimester and every 6–12 wk thereafter. After delivery, the L-T4 dose returns to the prepartum level, and overreplacement will ensue if the dose is not decreased at the time of delivery.

TRANSIENT HYPOTHYROIDISM

Patients with postpartum thyroiditis or subacute thyroiditis may have transient hypothyroidism as part of the evolution of their illness (64). The majority of patients have mild hypothyroidism and remain asymptomatic. Occasionally, however, the hypothyroidism is severe enough to warrant treatment with L-T4. In this situation, treatment is continued for 3–6 mo and is then discontinued. In most instances, a euthyroid state will be found; however, approx 25% of patients with postpartum thyroiditis will require continued L-T4 therapy because of permanent impairment in thyroid function. The vast majority of patients with Hashimoto's thyroiditis have permanent hypothyroidism, but a small fraction (in the range of 10%) may have recovery of thyroid function (65,66). However, most experts do not recommend a trial discontinuation of thyroxine in patients with long-standing typical primary hypothyroidism.

L-T4 Therapy in Patients with Ischemic Heart Disease

In the elderly (over age 65) or in patients with significant cardiac disease, it is prudent to begin with lower doses of L-T4 and to build up the dose gradually ("start low, go slow"). L-T4 therapy may increase myocardial oxygen requirements by enhancing myocardial contractility and heart rate. Theoretically, however, L-T4 therapy would simultaneously decrease systemic vascular resistance and end diastolic volume, both of which would tend to decrease myocardial oxygen consumption *(67)*. Indeed, the rate of development of angina was <5% in a large retrospective study of older hypothyroid individuals *(68)*. In the same study, 16% of patents with pre-existing angina had a worsening of symptoms with thyroid hormone, whereas 38% had improvement or disappearance of symptoms. This study was published in an era before the advent of β-blockers, calcium channel blockers, and TSH assays. Nowadays, it is possible to treat virtually all hypothyroid patients with coexisting cardiac disease effectively. It is appropriate to initiate therapy with L-T4 doses of 12.5–25 μg/d, with titration by 25-μg increments every 6–8 wk until the serum TSH levels are within the normal range. Occasional patients cannot be fully replaced with thyroxine because of exacerbation of angina, despite maximal anti-anginal medical therapy. In such patients, coronary revascularization or angioplasty should be considered. In hypothyroid patients who are in emergent need of myocardial revascularization or angioplasty because of myocardial infarction or crescendo angina, it is probably safer to proceed with the procedure rather than attempt to replace them with L-T4. The surgical mortality in untreated hypothyroidism is no higher than in euthyroid individuals *(69,70)*, and the myocardium may be further jeopardized when waiting for the patient to achieve a euthyroid state *(71)*. However, perioperative morbid events (e.g., ileus, hyponatremia) do occur more frequently in hypothyroid patients *(70)* than in euthyroid controls.

Myxedema Coma

Myxedema coma represents the ultimate degree of hypothyroidism and results in death in at least 50% of cases *(72)*. Often patients are elderly and are either undiagnosed or have discontinued L-T4 therapy for a protracted period of time. The management of myxedema coma is beyond the scope of this chapter, since the correction of abnormalities related to profound hypothyroidism (CO_2 retention, hyponatremia, ileus, sepsis, and so forth) is at least as important as therapy with thyroid hormones. There is controversy about the best treatment of myxedema coma, because of its rarity and the lack of controlled clinical trials. Most clinical reviews (e.g., *72–74*) recommend a 300–500 μg IV bolus of L-T4, which will raise the serum concentration of T4 to normal levels (based on a T4 volume of distribution of 0.1 L/kg body weight, 500 μg will raise the serum T4 concentration by about 7 μg/dL). Patients appear to have few adverse cardiovascular effects, despite receiving what seem to be very large L-T4 doses *(75)*. Because patients are critically ill, however, conversion of T4 to T3 in peripheral tissues will be diminished. Some feel that this is a beneficial protective mechanism, whereas others have advocated the use of T3 in this situation to more quickly treat the underlying hypothyroidism *(76–78)*. In the absence of a consensus, it is reasonable to recommend initial therapy with a bolus of IV L-T4, followed by daily IV L-T4 in doses of 75–125 μg/d. The IV route is preferred, because of uncertain L-T4 absorption in any severe illness; the IV dose should be 20% lower than the oral dose, since oral L-T4 is only 60–80% absorbed. If a clinical response fails to occur after a few days, intravenous T3 can be added in doses of 5 μg every

6 h or 10 µg every 8 h. Oral L-T4 can be resumed when gastrointestinal function has returned to normal. As previously noted, scrupulous attention to the host of attendant medical problems is of vital importance, and most authorities recommend he use of stress doses of glucocorticoids.

THYROXINE "ALLERGY"

Occasional patients develop anxiety, palpitations, sweating, and other symptoms suggestive of hyperthyroidism on doses of L-T4 that do not produce biochemical hyperthyroidism. Typically, these complaints develop early in the course of treatment. The best way of treating these symptoms is to decrease the L-T4 dose and to progress with dose increases more slowly. True allergy to L-T4 has been documented in one case report *(79)*, but numerous instances of urticaria or rash, possibly related to tartrazine or other dyes, have been reported *(80)*. The 50 µg tablets do not contain any dye and could be substituted if dye allergy is suspected. Lactose is present in thyroxine and many other drugs as a diluent. It is unlikely that the small amount of lactose present in a single tablet would cause problems even in lactose-sensitive individuals.

TREATMENT OF SECONDARY HYPOTHYROIDISM

The treatment of secondary hypothyroidism is less straightforward than that of primary disease. First, the presence of coexistent secondary adrenal insufficiency must be considered, and if present, glucocorticoid therapy should be initiated first. In addition, serum TSH levels cannot be used as a benchmark for the adequacy of therapy; it is reasonable to strive to keep the fT4 or FTI in the upper half of the normal range and to monitor the patient's clinical response. The replacement dose of L-T4 in central hypothyroidism will be roughly the same as would be calculated in a patient with primary hypothyroidism *(81)*.

REFERENCES

1. Vanderpump MPJ, Tunbridge WMG, French JM, et al. The incidence of thyroid disorders in the community: a twenty-year follow-up of the Whickham Survey. Clin Endocrinol (Oxf) 1995;43:55–68.
2. Wiersinga WM. Subclinical hypothyroidism and hyperthyroidism. I. Prevalence and clinical relevance. Neth J of Med 1994;46:197–204.
3. Faglia G, Bitensky L, Pinchera A, Ferrari C, Parachi A, Beck-Peccoz P, et al. Thyrotropin secretion in patients with central hypothyroidism: evidence for reduced biological activity of immunreactive thyrotropin. J Clin Endocrinol Metab. 1979;48:989–998.
4. Beck-Peccoz R, Amir S, Menezes-Ferreira MM, Faglia G, Weintraub BD. Thyrotropin secretion in patients with central hypothyroidism: evidence for reduced biological activity of immunoreactive thyrotropin. J Clin Endocrinol Metab 1985;312:1085–1090.
5. Mandel SJ, Brent GA, Larsen PR. Levothyroxine therapy in patients with thyroid disease. Ann Intern Med 1983;119:492–502.
6. Roti E, Minelli R, Gardini E, Braverman LE. The use of misuse of thyroid hormone. Endocrine Rev 1993;14:401–423.
7. Toft AD. Thyroxine therapy. NEJM 1994;331:174–180.
8. USP Dispensing Information: Volume 1—Drug Information for Health Care Professionals. The United States Pharmacopeial Convention, Rockville, MD, 1997.
9. Kaufman SC, Gross GP, Kennedy DL. Thyroid hormone use: trends in the United States from 1960 through 1988. Thyroid 1997;1:285–291.
10. Sawin CT, Geller A, Hershman JM, Castelli W, Bacharach P. The aging thyroid: the use of thyroid hormone in older persons. JAMA 1989;261:2653–2655.

11. Fish LH, Schwartz HL, Cavanaugh J, Steffes MW, Bantle JP. Replacement dose, metabolism, and bioavailability of levothyroxine in the treatment of hypothyroidism. Role of triiodothyronine in pituitary feedback in humans. N Engl J Med 1987;316:764–70.

12. Choe W, Hays MT. Absorption of oral thyroxine. 1993;5:22–228.

13. Hays MT, Nielsen KRK. Human thyroxine absorption: age effects and methodological analyses. Thyroid 1994;4:55–64.

14. Wenzel KW, Kirscheiper HE. Aspects of the absorption of oral l-thyroxine in normal man. Metabolism 1977;26:1–8.

15. Benvenga S, Bartolone L, Squadrito S, Lo Giudice F, Trimarchi F. Delayed intestinal absorption of levothyroxine. Thyroid 1995;5(4):249–253.

16. Read DG, Hays MT, Hershman JM. Absorption of oral thyroxine in hypothyroid and normal man. J Clin Endocrinol Metab 1970;30:798–799.

17. Azizi F, Belur R, Albano J. Malabsorption of thyroid hormones after jejunoileal bypass for obesity. Ann Intern Med 1979;90:941–942.

18. Bevan JS, Munro JF. Thyroxine malabsorption following intestinal bypass surgery. Int J Obes 1986;10:245,246.

19. Stone E, Leiter LA, Lambert JR, Silverberg JDH, Jeeyeebhoy KN, Burrow GN. L-Thyroxine absorption in patients with short bowel. J Clin Endocrinol Metab 1984;59:139–141.

20. Ain KB, Refetoff S, Fein HG, Weintraub BD. Pseudomalabsorption of levothyroxine. JAMA 1991;266:2118–2120.

21. Northcutt RC, Stiel JN, Hollifiels JW, Stant EG. The influence of cholestyramine on thyroxine absorption. JAMA 1969;208:1857–1861.

22. Harmon SM, Siefert CF. Levothyroxine-cholestyramine interaction reemphasized. Ann Intern Med 1991;115:658–659.

23. Sperber AD, Liel Y. Evidence for interface with the intestinal absorption of levothyroxine sodium by aluminum hydroxide. Arch Intern Med 1992;152:183,184.

24. Campbell NR, Hasinoff BB, Stalts H, Rao B, Wong NC. Ferrous sulfate reduces thyroxine efficacy in patients with hypothyroidism. Ann Intern Med. 1992;117:1010–1013.

25. Sherman SI, Tielens E, Ladenson PW Sucralfate causes malabsorption of L-thyroxine. Am J Med 1994;96:531–535.

26. Liel Y, Harman-Boehm I, Shany S. Evidence for a clinically important adverse effect of fiber-enriched diet on the bioavailability of levothyroxine in adult hypothyroid patients. J Clin Endocrinol Metab 1996;80:857–859.

27. Browning MC, Bennet WM, Kirkaldy AJ, Jung RT. Intra-individual variation of thyroxine, triiodothyronine, and thyrotropin in treated hypothyroid patients: implications for monitoring replacement therapy. Clin Chem 1988;34:696–699.

28. Ain KB, Pucino F, Shiver TM, Banks SM. Thyroid hormone levels affected by time of blood sampling in thyroxine-treated patients. Thyroid 1993;3:81–85.

29. Faber J, Lumholtz IB, Kirkegaard C, Poulsen S, Jorgensen PH, Siersback-Nielsen K, et al. The effects of phenytoin (diphenylhydantoin) on the extrathyroidal turnover of thyroxine, 3,5,3'-triiodothyronine, 3,3',5'-triiodothyronine, and 3'5'-diiodothyronine in man. J Clin Endocrinol Metab 1985;61:1093–1099.

30. DeLuca F, Arrigo T, Pandullo E, Siracusano MF, Benvenga S. Changes in thyroid function tests induced by 2 month carbamazepine treatment in L-thyroxine-substituted hypothyroid children. Eur J Pediatr 1986;145:77–79.

31. Isley WL. Effect of rifampin therapy on thyroid function tests in a hypothyroid patient on replacement L-thyroxine. Ann Intern Med 1987;107:517,518.

32. Figge J, Dluhy RG. Amiodarone-induced elevation of thyroid stimulating hormone in patients receiving levothyroxine for primary hypothyroidism. Ann Intern Med 1990;113:553–355.

33. Arafah BM. Decreased levothyroxine requirement in women with hypothyroidism during androgen therapy for breast cancer. Ann Intern Med 1994;121:247–251.

34. Rosenbaum RL, Barzel US. Levothyroxine replacement dose for primary hypothyroidism decreases with age. Ann Intern Med 1982;96:53–55.

35. Sawin CT, Herman T, Molitch ME, London MH, Kramer SM. Aging and the thyroid. Decreased requirement for thyroid hormone in older hypothyroid patients. Am J Med 1983;75:206–209.

36. Fisher DA. Management of congenital hypothyroidism. J Clin Endocrinol Metab 1991;72:523–529.

37. Bearcoft CP, Toms GC, Williams SJ, Noonan K, Monson JP. Thyroxine replacement in post-radioiodine hypothyroidism. Clin Endocrinol 1991;34:115–118.

38. Ridgway EC, McCammon JA, Benotti J, Maloof F. Acute metabolic responses in myxedema to large doses of intravenous L-thyroxine. Ann Intern Med 1972;77:549–555.
39. Helfand M, Crapo LM. Monitoring therapy in patients taking levothyroxine. Ann Intern Med 1990;113:450–454.
40. Stefan K, Grebe G, Cooke RR, Ford HC, Fagerstrom JN, Cordwell DP, et al. Treatment of hypothyroidism with once weekly thyroxine. J Clin Endocrinol Metab 1997;82:870–875.
41. Paul TL, Kerrigan J, Kelly AM, Braverman LE, Baran DT. Long-term L-thyroxine therapy is associated with decreased hip bone density in premenopausal women. JAMA 1988;259:3137–3141.
42. Stall GM, Harris S, Sokoll LJ, Dawson-Hughes B. Accelerated bone loss in hypothyroid patients overtreated with contemporary preparations. Ann Intern Med 1990;105:11–15.
43. Greenspan SL, Greenspan FS, Resnick NM, Block JE, Friedlander AL, Genant HK. Skeletal integrity in premenopausal and postmenopausal women receiving long-term L-thyroxine therapy. Am J Med 1991;91:5–14.
44. Franklyn JA, Betteridge J, Daykin J, Holder R, Oates GD, Parle JV, et al. Long-term thyroxine treatment and bone mineral density. Lancet 1992;340:9–13.
45. Schneider DL, Barrett-Connor EL, Morton DJ. Thyroid hormone use and bone mineral density in elderly women. JAMA 1994;271:1245–1249.
46. Sawin CT, Geller A, Wolk PA, et al. Low serum thyrotropin concentration as a risk factor for atrial fibrillation in older persons. N Engl J Med 1994;331:1249–1252.
47. Carr D, McLeod DT, Parry G, Thornes HM. Fine adjustment of thyroxine replacement dosage: comparison of the thyrotrophin releasing hormone test using a sensitive thyrotropin assay with measurement of free thyroid hormones and clinical assessment. Clin Endocrinol (Oxf). 1988;28:325–333.
48. Oppenheimer JH, Braverman LE, Toft A, Jackson, IM, Ladenson, PW. Thyroid hormone treatment: when and what? J Clin Endocrinol Metab 1995;80:2873–2883.
49. Dong BJ, Brown CH. Hypothyroidism resulting from generic levothyroxine failure. J Am Board Fam Pract 1991;4:167–170.
50. Escalante DA, Arem N, Arem R. Assessment of interchangeability of two brands of levothyroxine preparations with a third generation TSH assay. Am J Med 1995;98:374–378.
51. Dong BJ, Hauck WW, Gambertoglio JG, Gee L, White JR, Bubp JF, et al. Bioequivalence of generic and brand-name levothyroxine products in the treatment of hypothyroidism. JAMA 1997;277(15):1205–1213.
52. Singer PA, Cooper DS, Levy EG, Ladenson PW, Braverman LE, Daniels G, et al. Treatment guidelines for patients with hyperthyroidism and hypothyroidism. JAMA 1995;273(10):808–812.
53. Cooper DS, Halpern R, Wood LC, Levin AA, Ridgway EC. Thyroxine therapy in subclinical hypothyroidism. A double-blind, placebo-controlled trial. Ann Intern Med. 1984;101:18–24.
54. Nystrom E, Caidahl K, Fager G, Wikkelso C, Lundberg PA, Lindstedt G. A double-blind cross-over 12 month study of L-thyroxine treatment of women with 'subclinical' hypothyroidism. Clin Endocrinol (Oxf) 1988;29:63-75.
55. Althaus BU, Staub JJ, Ryff-De Leche A, Oberhansil A, Stabelin HB. LDL/HDL changes in subclinical hypothyroidism: possible risk factors for coronary heart disease. Clin Endocrinol (Oxf) 1988;28:157–163.
56. Caron P, Calazel C, Parra HJ, Hoff M, Louvet JP. Decreased HDL cholesterol in subclinical hypothyroidism: the effect of L-thyroxine therapy. Clin Endocrinol (Oxf) 1990;33:519–523.
57. Arem R, Patsch W. Lipoprotein and apolipoprotein levels in subclinical hypothyroidism. Effect of levothyroxine therapy. Arch Intern Med. 1990;150:2097–2100.
58. Tunbridge WM, Brewis M, French JM, Appleton D, Bird T, Clark T, et al. Natural history of autoimmune thyroiditis. Br Med J 1981;282:258–262.
59. Sawin CT, Castelli WP, Hershman JM, McNamara P, Bacharach P. The aging thyroid. Thyroid deficiency in the Framingham Study. Arch Intern Med 1985;145:1386–1388.
60. Rosenthal MJ, Hunt WC, Garry PJ, Goodwin JS. Thyroid failure in the elderly. Microsomal antibodies as discriminant for therapy. JAMA 1987;258:209–213.
61. Kabadi UM. Optimal daily levothyroxine dose in primary hypothyroidism. Its relation to pretreatment thyroid hormone indexes. Arch Intern Med 1990;149:2209–2212.
62. Mandel SJ, Larsen PR, Seely EW, Brent GA. Increased need for thyroxine during pregnancy in women with primary hypothyroidism. N Engl J Med 1990;323:91–96.
63. Kaplan MM. Monitoring thyroxine treatment during pregnancy. Thyroid 1992;2:147–152.
64. Singer PA. Thyroiditis acute, subacute, and chronic. Med Clin North Am 1991;75:61–77.

65. Takasu N, Yamada T, Takasu M, Komiya I, Nagasawa Y, Asawa T, et al. Disappearance of thyrotropin-blocking antibodies and spontaneous recovery from hypothyroidism in autoimmune thyroiditis. N Engl J Med 1992;326:513–518.

66. Comtois R, Faucher L, Lafleche. Outcome of hypothyroidism caused by Hashimoto's thyroiditis. Arch Intern Med 155:1404–1408.

67. Klein I, Ojamaa K. Thyroid hormone and the heart. Am J Med 1996;101:459-460.

68. Keating FR, Parkin TW, Selby JB, Dickinson LS. Treatment of heart disease associated with myxedema. Prog Cardiovasc Dis 1960;3:364–381.

69. Weinberg AD, Brennan MD, Gorman CA, Marsh HM, O'Fallon WM. Outcome of anesthesia and surgery in hypothyroid patients. Arch Intern Med 1983;143:893–897.

70. Ladenson PW, Levin AA, Ridgway EC, Daniels GH. Complications of surgery in hypothyroid patients. Am J Med 1984;77:261–266.

71. Hay ID, Duick DS, Vliestra RE, Maloney JD, Pluth JR. Thyroxine therapy in hypothyroid patients undergoing coronary revascularization: a retrospective analysis. Ann Intern Med 1981;95:456–457.

72. Nicoloff JT. Thyroid storm and myxedema coma. Med Clin North Am 1985;69:1005–1017.

73. Arlot S, Debusche X, Lalas JD, Mesmacque A, Tolani M, Quichaud J, et al. Myxoedema coma: response of thyroid hormones with oral and intravenous high-dose L-thyroxine treatment. Intensive Care Med 1991;17:16–18.

74. Hylander B, Rosenquist U. Treatment of myxoedema coma - factors associated with fatal outcome. Acta Endocrinol (Copenh) 108:65–71.

75. Kaptein EM, Quion-Verde H, Swinney RS, Egodage PM, Massry SG. Acute hemodynamic effects of levothyroxine loading in critically ill hypothyroid patients. Arch Intern Med 1986;146:662–666.

76. Pareira VG, Haron ES, Lima-Neto N, Medeiros-Neto GA. Management of myxedema coma: report on three successfully treated cases with nasogastric or intravenous administration of triiodothyronine. J Endocrinol Invest 1982;5:331–334.

77. Chernow B, Burman KD, Johnson DL, McGuire RA, O'Brian T, Wartofsky L, et al. T3 may be a better agent than T4 in the critically ill hypothyroid patient: evaluation of transport across the blood-brain barrier in a primate model. Crit Care Med 1983;2:99–104.

78. Arlot S, Debusche X, Lalas JD, Mesmacque A, Tolani M, Quichaud J, et al. Myxoedema coma: response of thyroid hormones with oral and intravenous high-dose L-thyroxine treatment. Intensive Care Med 1991;17:16–18.

79. Shibata H, Hayakawa H, Hirukawa M, Tadokoro K, Ogata E. Hypersensitivity caused by synthetic thyroid hormones in a hypothyroid patient with Hashimoto's thyroiditis. Arch Intern Med 1986;146:1624–1625.

80. Magner J, Gerber P. Urticaria due to blue dye in Synthroid tablets. Thyroid 1994;4:341.

81. Banovac K, Carrington SAB, Levis S, Fill MD, Bilsker MS. Determination of replacement and suppressive doses of thyroxine. J Intern Med Res 1990;18:210–218.

7

Thyroid Hormone Replacement During Pregnancy

Jorge H. Mestman, MD

INTRODUCTION

Thyroid diseases are five to seven times more common in women than men. It has been suggested—although never proven—that multiparity could be a risk factor for such increased prevalence in thyroid pathology. In a follow-up study of women with mild thyroid abnormalities in pregnancy, thyroidal abnormalities never returned to complete normalcy following pregnancies *(1)*. Chronic autoimmune disease, the most common etiology of thyroid pathology in areas of sufficient iodine supply, occurs frequently; however the incidence varies with the criteria for diagnosis, the decade when the study was performed and the patients studied *(2)*. In autopsy studies, the prevalence of chronic thyroiditis varies form 5–45% in women and 1–20% in men, according to the severity of the pathologic findings *(3)*. When thyroid antibodies are measured, the incidence is 10–13% in women and 3% in men and increases with age *(4)*. The incidence rate of positive thyroid antibodies in asymptomatic pregnant women is between 6–19.6% *(5,6)*. It is two to three times higher in women with type 1 diabetes mellitus *(7)*. Immunologic changes occurs throughout normal pregnancy, and it explains the frequent alterations in the natural history of thyroid diseases during and up to 1 yr after delivery *(8)*. Pregnancy is associated with significant—and in most cases reversible—changes in thyroid function.

From: *Contemporary Endocrinology: Hormone Replacement Therapy*
Edited by: A. W. Meikle © Humana Press Inc., Totowa, NJ

Table 1
Factors Affecting Thyroid Economy in Early Pregnancy

Thyroxine binding globulin (TBG)
Human chorionic gonadotropin (hCG)
Iodine supply in diet and water
Iodine renal clearance
Placenta deodinase enzymes

Although never demonstrated with certainty that there is an increase in thyroid production from early pregnancy, laboratory parameters suggest very strongly that such an increase occurs in response to physiologic changes in thyroid economy. In most cases, there is a complete adaptation to this challenge; however, in patients with thyroid pathology, changes in thyroid tests are clearly demonstrated *(9,10)*. The reason(s) for this increase in thyroid demands from very early in pregnancy is not clear; however, there is increasing evidence, that maternal thyroid hormones are important for development of the embryo before fetal thyroid gland becomes functional, which occurs after the 10th wk of gestation.

In this chapter, I will discuss the present understanding of the changes in thyroid physiopathology during and after gestation, with the intent to develop a rational approach to thyroid hormone replacement during pregnancy. The following topics will be covered:

1. Physiologic changes in thyroid economy during and following normal pregnancy.
2. Interpretation of thyroid test early in pregnancy.
3. Etiology of hypothyroidism.
4. The clinical spectrum of maternal, fetal and neonatal complications of hypothyroidism in pregnancy.
5. Thyroid hormonal requirements in hypothyroid women in the different trimesters of pregnancy and postpartum.
6. Indications for thyroid therapy in euthyroid pregnancy.
7. Postpartum thyroiditis.

PHYSIOLOGICAL CHANGES IN THYROID ECONOMY DURING AND FOLLOWING NORMAL PREGNANCY

A series of changes in thyroid metabolism follow conception. The maternal hypothalamic-pituitary-thyroid axis adapts to these demands, and in most women, maternal-placenta-fetal interrelationship remains within the norms for pregnancy *(9–11)*. Several factors described here are responsible for these changes in thyroid economy during pregnancy (Table 1).

Thyroxine Binding Globulin (TBG)

Serum thyroid hormones, both thyroxine (T4) and triiodothyronine (T3), circulate in blood bound to several proteins. Seventy percent of T4 is bound to TBG and the rest to transthyretin (thyroxine binding prealbumin) and to albumin. Only 0.02% of T4 and 0.3% of T3 circulates in the free or biologically form. Very early in pregnancy, serum TBG concentration increases, owing to a reduced clearance by the liver because of an estrogen-induced increase in sialylation of TBG and an estrogen-stimulated increase in its synthesis *(12)*. The elevation in serum TBG is seen by the third week of pregnancy, and the levels plateau by the 20–24 wk gestation until delivery. It is speculated that this increased in TBG produces a very transient decrease in serum-free T4 with a concomitant stimulation of pituitary thyroid stimulating hormone (TSH) to restore the normal equilibrium. These changes go unnoticed from the clinical point of view.

Human Chorionic Gonadotropin (hCG)

Levels of hCG increase shortly after conception reaches a maximum concentration by 12–14 wk gestation, and its levels decrease thereafter *(13)*. hCG binds to the thyroid TSH receptors and stimulates the secretion of T4 *(14)*. Its thyrotropic activity is explained by the structural homology between the hCG and TSH molecules and its receptors *(15)*. The magnitude of the stimulation depends on the hCG concentration and also on molecular changes in its structure. It has been shown that changes in the sialic content of the molecule increases its bioactivity. This transient elevation in free T4 hormone levels in serum, in turn feed back to the pituitary gland with a decrease in TSH production. There is an inverse correlation between serum hCG and TSH levels. In situations with high production of hCG *(16)*, such as hydatidiform mole, multiple gestation, and hyperemesis gravidarum, one finds an elevation of serum FT4 concentration with suppression on TSH levels characteristic of hyperthyroidism. In some cases, few signs of thyrotoxicosis are detected on physical examination along with mild symptoms of hypermetabolism; however, palpable goiter is an exceptional finding in these patients. In a few cases, severe hyperthyroid symptoms, including pulmonary edema, have been reported *(17)*.

The need for the increase demand in free T4 in the first trimester of pregnancy, as shown by the increase requirements of thyroxine in hypothyroid women, is not well understood. Several reasons have been suggested *(9)*: the increase in serum TBG production increasing the extra thyroidal T4 pool, the degradation of T4 by the placenta, the transfer of T4 from mother to fetus, and an increase in maternal clearance of T4.

The importance of maternal thyroxine transfer to the embryo in the few weeks following conception has been debated by many investigators. Human fetal thyroid function is demonstrable by 10 wk gestation with the synthesis, albeit limited, of thyroxine. The hypothalamic pituitary axis develops by 18–20 wk gestation *(18)*. The transfer of maternal thyroid hormones to the fetus in normal pregnancy is limited; the maturation of the fetal-thyroid system is largely independent of maternal influence. In the human, a role in early fetal development has been suggested, because T4 has been shown to be present in amniotic fluid before the fetal thyroid is able to secrete thyroid hormones. Centempre et al. *(19)* has shown the presence of thyroxine in the coelomic and amniotic fluid before the maturation of the fetal thyroid system. Nuclear T3 receptors in the brain of human fetus early in gestation has been demonstrated, supporting the role for maternal thyroid hormones in the maturation of the fetal brain. From the clinical point of view, the effect of maternal hypothyroidism on the intellectual development of the infants is controversial. In areas of sufficient iodine supply, low and normal IQs have been found. Man et al. described a group of children of mothers with hypothyroxinemia with low IQs *(20)*; Liu et al. *(21)*, in a controlled study of hypothyroid mothers in the first trimester of their pregnancies, found no difference in the IQs of their children, as compared to their siblings conceived when the mother was euthyroid.

Iodine-Renal Clearance

Renal iodine clearance is increased from early pregnancy, and this could explain reports of high 24 h RAIU early in pregnancy *(22)*. Furthermore, in the second half of gestation, iodine is transferred to the fetus for thyroid hormonogenesis. In areas of iodine deficiency, this insufficient supply to mother may be the cause of maternal goiter. Severe iodine deficiency results in the development of cretinism and other syndromes of iodine deficiency *(23)*. This is not seen in the US, Japan, and some countries in Europe, where there is sufficient supply of iodine in water and food. However in other areas of the world, it is estimated that 1–1.5 billion people are at risk of iodine deficiency *(24)*. In areas of marginal iodine intake, between 50 and 100 µg/d, thyromegaly as measured by ultrasonography is detected from the first trimester of pregnancy. In an elegant study by Smyth et al. *(25)*, thyroid volume was measured by ultrasound in each trimester and in the postpartum period. The thyroid volume increased from a baseline of 11.3 mL before conception to a maximum of 16.0 mL in the third trimester—an overall increase of 47%. Enlarged thyroid volumes, defined as > 18 mL, were detected in 6.3% of prepregnancy control, 19.5% in the first trimester, and 32% in the third, which was maintained up to 40 d postpartum. The authors also noted an increase in iodine excretion since early in pregnancy, but a sharp drop in the first days after delivery. This increase in renal loss of iodine may contribute to thyroid enlargement, because iodine replacement during pregnancy may prevent the formation of goiter *(26)*. The rapid decline in iodine excretion soon after delivery could reflect rapid normalization of renal clearance or even placental loss. The authors confirmed previous estimation of decrease in thyroidal iodine stores of approx 40% during gestation; they asked if this iodine lost throughout consecutive pregnancies could explain the female preponderance of thyroid disease *(25)*. The increased in volume of the thyroid gland during pregnancy, reported by other authors in area of iodine deficiency, is seen to a much lesser degree in areas of sufficient supply of iodine *(27,28)*.

Serum thyroglobulin (TG) levels normally secreted by the thyroid gland, are increased with progression of pregnancy, particularly in areas of iodine deficiency. Glinoer et al., has shown, in an area of mild iodine deficiency in Belgium, an elevation in TG concentration with progression of pregnancy, ultrasonographic enlargement of the thyroid gland, and the development of clinical goiter in 18% of patients *(29)*. When iodine plus T4 were given to patients, initial high TG levels were normalized, along with a slight reduction in serum TSH concentrations *(30)*.

5-Deiodinase Activity

The enzyme 5-deiodinase (type III) regulates the metabolism of T4. It converts T4 to the biologically inactive metabolite reverse T3 (rT3). This enzyme is present in the human placenta, but the extent to which it affects changes in the metabolism of thyroid hormones during pregnancy is presently unclear *(10,31)*.

All of the aforementioned changes occurring in pregnancy support the clinical observation for increased thyroid hormonal need in early and late pregnancy. Glinoer *(10)* suggests that several biochemical markers are indicative of increase thyroid production in pregnancy:

1. Lower total serum T4/TBG ratio.
2. Preferential T3 secretion, reflected in an elevated T3/T4 molar ratio.

3. Elevation in serum TSH, albeit within the normal range in the second half of pregnancy.
4. Increase in TG concentrations.

He was able to demonstrate these changes in areas of iodine deficiency. In the US and other countries with sufficient iodine supply, these parameters are much less affected unless the patient suffers from thyroid pathology. The typical example, which will be discussed in more detail, is the women on thyroid replacement therapy following ablation of the thyroid gland; significant number of them require an increased dose of thyroid hormone from early pregnancy in order to prevent the development of hypothyroidism *(32,33)*.

It appears that in early pregnancy, the maternal thyroid gland is stimulated to increase the production of T4, perhaps to assist in the early development of the embryo or for other unclear reasons. In a normal situation, the adaptation occurs without clinical repercussions. However, in those patients with thyroid disease, an elevation in serum TSH will be indicative of a need for increasing the dose of thyroid hormone. In a study by Kamijo *(34)*, a few patients with an elevation of serum TSH and other markers for autoimmunity early in pregnancy spontaneously normalized serum TSH with progression of pregnancy. It is tempting to speculate that, in cases of borderline thyroid pathology, the thyroid gland is unable to compensate for the stimulation of hCG early in pregnancy, but with progression of pregnancy and decreasing hCG production, the need for thyroxine diminishes and, in some patients, the initial elevated TSH returns to normal values.

One other speculation regarding thyroid stimulation and TSH response early in pregnancy is related to normal values of serum TSH early in pregnancy. It has been shown by many investigators, that serum TSH levels are lower in the first trimester of pregnancy, increasing with progression of pregnancy albeit remaining within normal limits *(11)*. It is possible, although unproven, that a serum TSH level over 3 U/L in the first half of pregnancy could be abnormal and indicative of early thyroid failure.

INTERPRETATION OF THYROID TESTS EARLY IN PREGNANCY

Thyroid function testing in pregnancy is indicated by the presence of a history or physical findings suggestive of thyroid dysfunction, for adjusting the dose of thyroid medication, or in cases of hyperthyroidism to assess dosage of antithyroid medication. A simple algorithm for thyroid function tests is shown in Fig. 1. The interpretation of thyroid tests early in pregnancy may be confusing to the physician. Second- and third-generation serum TSH concentration, an excellent screening test in the outpatient setting, may be low or suppressed in up to 15% of normal pregnancies in the first trimester *(29)*, as well as in cases of multiple gestation *(35)*, hydatidiform mole *(36)*, hyperemesis gravidarum *(37,38)*, or even in cases of mild nausea and vomiting *(39)*. In addition to the low serum TSH value, free thyroxine concentration may be also in the hyperthyroid range, with spontaneous normalization with progression of pregnancy or correction of the obstetric pathology, as in the case of hydatidiform mole. These transient thyroid abnormalities are explained by high levels of serum hCG, known to occur in the aforementioned situations, which, with its thyrotropic biologic activity acting on the TSH thyroid receptor, stimulates the secretion of thyroxine. By midgestation, thyroid tests normalize and remain within normal limits throughout pregnancy.

Thyroid autoantibodies are present in 6–19.6% of pregnant women *(5,6)*, as compared to 5% of nonpregnancy. They are markers of thyroid autoimmune disease. Antibodies to

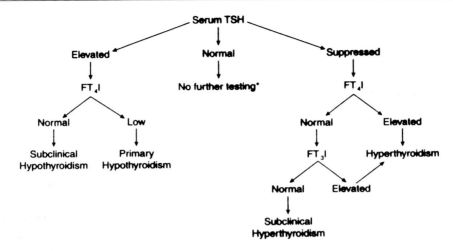

Fig. 1. Algorithm for the diagnosis of thyroid disease. If there is a clinical suspicion of secondary thyroidism a determination of FT_4I is indicated. In this situation, the serum TSH is normal in the presence of low FT_4I. FT_4I, free thyroxine index or its equivalent, free thyroxine; FT_3I, free triiodothyronine index or its equivalent, free triiodothyroine; TSH, thyroid stimulating hormone.

thyroglobulin and thyroid peroxidase (PTO) are measured by radioassay techniques that have replaced in most commercial laboratories hemagglutination and immunofluorescence assays. Anti-TPO antibodies (formerly know as microsomal antibodies [AMA]) and antithyroglobulin antibodies (ATA) titers decrease with progression of pregnancy, rebounding after delivery *(40)*. Both antibodies are present in 95–100% of persons with autoimmune thyroiditis and in 60–90% of Graves' disease patients. Anti-TPO thyroid antibodies, and antithyroglobulin antibodies cross the placenta and are detected in cord blood in concentrations similar to maternal values. However, they are not cytotoxic to the fetal thyroid, and their presence and titer are not related to neonatal thyroid hypothyroidism *(41)*. High titers in the first trimester of pregnancy are predictive for the development of the syndrome of postpartum thyroiditis *(42)*. The incidence of spontaneous miscarriages is also increased in euthyroid chronic thyroiditis women *(6,43,44)*. From a practical and cost-effective point of view, there is no reason to determine both antibodies; measurement of anti-TPO antibodies is sufficient to make the diagnosis of autoimmune thyroiditis, since it is present in almost every patient with chronic thyroiditis. ATA may be ordered in cases of negative anti-TPO titers and strong clinical suspicion of chronic thyroiditis. Indications for measuring anti-APO antibodies include the presence of goiter, patients with unexplained miscarriages, family history of thyroid disease, to establish the etiology of hypothyroidism and in other autoimmune diseases, such as type 1 diabetes mellitus.

TSH Receptors antibodies, are IgG antibodies acting on TSH receptors. These antibodies, binding to different sites of the TSH receptor, may stimulate or block the production of thyroid hormones *(45)*. The nomenclature is confusing, and many terms have been applied *(46)*. In Table 2, the name, abbreviation, method of detection, and frequency are shown. Basically, these antibodies may be measured by a radioreceptor assay or by a bioassay. The radioreceptor assay is simple to perform and more economical; it is known as TSH receptor antibody (TRAbs) or TSH-binding inhibitory immunoglobulin (TBII).

Table 2
Nomenclature, Method of Detection,
Frequency, and Abbreviation of TSH Receptor Antibodies

Name	Abbreviation	Method of detection	Frequency
TSH receptor antibodies	TRAbs	Radioreceptor assay	80–90% Graves' disease
TSH-binding inhibitory immunoglobulins	TBIIs	Radioreceptor assay	80–90% Graves' disease 30–50% Chronic Thyroiditis
A. STIMULATORY			
Thyroid-stimulating antibodies	TSAbs	Bioassay: Stimulation of adenyl-cyclase	
Thyroid-stimulating immunoglobulins	TSIs	Bioassay: Stimulation of adenyl-cyclase	80–90% Graves' disease
B. BLOCKING			
TSH receptor-blocking antibodies	TRBAbs	Bioassay: Inhibition of TSH-induced adenyl-cyclase stimulation	10% Hashimoto's 20–40% Primary myxedema

[a]Adapted with permission from ref. 46.

This technique measures the inhibition of the binding of TSH to thyroid membranes. It does not discriminate between the stimulating or blocking action of the antibodies and therefore does not provide functional information. The bioassay, based on the stimulation of adenyl cyclase, discriminate between their stimulation and blocking effect. It is technically more cumbersome and expensive to perform than the radioreceptor assay. They are known as thyroid-stimulating antibodies (TSAbs) or thyroid stimulating immunoglobulin (TSI); TSH receptor-blocking antibodies (TRBAbs) or TSH stimulation-blocking antibodies (TSI-Block) for those inhibiting TSH-induced adenyl cyclase stimulation.

TSAbs or TSI are present in almost 90% of patients with Graves' disease. IgG antibodies cross the placenta, starting at about 24 wk gestation; by the end of pregnancy, the fetal concentration of IgG is close to maternal values. Maternal high titers of TSI may affect the fetal thyroid gland, causing fetal and/ or neonatal hyperthyroidism, which occurs in less than 2% of pregnancies complicated by Graves' disease (45).

Antibodies to the TSH receptor that block TSH-induced thyroid stimulation and growth, TRBAbs, are detected in 10% of patients with goitrous or Hashimoto's thyroiditis (47), and in 20–40% of patients with primary myxedema or nongoitrous thyroiditis (48,49). The biologic half-life of these antibodies is of a few months; transfer to the fetus in high titers may cause transient neonatal hypothyroidism (48). Brown et al. (50) measured TBII in dried-blood specimens obtained from 788 neonates identified as having possible congenital hypothyroidism. Eleven of them with titers > 132 U/L were hypothyroid, confirmed by low-serum T4 and high-serum TSH levels. The incidence of transient or neonatal hypothyroidism was estimated by this author to be 1 in 180,000 of normal infants and accounts for approx 2% of babies born with congenital hypothyroidism (50). Tamaki et al. (51) studied 104 mothers with chronic thyroiditis, 92 of them with goiter

Table 3
Clinical Indications for TSHRAbs in Pregnancy

1. Suspicious of fetal or neonatal hyperthyroidsm–women with active or postablation Graves' disease.
   a. Previous pregnancy with fetal or neonatal hyperthyrodism.
   b. Presence of fetal tachycardia or intrauterine growth retardation.
   c. Incidental fetal goiter on ultrasound.
   d. Treatment with antithyroid drugs.
2. Women with primary myxedema or Hasimoto's thyroiditis.
   a. Previous pregnancy with neonatal hypothyrodism.
   b. Infant born with neonatal hypothyroidism.
3. Any woman in the postpartum period.
   a. Infant born with neonatal hypothyroidism.
   b. Neonatal thyroid gland is presen on ultrasound in a hypothyroid infant.

and 12 of them with primary atrophic hypothyroidism or nongoitrous thyroiditis. TBII was present in 4 of 12 mothers (33%) with primary atrophic hypothyroidism, none in mothers with goitrous or Hashimoto thyroiditis. Three of the four infants were born with hypothyroidism that was transient, with the antibodies titer disappearing in 5–7 mo postpartum. Because the differential diagnosis of congenital hypothyroidism caused by thyroid dysgenesis vs blocking antibody-induced is almost impossible to make clinically (18), measuring TBII in infants born with congenital hypothyroidism is mandatory. Prompt treatment with thyroxine is essential to prevent mental retardation; therapy is continued until subsequent measurement of TBII becomes negative, usually in a few months.

There are few indications for ordering TSH Receptor Antibodies in pregnancy. They are shown in Table 3. In order for these antibodies to cause thyroid dysfunction in the fetus and neonate, their titer concentration in maternal blood needs to be significantly elevated. There is a tendency for the titers to decrease with progression of pregnancy. In women with Graves' disease, it is measured by the end of pregnancy to predict neonatal hyperthyroidism; one other approach is to measure the antibody in infants born to mothers with Graves' disease, since a high titer predicts neonatal hyperthyroidism (52). In euthyroid mothers with a previous history of Graves' disease, it is measured only if the fetus shows manifestation of fetal thyrotoxicosis, such as fetal tachycardia, uterine growth retardation, or if the mother had delivered previously an affected infant. In the case of a mother with chronic thyroiditis, it should be measured if the neonate is born with congenital hypothyroidism, if previous siblings were affected, and if the thyroid gland is present on ultrasonography.

ETIOLOGY OF HYPOTHYROIDISM

Thyroid requirement increases in pregnancy, and it is normally compensated by the secretion of thyroid hormones by the thyroid gland. In many hypothyroid women on replacement therapy, however, subclinical or even clinical hypothyroidism may be diagnosed at some time in pregnancy because of the inability of the thyroid gland to compensate for this increase in thyroxine demands. This is the most common cause of hypothyroidism diagnosed in pregnancy. In about 10% of patients, the diagnosis of

Table 4
Indications for Thyroid Testing in Pregnancy

High Risk
    Previous therapy for hyperthyroidism
    Previous high-dose neck irradiation
    Previous postpartum thyroiditis (evidence of thyroid autoimmunity)
    Goiter (diffuse or nodular)
    Family history of thyroid disease
    Treatment with amiodarone
    Suspected hypopituitarism
    Type 1 diabetes mellitus
    Hyperlipidemia
Moderate Risk
    Any endocrinopathy
    Any autoimmune disorder
    Various medications (see Table 6)
    Exposure to industrial/chemical substances (e.g., polybrominated biphenyl compounds)

hypothyroidism is made for the first time in pregnancy; the patient presents with hypothyroid symptoms, or the diagnosis is made because of the detection of goiter on physical examination, or because of a family history of thyroid disease. In some cases, the women had been treated with ablation therapy for Graves' hyperthyroidism and had never received replacement therapy. Table 4 shows the different clinical situations in which thyroid tests are indicated in pregnancy. We discourage the routine use of thyroid tests for screening purposes in pregnancy.

Hypothyroidism may be because of intrinsic disease of the thyroid gland (primary hypothyroidism) or secondary to pituitary or hypothalamic pathology (secondary hypothyroidism) (53). The majority of cases are a result of primary thyroid failure. Other causes are shown in Table 5.

Primary hypothyroidism is classified as clinical hypothyroidism, characterized by an elevated serum TSH concentration and low-serum free thyroxine levels or as subclinical hypothyroidism, normal free thyroxine and elevated TSH, usually below 20 U/mL. In the latter, hypothyroid symptoms are usually absent.

When the diagnosis of hypothyroidism is made for the first time in pregnancy, symptomatology is present in about 60% of cases, and the in the rest, symptoms are very mild or absent (54–56).

Secondary hypothyroidism is rare in pregnancy. Most common etiology is pituitary or hypothalamic disease, following hypophysectomy for pituitary tumor or following brain radiation therapy. In most cases, there is more than one pituitary hormone deficiency. Isolated TSH deficiency has been reported in few isolated cases. Onset of partial or panhypopituitarism have been reported in pregnancy; in such cases, an acute bleeding develops within a pre-existing pituitary tumor or the rare case of autoimmune hypophysitis, a syndrome that presents in most cases in the postpartum period (57).

Congenital hypothyroidism occurred in 1:4000 births, and it is an uncommon etiology in pregnancy. Peripheral resistance to thyroid hormones, another rare cause of hypothyroidism, has been occasionally reported in pregnancy. In the patient reported by Weiss et al. (58), the mother suffered from generalized resistance to thyroid hormone (GRTH);

Table 5
Etiology of Hypothyroidism

More common causes of primary hypothyroidism
    Chronic autoimmune thyroid disease
        Goitrous
        Atrophic
    Radioiodine 131 ablation
    Thyroidectomy
Less common causes of primary hypothyroidism
    Transient hypothyroidism
        Silent ("painless") thyroiditis
        Subacute thyroiditis
    Drug-induced (*see* Table 6)
    High-dose external neck radiation
    Congenital hypothyroidism
    Inherited metabolic disorders of the thyroid
    Thyroid hormone resistance syndrome
Secondary hypothyroidism
    Pituitary or hypothalamic disease

the infant was detected by analysis of blood obtained during routine neonatal screening; serum TSH level of 26 U/L and an inappropriate thyroxine concentration of 656 nm/L (normal 84–232). The authors pointed out that the diagnosis may be missed when serum TSH is used as the only screening test for congenital hypothyroidism.

Medications that interfere with the synthesis, release, or peripheral action of thyroid hormone may cause hypothyroidism, as well as those drugs interfering with l-thyroxine absorption in the gastrointestinal system (Table 6). In this regard it is important to point out that ferrous sulfate should be given 2 h apart from l-thyroxine, because it may interfere with thyroxine absorption *(59)*.

In countries with sufficient iodine supply, the two most common causes of primary hypothyroidism in pregnancy are post ablation therapy for Graves' disease (131I or surgery) or thyroid carcinoma, and chronic autoimmune or Hashimoto's thyroiditis. Chronic autoimmune thyroiditis may present with goiter; in other cases, no goiter is palpable, which is known as primary atrophic thyroiditis or primary mxedema. Thyroidectomy and postablation with 131 iodine were the cause of hypothyroidism in 65% of patients in one series *(55)* and in 25 out of 68 women (37%) in another series *(56)*. In most cases, hypothyroidism antedate pregnancy. Overt hypothyroidism was diagnosed de novo in 3 out of 23 cases *(56)* and 1 out of 14 patients *(55)*. Not uncommonly, patients may have stopped taking thyroid medications when learning of their pregnancy because of misconceptions or being ill-advised.

THE CLINICAL SPECTRUM AND MATERNAL, FETAL, AND NEONATAL COMPLICATIONS OF HYPOTHYROIDISM IN PREGNANCY

Until recently, it was stated that pregnancy in untreated hypothyroid women was a rare event because of anovulation, and if conception occurred, fetal and neonatal morbidity

Table 6
Drugs That May Affect Bioavailability of l-Thyroxine

Interference with thyroid hormone synthesis and/or release
　　Antithyroid medications (methimazole, PTU)
　　Iodine
　　Lithium
Increased thyroxine clearance
　　Carbamazipine
　　Phenytoin
　　Rifampin
Decreased conversion from T4 to T3 and possible inhibition of T3 action
　　Amiodarone
Inference with intestinal absorption
　　Aluminum hydroxide
　　Cholestyramine
　　Ferrous sulfate
　　Sucralfate

PTU, Propylthiouracil.

and mortality were significant *(65)*. Impaired mental and somatic development were also reported in 50–60% of the surviving children *(61,62)*. Many of the original series of hypothyroxinemia in pregnancy were reported before specific tests (such as free T4 or serum TSH) for the diagnosis of hypothyroidism were available. In many cases the diagnosis was based on the clinical picture of hypothyroidism or myxedema *(63)*; in other cases, serum PBI or BEI were used *(64)*; furthermore, thyroid extract or proloid was used as the only form of replacement therapy that may give a low-serum thyroxine value *(62)*. Before 1981, only 36 cases of proven hypothyroidism in pregnancy from the English literature, most of them isolated cases, were reported *(54)*. Since then, published series *(54–56,65,66)*, albeit of a relatively small number of patients, have reported a better outcome as compared to early series. The explanation for this better perinatal results is not clear; however, early diagnosis of the disease, prompt correction of hypothyroxinemia, aggressive evaluation of fetal well-being, timely delivery, and better neonatal care could have affected and resulted in an improved neonatal outcome *(67)*. Montoro et al. *(54)* reported in 1981 the neonatal outcome of 11 pregnancies in 9 severely hypothyroid women, with a mean serum TSH value of 105 U/mL when first seen in pregnancy (40–293 U/mL) and mean serum T4 of 2.3 µg/dL (0.2–4.4 µg/dL). The perinatal outcome was significantly better that previously reported, and in nine pregnancies, thyroxine treatment brought serum TSH to nearly normal values at delivery. There was one intrauterine death at 29 wk of gestation in an untreated mother with a serum TSH of 293 U/mL who developed severe preeclampsia. Another patient, euthyroid at birth, delivered an infant with Down's syndrome, the mother's age was 41 yr. Seven children, followed up to 2.7 yr of age, developed normally. The neonatal outcome in this small series was in marked contrast with previous reports of high abortion rate, congenital malformations and perinatal mortality.

　　The clinical diagnosis of hypothyroidism is based on symptoms of fatigue, sleepiness, cold intolerance, depression, deeper voice or hoarseness, arthralgia, morning hand stiffness, constipation. On physical examination a goiter is present in a significant number of patients, the skin is dry, there is a delayed in the relaxation phase of deep tendon reflexes, periorbital edema is frequently seen. However, not always the diagnosis is clinically obvious. In three of the largest series reported in pregnancy (54–56), classical symptoms of hypothyroidism were present in one third of the patients, another third had mild symptomatology and in the remaining third, no symptoms could be elucidated in spite of significant hypothyroid values. In the cases of subclinical hypothyroidism, the symptomatology is usually absent. Therefore, the physician should have a high index of suspicion in order to detect the disease in its early states. This is an important issue particularly in pregnancy, because perinatal outcome is directly related to prompt thyroid therapy.

It is estimated that the diagnosis of hypothyroidism is made in one of 1000 to 2000 pregnancies (56,65). In population screening studies, however, the incidence of elevated serum TSH is much higher; in Belgium, 2.2% has been reported (10) in an area of low iodine intake. In this study, 1900 consecutive pregnant women were screened by a determination of serum TSH and thyroid antibodies; in most of the 41 women (2.2%) with elevated serum TSH, the range was between 4 and 10 U/L, with a few having values between 10 and 20 U/L. Positive thyroid antibodies were detected in 40% of the 41 women. Klein et al. (68) in the US, measured serum TSH between 15 and 18 wk gestation in a group of 2000 women; 49 (2.5%) of them had serum TSH levels above 6 U/L. Six of the 49 patients had overt hypothyroidism, with low serum thyroxine and mean serum TSH value of 17.9 U/L with a range of 6.9 to 54.2 U/L. Positive thyroid antibodies were detected in 58% in those women with serum TSH over 6 U/L, as compared to 11% of control euthyroid pregnant women. The authors also found a direct correlation between TSH concentration and patient's age. A screening study was carried out during the first trimester of pregnancy in a group of 9453 Japanese women (31), 28 of them (0.29%) had an elevated serum TSH level, mean value of 11.7 ng/dl (7.7–26.3) at a mean gestational age of 8.5 wk; in 18 of them, the elevations of serum TSH were transient. Sixteen of the 18 patients had positive thyroid antibodies titers. The authors were able to follow 12 of these women throughout gestation, the serum TSH returning to normal spontaneously by 18 wk gestation (mean 3.5 ng/dl ranging from 1.5–4.9). Small goiters were palpable in 11 out of the 12 women; examination of seven of the neonates showed no evidence of physical abnormalities. In the report by Leung et al. (56) from Los Angeles County/USC Women's hospital, 101 pregnant women with hypothyroidism were identified between 1981 and 1990; 23 with overt hypothyroidism, 45 with subclinical hypothyroidism, and 33 euthyroid on thyroxine replacement therapy. The incidence was of 1:1,629 deliveries; similar to the incidence reported from Mercy Hospital for Women in Melbourne, Australia (editorial comment in 65). The prevalence of high serum TSH in the few screening programs reported is much greater than the incidence of actual cases reported in relatively large series. Since in the majority of the screening studies, no medical history or physical examination were obtained, it is possible that in many cases, the women had discontinued the use of thyroid therapy at the time of conception or the usual increase in thyroid requirements were not met at the time of testing. In most of the series reported in the literature, the diagnosis of overt hypothyroidism was rarely made for the first time during pregnancy; 3 out of 23 cases (56), 2 out of 25 (55), 2 out of 26 (65); in the majority of cases when the diagnosis of overt hypothyroidism is made in pregnancy, the patients were non compliant with thyroxine therapy or had discontinued thyroid therapy at the time of conception.

Maternal complications and perinatal morbidity is high when hypothyroidism is not well controlled. In the combined series of 50 proven overt hypothyroid pregnant women

Table 7
Maternal and Neonatal Complications of Hypothyroidism in Pregnancy

| | Overt Hypothyroidism | | | | Subclinical Hypothyroidism | | |
| | | | | Total | | | Total |
No. of patients	16^{26}	23^{63}	11^{66}	50 (%)	12^{26}	45^{53}	57 (%)
PIH	7	5	1	13 (26)	2	7	9 (15)
Placenta abruptio	3	0	0	3 (6)	0	0	0
PPH	3	1	0	4 (8)	2	0	2 (3.5)
Stillbirths	2	1	1	4 (8)	1^c	0	1 (1.7)
Cong							
Malf	0	1	1	2 (4)	0	0	
LBW	5^a	5^b	0	10 (20)	$1^{a,d}$	4	5 (8.7)
Anemia							
(HCT < 26%)	5	0	0	5 (10)	0	1	1 (1.7)

Cong Malf, congenital malformations; HCT, hematocrit; PIH, pregnancy-induced hypertension; PPH, postpartum hemorrhage; LBW, low birth weight. Adapted with permission from refs. *26, 63,* and *86.*
[a]LBW < 2000 g.
[b]LBW < 2500 g.
[c]Congenital syphillis.
[d]Class F diabetes.

(Table 7) by Davis et al. *(55)* and Leung et al. *(56)* significant findings were a 26% incidence of pregnancy-induced hypertension (PIH), intrauterine death in 8%, low birth weight (LBW) in 20% and 6% of placenta abruptio. In the subclinical hypothyroid combined group of 57 patients, the incidence of PIH was 15%, LBW 8.7%, and there was only one intrauterine death, the infant affected by congenital syphilis. The high incidence of LBW is related to premature delivery as a result of PIH.

Pregnancy-induced hypertension is the most common and serious complication in most of the series reported, with one exception *(66)*. In the latter, the outcome of nine overt hypothyroid pregnancies were compared with the outcome in 34 women with mild hypothyroidism or euthyroid on replacement therapy. In five of the nine overt hypothyroid women cesarean section was performed for fetal distress; none of the nine women developed pre-eclampsia/eclampsia, although the authors could not rule out mild pre-eclampsia in some of their patients. The patients developing fetal distress at term were more hypothyroid than those having no fetal distress. The incidence of anemia was also significant. In the group with mild hypothyroidism or euthyroid on replacement therapy, there was only one cesarean section caused by fetal distress. In reviewing the series reported, one note of caution need to be address; in some series *(56,66)*, patients with chronic diseases were not included, in order to prevent other confounding factors in the incidence of complications; in other series *(55,65)* patients with chronic hypertension, anemia, diabetes mellitus were included. In Davis et al. *(55)* report, five hypothyroid patients with poor neonatal outcome were studied in subsequent pregnancies, while they remained euthyroid on replacement therapy. Four of them delivered prematurely, one of them complicated by pre-eclampsia. As stated by the authors, perhaps other factors in addition to hypothyroidism may have influenced these outcomes. In the series reported by Buckshee et al. *(65)*, only in two patients out of 26 the diagnosis of overt hypothyroidism was made in pregnancy. The other 24 cases were on replacement therapy; thyroxine needed to be adjusted in seven of them, five with an increase in doses and in the other two a decrease was needed. It is difficult to assess perinatal complications in this report, because many patients had coexisting chronic medical problems such as diabetes mellitus, epilepsy, bronchial asthma, glomerulonephritis, and pulmonary tuberculosis. The overall incidence of pregnancy-induced hypertension in the 26 patient was 27%. In Leung et al. *(56)*, gestational hypertension complicated 12 cases, five out of 23 with overt hypothyroidism and seven out of 45 with subclinical hypothyroidism. Eight out of 12 (67%) were hypothyroid at the time of delivery, the more severe toxemia in those patients with the most abnormal hypothyroid tests. In those developing toxemia, the mean serum TSH at delivery was 106 U/L, as compared to a TSH of 11.1 U/L in those without toxemia; in the subclinical hypothyroid group, the mean serum TSH at delivery was 18.4 U/L in those with toxemia as compared to 4.3 U/L in the group without toxemia. Of the five infants born to mothers with severe hypertension, the birth weight was less than 2000 g because of prematurity; one intrauterine death occurred in an woman at 28 wk gestation, untreated, with a serum TSH at delivery of 288.5 U/mL and serum FT4I of 1.4.

Autoimmune thyroid diseases are seen more frequently in type 1 diabetes mellitus. The incidence of chronic thyroiditis, diagnosed by the presence of positive antibodies has been reported to be as high as 40% *(69,70)*. The incidence of subclinical hypothyroidism may be as high as 17% in women with type 1 diabetes *(7,71)*. Furthermore the incidence of postpartum thyroiditis is threefold increased in type 1 patients *(72,73)*. Therefore, women with type 1 diabetes should be screened for thyroid dysfunction at regular intervals, and ideally before conception or early in pregnancy. A group of 51 type 1 women were evaluated in the first trimester of pregnancy for thyroid dysfunction *(74)*. Twenty-six of them had positive thyroid antibodies; eight of them were diagnosed with subclinical hypothyroidism and had moderate proteinuria (mean 1.22 g/d) ; overt hypothyroidism aggravated by significant proteinuria (>4 g/d) developed by the second trimester of pregnancy in all of them. In a similar group of 18 women with mild thyroid tests abnormalities, but without proteinuria (mean 0.14 g/d), overt hypothyroidism did not develop; in a third group of eight patients with mild proteinuria (mean 0.80 g/d) in the first trimester and no laboratory indicators of thyroid autoimmunity, significant proteinuria developed with progression of pregnancy, however none of them developed overt hypothyroidism. In summary, in a group of patients with subclinical hypothyroidism in the first trimester of pregnancy, only those with moderated proteinuria progressed into overt hypothyroidism. In these patients, insulin requirements increased to the usual daily dose, once thyroid therapy was started and thyroid tests normalized. Unfortunately there was not post partum follow up. No decrease in thyroid antibodies titer were seen with progression of pregnancy, at variance with most reports in the literature showing a decrease in titers to even undetectable titers in almost 30% of patients with chronic thyroiditis *(75)*. In a recent report of 20 type 1 pregnant women *(76)*, seven had positive anti-TPO antibodies. Of these, three developed subclinical hypothyroidism in the second trimester of pregnancy requiring thyroid therapy. Patients with autoimmune thyroid disease required more insulin during pregnancy. In contrast to previous observation in women with type 1 diabetes mellitus *(74)* the titers of antibodies decrease with progression of pregnancy, as reported in nondiabetic pregnant women. Bech et al. *(77)* measured thyroid antibodies in a group of 85 type 1 diabetic women in each trimester of pregnancy. The incidence of positive antibodies titer was 20%, and serum TSH was normal in all of them; an slight elevation in serum TSH concentration was seen with progression of pregnancy as compared to antibody negative patients; however none of them developed subclinical or clinical hypothyroidism. Postpartum thyroid dysfunction developed in 6 out of 10 women with diabetes, of which five were antibody positive both in pregnancy and postpartum and in one patient that was antibody negative.

A controversial issue in the literature evolves in the effect of maternal hypothyroidism on the physical and intellectual development of the offspring. Early studies in the literature associated maternal hypothyroidism with mental retardation in the euthyroid offspring, as well as an increase in fetal and neonatal losses. A significant difference in IQ of children whose mothers were treated inadequately was reported (62); the score was 92 as compared to an IQ of 105 in infants whose mothers were properly treated. Poor obstetric outcomes were reported in some of early series. The question of mental retardation was recently studied by Liu et al. (21). They carefully examined the IQs of children whose mothers were hypothyroid early in pregnancy and compared to their siblings born when mothers were euthyroid during gestation. The mean serum maternal TSH was 106.4 U/L at 6.9 wk gestation, and the FT4 was 4.227 pmol/L (normal 11.6–24.5). The IQ of the siblings born when mothers were hypothyroid was not different from the siblings born when mothers were euthyroid. In all but one of the patients the hypothyroidism was corrected by 20 wk gestation. Montoro et al. (54) evaluated seven children of hypothyroid mothers between 1 mo and 2.7 yr after birth. Developmental milestones were reached at the appropriate time, and development was normal for age at the time of the examination.

The goal in the management of hypothyroidism is to normalize thyroid tests, both serum TSH and free thyroxine. Increased risk of toxemia, placenta abruptio, and prematurity caused by early pre-eclampsia has been reported in poorly controlled hypothyroidism in pregnancy. Even women with subclinical hypothyroidism, not properly treated, had an incidence of pre-eclampsia two times greater than a control group (56). The incidence of congenital malformations is not increased. In one study, cesarean section was more frequent because of fetal distress in the group of women with high serum TSH compared to a hypothyroid group with mild elevation in serum TSH (66).

An increased incidence of spontaneous miscarriages have been reported in women with positive titers of thyroid antibodies. Whether hypothyroidism by itself is a cause for spontaneous abortions is not clear at present.

THYROID HORMONAL REQUIREMENTS IN HYPOTHYROID WOMEN IN THE DIFFERENT TRIMESTERS OF PREGNANCY AND POSTPARTUM

As discussed briefly, in the previous section, thyroid hormone requirements increase during pregnancy. In normal pregnancy, there are no changes in thyroid tests, and the adjustment of thyroid needs goes on unnoticed. However, in situations of decrease thyroid reserve, such as in hypothyroid patients on thyroxine therapy, chemical hypothyroidism develops in a significant number of women. With very few exceptions, there are no clinical indicators of thyroid deficiency. A careful history obtained at the time of first booking allows the health care professional to order the proper thyroid tests and assess thyroid requirements. The physician may be presented with two different situations regarding thyroid replacement therapy in pregnancy; one is the evaluation and adjustment of thyroxine in patients already taking daily thyroxine; the second challenge is the management of the woman in whom the diagnosis of hypothyroidism is made for the first time during pregnancy.

Women on Replacement Therapy Before Pregnancy

Thyroid therapy is usually given for the treatment of hypothyroidism; chronic thyroiditis and postthyroid ablation caused by Graves' disease or thyroid carcinoma are the most common causes. In the last few years, the concept of increased thyroid requirements in pregnancy is being accepted by almost every investigator in the field. Mandel et al. *(32)* reported such a finding in a small group of hypothyroid women studied, in early pregnancy, and postpartum period. Previous to their study, the need for adjusting thyroid medication in pregnancy was reported in a minority of cases; the general consensus was that thyroxine doses rarely require an adjustment in pregnancy. Pekonen et al. *(78)* reported on 34 hypothyroid women followed during 37 pregnancies. Serum FT4I and TSH (first generation) were measured. In seven patients an increased in the dose of thyroxine was necessary because of serum TSH values of over 7 U/L. The mean increase in thyroxine dose was 62 μg/d. At delivery the patients were receiving a mean thyroxine dose of 141 ± 47 μg/d. In Mandel et al. *(31)*, serum TSH was measured by a immunoradiometric assay with a sensitivity of 0.1 U/L. Therefore they were able to adjust the thyroxine dose in order to prevent overdosage. The prepregnancy mean thyroxine dose in their 12 patients was 0.102 mg/d (range 0.05–0.175). Mean serum TSH was 2.0 U/L. Most patients, with two exceptions, were studied between 6 and 25 wk gestation, at which time the serum FT4I was lower as compared to prepregnancy values, but in only one patient it fell below the normal range. Serum TSH increased in every single patient, and in nine of them the level was in the hypothyroid range, mean 13.5 U/L (1.2–36). Thyroxine dosage needed to be increased to a mean maximal dose of 0.148 mg/d, similar to the dose received by Pekonen's patients *(78)*. There is a logical explanation for the delay in previous studies in the recognition for the need in the increase in thyroxine requirement in pregnancy. In Mandel's study, adjustment of thyroxine dose was based on a sensitive TSH assay not available in previous studies. Since the advent of such sensitive test, it has been observed that the amount of thyroxine to maintain euthyroidism was lower than before the use of sensitive TSH testing. This is exemplified comparing thyroxine dose in Pekonen et al. *(78)* and Mandel et al. *(31)* patients; both groups received similar daily doses of thyroxine; however, it was the same prepregnancy dose in the majority of patients in one study *(78)*; whereas the dose has to be increased in Mandel's patients from prepregnancy dose. Furthermore, following delivery, the dose of thyroxine had to be reduced to the prepregnancy dose. This original study was later confirmed by several authors *(79,80)*; it is well-accepted today that a significant number of patients will require an adjustment of thyroid doses at some time in pregnancy.

The causes for this increment in thyroxine need is not well understood, but several events early in pregnancy, discussed in the first section, may explain this phenomenon; the stimulation of the normal thyroid gland by two mechanisms: a slight decrease in free hormone secretion due to the early increase in serum TBG concentration, and by hCG stimulation. In situations of decreased thyroid reserve, such as chronic thyroiditis or following ablation therapy, the thyroid gland is unable to respond to this challenge, and hypothyroidism, mild in most cases, ensues. In addition, early in pregnancy, the renal clearance for iodine is increased, which may affect thyroid economy in areas of iodine deficiency. The need for more thyroxine continues throughout pregnancy; other factors, although still speculative, may be responsible. Later in pregnancy, iodine is transferred from mother to fetus, depriving the maternal thyroid of available iodine. In areas of iodine deficiency, this results in an enlargement of the thyroid gland with the production of goiter and even mild hypothyroidism. This also may affect the fetus with the development of cretinism in areas of severe iodine deficiency (23). Placental 5-deiodinase, an enzyme responsible for inner ring T4 deiodination, is markedly increased with decrease in the availability of serum thyroxine with the progression of pregnancy. The importance of this enzyme in maternal thyroid economy is unclear at present (31).

All of the aforementioned factors present a challenge to the thyroid gland, which compensates normally with an increased in production of thyroid hormones; however in situations of thyroid pathology this adjustment can not take place and hypothyroidism may occur the novo. In the most common case of a women on replacement therapy, the need for increasing the dose is seen in about 50% of them. Since the introduction of sensitive serum TSH tests (81), it is possible to assess and adjust the dose of thyroid hormone in a more precise way.

This subject has been recently reviewed by Kaplan (79,82). He analyzed 77 pregnancies in 65 hypothyroid women on replacement therapy from his own practice. Serum TSH became abnormal in 76% of 36 women with previous ablation therapy and in 47% of 29 women with chronic thyroiditis. The increase in thyroid replacement occurred in the majority of patients from early pregnancy, but in some, eight out of 27 women, serum TSH levels became abnormal later in pregnancy. He pooled the data from other four reports for a total of 125 hypothyroid women. In all but one study, a highly sensitive TSH assay was used for assessing need of thyroxine. Overall, serum TSH values increased above normal in 45% of patients, and the mean daily dose of l-thyroxine was 146 µg daily.

The adjustment in dose varies from patient to patient; it was estimated that the dose could be adjusted according to the original TSH value: the increment in l-thyroxine dose is 41 ± 24 µg a day if the initial TSH is less than 10 U/L; 65 ± 19 µg/d when TSH levels are between 10 and 20 U/L, and 105 ± 19 µg/d for TSH values greater than 20 U/L. It is also recommended to repeat TSH determination 4–6 wk after adjusting the dose. If the patient is seen early in pregnancy, serum TSH should be done at the first visit, 4–8 wk later and the last determination between 30 and 32 wk gestation. Soon after delivery, the dose is reduced to prepregnancy dose. Patients with ablation therapy for thyroid cancer need a larger thyroxine dose, because the serum TSH should remain suppressed (83).

Hypothyroidism Diagnosed During Pregnancy

In women in whom hypothyroidism is diagnosed *de novo* during pregnancy, it is recommended to start with 150 µg/d of l-thyroxine. These young women tolerate this initial dose well. Thyroid tests should be repeated in 4–6 wk and thyroxine dose adjusted accordingly. Postpartum thyroid patients are followed at regular intervals, since they may need a reduction in doses.

INDICATIONS FOR THYROID THERAPY IN EUTHYROID PREGNANCY

There are few indications for the use of thyroid therapy in euthyroid patients. This is more relevant in pregnancy when there is a sense of reservation from the patient, her family, and the health care professional to use drug therapy unless it is medically indicated. Perhaps the most common situations are women on long-term thyroid therapy in whom the original diagnosis or indications for thyroid therapy are not clear. The most frequent reason for initiation of therapy is obesity or chronic fatigue. On physical examination, a goiter is not detected, thyroid tests are within normal limits, and thyroid antibodies are not detected. It is our advice and practice to continue with thyroid therapy, keeping the thyroid tests within normal limits. In the nonpregnant state, a common option is to offer the patient to discontinue thyroid medication and to recheck thyroid tests between 1 and 3 mo according to the initial serum TSH. If the TSH is suppressed when on thyroid therapy, it will take at least 2 mo for recovery of pituitary TSH secretion.

Diffuse euthyroid or nontoxic goiter with negative thyroid antibodies is common in areas of iodine deficiency; however, sporadic cases are not uncommon. Thyroxine therapy may be used for a few months in order to reduce the size of the gland.

In euthyroid women with chronic thyroiditis, occasionally hypothyroidism may develop late in pregnancy *(44)*. On the contrary, rarely hyperthyroidism may occurred; the author followed a women with euthyroid chronic thyroiditis who developed hyperthyroidism by 32 wk gestation. It has been suggested, in areas of mild iodine deficiency that thyroid therapy may avoid the development of hypothyroidism during gestation and may prevent the formation of goiter *(30)*. It is our practice in pregnancy not to use thyroid therapy in euthyroid women with diffuse goiters, regardless of the presence of thyroid antibodies. Those with positive thyroid antibodies are followed at regular intervals, and thyroid tests are repeated every trimester and every 2–3 mo postpartum, because of the higher probability of developing postpartum thyroiditis.

Thyroid nodular disease is found in about 5% of women of childbearing age *(84)*. The presence of a single thyroid nodule or a predominant nodule in a multinodular gland during pregnancy is of concern to both future parents and physician. In the last few years, several articles on the subject have been published *(84–87)*. Most thyroid malignancies diagnosed during pregnancy are caused by papillary or follicular lesions. Thyroid medullary carcinoma is a rare event, and no case of undifferentiated thyroid carcinoma has been reported in pregnancy. The diagnostic workup depends mainly on gestational age *(85)*. A practical approach to the diagnosis and management of thyroid nodular disease is shown in Fig. 2. If a single thyroid nodule or predominant thyroid nodule in a multinodular gland is detected before 20 wk gestation, most publications on the subject elect ultrasonography, followed by (FNAB) as the first diagnostic tool *(84,85)*. If the lesion is benign, the choice of observation vs thyroid therapy to prevent further growth of the lesion is decided, based on the physician's clinical experience and patient choice. It is controversial in the literature the beneficial effect of thyroid suppression therapy *(88,89)*, but a few months of thyroid administration during pregnancy, provided the thyroid tests are kept within normal limits, may be indicated, and in some patients may be beneficial in reducing the size of the lesion. If the lesion is malignant or microfollicular, partial or almost total thyroidectomy should be discussed with the patient. Some of them will accept this form of therapy, whereas others will favor surgery after delivery, in which case thyroid suppressive therapy during pregnancy is recommended, although the degree to suppression of the serum TSH is controversial *(90)*. If there is evidence of local metastasis, surgery should not be postponed. For those women after 20 wk gestation, the risk of surgery, mainly premature delivery, should be considered when making the therapeutical decision. FNAB may be postponed until after delivery, with the option of suppression therapy. The presence of a single thyroid nodule, always create a feeling of

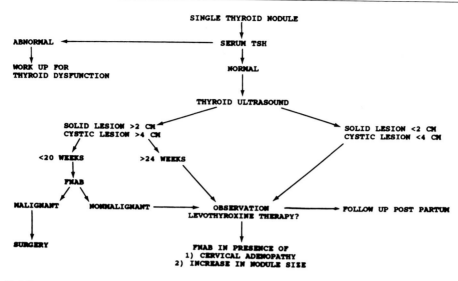

Fig. 2. Management of the single thyroid nodule during pregnancy.

anxiety in the patient, particularly in pregnancy. Therefore, the physician should be aware of the information in the literature, which indicates that postponement of surgery for a few months until delivery does not modify the natural history of these lesions *(8)*. It is very rare in our experience to observe a rapid change in size of a nodular lesion during pregnancy.

Finally, patients treated with thyroid ablation for thyroid carcinoma need to have their serum TSH in the low or undetectable level, similar to the nonpregnant state. Because most of these women have had a complete ablation of the thyroid gland, they may need an increment of their usual dose by at least 50–75 μg of l-thyroxine a day. Thyroid test are recommended at the first visit and every 4–8 wk thereafter, with return to the prepregnancy dose after delivery. Serum thyroglobulin determinations should be interpreted with caution, since its value may increased slightly in pregnancy.

Postpartum Thyroiditis

Postpartum thyroid dysfunction occurs in 5–10% of all pregnancies. Patients with autoimmune thyroid disease, both Graves' disease and Hashimoto's or chronic thyroiditis have a higher risk to develop the condition. Hypothyroidism, secondary to pituitary disease, is an uncommon cause of thyroid dysfunction in the postpartum period; Sheehan's syndrome and lymphocytic hypophysitis being the most common etiologies *(91)* (Table 8). The scope of this presentation, does not allow for a complete description of the postpartum thyroid dysfunction syndrome. A brief summary is to be presented; the reader is referred to excellent reviews published within the last few years *(42,92,93)* (*See also* Fig. 3).

The first description of hypothyroid symptoms occurring in the postpartum period was by Robertson *(94)*. He described symptoms of depression, irritability and fatigue in a large number of postpartum women. Amino et al. *(95,96)*, defined the frequency and characteristics of the syndrome. It affects women with autoimmune thyroid disease, and indeed the presence of high thyroid antibodies titers in the first trimester of gestation is predictive of the development of postpartum thyroiditis. The clinical course is character-

Table 8
Postpartum Thyroid Dysfunction

Chronic thyroiditis
    Transient hyperthyroidism (low RAIU)
    Transient hypothyroidism
    Permanent hypothyroidism
Graves disease
    Exacerbation of hyperthyroidism (high RAIU)
    Transient hyperthyroidism of chronic thyroiditis (low RAIU)
Hypothalamic-pituitary disease
    Sheehan's syndrome
    Lymphocytic hypophysitis

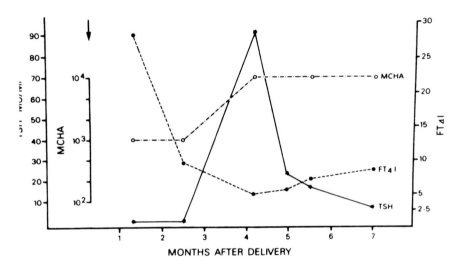

Fig. 3. Transient hyperthyrodism and hypothyroidism in the postpartum period in a patient with chronic autoimmune thyroditis with spontaneous recovery. TSH, thyroid stimulating hormone; MCHA, microsomal hemagglutination antibodies; FT$_4$I, free thyroxine index.

ized in about one third of patients by mild hyperthyroid symptoms developing in the first 2–4 mo postpartum, sometimes with an increase in the size of a present goiter. In general, the symptoms are mild and difficult to differentiate from the tiredness, irritability, and weight loss that frequently occurs after delivery. Fatigue is the common complaint of most patients. This initial phase is followed in some patients by a hypothyroid phase, in which symptoms of depression may be significant. In most patients the hypothyroid phase resolves spontaneously in a few months, returning to euthyroidism in the majority of patients However, 5–10% of women remained permanently hypothyroid (97). Along with the changes in thyroid size, there is an increase in thyroid antibodies titer.

    The clinical course may be manifested by a hypothyroid stage without the initial hyperthyroid phase; in other patients, remission occurs following the initial hyperthyroid phase without developing hypothyroidism. Diagnosis of postpartum thyroiditis is important because in some patients, treatment with β-blockers in the hyperthyroid phase or thyroxine in the hypothyroid phase is necessary because of the patient's symptoms.

Furthermore, these patients need to be followed, because the incidence of permanent hypothyroidism years after the first episode is high *(97)*, and there is a high recurrence rate in subsequent pregnancies *(98)*.

Women with Graves' disease often have a recurrence of hyperthyroidism in the postpartum period. It occurs earlier than in the hyperthyroid phase of chronic thyroiditis; however, both conditions may occur in a given patient *(99)*. In such cases a 6–24 h thyroid radioactive uptake, if not contraindicated because of breast feeding, is helpful in the differentiation of both entities; RAIU is elevated in hyperthyroidism because of Graves' disease; it is suppressed in the hyperthyroid phase of thyroiditis.

In summary, postpartum thyroiditis should be suspected in any woman who has fatigue, palpitations, emotional liability, symptoms of mental depression, or, in the presence of a goiter during the first year after delivery.

ACKNOWLEDGMENTS

The author thanks Mrs. Elsa Ahumada for her excellent secretarial assistance.

REFERENCES

1. Glinoer D, Lemone M, Bourdoux P, De Nayer P, Delange F, Kinthaert J, et al. Partial reversibility during late postpartum of thyroid abnormalities associated with pregnancy. J Clin Endocrinol Metab 1992;74:453–457.
2. Dayan CM, Daniels GH. Chronic autoimmune thyroiditis. N Engl J Med 1996;335:99–107.
3. Williams ED, Doniach I. The post mortem incident of focal thyroiditis. J Pathol Bacteriol 1962;83:255–264.
4. Tunbridge WMG, Evered DC, Hall R, et al. The spectrum of thyroid disease in a community. The Whickham survey. Clin Endocrinol (Oxf) 1977;7:481–493.
5. Glinoer D, Fernandez-Soto M, Bourdoux P, Lejeune B, Delange F, Lemone M, et al. Pregnancy in patients with mild thyroid abnormalities. Maternal and neonatal reprecussions. J Clin Endocrinol Metab 1991;73:421–427.
6. Stagnaro-Green A, Roman SH, Cobin RH, et al. Detection of at-risk pregnancy by means of highly sensative assays for thyroid antibodies. JAMA 1990;264:1422–1425.
7. Riley J, MacClaren NK, Lezzote DC, et al. Thyroid autoimmunity in insulin dependent diabetes mellitus. The case of routine screening. J Pediatr 1981;98:350–357.
8. Mestman JH, Goodwin TM, Montoro MN. Thyroid disorders of pregnancy. Endocrinol Metab Clin N Am 1995;24:41–71.
9. Burrow GN, Fisher DA, Larsen PR. Maternal and fetal thyroid function. N Engl J Med 1994;331:1072–1078.
10. Glinoer D: The regulation of thyroid function in pregnancy: pathways of endocrine adaption from physiology to pathology. Endocr Rev 1997;18:404–433.
11. Brent GA. Maternal thyroid function. Interpretation of thyroid function tests in pregnancy. Clin Obstet Gynecol 1997;40:3–15.
12. Ain KB, Mori Y, Refeteoff S. Reduced clearance rate of thyroxine-binding globulin (TBG) with increased sialylation. A mechanism for estrogen-induced elevation of serum TBG concentration. J Clin Endocrinol Metab 1987;65:686–698.
13. Braunstein GD, Hershmann JM. Comparison of serum pituitary thyrotropin and chorionic gonadotropin concentrations throughout pregnancy. J Clin Endocrinol 1976;42:1123–1126.
14. Ballabio M, Poshyachinda M, Ekins RP. Pregnancy induced chnages in thyroid function. Role of human chorionic gonadotropin as putative regulator of maternal thyroid. J Clin Endocrinol Metab 1991;73:824–831.
15. Yoshimura M, Hershman JM. Thyrotropic action of human chorionic gonadotropin. Thyroid 1995;5:425–434.
16. Goodwin TM, Hershman JM. Hyperthyroidism due to inappropriate production of human chorionic gonadotropin. Clin Obstet Gynecol 1997;40:32–44.
17. Hershman JM, Higgins HP. Hydatidiform mole: a cause of clinical hyperthyroidism. N Engl J Med 1971;284:573–577.

18. Fisher DA. Fetal thyroid function. diagnosis and management of fetal thyroid disorder. Clin Obstet Gynecol 1997;40:16–31.
19. Centempre B, Jauniaux E. Calvo R, Jurkovic D, Campbell S, Morreale de Escobar G. Detection of thyroid hormone in human embryonic cavities during the first trimester of pregnancy. J Clin Endocriol Metab 1993;77:1719–1722.
20. Man EB, Holden RH, Jones WS. Thyroid function in human pregnancy. Am J Obstet Gynecol 1971;109:12–19.
21. Lui H. Momatani N, Noh JA, et al. Maternal hypothyroidism during early pregnancy and intellectual development of the progeny. Arch Intern Med 1994;154:785–787.
22. Halnan KE. The radioiodine uptake of the human thyroid in pregnancy. Clin Sci 1958;17:281–290.
23. Pharoah POD, Connolly KJ, Ekins RP, Harding AG. Maternal thyroid hormone levels in pregnancy and the subsequent congnitive and motor performance of the children. Clin Endocrinol 1984;21:265–270.
24. Laurberg P. Iodine intake - what are we aiming at? J Clin Endocrinol Metab 1994;79:17–19.
25. Smyth PPA, Hetherton AMT, Smith DF, Radcliff M, O'Herlihy C. Maternal iodine status and thyroid volume during pregnancy. Correlation with nonatal iodine intake. J Clin Endocrinol Metab 1997;82:2840–2843.
26. Pedersen KM, Laurberg P, Iverson E, et al. Amelioration of some pregnancy associated variations in thyroid function by iodine supplementation. J Clin Endocrinol Metab 1993;77:1078–1083.
27. Levy RP, Newman DM, Rejall LS, Barford DAG. the myth of goiter in pregnancy. Am J Obstet Gynecol 1980;137:701–703.
28. Berghout A, Endert E, Ross A, Hozerzeil HV, Smits NJ, Wiersinga WM. Thyroid function and thyroid size in normal pregnant women living in an iodine replete area. Clin Endocrinol (Oxf) 1994;41:375–379.
29. Glinoer D, DeNayer P, Bourdoux P, et al. Regulation of maternal thyroid during pregnancy. J Clin Endocrinol Metab 1990;71:276–287.
30. Glinoer D, De Nayer P, Delange F, et al. A randomized trial for the treatment of mild iodine deficiency during pregnancy: Maternal and neonatal effects. J Clin Endocrinol Metab 1995;80:158–169.
31. Roti E, Gnudi A, Braverman LE. The placental transport, synthesis, and metabolism of hormones and drugs which affect thyroid function. Endocr Rev 1983;4:131–149.
32. Mandel SL, Larsen PR, Seely EW, et al. Increased need for thyroxine during pregnancy in women with primary hypothyroidism. N Engl J Med 1990;323:91–96.
33. Kaplan MM. Management of women on thyroxine therapy during pregnancy. Endocr Prac 1996;2:281–286.
34. Kamijo K, Saito T, Sato M, et al. Transient subclinical hypothyroidism in early pregnancy. Endocrinol Jpn 1990:37:397–403.
35. Grun JP, Meuris S, De Nayer P, Glineor D. The thyrotropic role of human chorionic gonadotropin (hCG) in the early stages of twin (vs. single) pregnancy. Clin Endocrinol (Oxf) 1997;46:719–725.
36. Hershman JM, Higgins HP. Hydatidiform mole: a cause of clinical hyperthyroidism. N Engl J Med 1971;284:573–577.
37. Bouillon R, Naesens M, Van Assche, et al. Thyroid function in patients with hyperemesis gravidarum. Am J Obstet Gynecol 1982;143:922–926.
38. Goodwin TM, Montoro MN, Mestman JH. Transient hyperthyroidism and hyperemesis gravidarum. Clinical aspects. Am J Obstet Gynecol 1992;167:648–652.
39. Goodwin TM, Montoro M, Mestman JH, et al. The role of chorionic gonadotropin in transient hyperthyroidism of hyperemesis gravidarum. J Clin Endocrinol Metab 1992;75:1333–1337.
40. Amino N, Kuro R, Tanizawa O, et al. Changes of serum anti-thyroid antibodies during and after pregnancy in autoimmune thyroid disease. Clini Exp Immunol 1978;31:30–37.
41. Dussault JH, Letarte J, Guyda H, et al. Lack of influence of thyroid antibodies on thyroid function in the newborn infant on a mass screening program for congenital hypothyroidism. J Pediatr 1980;96:385–389.
42. Brown-Martin K, Emerson CH. Postpartum thyroid dysfunction. Clin Obstet Gynecol 1997;40:90–101.
43. Branch DW. Autoimmunity and pregnancy loss. JAMA 1990;264:1453–1454.
44. Lejeune B, Grun P, de Nayer PH, Servais G, Glinoer D. Anithyroid antibodies underlying thyroid abnormalities and miscarriage or pregnancy induced hypertension. Brit J Obstet Gynecol 1993;100:669–672.
45. NcKenzie JM, Zakarija M. Fetal and neonatal hyperthyroidism and hypothyroidism due to maternal TSH receptor antibodies. Thyroid 1992;2:155–160.
46. Brown RS. Autoimmune thyroid disease in pregnant women and their offspring. Endocr Pract 1996;2:53–61.
47. Tamaki H, Amino N, Yukihiko W, et al. Radioreceptor assay of anti-TSH receptor antibody activity. Comparision of assays using unextracted serum and immunoglobulin fractions, and standardizaiton of epxression in activity. J Clin Lab Immunol 1985;20:1–6.

48. Konishi J, Yasuhiro I, Kasagi K, Misaki T, Nakashima T, Endo K, et al. Primary Myxedema with thyrotropin-binding inhibitor immunoglobulins. Ann Int Med 1985;103:26–31.
49. Tamaki N, Yamada T, Takasu M, et al. Disappearance of thyrotropin blocking antibodies and spontaneous recovery from hypothyrodism in autoimmune thyroiditis. N Eng J Med 1992;326:513.
50. Brown R, Bellisario RI, Botero D, Fournier L, Abrams CAL, Cowger M. Incidence of transient congenital hypothyroidism due to maternal thyrotropin receptor-blocking antibodies in over one million babies. J Clin Endocrinol Metab 1996;81:1147–1151.
51. Tamaki H, Amino N, Aozasa M, et al. Effective method for prediction of transient hypothyroidism in neonates born to mothers with chronic thyroiditis. Am J Perinatol 1989;6:296–303.
52. Skuza KA, Sills IN, Stene M, Rapaport R. Prediction of neonatal hyperthyroidism in infants born to mothers with Graves' disease. J Pediatr 1996;128:264–267.
53. Mestman JH. Thyroid disease. In: Sciarra JJ, ed. Gynecology and Obstetrics. Lippincott-Raven, Philadelphia, 1996.
54. Montoro MN, Collea JV, Frasier SD, et al. Successful outcome of pregnancy in women with hypothyroidism. Ann Intern Med 1981;94:31–34.
55. Davis LE, Leveno KJ, Cunningham FG. Hypothyroidism complicating pregnancy. Obstet Gynecol 1988;72:108–112.
56. Leung AS, Millar LK, Koonings PP, et al. Perinatal outcome in hypothyroid pregnancies. Obstet Gynecol 1993;81:349–353.
57. Mestman JH. Endocrine diseases in pregnancy. In: Sciarra JJ, ed. Gyncology and Obstetrics. Lippincott-Raven, Philadelphia, 1997, pp. 1–41.
58. Weiss RE, Balzano S, Scherberg NH, Retetoff S. Neonatal detection of generalized resistance to thyroid hormone. JAMA 1990;264:2245–2250.
59. Campbell NRC, Hassinoff BB, Stalts H, et al. Ferrous sulfate reduces thyroxine efficacy in patients with hypothyroidism. Ann Intern Med 1992;117:1010–1013.
60. Thomas R, Reid RL. Thyroid disease and reproductive dysfunction. A review. Obstet Gynecol 1987;70:789–798.
61. Grennman GW, Gabrielson MD, Howard-Flanders J, Wessel MA. Thyroid dysfunction in pregnancy. Fetal loss and follow up of surviving infants. N Engl J Med 1962;267:426–431.
62. Man EB. Maternal hypothyroxiinemia development of 4 and 7 year old offspring. In: Fisher DA, Burrows GN, eds. Perinatal Thyroid Physiology and Disease. Raven Press, 1975, pp. 177.
63. Burk K, Kerr A. Pregnancy in a patient with myxedema. Am J Obstet Gynecol 1954;68:1623–1626.
64. Man EB, Reid WA, Hellegers AE, Jones WS. Thyroid function in human pregnancy. Am J Obstet Gynecol 1969;103:328–337.
65. Buckshee K, Kriplani A, Kapil A, Bhargava VL, Takkar D. Hypothyroidism complicating pregnancy. Aust NZ J Obstet Gynecol 1992;32:240–242.
66. Wasserstrum N, Anania CA. Perinatal consequences of maternal hypothyroidism in early pregnancy and inadequate replacemnts. Clinical Endocrinology 1995;42:353–358.
67. Montoro MN. Management of hypothyroidism during pregnancy. Clin Obstet Gynecol 1997;40:65–80.
68. Klein RZ, Haddow JE, Faix JD, et al. Prevalence of thyroid deficiency in pregnant women. Clin Endocrinol (Oxf) 1991;35:41–46.
69. Irvine WJ. Autoimmunity in endocrine disease. Clin Endocrinol Metab 1979;4:227–235.
70. Bright GM, Blizzard RM, Kaiser DJ, et al. Organ specific autoantibodies in children with common endocrine diseases. J Pediatr 1982;100:8–12.
71. Gray RS, Dorsey DQ, Seth J, et al. Prevalence of subclinical thyroid failure in insulin dependent diabetes. J Clin Endocrinol 1980;50:1034–1045.
72. Gerstein HC. Incidence of postpartum thyroid dysfunction in patients with type I diabetes mellitus. Ann Int Med 1993;118:419–423.
73. Alvarez-Marfany M, Roman SH, Drexler AJ, et al. Long term prospective study of postpartum thyroid dysfunction in women with insulin dependent diabetes mellitus. Clin Endocrinol Metab 1994;79:10–16.
74. Jovanovic-Peterson L, Peterson CM. De novo clinical hypothyroidism in pregnancies complicated by type I diabetes, subclinical hypothyroidism, and proteinuria: a new syndrome. Am J Obstet Gynecol 1988;159:442–446.
75. D'Armiento M, Salabe H, Vetrano G, Scucchia M, Pachi A. Decrease in thyroid antibodies during pregnancy. J. Endocrinol Invest 1980;4:437–438.
76. Fernandez-Soto L, Gonzalez A, Lobon JA, Lopez JA, Peterson CM, Escobar-Jimenez F. Thyroid peroxidase autoantibodies predict poor metabolic control and need for thyroid treatment in pregnant IDDM women. Diabetes Care 1997;20:1524–1528.

77. Bech K, Hoier-Madsen M, Feldt-Rasmussen U, Moler-Jensen B, Molsted-Pedersen L, Kuhl C. Thyroid function and autoimmune manifestations in insulin dependent diabetes mellitus during and after pregnancy. Acta Endocrinologica (Copenh) 1991;124:534–539.

78. Pekonen F, Teramo K, Ikonen E, Osterlund K, Makinen T, Lamberg BA. Women on thyroid hormone therapy: Pregnancy course, fetal outcome, and amniotic fluid thyroid hormone level. Obstet Gynecol 1994;63:635–638.

79. Kaplan MM. Monitoring thyroxine treatment during pregnancy. Thyroid 1992;2:147–152.

80. Girling JC, de Swiet M. Thyroxine dosage during pregnancy in women with primary hypothyroidism. Br J Obstet Gynecol 1992;99:368–370.

81. Spencer CA, Takeuchi M, Kasarosyan M. Current status and performance goals for serum thyrotropin (TSH) assays. Clin Chem 1996;42:140–145.

82. Kaplan MM. Management of women on thyroxine therapy during pregnancy. Endocr Prac 1996;2:281–286.

83. Mandel SJ, Brent GA, Larsen PR. Levothyroxine therapy in patients with thyroid disease. Ann Intern Med 1993;119:492–502.

84. Rosen JB, Walfish PG, Nikore V. Pregnancy and surgical thyroid disease. Surgery 1985;98:1135–1140.

85. Doherty CM, Shindo ML, Rice DH, Montoro MN, Mestman JH. Management of thyroid nodules during pregnancy. Laryngoscope 1995;105:251–255.

86. Hamburger JI. Thyroid nodules in pregnancy. Thyroid 1992;2:165–168.

87. Tan GH, Gharib H, Goellner JR, van Heerden JA, Bahn RS. Management of thyroid nodules in pregnancy. Arch Intern Med.1996;156:2317–2320.

88. Gharib H, James EM, Charboneau JQ, Naessens JM, Offord KP, Gorman CA. Supresive therapy in levothyroxine for solitary thyroid nodules. A double blind controlled clinical study. N Engl J Med 1987;31,770–31,775.

89. Cheung PS, Lee JM, Boey JH. Thyroxine suppressive therapy of benign solitary thyroid nodules. A prospective randomized study. World J Surg 1989;13:818–822.

90. Singer PA, Cooper DS, Daniels G, et al. Guidelines for the diagnosis and management of thyroid nodules and well differentiated thyroid cancer. Arch Intern Med 1996;156:2165–2172.

91. Asa SL, Bilbao JM, Kovacs K, et al. Lymphocytic hypophysitis of pregnancy resulting in hypopituitarism. A distinct clinicopathological entity. Ann Intern Med 1981;95:166–171.

92. Lazarus JH, Hall R, Othman S, Parkes AB, Richards CJ, McCullouch B, Harris B. The clinical spectrum of postpartum thyroid disease. Q J Med 1996;89:429–435.

93. Amino N, Tada H, Hidaka Y. The spectrum of postpartum thyroid dysfunction. Diagnosis, management, and long term prognosis. Endocr Pract 1996;2:406–410.

94. Robertson HEW. Lassitude, coldness, and hair changes following pregnancy and their responses to treatment with thyroid extract. Br Med J 1948;2(suppl):93–103.

95. Amino N, Miyai K, Yamamoto T, et al. Transient recurrence of hyperthyroidism after delivery in Graves' disease. J Clin Endocrinol Metab 1977;44:130–136.

96. Amino N, Kuro R, Tanizawa O, et al. Changes of serum anti-thyroid antibodies during and after pregnancy in autoimmune thyroid disease. Clin Exp Immunol 1978;31:30–37.

97. Tachi J, Amino N, Tamaki H, Aozasa M, Iwatani Y, Miyai K. Long term follow up and HLA association in patients with postpartum hypothyroidism. J Clin Endocrinol Metab 1988;66:480–484.

98. Lazarus JH, Ammari F, Orett R, Parkes AB, Richards CJ, Harris B. Clinical aspects of recurrent postpartum thyroiditis. Br J Gen Pract 1997;47:305–308.

99. Ekel RH, Green WL. Postpartum thyrotoxicosis in a patient with Graves' disease. Association with low radioactive iodine uptake. JAMA 1980;243:1554–1456.

IV DIABETES

8

Insulin Management of Insulin-Dependent Diabetes Mellitus
Core Concepts of Insulin Management

R. Philip Eaton, MD, and Martin Conway, MD

CONTENTS

INTRODUCTION

Insulin treatment of insulin-dependent diabetes mellitus (IDDM) requires the following core concepts:

1. A knowledge of pancreatic beta cell insulin secretion in the nondiabetic person, which is the goal of management;
2. A knowledge of the timing of our insulin-delivery preparations and methods of injection, which will provide the tools to achieve approximation of normal insulin delivery;
3. A knowledge of how to observe the effects of insulin delivery in terms of the changes in concentration of blood glucose achieved by home glucose monitoring.

With these three concepts, the goal, the tools, and the monitor, the patient and the clinician are in position to manage IDDM even in the presence of imbalances in normal glucose regulation induced by diet, exercise, and stress. To achieve an appropriate orchestration of these concepts in the management of an individual patient, education of the patient with informed health professionals is essential.

From: *Contemporary Endocrinology: Hormone Replacement Therapy*
Edited by: A. W. Meikle © Humana Press Inc., Totowa, NJ

Matching the Normal β-Cell

Matching the normal function of the pancreatic β-cell is the core concept of insulin management in insulin-dependent diabetes mellitus (IDDM). From insulin kinetic studies in humans, it has been established that in the absence of eating, the β-cell produces approximately 1 U/h all day and all night. This translates into a continuous delivery of 24 U/24-h/d, which may be provided by a variety of modalities depending upon patient and physician preference.

BASAL INSULIN DELIVERY

1. Divided injections of long-acting insulin at approximately 12 U every 12 h.
2. Continuous pump infusion of 1 U/h.

It is important to instruct the patient that this "basal" insulin management must be continued even when no meals are eaten, and/or when the patient is sick and unable to eat. Clearly, the actual dosage in a given patient may be somewhat more or less than 1 U/hr all day and all night depending on body size, physical activity, illness, and medications (such as steroids). These issues are discussed in later sections in detail. But the general concept of continuous insulinization independent of food ingestion that is always required by the human body is a fundamental core concept of insulin management in IDDM. The major physiologic role of this basal insulin is to restrain glucose production from the liver to prevent basal hyperglycemia, and inhibit lipolysis and ketone production from the liver to prevent ketoacidosis.

The second core concept from insulin kinetic studies in humans, describes the insulin secretion in response to meals as 1 U/100 calories. This translates into 25 U for a daily consumption of 2,500 calories, taken in divided dosages concurrently with eating. As in the case of basal insulin management, this meal related insulin dosage might be provided by a variety of modalities depending on patient and physician preference.

MEAL-TIME INSULIN DELIVERY

1. Regular insulin or lispro (Humalog®, Eli Lilly & Co., Indianapolis, IN) insulin given as pre-meal injections at 1 Ut/100 calories, based on individual meal calorie content (i.e., 400 calories breakfast requires 4 U injected pre-meal, and so forth).
2. Bolus insulin delivery from a pump during each meal at 1 U/100 calories ingested.

As in the case of basal insulin, the actual determination of U/100 calories will depend upon the relative mix of caloric contributions from simple carbohydrates, complex carbohydrates, protein, and fat contained within a meal. In general, more insulin may be required for larger contributions of simple carbohydrate, with a relatively lower amount of insulin for increasing amounts of the other food categories. Each patient must determine this estimation based on his or her individual food selection and using his or her own blood glucose testing in the postprandial period. The major physiologic role of the "meal" insulin administration is to restrain the glycemic surge of blood sugar as the meal carbohydrate load is digested and absorbed.

The balance between the pre-meal "rapid-acting" insulin administration to control the glycemic response to meals, and the basal "long-acting" insulin administration to control the glycemic and ketogenic secretions from the liver form the core concepts of "split-mixed" insulin injection.

SPLIT-MIXED INSULIN DELIVERY FOR BOTH BASAL AND MEAL-TIME

1. The splitting of insulin shots at multiple times of the day and mixing long-acting with rapid-acting insulin is the clinical application of meeting basal and mealtime insulin management by syringe injections.
2. The pump delivery of basal rates of insulin infusion with multiple bolus deliveries prior to meals is the clinical application of meeting basal and mealtime insulin management by implanted or external pump infusion.

In both approaches, the method of calculating from an initial estimate of 1 U/hr all day and all night for hepatic regulation, and 1 U/100 calories from the meal-induced glycemic response remain fundamental to the management of IDDM with insulin.

INSULIN DOSING STRATEGIES

Regardless of what is happening with the patient (i.e., not eating, having surgery, exercising, and so forth) insulin coverage must be provided throughout the entire 24 h. In most Type I patients, this is most easily achieved by using intermediate acting (as NPH) (Humulin N.®, Eli Lilly & Co., Indianapolis, IN) or long acting (as Ultra-Lente) (Humulin U.®, Eli Lilly & Co., Indianapolis, IN) semisynthetic human insulin preparations. It is also important to remember that, whereas the β-cell delivers insulin directly into the portal circulation, clinically, we are largely limited to subcutaneous delivery. Because of the vagaries of insulin absorption, differences in body weight, and physical activity, we are usually faced with the need for an insulin dose greater then those values indicated in the kinetic studies previously noted. Nonetheless, we still attempt to mimic the beta cell in developing an insulin prescription to achieve fasting and preprandial blood sugars of 70–140 mg/deciliter (dL), and post prandial levels less than 200 mg/dL.

Extended Acting Insulin for Basal Replacement

NPH INSULIN (INTERMEDIATE-ACTING)

Current preparations of NPH are characterized by an onset of action approximately 2 h after injection, achieving peak effect at 5–8 h, and a total duration of action of 14–16 h. Consequently, for effective basal coverage NPH must be given at least twice daily. One of the simpler schedules is to administer it before breakfast and before the evening meal, presuming these are separated by an interval of 10–12 h. In this strategy, the NPH can be mixed with pre-meal regular insulin and in many instances provide basal and meal coverage with 2 shots/d. In about one-third of patients, however, this does not provide adequate coverage overnight; by administering the second dose at bedtime, better glycemic control is achieved. Because of increased insulin resistance in the morning, most practitioners divide the total basal dose by giving two-thirds before breakfast and one-third before the evening meal or at bedtime. Again, because of variation in insulin absorption, body fat, and physical activity, most patients will need to have their dose individualized beyond the calculated 24 U/24 h.

ULTRA-LENTE INSULIN (LONG-ACTING)

The prolonged duration of action of this preparation is accomplished by utilizing a suspension of insulin crystals, the size of which is controlled by adding excess zinc to an insulin solution. The preparation was designed to provide a continuous reservoir of insulin for a 24-h period. However, pharmacokenetic studies have demonstrated a variable absorption pattern, as well as patient-to-patient variation in duration of action. Despite these difficulties, this insulin can be quite helpful in a subset of Type I diabetic patients, especially those who display considerable instability despite careful attention to diet, exercise, and overall compliance. Ultra-Lente has an onset of action about 2 h following injection, does not display a clear "peak" effect and has a duration of action of 16–24 h. Whereas a small number of patients will achieve adequate glycemic control with a single injection of Ultra-Lente and 3–4 pre-meal injections of short-acting insulin/d, our experience suggests most will need two doses of ultra-lente for adequate basal insulin replacement. Some clinicians choose to split the dose evenly between the morning and evening injections; however, we have found it more effective to give about 60% of the dose on arising and the remaining 40% before the evening meal. The same considerations regarding individualization of dose noted for NPH also apply to Ultra-Lente.

Short-Acting Insulin for Use with Meals

REGULAR INSULIN (RAPID-ACTING)

This preparation has an onset of action of 30–60 min following injection, with a peak action at 2 h and a duration of 4–6 h. The delay in onset of action appears to be owing to the formation of insulin dimers and hexamers, which must be broken up before the insulin is transported into the blood. The purpose of premeal regular insulin is to limit the postprandial rise in blood sugar following food ingestion. For these reasons, it is most effectively administered 30–60 min before beginning food intake. Generally speaking, the dose selected should be approximately 1 U/100 calories, assuming a mixed meal containing about 55% carbohydrates, 15–20% protein, and 25–30% fat. If the patient's blood sugar at this time is in excess of 200 mg/dL, the patient should be instructed to wait at least 1 h after injecting the insulin before starting to eat. Frequently, if the patient is using a mixture of regular and NPH insulin, it is not necessary to add regular insulin before lunch or at bedtime because of the peaking effects of NPH action during the lunchtime from the pre-breakfast injection, and the peaking effects of NPH action near the hour of bedtime from the pre-dinner NPH injection. Because of the flat action curve of Ultra-Lente insulin, with no peaking during lunch or at bedtime, it is necessary to administer regular insulin before all meals and frequently at the time of bedtime snack as well.

GLYCEMIA INJECTION (VARIABLE SCALE)

Because of the lability of blood sugar levels in the Type I patient, we have found it quite helpful to develop a variable-scale "Glycemia Injection" for additional short-acting insulin use beyond that necessary to cover the requirements of the calories in a meal. Because of decreased insulin sensitivity in the morning, such a scale provides for a larger amount of insulin for any given level of blood sugar at that time, and a lower dose for the same level later in the day and at bedtime. An initial variable scale recommends an additional unit of regular insulin for every 50 mg/dL of blood glucose above 150 mg/dL as determined by the patient's home-glucose monitoring self evaluation. This extra insulin is added to the pre-meal dosage so that the patient actually combines the meal injection with the glycemia injection.

COMBINED GLYCEMIA INJECTION AND MEAL-TIME INJECTION

1. Short-acting insulin injections are given in the pre-meal time period, and calculated as the sum of 1 U/100 calories to be eaten with 1 U per every 50 mg/dL of blood glucose

above the measured value of 150 mg/dL (i.e., 400 calorie breakfast requires 4 U, and a measured blood glucose of 250 mg/dL at 7:00 am requires a glycemia dosage of 2 U, so a total of 6 U of short-acting insulin would be given in the pre-breakfast injection)

2. Bolus insulin delivery from a pump in the aforementioned example would also be calculated as the meal dosage based on 1 U/calorie ingested, and 1 U/50 mg/dL increment in measured blood glucose above the 150 mg/dL goal.

Insulin Lispro (Very Rapid-Acting)

This recent addition to our armamentarium is an analog of human insulin produced by reversing the sequence of proline and lysine in the beta chain of the molecule. The result of this rearrangement is a molecule that retains the biologic effects of insulin, but does not form dimers and hexamers. Consequently, it is absorbed much more rapidly than regular insulin and begins to lower blood sugar within 5 min of injection. It achieves peak effect within 30–40 min following injection and has a duration of action of 3–4 h. The advantage of this rapid onset of action is a more predictable limitation of the rise in blood sugar following a meal. The shorter duration of action provides added flexibility for those patients whose day-to-day schedules are variable, resulting in variation in meal times with more true reliance on extended action insulin to maintain basal euglycemia. This insulin formulation can more easily be visualized as actually controlling predominantly the glycemic excursion following a meal. It has also been reported to result in fewer hypoglycemic episodes in Type I patients. As in the case of regular insulin, it may be helpful to construct a variable-scale dosage schedule linked to pre-meal blood sugar level for patients using this preparation, though emphasis should be directed toward the extended-acting insulin injections to maintain basal euglycemia and rely on the Lispro insulin to manage the glycemic rise induced by meal ingestion.

Insulin Pumps for Basal and Meal-Time Insulin Coverage

Since the introduction of a pump designed to deliver continuously subcutaneous insulin some two decades ago, these devices have undergone remarkable technologic improvement, as have the insulin preparations designed for them. Current models provide the user with up to four programmable basal infusion rates and several options for pre-meal bolus doses of insulin. Buffered solutions of both regular insulin and lyspro insulin are available for pump use. However, pumps are not trouble-free. Although most problems related to batteries and alarm systems have been resolved, problems with delivery tubing, infusion needles, and infusion sites persist. As a consequence, the user must be willing to monitor blood sugars more frequently (up to eight times daily) and regularly evaluate tubing and needle sites to assure they are problem-free. It should be pointed out that use of an insulin pump has no effect on patient compliance; patients who are noncompliant using injections do not become compliant when they are using a pump. Moreover, pump use in a noncompliant patient can result in serious complications (such as ketosis) much more quickly than in one using injections. However, with proper patient selection, pump use can significantly improve glycemic control. Initiation and maintenance of insulin-pump therapy is best carried out by an experienced diabetes team with readily available access to the patient, especially in the first few months of use.

INJECTION SITE SELECTION

Insulin injection site plays an important role in the rate and extent of insulin absorption from the subcutaneous space. Although a number of factors—such as size of dose and depth of injection—mediate these differences, most data suggest that local blood flow plays a central role in the rate and completeness of insulin absorption into the blood stream. It should also be noted that the extent of insulin absorption from the same site on a day-to-day basis may have a coefficient of variance of up to 25%. Recognizing these variables, a number of studies have shown that at-rest insulin absorption is most rapid and complete from the abdominal wall; next best from the upper arm, and least from the thigh/upper leg. However, when the leg is exercised, absorption rates equals or exceeds that from the abdomen, and the same holds true for the upper arm. Thus, when a period of rest or inactivity is expected, the site that will give most reliable absorption is the abdominal wall. When moderate activity or exercise is expected, the upper arm or thigh can be used effectively. In the very unstable/labile patient, we have found use of the abdominal wall as the exclusive injection site seems to be associated with some reduction in blood sugar lability.

It is also important to emphasize to the patient to rotate injection sites. Repeated insulin injection into the same site may be associated with local fat hypertrophy resulting in a local fatty "hump," or the loss of subcutaneous fat, leaving an area of subcutaneous atrophy that may be disfiguring.

HOME GLUCOSE MONITORING

Perhaps the most significant advance in the management of insulin-dependent diabetes, since the discovery of insulin in 1923, has been the development of the capability of home glucose monitoring of blood glucose. In the 75 years since the availability of insulin in the treatment of diabetes, we have progressed from no monitoring, urine monitoring of excreted glucose, and finger-stick blood monitoring, utilized widely today. Further technological capabilities are beginning to emerging for tissue fluid monitoring and noninvasive tissue monitoring; these should be available by the turn of this century. This capability has placed the patient in the position of total control of his or her own sugar management. The ability to monitor one's own blood glucose is similar to driving a car with a speedometer; a patient with this information can adjust his/her insulin levels appropriately, as a driver adjusts the speed of a car.

Methodology

The performance of home glucose monitoring requires creating a prick in the skin of the finger using a stylet. Only a drop of blood is required, and this is placed upon the glucose "strip." When the strip with its drop of blood is placed within the glucose-testing instrument, the value of blood glucose is quickly available on a digital screen, and the value electronically stored within the memory of the device.

Evaluation of Consistency of Values

A change in insulin management should rarely be made on the evaluation of a single abnormal value by home glucose monitoring. The concept of "consistent" abnormal value at a given time of day is critical to the management of IDDM with insulin. To develop consistent information, all patients should perform home glucose monitoring daily on a regular basis throughout all 7 d of each week. The time-honored method of determining a consistent abnormality is then to examine the blood glucose value at a given time of day, over a period of at least a week, and determine whether it is consistently either too high or too low relative to an ideal value of 120 mg/dL.

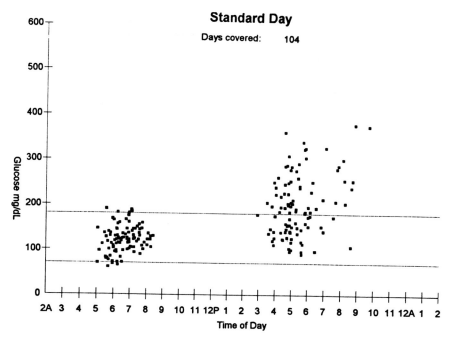

Fig. 1. Typical computer-generated graphical depiction of twice-a-day home glucose testing of monitor-saved values over 104 d in a patient with IDDM. Data demonstrate cumulative information from all pre-breakfast tests and all pre-dinner tests, and illustrate poor regulation in the pre-dinner data on a consistent basis.

The determination of consistency is significantly enhanced by the use of a glucose-testing device, which has the ability to retain in memory the values from the previous 30 d. Using such an instrument, the patient brings the unit to the physician, where readily available computer programs permit downloading of the information and graphical representation of the blood glucose values. The most useful printout of such data provides a cumulative graph of all data points represented over a 24-h day. In this way, all values for a given time of day are readily appreciated, and both the patient and the health professional can appreciate any deviation from ideal glucose values.

An example of a typical electronic summary of the data retained in the memory of a home-glucose monitor is shown in Fig. 1. In this example, the twice-daily values from a patient over 104 d have been printed cumulatively in the format of the 24-h day. It is apparent that the basal pre-breakfast data cluster within the 75–175 mg/dL range. In contrast, the pre-evening dinner data demonstrate a broad spread between 100–400 mg/dL. The physician and patient can readily appreciate from this graphical depiction of the data that attention to a change in management must be directed toward the escape from glycemic control that is developing throughout the afternoon on a consistent basis over more than 3 mo. Using this information, the patient and physician can now adjust the insulin dosage as described in the next section.

Timing of Home Glucose Testing

1. Basal glucose testing. The most useful testing time is the pre-breakfast or basal state, each morning. The blood glucose at this time represents production from the liver all night,

because ordinarily no food has been ingested since the previous evening at bedtime. If this value approximates a normal basal value of 120 mg/dL on a consistent basis, then the patient can be confident that a regular regimen of basal and mealtime insulin will control the glucose throughout the waking hours of the day with its three meals. However, if the pre-breakfast glucose value is elevated on a consistent basis, then the patient can anticipate persistent hyperglycemia throughout the subsequent day. For this reason, considerable effort should be made to start the day with a "normal" basal pre-breakfast blood sugar value.

If the patient is experiencing basal hyperglycemia on a consistent basis, then an increase in the evening long-acting basal insulin delivery should be instituted. Ordinarily, an increase of 2 U is a reasonable change, and the effects should be monitored by serial pre-breakfast home glucose monitoring at this new evening dosage level for 3–7 d. If this change is insufficient to correct the basal glycemia, then a further increment of 2 U in the evening long-acting insulin delivery should be introduced and the monitoring process repeated. This process should proceed until basal euglycemia is achieved.

2. Pre-evening dinner glucose testing. If the pre-evening dinner home glucose monitoring reveals hyperglycemia above 150 mg/dL before the evening meal on a consistent basis, then further adjustment of the morning long-acting basal insulin delivery needs to be considered. As in the case of changing the evening delivery to influence the morning basal glucose value, an increment of 2 U to the morning long-acting basal insulin can be expected to reduce the pre-dinner glucose value. Again, testing serial values over 5–7 d with this new dosage is required to assess the influence of this change in management. It should be noted that as the pre-dinner glucose value is reduced, the effect of the evening long-acting insulin injection will be greater, and may be expected to lead to further reduction in the subsequent morning blood-glucose value. Thus, resolving the most appropriate long-acting insulin dosage in both the morning and the evening will require prolonged effort by the patient with regular twice-daily blood monitoring in the pre-breakfast and pre-dinner times.

3. Pre-lunch glucose testing. The third most helpful time of home glucose monitoring is pre-lunch, which will provide information about the combined effects of the morning long-acting basal and short-acting meal-time insulin delivery and the caloric load of breakfast and/or midmorning snack ingestion. If the pre-lunch blood glucose value is below 90 mg/dL on a consistent basis, then the patient might reduce the pre-breakfast short-acting insulin by 1 U, or consider reducing the long-acting basal insulin by 1 U. A patient would ordinarily evaluate both options.

DIET AND NUTRITIONAL CONSIDERATIONS

This component of diabetes care is frequently under appreciated and inadequately utilized. It should be considered the cornerstone of the diabetic prescription. The approach to nutrition/diet management in the Type 1 patient is designed to assure maintenance of growth and development, as well as ideal body weight. Diet planning must be integrated with the insulin dosage schedule because the insulin dose is calculated per Kcal ingested in each meal. Currently the recommended diet is made up of approximately 55% carbohydrate (both complex and simple), 15–20% protein, and 20–25% fat. These proportions may need to be modified for special circumstances such as increasing the percentage of protein during the adolescent growth spurt, or decreasing the percentage of fat in the face of evidence of atherosclerotic vascular disease.

Total caloric allowance should be sufficient to maintain ideal body weight. This obviously will vary depending on body size, gender, and usual activity. A number of formulae have been designed to calculate this, though in general one allows 1200–1500 calories for basal needs, adds 500–600 calories for moderate physical activity (such as office work, school teaching) and another 500–1000 calories for more physically demanding work such as construction, and so forth. These are usually distributed into four feedings as 1/7 for breakfast, 2/7 for lunch, 3/7 at supper, and 1/7 for a bedtime snack. This is, at best, a general rule; dietary plans are developed on an individual basis, preferably with the assistance of a registered dietitian.

One should also recognize that day-to-day adjustments will be necessary depending on changes in activity. For example, the usually sedentary office worker who becomes a "weekend warrior" every Saturday may require adjustments of both insulin and diet for the weekend. As previously noted, it is important to integrate changes in diet with changes in insulin dose. Short-term changes in dietary intake, such as holidays, can frequently be managed by simple adjustments in short-acting insulin. Longer-term changes in diet, however, usually require changes in both basal and pre-meal insulin dosage. For example, if the patient is actively involved with seasonal sports such as high school or college football, it is frequently necessary to decrease total insulin dose while increasing total caloric intake because of exercise-induced lowering of blood glucose level independent of insulin. When the season is over, the patient then returns to the pre-season diet and insulin prescription.

A more recent approach to matching insulin dose with diet is referred to as "carbohydrate counting." In this method, the patient is taught to estimate the number of grams of carbohydrate they expect to eat in any meal. This is then matched with an insulin dose that has been determined to "cover" that amount of carbohydrate. Usually this amounts to 1–2 U of short-acting insulin/100 g of carbohydrate. Although this can be a valuable program in the Type I patient, it requires a considerable time commitment from the patient to learn, as well as a dietitian who is very familiar with the method.

EXERCISE

Currently, it is recommended that a regular exercise program be an integral part of diabetes care. Such a program not only enhances a patient's sense of well being, muscle tone, and cardiovascular fitness, it also increases the patient's basal metabolic rate, thereby improving blood sugar regulation and lipid metabolism. Such a program can be quite simple, such as a brisk 35–40-min walk on alternate days, to a very comprehensive, instructor-guided program. The most important aspect of an exercise program is that it is something the patient will do a continuing, regular basis. Walking is usually an easy way to get started, because almost all patients can do it and it requires no special equipment. To effectively increase basal metabolic rate, the duration of the walk or other exercise should be at least 40 min. Once basal rate is increased, it remains at the higher level for 36–40 h. Thus an exercise program can be carried out on alternate days and achieve most of the positive effects previously noted. Again, it is important to integrate exercise with diet and insulin prescriptions, and modify them accordingly.

Some caveats regarding exercise in the Type I patient: Although in general, exercise increases insulin sensitivity and muscle glucose uptake, this rule applies to the patient who is reasonably well insulinized; that is, they have their blood sugar in a range between

100 and 200 mg/dL and no ketones in their urine. If that is not the case, exercise may make matters worse by increasing fat mobilization and, in turn, the development of ketosis. Therefore the patient should be instructed to test their blood sugar before starting to exercise and if blood sugar is elevated over 250 mg/dL, to test their urine for ketones. If present, the patient should take additional short acting insulin and delay exercising until blood sugar is in the range of 125–180 mg/dL, and urine ketones have cleared. If urine ketones are negative and only the blood sugar is elevated, the patient should be advised to take additional short-acting insulin and wait at least 1 h before beginning to exercise, preferably retesting blood sugar at that time.

Another situation related to exercise that puts the Type I patient at risk is prolonged strenuous physical activity such as cross-country skiing, long distance running, and so forth. In this setting, the effect of such exercise is to deplete muscle glycogen, a situation which obligates repair over the next 36–48 h regardless of whether the blood sugar is 50 mg/dL or 300 mg/dL. Therefore, it is important that patients who undertake these activities be provided with directions as to how to prevent severe hypoglycemia, especially at night when the usual warning signals of low blood sugar are obscured by sleep. Usually, severe hypoglycemia can be avoided by reducing the evening insulin dose on the day of exercise and increasing both the evening meal and bedtime snack by adding complex carbohydrate such as pasta. The patient should also be instructed to be awakened at 2:00 or 3:00 AM for a blood-sugar test, with additional food intake if the blood sugar is less than 120 mg/dL. It is also necessary to increase food intake on the day following strenuous exercise to prevent hypoglycemia on that day as well. Additional blood sugar monitoring during the 48 h following the activity is also strongly recommended.

INSULIN DOSAGE CHANGES WITH STRESS

There are four classic situations in which the hormones secreted in counter-regulation to the actions of insulin require altering both the insulin dosage and the balance between basal and meal-time insulin delivery:

1. Sickness
2. Surgery
3. Trauma
4. Emotional Crises

Physiology

STRESS HYPERGLYCEMIA

The physiological effect of stress leads to the acute secretion of catecholamines and glucagon, which rapidly increase glucose release from the liver. This stress response is related to the "flight or fight" survival response, which may be important for a variety of physiological survival changes in many body organs. However, the problem in IDDM is that this response causes glucose production from the liver by both glycogenolysis and gluconeogenesis, resulting in a defacto "counter-regulation" of the actions of insulin to reduce blood glucose concentration.

If the stress persists, then the longer acting secretion of growth hormone and cortisol from the pituitary and adrenal gland will result is still further release of glucose from the liver. The combined effects of these four counter-regulatory hormones will clearly work against the insulin management of blood glucose control, which was satisfactory in the non-stressed state.

STRESS KETOSIS/KETOACIDOSIS

These four counter-regulatory hormones also result in free fatty acid (FFA) mobilization from fat depots, and their conversion to ketones in the liver. If unchecked, this disturbance in fat metabolism will lead to the evolution of ketosis and then to diabetic ketoacidosis. This event occurs independent of the effects of the hormones on glucose metabolism, so that the physician and patient must be alert to the fact that diabetic ketoacidosis (DKA) can evolve purely from disturbance in this lipid-axis of insulin action, independent of the presence of a disturbance of the glucose-axis.

Response

INITIATE INCREASED MONITORING OF BLOOD GLUCOSE

Clearly, the patient must introduce increased home glucose monitoring of the response to stress and record the values on an appropriate "follow-up management " sheet. This sequential information on the change in blood-glucose values as treatment is introduced will both educate the patient as to their own response to stress, and make it possible for the physician and health-care team to participate in the educational and management challenge.

INCREASE BASAL INSULIN DELIVERY

The loss of control is exerted at the level of "basal insulin delivery," so that a fundamental increase in the continuous state of basal insulin exposure must be introduced. There are commonly two strategies to address this relative insufficiency of basal insulin delivery.

The first strategy entails increasing basal insulin delivery by 20% each 24 h. In this response, the patient is advised to increase the long-acting insulin by approximately 10% at both the morning and the evening injections. Thus if the patient is receiving 1 U/h all day and all night as two injections of 12 U of NPH insulin, then this would be increased to 15 U of NPH insulin twice a day. If after 12 h, this is clearly insufficient, then the patient—on the physician's advice, introduces a further increase in each of the two long-acting insulin shots.

The second strategy entails supplementing basal insulin delivery with "short-acting" insulin. In this response, the patient is advised to administer bursts of a rapid acting form of insulin, Regular or lispro, at intervals of 4–6 h. Ordinarily, this approach would be introduced if the blood glucose were in excess of 300 mg/dL for more than 6 h duration by home glucose monitoring. Although the exact dosage of such a supplement will vary depending on the individual's response, a dosage of 5 U of lispro or regular insulin would be typical at 4-h intervals if the glucose values remain above 300 mg/dL. This strategy is utilized in addition to that of increasing the basal insulin delivery previously described. If the patient is using a variable scale for short-acting insulin dosing, the scale may be modified upward for the duration of the period of increased stress.

AUGMENT MEAL-TIME INSULIN DELIVERY

Because there may be resistance to insulin action imposed by stress and by hyperglycemia (glucose toxicity), it may be necessary to augment the usual mealtime insulin dosage during stress-induced hyperglycemia. Typically, an increase of 2 U of regular or lispro insulin given with meals will provide adequate insulin coverage for a meal glycemic surge. This is based on the assumption of 1 U/100 calories of ingested food, and a typical meal of approximately 1000 calories. Each patient will need to identify the augmented dosage, which works to control his or her own glycemic surge during times of stress.

The stress of sickness, surgery, trauma, or emotional crises are typically accompanied by hyperglycemia, which will last as long as the episode is sustained, but other stress-inducing situations may be proposed that will clearly initiate these processes and require the same management approach in changing insulin dosages and balance.

DIABETIC EDUCATION

One of the more important lessons learned during the Diabetes Control and Complications Trial was the importance of a team approach to diabetes management that included a considerable amount of education for the individual patient. The goal of education is to teach the patient how to incorporate diabetes management skills into daily life and thus become more self-sufficient and less dependent on the physician. Ideally, the diabetes team consists of at least a physician, nurse educator, and dietitian. If access to such a team is not feasible, other resources can be used, such as other patients with diabetes who have mastered self-management skills, local chapters of the American Diabetes Association, or local hospitals.

At the very least, the patient must be instructed in "survival skills," such as insulin injection, meal planning, self glucose monitoring, information about hypo and hyperglycemia, ketoacidosis, necessary supplies, management of sick days, and some basic pathophysiology of the disease. More advanced training might include self insulin adjustment, maintaining balance, and understanding complications of the disease, as well as their prevention. Further in-depth teaching is necessary in the case of pregnancy or other special circumstances, such as long-distance travel that involves crossing several time zones. It is also helpful to include other family members in the teaching sessions so that they may serve as a more effective support system. Finally, if the patient is still in school, instruction might be provided to the patient's teachers so they can be of assistance should an adverse event like hypoglycemia occur during the school day. School nurses or teachers should also be provided with a list of individuals to be contacted in such an event.

REFERENCES

1. Eaton RP, Allen RC, Schade DS, Standefer JC. "Normal" insulin secretion: the goal of artificial insulin delivery systems. Diabetes Care 1980:270–273.

9

Type 2 Diabetes Mellitus

David G. Johnson, MD, and Rubin Bressler, MD, PhD

CONTENTS

INTRODUCTION

Type 2 diabetes mellitus is a disease characterized by both abnormalities in insulin secretion and target-tissue resistance to the actions of insulin. Therefore, it is not surprising that replacement therapy with insulin alone is not sufficient to control blood glucose and many of the other metabolic abnormalities in patients with type 2 diabetes. Drugs, such as the sulfonylurea agents can enhance insulin secretion. Other agents, such as metformin, decrease hepatic glucose production (glycogenolysis and gluconeogenesis) in patients with type 2 diabetes. The thiazolidinediones act mainly by sensitizing peripheral tissues (e.g., muscle) to the action of insulin. The disaccharidase inhibitors slow down the absorption of starch from the intestine, leading to smaller rises in blood glucose after meals. Nevertheless, deficient secretion of insulin in many patients with type 2 diabetes may require injection of exogenous insulin, just as it does in patients with type 1 diabetes. In fact, the resistance to insulin's action in patients with type 2 diabetes often requires the use of large doses of insulin to achieve adequate glycemic control. The goals of insulin therapy in patients with type 2 diabetes are slightly different than in patients with type 1 diabetes and often necessitate some adjustment in the types of insulin preparations that are used, as well as the timing of insulin injections (Table 1).

INSULIN THERAPY IN TYPE 2 DIABETES

Insulin is indicated to treat the following conditions occurring in patients with type 2 diabetes.

1. Ketoacidosis.
2. Nonketotic hyperosmolar coma.
3. Daily maintenance of patients with unintentional weight loss.
4. Poor glycemic control on diet, exercise, and oral agents.
5. Serious or chronic bacterial or fungal infections.

From: *Contemporary Endocrinology: Hormone Replacement Therapy*
Edited by: A. W. Meikle © Humana Press Inc., Totowa, NJ

Table 1
Insulin Preparations

	Usual daily dosage (U)	Doses/d	Combination therapy
NPH insulin	4–40	Bedtime	Can use with AM dose of sulfonylurea, QD or BID metformin, or AM troglitazone
NPH insulin	4–100	1–2, Usually before breakfast and before supper	Similar combinations as with bedtime NPH
Ultralente	4–100	1–2	Similar combinations as with NPH
Lente	4–100	1–2	Similar combinations as with NPH
Semilente	2–30	1–2	Usually mixed with ultralente
Regular	2–30	1–2	Usually mixed with NPH and given before meals
Lispro	2–30	1–2	Given before meals for post-prandial glycemic control

Ketoacidosis

People with either type 1 or type 2 diabetes mellitus can develop ketoacidosis. Usually, individuals with type 2 diabetes develop ketoacidosis in association with precipitating stresses, such as infection, ischemia or physical or emotional trauma. The primary patho-physiologic event in the genesis of ketoacidosis occurs in the fat cell, where there is a disruption of the normal balance between insulin, which is antilipolytic, and the counter-regulatory hormones (especially catecholamines and glucagon), which are lipolytic. This altered hormonal balance (too little insulin vs excessive counter-regulatory hormones) causes free fatty acids (FFA) to be released into the circulation. In the liver FFA are taken up, and under the conditions of deficient insulin and excessive counter-regulatory hormones, the FFA are preferentially directed into the metabolic pathway leading to ketone body production. This occurs because insulin normally inhibits FFA oxidation in the liver by stimulating mitochondrial acetyl CoA carboxylase, which increases malonyl CoA formation. Malonyl CoA normally inhibits long-chain FFA oxidation. Under the conditions of deficient insulin and excessive counter-regulatory hormones, the levels of hepatic carnitine rise, promoting the transfer of long-chain FFA into the mitochondria, where they are oxidized to form ketone bodies. The ketone bodies are secreted from the liver into the circulation, accumulating to high levels and appearing in the urine with the accompanying loss of cations and water. Because the ketone bodies (acetoacetate, beta-hydroxybutyrate, and acetone) are mainly organic acids, the body's bases are consumed, and a metabolic acidosis ensues.

In addition to the abnormalities in fatty-acid metabolism occurring in diabetic ketoacidosis, glucose metabolism is also defective. Hepatic glucose production from glycogenolysis and gluconeogenesis is increased, whereas glucose uptake in peripheral tissues, such as muscle and fat, is decreased. The rising concentrations of glucose eventually exceed the renal threshold, resulting in the loss of glucose and water in the urine and subsequent dehydration.

The primary goal of insulin therapy is to stop the excessive production of ketones and thus allow the ketoacidosis to be corrected. Insulin does this by:

1. Inhibiting FFA mobilization (fat cell).
2. Decreasing ketone body formation (liver).
3. Increasing ketone body metabolism (heart and skeletal muscle).

Only short-acting soluble forms of insulin should be used to treat diabetic ketoacidosis. Traditionally, this has been regular insulin, although lispro insulin is also effective. Insulin is usually administered intravenously by a continuous infusion in severely ill patients to ensure systemic delivery, but it can also be given intramuscularly or subcutaneously in patients with less severe ketoacidosis. Despite the resistance to insulin's action in patients with type 2 diabetes, most patients with ketoacidosis respond to insulin doses in the range of four to seven units per hour. When the plasma glucose falls to less than 250 mg/dL, glucose should be added to the intravenous fluid therapy to prevent hypoglycemia. Insulin therapy must be continued until ketosis has resolved (little or no ketones in the urine), the acidosis has been reversed (serum bicarbonate greater than 17 meq/L), and the patient's gastrointestinal system has recovered (no nausea, signs of normal bowel activity).

Several aspects of the treatment of ketoacidsosis in patients with type 2 diabetes deserve special attention:

1. Development of ketoacidosis does not indicate in any way that the patient has become "insulin dependent" or that the patient's diabetes is actually type 1.
2. The severity of the ketoacidosis is mainly determined by the severity of the accompanying medical disorders and the length of time that the ketoacidosis proceeded before effective treatment to reverse it was initiated. Patients with otherwise mild type 2 diabetes can develop severe diabetic ketoacidosis.
3. Use of insulin in the treatment of the ketoacidosis does not mean that the patient will require insulin later in the form of daily maintenance therapy.

Nonketotic Hyperosmolar Coma

This disorder of glucose metabolism is seen mainly in patients with type 2 diabetes rather than type 1 diabetes because it requires that the patient have enough insulin secretory reserve to resist development of ketoacidosis. Adipose tissue is more sensitive to insulin than muscle. Consequently, excessive lipolysis leading to ketosis can be prevented by insulin levels that are insufficient to control hyperglycemia. The fundamental pathophysiologic abnormalities in hyperosmolar coma are the overproduction of glucose by the liver and the underutilization of glucose by insulin-sensitive peripheral tissues (such as muscle). The extremely high glucose concentrations that develop cause an osmotic diuresis, with profound renal losses of water and electrolytes (such as potassium). Because of severe dehydration, many patients with hyperosmolar coma develop arterial or venous thrombosis. The overall mortality rate is still approx 40%. Initial treatment of hyperosmolar coma involves the use of insulin in doses similar to those used in the treatment of ketoacidosis. However, the main goal of this insulin therapy is to inhibit hepatic glucose production and to promote the uptake and metabolism of glucose in peripheral tissues. Vigorous fluid and electrolyte replacement using hypotonic solutions, such as half-normal saline, is essential for successful treatment of hyperosmolar coma. As mentioned in the treatment of ketoacidosis, use of insulin to reverse hyperosmolar coma in patients with type 2 diabetes does not imply that insulin will be required in the form of maintenance therapy after the acute symptoms have resolved.

Type 2 Diabetes with Unintentional Weight Loss

Approximately 80% of patients with type 2 diabetes in the US are obese at the time of diagnosis of the condition. Many of these patients remain obese, despite efforts to lose weight to restore sensitivity to insulin and improve glycemic control. However, some patients with type 2 diabetes develop a condition or syndrome characterized by gradual (weeks or months) unintentional weight loss and fatigue. Glycemic control may worsen, but these individuals do not become ketotic, presumably because insulin levels are sufficient to prevent severe ketosis. Not surprisingly, as these individuals become thin, they become sensitive to insulin and can be treated effectively with small doses of intermediate-acting insulin, such as a morning injection of 10–20 units of (NPH) insulin. Initiation of insulin therapy halts the progression of weight loss and fatigue. Although the underlying basis for this syndrome is probably a further deterioration in insulin secretory capacity, many patients achieve better glycemic control after they are forced to start insulin injections with subsequent retardation of diabetic complications. It is important that this syndrome be recognized, so that expensive, uncomfortable, and fruitless searches for other etiologies (e.g., malignancy) can be avoided or minimized. Adding to the complexity of diagnosing this syndrome are those patients who develop what appears to be type 2 diabetes in association with pancreatic carcinoma. The latter group usually have not been diabetic for very long, and the doses of insulin needed to control the blood glucose are higher at the time when insulin treatment is begun.

Insulin Therapy in Patients with Poor Glycemic Control on Diet, Exercise, and Oral Agents

Some patients with type 2 diabetes cannot be controlled with diet, exercise, and combination therapy with oral agents. This may cause chronic fatigue in addition to the classic symptoms of polydipsia, polyuria, and loss of visual acuity. The fasting blood glucose remains greater than 120 mg/dL, and the glycosylated hemoglobin A1c is greater than 7%, even on maximum effective doses of two or more oral agents. (Some patients may not be candidates for one or more of the oral agents because of contraindications, side effects, and allergies.) In this situation insulin therapy is indicated. In the past, patients who were not controlled on diet, exercise, and oral therapy were usually treated by discontinuing the oral agents and starting insulin injections once or twice a day with intermediate or long-acting forms of insulin (NPH, lente, or ultralente insulin). However, many studies have demonstrated that combination therapy with insulin and sulfonylurea agents may be superior to insulin monotherapy in patients with primary or secondary failure to sulfonylurea therapy *(1,2)*. The studies of Riddle et al. *(3,4)* recommended the use of bedtime intermediate-acting insulin together with a morning dose of sulfonylurea, to suppress hepatic glucose output at night with insulin, while allowing the sulfonylurea to enhance meal-stimulated insulin secretion and peripheral glucose utilization during the daytime. The usefulness of this technique has been confirmed by other investigators *(5–7)*. Although some studies *(8)* have not demonstrated any advantage of bedtime vs daytime insulin in combination with sulfonylurea agents with regard to glycemic control, most studies show that bedtime insulin with morning sulfonylurea leads to less weight gain *(9)*, lower daytime insulin levels *(9)*, and fewer daytime hypoglycemic reactions. Compared with using insulin alone, combination therapy with insulin and a sulfonylurea agent does not require as high doses of insulin and, in some studies, causes less weight gain *(10)*. As expected, type 2 patients who respond to combination therapy using sulfonylurea and insulin are those with residual C-peptide secretion (i.e., those patients with residual endogenous insulin secretion) *(11)*. Perhaps the most attractive aspect of bedtime insulin compared to daytime insulin is the simplicity of its goals. Patients can be instructed to increase the dosage gradually (for example, with weekly adjustments of 1–4 U/dose) until normal morning fasting blood glucose levels are achieved, without consideration of mealtime insulin needs.

The use of insulin, in combination with metformin therapy, in patients with type 2 diabetes has been found to improve glycemic control and to require lower doses of insulin *(12)*. Some investigators *(13,14)* have used insulin in combination with both a sulfonylurea agent and metformin with good results. Similarly, acarbose has been combined with insulin in the treatment of patients with type 2 diabetes with improvement in glycemic control *(15)*. The thiazolidinedione, troglitazone, has been approved by the Food and Drug Administration (FDA) for use with insulin in type 2 diabetic patients. This combination of troglitazone and insulin has led to improvement in glycemic control with lower doses of insulin. In the future, it is likely that other combinations of thiazolidinediones, metformin, sulfonylureas, and insulin will be used.

The treatment of patients with type 2 diabetes should be focused on normalization of the blood glucose during fasting and postprandial periods. This reverses the adverse effects of glucose toxicity on both insulin secretion and insulin action in peripheral tissues. The propensity for weight gain caused by insulin should not deter the use of insulin when it is needed to achieve adequate control of the blood glucose. Short-term or even intermittent use of insulin during periods of stress-induced hyperglycemia is safe and effective. Concern for creating insulin antibodies by this use of intermittent insulin injection has lessened considerably with the use of highly purified human insulin.

Insulin Therapy in Serious or Chronic Bacterial or Fungal Infections

Some patients with type 2 diabetes can develop serious and/or chronic bacterial or fungal infections that do not respond to conventional antibiotic agents. Often, this will lead to worsening glycemic control that mandates the use of insulin. However, even in those patients with satisfactory glycemic control, it is advisable to add insulin, which may improve the body's host defense mechanisms *(16)*.

Traditionally, insulin therapy has been initiated in the daily maintenance of patients with type 2 diabetes, mainly when diet, exercise, and oral agents have failed. This was a result, at least in part, of the pain and inconvenience of insulin administration. However, the numerous improvements in insulin syringes and other injectors—together with the increased purity and stability of modern insulin preparations—have made insulin therapy much more convenient and acceptable for many patients with type 2 diabetes. Most type 2 patients can be treated with only one or two injections of insulin a day, especially if the insulin is given in combination with one or more oral agents. Unless endogenous insulin secretion is extremely deficient or the patient has a high rate of gluconeogenesis (for example, in patients on large doses of glucocorticoids), most patients with type 2 diabetes can be treated with intermediate or long-acting insulin alone. Even those patients who require the addition of regular or lispro insulin to control postprandial hyperglycemia, the amounts of such short-acting insulin that are required are usually low. Therefore, fixed mixtures of intermediate and short-acting insulin, such as "70:30" or "50:50," are seldom necessary or of much benefit. In the future, it is likely that more patients will opt for

Table 2
Sulfonylurea Agents

	Usual daily dosage (mg)	Doses/d	Dosage forms available (mg)
Tolbutamide	500–3000	2–3	500
Tolazamide	250–1000	1–2	250, 500
Chlorpropamide	100–500	1	100, 250
Glipizide	2.5–40	1–2	5,10
Glyburide	1.25–20	1–2	1.25, 2.5, 5
Glyburide (micronized)	0.75–12	1–2	1.5, 3, 6
Glimepiride	1–8	1	1, 2, 4

low-dose insulin therapy in combination with oral agents earlier in the course of their disease in order to achieve good glycemic control.

ORAL HYPOGLYCEMIC DRUGS

Sulfonylureas

The sulfonylureas remain the most popular oral hypoglycemic agents in use in the US and throughout the world (Table 2). Their main mechanism of action is to enhance the acute or "first-phase" release of insulin from the pancreas as a result of binding to specific pancreatic B-cell receptors (17,18). When the sulfonylureas bind to their receptors an adenosine triphosphate-dependent potassium channel is inhibited, which determines the resting B-cell membrane potential. The resultant decrease in potassium efflux causes B-cell depolarization, activation of calcium channels, calcium influx, and insulin secretion through exocytosis. The sulfonylureas do not stimulate insulin biosynthesis; so they act only on the early phase of stimulated insulin secretion (19,20). Because the acute or first phase of insulin secretion is not seen in diabetic subjects with fasting hyperglycemia, it is not surprising that sulfonylureas lose their efficacy in patients with fasting hyperglycemia. Responsiveness to sulfonylureas can be restored by diet, weight loss, other oral agents, or insulin, which lowers the fasting blood glucose below 115–120 mg/dL. Some studies have investigated proposed extrapancreatic effects of the sulfonylureas that might contribute to their antidiabetic efficacy (17).

Although the sulfonylurea agents are not replacement therapy for insulin (they are ineffective in type 1 diabetes), they do replace or restore the defective or insufficient release of first-phase insulin secretion that occurs in patients with type 2 diabetes. The sulfonylureas remain popular agents because of their efficacy, reasonably low cost, and acceptably low incidence of side effects. In general, the sulfonylureas are absorbed well from the gastrointestinal tract, although absorption may be delayed in elderly patients with gastroparesis and in the presence of food (21–23). The sulfonylureas differ from one another mainly in their potency, duration of action, metabolism, and excretion. All of the sulfonylureas are highly bound to plasma proteins by both ionic and nonionic binding. Some of the sulfonylureas are metabolized in the liver to inactive or weakly active metabolites. The metabolite of acetohexamide is more active than the parent compound. Hepatic inactivation of sulfonylureas may be impaired in elderly patients or those with liver disease. Therefore, doses of sulfonylureas need to be decreased or given less frequently to prevent hypoglycemia. Similarly, renal disease can interfere with the elimination of those sulfonylureas with active or partially active metabolites. The long-acting sulfonylurea, chlorpropamide, is contraindicated in patients with renal disease. Despite the greater potency of the second-generation sulfonylureas (glyburide, glipizide, and glimepiride) compared to the first-generation agents (tolbutamide, tolazamide, acetoheximide, and chlorpropamide), the maximal efficacy of all of the sulfonylureas is approx the same *(24,25)*.

The duration of action of the sulfonylureas varies considerably, with short-acting agents, such as tolbutamide, requiring two to three doses a day, whereas the longer-acting agents (e.g., glyburide, glipizide, and glimepiride) are usually given only once daily. The slower hepatic metabolism and renal excretion seen in many elderly patients may require lower doses or less frequent dosing schedules. The longer-acting sulfonylureas are more likely to cause hypoglycemia *(26)*.

The sulfonylureas are most effective in patients with diabetes of less than 5-yr duration *(27,28)*. They remain the most popular first-line drug for the treatment of patients who have inadequate control of diet, exercise, and weight reduction. Because of the tendency for sulfonylureas to cause weight gain, extremely obese patients may be treated better with agents that do not promote weight gain, such as metformin or acarbose. It is common for the dosage of sulfonylurea to need to be lowered after several days or weeks of therapy to prevent hypoglycemia. This is probably because of the favorable effects of normalizing the blood glucose on peripheral tissue sensitivity to insulin-induced glucose uptake and utilization. Approx 15% of patients with the recent onset of type 2 diabetes fail to obtain a significant decrease in blood glucose levels with sulfonylurea therapy (primary sulfonylurea failure) *(29)*. Even among those patients who obtained a satisfactory response to sulfonylureas when they first started taking them, failure to respond occurs after months or years of use (secondary failure). The rate of secondary failure has been estimated at high as 3–5% *(30,31)*.

When patients' blood sugar is not controlled adequately with sulfonylurea alone, there are several pharmacologic choices that can be tried. The addition of another oral agent of a different class, such as metformin, acarbose, or troglitazone, may lower the blood glucose to acceptable levels. As discussed earlier, combination therapy with insulin—particularly bedtime NPH insulin—may be very effective. Some patients may respond to this combination therapy with oral agents or insulin so well that the "second" agent can be discontinued again. Therefore, the terminology of primary or secondary "failure" of sulfonylurea therapy has lost much of its impact, compared to the era when this usually meant discontinuation of oral therapy and insulin injections for the rest of the patients' lives.

The incidence of adverse effects from sulfonylureas is low. The most common adverse effects are gastrointestinal disorders and skin eruptions. These are often seen in individuals with known allergy to other sulfa-like compounds. Rare cases of hepatic, hematologic, and immunologic complications have been reported *(17)*. Chlorpropamide can cause hyponatremia and water retention because of its ability to increase secretion and activity of antidiuretic hormone *(32,33)*. This problem is exacerbated by thiazide diuretics and is seen most often in elderly patients. Some individuals taking chlorpropamide develop an intense flush in their face and upper torso area after alcohol consumption. This effect is not shared by other sulfonylurea agents.

Table 3
Nonsulfonylurea Oral Agents

	Usual daily dosage (mg)	Doses/d	Dosage forms available (mg)	Usual combinations
Metformin	500–2550	1–3	500, 850	Sulfonylurea
Acarbose	25–300	1–3	50, 100	Sulfonylurea, metformin, or insulin
Troglitazone	200–600	1	200, 400, 600	Sulfonylurea or insulin

The most serious adverse effect of sulfonylureas is hypoglycemia. Symptomatic hypoglycemia was noted in 20.2% of 40- to 65-yr-old patients with type 2 diabetes treated with sulfonylureas during a 6-mo period *(34)*. The risk of sulfonylurea-induced hypoglycemia is greater in the elderly, patients with liver or renal disease, patients with poor nutrition, and ingestion of multiple drugs, including alcohol. The long-acting sulfonylureas (chlorpropamide and glyburide), can cause prolonged hypoglycemia *(35)*.

Metformin

Metformin is a biguanide drug that has been used to treat patients with type 2 diabetes since 1957 (Table 3). Like other biguanides, metformin reduces hyperglycemia primarily by inhibition of hepatic glucose production, although it also facilitates glucose uptake in peripheral tissues *(36)*. Metformin reduces hyperglycemia but does not induce hypoglycemia. Therefore, metformin is a particularly advantageous agent in the management of patients with type 2 diabetes who have hypoglycemic reactions when taking agents (such as sulfonylureas or insulin) that can cause hypoglycemia. From the perspective of hormone replacement therapy, metformin can be regarded as an agent that can replace the effects of insulin to inhibit gluconeogenesis and glycogenolysis in the liver. Metformin has a lower degree of lipid solubility than most other biguanides *(37)*, which is the plausible explanation for its decreased tendency to produce lactic acidosis. Metformin does not distribute into the membranes of mitochondria to the same extent as other biguanides, such as phenformin, which was withdrawn from clinical use because of the increased rate of lactic acidosis. Metformin has similar efficacy as the sulfonylureas when used as monotherapy in the treatment of patients with type 2 diabetes *(38)*. It is also a valuable agent in combination with sulfonylureas *(39)* or insulin *(12,40)* in the treatment of patients who are not controlled by single drug therapy alone.

The exact mechanism of action for metformin to reduce hepatic glucose output is unknown. Metformin has also been shown to decrease the rate of glucose absorption in the gastrointestinal tract and to improve peripheral glucose disposal *(41,42)*. Since these effects of metformin do not mimic the effects of sulfonylurea agents, it is not surprising that the use of both agents in combination has been shown to lower blood glucose better than the use of either agent alone *(43)*. Metformin is absorbed within 6 h of ingestion. The oral bioavalability is approx 50–60%, with peak plasma concentrations occurring at 2–3 h after ingestion. Metformin is not protein-bound in the circulation and is excreted unmetabolized in the urine *(44)*. Therefore, metformin is contraindicated in patients with renal insufficiency (plasma creatinine > 1.5 mg/dL or glomerular filtration rate less than 65 mL/min). Although the propensity for lactic acidosis is much less with metformin than other biguanides, metformin should not be used in patients with severe cardiac, pulmonary, renal, and liver disease, because of the risk of lactic acidosis associated with these conditions. Metformin overdoses can be treated by hemodialysis, which has been used when such patients have developed lactic acidosis *(45)*.

Unlike sulfonylureas and insulin, metformin does not cause weight gain in most patients. In addition, metformin has been shown to decrease plasma triglyceride, VLDL, and LDL levels and increase HDL cholesterol levels, which are risk factors for atherosclerotic heart disease. These properties of metformin are particularly useful in treating obese patients or those with hyperlipidemia *(46)*.

The most common adverse effects of metformin are gastrointestinal. Approx 5–20% of patients receiving metformin develop anorexia, nausea, and diarrhea. These effects can be minimized by ingestion of the drug with meals and by gradually increasing doses. Less than 5% of patients treated with metformin have discontinued it because of gastrointestinal side effects *(47)* The range of effective doses of metformin is from 500 to 2550 mg daily. (It is available in 500 mg and 850 mg tablets.) Metformin decreases the absorption of vitamin B12 *(48,49)*, but this is seldom of clinical importance.

It is very important to recognize that the lowering of blood glucose with metformin takes from 1–4 wk to develop in patients with type 2 diabetes, despite the relatively rapid absorption and excretion of the drug. This slower pharmacodynamic response is also seen when increasing a patient's dose of metformin. Likewise, if hypoglycemia occurs during the concomitant use of metformin with either a sulfonylurea or insulin, it is usually preferable to reduce the dose of sulfonylurea or insulin rather than metformin, since metformin does not induce hypoglycemia when used alone.

Acarbose

One of the important goals of dietary therapy in patients with type 2 diabetes is to distribute the ingestion of carbohydrate throughout the day. Multiple small meals have been shown to be superior to fewer large meals in achieving better blood glucose control in diabetic patients *(50,51)*. Similarly, pharmacologic agents that can delay the digestion and absorption of complex carbohydrates have been developed over the past several decades *(52)*. Acarbose is currently the only agent of this class of disaccharidase inhibitors in clinical use in the US (Table 3). However, miglitol has been demonstrated to have similar safety and efficacy, and several other similar compounds are in earlier stages of clinical investigation.

Acarbose is an oligosaccharide produced by cultured strains of actinomycetes. It acts as a competitive inhibitor of several intestinal brush-border glucosidases *(53)*. It has a high affinity for sucrase and lesser affinity for glucoamylase and pancreatic amylase *(53)*. Absorption of glucose and other monosaccharides is not affected. When ingested with meals, acarbose decreases the rise in postprandial blood glucose *(54)*. Studies in diabetic patients with both type 1 and type 2 diabetes have demonstrated improvements in postprandial blood glucose control *(55,56)*. When given chronically, acarbose decreases glycosylated hemoglobin in diabetic patients, indicative of improved overall glycemic control.

The doses of acarbose that are used most commonly in clinical practice vary from 25–100 mg before or with each meal or snack. The main side effects are due to production of gas by bacterial metabolism of undigested carbohydrate in the large intestine. This leads to abdominal distention, flatulence, and, occasionally, diarrhea. By starting patients on lower doses, such as 25 mg and gradually increasing the dosage, gastrointestinal symptoms can be minimized. In addition to monotherapy, acarbose is effective when added to treatment with other drugs, such as sulfonylureas, metformin, or insulin *(57)*. Like metformin, acarbose is a useful agent in treating patients with type 2 diabetes who develop hypoglycemia on even low doses of sulfonylureas. Because acarbose is absorbed to a minimal extent from the gastrointestinal tract, it is a safe agent for patients with impaired liver and/or renal function.

Thiazolidinediones

The thiazolidinediones have been investigated as antidiabetic antihyperglycemic agents for many years in a number of animal models of insulin resistance, including both obese, nondiabetic (ob/ob mouse and Wistar and Zucker fatty rats) and obese diabetic (KK and db/db mouse) *(58,59)*. The early compounds had toxic side effects that precluded clinical use. However, one of these agents, troglitazone, was found to be effective in patients with type 2 diabetes with a low incidence of adverse effects (Table 3). The main toxic side effect that has been noted with troglitazone is a less than 2% incidence of elevation of liver enzymes. This was reversible in most patients after discontinuation of troglitazone. In rare instances, patients have developed liver failure while taking troglitazone (less than one case per 100,000 patients) *(60)*. Other thiazolidinediones are in late stages of clinical development, and it is likely that there will soon be additional drugs available.

The thiazolidinediones act primarily in peripheral tissues such as muscle and fat by improving glucose uptake. This effect appears to be due to interaction with a protein that regulates transcription of glucose transporter DNA in the nucleus *(61)*. The protein regulator is called peroxisome proliferator activated receptor (PPAR), and the thiazolidinediones interact with the gamma-subunit of PPAR. The thiazolidinediones also decrease hepatic glucose production through effects that have not been elucidated *(62,63)*. Of interest, troglitazone and other thiazolidinediones have no effect on blood glucose in insulinopenic diabetic animals *(64)*. This suggests that insulin must be present for the thiazolidinediones to exert their favorable effects in target tissues. In the presence of adequate insulin, the thiazolidinediones act as "insulin sensitizers" by amplifying the target tissue responses to insulin, particularly enhanced glucose transport.

Troglitazone has been used to lower the blood glucose in patients with type 2 diabetes *(65,66)*. It was first approved for use in the US in the treatment of patients with type 2 diabetes that were already receiving insulin injections. Addition of troglitazone to these patients' therapy resulted in improved glycemic control with lower doses of insulin. After additional studies were reported, troglitazone was approved for use as monotherapy and as combination therapy with sulfonylureas. The efficacy of troglitazone as monotherapy in patients with type 2 diabetes does not appear to be as great as sulfonylureas or metformin *(67)*. However, additive or slightly synergistic effects are seen when troglitazone is combined with other agents, such as sulfonylureas or insulin. Troglitazone is effective in doses from 200–600 mg. Like metformin, troglitazone lowers the blood glucose gradually over the course of several weeks.

The rational use of different oral agents with or without insulin injections now provides a means of treating most patients with type 2 diabetes. It is likely that new agents will be discovered in future years that will improve the treatment of these patients. It is encouraging to note the increased interest in this area by academic scientists, the pharmaceutical industry, practicing physicians, and the large population of individuals with type 2 diabetes.

REFERENCES

1. Pugh J, Wagner ML, Sawyer J, et al. Is combination sulfonylurea and insulin therapy useful in NIDDM patients? Diabetes Care 1992;15:953–959.
2. Johnson JL, Wolf SL, Kabadi UM. Efficacy of insulin and sulfonylurea combination therapy in type II diabetes. Arch Intern Med 1996;156:259–264.
3. Riddle M, Hart J, Bouma D, et al. An effective new regimen for type II diabetes: bedtime insulin with daytime sulfonylurea. Diabetes 1986;35(suppl):263. Abstract.
4. Riddle MC, Hart JS, Bjouma DJ, et al. Efficacy of bedtime NPH insulin with daytime sulfonylurea for subpopulation of type II diabetic subjects. Diabetes Care 1989;12:623–629.
5. Trischitta V, Italia S, Borzi V, et al. Low-dose bedtime NPH insulin in treatment of secondary failure to glyburide. Diabetes Care 1989;12:582–585.
6. Groop L, Widen E 1991 Treatment strategies for secondary sulfonylurea failure. Diabetes Metab 17:218–223.
7. Vigneri R, Trischitta V, Italia S, et al. Treatment of NIDDM patients with secondary failure to glyburide: comparison of the addition of either metformin or bed-time NPH insulin to glyburide. Diabete Metab 1991;17:232–234.
8. Soneru IL, Agarwal L, Murphy JC, et al. Comparison of morning or bedtime insulin with and without glyburide in secondary sulfonylurea failure. Diabetes Care 1993;16:896–901.
9. Landsted–Hallin L, Adamson U, Arner P, et al. Comparison of bedtime NPH or preprandial regular insulin combined with glibenclamide in secondary sulfonylurea failure. Diabetes Care 1995;18:1183–1186.
10. Chow CC, Tsans LW, Sorensen JP, et al. Comparison of insulin with or without continuation of oral hypoglycemic agents in the treatment of secondary failure in NIDDM patients. Diabetes Care 1995;18:307–314.
11. Quatraro A, Giugliano D. The combination of insulin and oral hypoglycemic drugs: a continuoous challenge. Diabetes Metab 1993;19:219–224.
12. Golay A, Guillet–Dauphine N, Fendel A, et al. The insulin-sparing effect of metformin in insulin–treated diabetic patients. Diabetes Metab Rev 1995;11(suppl 1):S63–S67.
13. Aguilar CA, Wong B, Gomez–Perez FJ, et al. Combination daytime chlorpropamide-metformin/bed-time insulin in the treatment of secondary failures in non–insulin dependent diabetes. Rev Invest Clin 1992;44:71–76.
14. diCianni G, Benzi L, Cliccarone AM, et al. Bedtime NPH-insulin plus combined sulfonylurea-biguanide oral therapy for treating refractory non–insulin dependent diabetic patients. Diabetes Metab 1992;18:468,469.
15. Chiasson JL, Josse RG, Hunt JA, et al. The efficacy of acarbose in the treatment of patients with non-insulin-dependent diabetes mellitus: a multi-center controlled clinical trial. Ann Intern Med 1994;121:928–935.
16. Nolan CM, Beaty HN, Bagdade JD. Further characterization of the impaired bactericidal function of granulocytes in patients with poorly controlled diabetes. Diabetes 1978;27:889–894.
17. Lebovitz HE, Melander A. Sulfonylureaas: basic and clinical aspects. In: Alberti KGMM, DeFronzo RA, Keen H, Zimmet P, eds. International Textbook of Diabetes Mellitus. Wiley, London, 1992, pp. 745–772.
18. Nelson TY, Gaines KL, Rajan AS, et al. Increased cytosolic calcium: a signal for sulfonylurea-stimulated insulin release from beta cells. J Biol Chem 1987;262:2608–2612.
19. Jackson JE, Bressler R. Clinical pharmacologoy of sulfonylurea hypoglycemic agents, I and II. Drugs 1981;22:211–245, 295–320.
20. Yalow RS, Black H, Villazon M, et al. Comparison of plasma insulin levels following administration of tolbutamide and glucose. Diabetes 1968;9:356–362.
21. Lebovitz H. Oral hypoglycemic agents. In: Kahn CR, Weir GC, eds. Joslin's Diabetes Mellitus. 13th ed. Lea & Febiger, Philadelphia, 1994, pp. 508–529.
22. Sartor G, Melander A, Schersten B, et al. Influence of food and age on the single dose kinetics and effects of tolbutamide and chlorpropamide. Eur J Clin Pharmacol 1980;17:285–293.
23. Antal EJ, Gillespie WR, Phillips JP, et al. The effect of food on the bioavailability and pharmacodynamics of tolbutamide in diabetic patients. Eur J Clin Pharmacol 1982;22:459–462.
24. Melander A, Lebovitz HE, Faber OK. Sulfonylureas: why, which, and how? Diabetes Care 1990;13(suppl):18–25.
25. Ferner RE, Chaplin S. The relationshgip between the pharmacokinetics and pharmacodynamic effects of oral hypoglycemic drugs. Clin Pharmacokinet 1987;12:379–401.
26. Seltzer HS. Drug–induced hypoglycemia: a review of 1418 cases. Endocrinol Metab Clin North Am 1989;18:163–183.

27. Melander A, Bitzen P–O, Faber O, et al. Sulfonylurea antidiabetic drugs: an update of their clinical pharmacology and rational therapeutic use. Drugs 1989;37:58–72.
28. Groop LC, Pelkonen R, Koskimies S, et al. Secondary failure to treatment with oral antidiabetic agents in non–insulin dependent diabetes. Diabetes Care 1986;9:129–133.
29. Shen SW, Bressler R 1977 Clinical pharmacology of oral antidiabetic agents. N Engl J Med.296:493–496,787–793.
30. Pontirolli AE, Calderara A, Pozza G. Secondary failure of oral hypoglycemic agents: frequency, possible causes and management. Diabetes Metab Rev 1994;10:31–43.
31. Turner RC, Holman RR, Matthews DR. Sulfonylurea failure and inadequacy. In: Cameron E, Colagiuri S, Heding L, et al., eds. Non-Insulin Dependent Diabetes Mellitus. Belle Mead, Excerpta Medica, Princeton, 1989, pp. 52–55.
32. Weissman PN, Shenkman L, Gregerman RI. Chlorpropamide hyponatremia: drug induced inappropriate antidiuretic hormone activity. N Engl J Med 1971;284:65–71.
33. Kadowaki T, Hagura R, Kajinuma H, et al. Chlorpropamide-induced hyponatremia: incidence and risk factors. Diabetes Care 1983;6:468–471.
34. Jennings AM, Wilson RM, Ward JD. Symptomatic hypoglycemia in NIDDM patients treated with oral hypoglycemic agents. Diabetes Care 1989;12:203–208.
35. Berger WL, Caduff F, Pasquel M, Rump A. Die relativ häufigkeit der schweren sulfonylharnstoff: hypoglykämie in den letzen 25 jahren in der Schweiz. Schweiz Med Wochenschr 1986;116:145–151.
36. Bailey CJ. Metformin: an update. Gen Pharmacol 1993;24:1299–1309.
37. Chow MSS. Focus on metformin. Formulary 1995;30:383–387.
38. Clarke BF, Campbell IW. Comparison of metformin and chlorpropamide in non-obese, maturity-onset diabetics uncontrolled by diet. BMJ 1977;2:1576–1578.
39. Reaven GM, Johnston P, Hollenbeck CB, et al. Combined metformin-sulfonylurea treatment of patients with noninsulin-dependent diabetes in fair to poor glycemic control. J Clin Endocrinol Metab 1992;74:1020–1026.
40. Giugliano D, Quatraro A, Consoli G, et al. Metformin for obese, insulin-treated diabetic patients: improvement in glycaemic control and reduction of metabolic risk factors. Eur J Clin Pharmacol 1993;44:107–112.
41. Bailey CJ 1992 Biguanides and NIDDM. Diabetes Care 15:755–772.
42. Klip A, Leiter LA. Cellular mechanism of action of metformin. Diabetes Care 1990;13:696–704.
43. DeFronzo RA, Goodman AM, and the Multicenter Metformin Study Group. Efficacy of metformin in patients with non-insulin-dependent diabetes mellitus. N Engl J Med 1995;333:541–549.
44. Tucker GT, Casey C, Phillips PJ, et al. Metformin kinetics in healthy subjects and in patients with diabetes mellitus. Br J Clin Pharmacol 1981;12:235–246.
45. Lalau JD, Andrejak M, Moniniere P, et al. Hemodialysis in the treatment of lactic acidosis in diabetics treated by metformin: a study of metformin elimination. Int J Clin Pharmacol Ther Toxicol 1989;27:285–288.
46. Vigneri R, Goldfine ID. Role of metformin in treatment of diabetes mellitus. Diabetes Care 1987;10:118–122.
47. Clarke BF, Duncan LJP. Biguanide treatment in the management of insulin independent (maturity-onset) diabetes: clinical experience with metformin. Res Clin Forums 1979;1:53–63.
48. Melchior WR, Jaber LA. Metformin: an antihyperglycemic agent for treatment of type II diabetes. [Review]. Ann Pharmacother 1996;30:158–164.
49. Lee AJ. Metformin in noninsulin-dependent diabetes mellitus. [Review]. Pharmacotherapy 1996; 16:327–351.
50. Jenkins DJA, Wolever TMS, Vuksan V, et al. Nibbling versus gorging: metabolic advantages of increased meal frequency. N Engl J Med 1989;321:929–934.
51. Jenkins DJA, Wolever TMS, Ocana AM, et al. Metabolic effects of reducing rate of glucose ingestion by single bolus versus continuous sipping. Diabetes 1990;39:775–781.
52. Taylor RH. Alpha–glucosidase inhibitors. In: Bailey CJ, Flatt PR, eds. New Antidiabetic Drugs. Smith–Gordon, London, 1990, pp. 119–132.
53. Puls W, Keup U, Krause HP, et al. Glucosidase inhibition: a new approach to the treatment of diabetes, obesity, and hyperlipoproteinaemia. Naturwissenschaften 1977;64:536–537.
54. Hillebrand I, Boehme K, Frank G, et al. The effects of the glucosidase inhibitor BAYg 5421 (acarbose) on postprandial blood glucose, serum insulin, and triglyceride levels: dose–time–response relationships in man. Res Exp Med 1979;175:87–94.

55. Walton RJ, Sherif IT, Noy GA, et al. Improved metabolic profiles in insulin-treated diabetic patients given an alpha-glucosidehydrolase inhibitor. BMJ 1979;1:220–221.
56. Hanefeld M, Fischer S, Schulze J. et al. Therapeutic potentials of acarbose as first-line drug in NIDDM insufficiently treated with diet alone. Diabetes Care 1991;14:732–737.
57. Chiasson JL, Josse RG, Hunt JA, et al. The efficacy of acarbose in the treatment of patients with non-insulin-dependent diabetes mellitus: a multi-center controlled clinical trial. Ann Intern Med 1994;121:928–935.
58. Fujiwara T, Yoshioka S, Yoshioka T, et al. Characterization of new oral antidiabetic agent CS–045: studies in KK and ob/ob mice and Zucker fatty rats. Diabetes 1988;37:1549–1558.
59. Chang AY, Wyse BM, Gilchrist BJ. Ciglitazone: a new hypoglycemic agent, I: studies in ob/ob and db/db mice, diabetic Chinese hamsters, and normal and streptozotocin-diabetic rats. Diabetes 1983;32:830–838.
60. Data on file, Sankyo/Parke–Davis.
61. Park KS, Ciaraldi TP, Abrams-Carter L, et al 1997 PPAR-gamma gene expression is elevated in skeletal muscle of obese and type II diabetic subjects. Diabetes 46:1230–1234.
62. Fujiwara T, Okuno A, Yoshioka S. Suppression of hepatic gluconeogenesis in long-term troglitazone treated diabetic KK and C57BL/KsJ-db/db mice. Metabolism 1995;44:486–490.
63. Henry RR. Effects of troglitazone on insulin sensitivity. [Review]. Diabetic Med 1996;13(suppl 6): S148–150.
64. Colca JR, Morton DR. Antihyperglycaemic thiazolidinediones: ciglitazone and its analogues. In: Bailey CJ, Flatt PR, eds. New Antidiabetic Drugs. Smith Gordon, London, 1990, pp. 255–261.
65. Iwamoto Y, Kuzuya T, Matsuda A, et al. Effects of new oral antidiabetic agent CS-045 on glucose tolerance and insulin secretion in patients with NIDDM. Diabetes Care 1991;14:1083–1086.
66. Suter SL, Nolan JJ, Wallace P et al. Metabolic effects of new and hypoglycemic agen CS–045 in NIDDM subjects. Diabetes Care 1992;15:193–203.
67. Iwamoto Y, Kosaka K, Kuzuya T, et al. Effects of troglitazone: a new hypoglycemic agent in patients with NIDDM poorly controlled by diet therapy. Diabetes Care 1996;19:151–156.

10

Management of Diabetes in Pregnancy

Kay F. McFarland, MD, and Laura S. Irwin, MD

Contents

INTRODUCTION

Intensive management of diabetes mellitus during pregnancy improves maternal and perinatal outcome. Maternal complications of diabetes during pregnancy include hypoglycemia, ketoacidosis, pre-eclampsia, pyelonephritis, polyhydramnios, and worsening of retinopathy and nephropathy. Untreated or conventionally managed diabetes significantly increases perinatal mortality from congenital anomalies, spontaneous abortions, and stillbirths *(1)*. Macrosomia, hypoglycemia, congenital anomalies, respiratory distress syndrome, hyperbilirubinemia, and hypocalcemia are causes of morbidity in the infant *(2,3)*. However, appropriate management of diabetes optimizes the outcome for both mother and the baby *(4–6)*.

CLASSIFICATION AND PREVALENCE

Gestational diabetes, carbohydrate intolerance first recognized during pregnancy, affects 4–15% of pregnancies *(7,8)*. The term gestational diabetes does not preclude the

From: *Contemporary Endocrinology: Hormone Replacement Therapy*
Edited by: A. W. Meikle © Humana Press Inc., Totowa, NJ

possibility that glucose intolerance antedated pregnancy; the designation simply means that hyperglycemia first became evident during pregnancy *(9)*. Also, the term applies whether or not diabetes persists after pregnancy. Subdividing gestational diabetes by treatment—diet-managed or insulin-treated—assists in timing the initiation of fetal surveillance and delivery.

The onset of diabetes prior to pregnancy, called pre-existing diabetes, occurs much less frequently than gestational diabetes. Further classification of preexisting diabetes into type 1—insulin-sensitive diabetes, and type 2—insulin-resistant diabetes, predicts the lability of glucose fluctuations, with the widest excursions occurring in type 1 diabetes. Pregnancy sometimes accelerates diabetic renal disease and retinopathy, which adds substantial risk to pregnancies associated with these complications. Therefore, diabetes-related complications warrant special notation. Some complications of past pregnancies, such a history of a stillbirth, also influence management of subsequent pregnancies. Therefore, classification of diabetes during pregnancy includes any diabetes-related complication or pregnancy-related complication, in addition to the designation: gestational diabetes (diet-managed or insulin-treated) or preexisting diabetes (type 1 or type 2).

PATHOPHYSIOLOGY

The placenta secretes insulin antagonistic hormones, including progesterone and human placental lactogen, which, along with elevated levels of prolactin and cortisol, contribute to the insulin resistance found during pregnancy. Usually, insulin secretion increases throughout gestation in proportion to the progressive decrease in insulin action. Hyperglycemia results when insulin secretion does not increase sufficiently to counterbalance the increasing insulin resistance characteristic of the second half of pregnancy. Thus, gestational diabetes results from a combination of insulin resistance and impaired insulin secretion *(10)*.

The insulin resistance leads to more rapid mobilization of maternal fat, which increases plasma and urinary ketones during the fasting state. Glucose utilization by the fetus contributes to lower maternal fasting plasma glucose levels and activation of hepatic glucose production. When insulin secretion does not keep pace with the increasing insulin resistance, maternal hyperglycemia results in an overabundant supply of glucose to the fetus. This causes increased fetal insulin production and macrosomia.

Both diabetes and pregnancy alter counterregulatory hormonal responses to hypoglycemia. This contributes to a higher incidence of hypoglycemia in insulin-treated women during pregnancy *(11)*. Immediately after delivery of the placenta, progesterone and human-placental lactogen levels fall and insulin requirements decline precipitously to levels present prior to pregnancy. By 6–8 wk postpartum, glucose tolerance returns to normal in more than three quarters of women with gestational diabetes *(12)*.

GLUCOSE LEVELS AND PREGNANCY OUTCOME

The Diabetes Control and Complication Trial, a multicenter study of the effect of intensive vs conventional management of type 1 diabetes, demonstrated less progression of retinopathy, nephropathy, and neuropathy in men and women using the insulin pump or taking three or more insulin injections/d compared to those taking less than three injections/d. One hundred eighty women completed 270 pregnancies during the Diabetes Control and Complications Trial, which resulted in 191 total live births. The mean glycated hemoglobin at conception differed between the intensively managed group and those using conventional therapy (7.4 vs 8.1%; $p = 0.0001$). After the onset of pregnancy, all women received intensive management and the glycated hemoglobin averaged 6.6% in both groups. Eight congenital malformations occurred in women assigned to conventional therapy before conception, and one occurred in the intensively managed group ($p = 0.06$) Thirty spontaneous abortions occurred—13.3% in the intensive group and 10.4% in the conventionally treated group. Overall, there was no significant difference in outcome between the women using conventional therapy prior to pregnancy and those on intensive therapy. The study suggests that timely institution of intensive therapy is associated with rates of spontaneous abortion and congenial malformation similar of those in the nondiabetic population *(13)*.

However, other retrospective studies show a significant difference in congenital anomalies in infants of women intensively managed compared to those receiving conventional therapy *(1)*. Type 1 diabetic women with initial glycated hemoglobin concentrations in pregnancy above 12% during the first trimester and those with preprandial glucose concentrations above 120 mg/dL have an increased risk for spontaneous abortion and malformations. Below these glycemic thresholds, the risks are comparable to those in nondiabetic women *(14)*. This may explain the lack of difference in the overall pregnancy outcomes in the Diabetes Control and Complications Trial, as the conventionally managed group had an 8.1% average glycated hemoglobin at conception.

Fetal size correlates with maternal glucose levels. Persson and coworkers *(2)* found that mothers with large-for-gestational-age infants had significantly higher fasting glucose levels between 27 and 32 wk gestation than mothers of average size for gestational age infants. Even in women without gestational diabetes, a continuum of risk related to maternal glucose levels exists for increased infant birth weight, an assisted delivery, and the likelihood of the baby being admitted to a special-care nursery *(15,16)*.

PRECONCEPTION PLANNING FOR WOMEN WITH DIABETES

The positive affect of preconception counseling on maternal and neonatal outcome hypothetically decreases total health care costs, though per-delivery costs increase *(17)*. Counseling before pregnancy provides an opportunity to discuss the benefits of intensive diabetes management on reducing diabetic retinopathy, nephropathy, and neuropathy, as well as on optimizing pregnancy outcomes *(18)*. However, only about one third of the women with established diabetes actually receive counseling before pregnancy *(19)*.

The heightened fears surrounding diabetes during pregnancy calls for tact during discussion of the risks associated with hyperglycemia during pregnancy. Nevertheless, women should know that high glucose levels during the first trimester increase the risk of congenital malformations and spontaneous abortion. Women with hypertension and diabetic renal disease need to know that pregnancy may induce or aggravate hypertension and that renal function worsens in 8–30% of women *(20)*. Additional incentives for intensive management that require discussion include the association of maternal hyperglycemia with fetal anomalies, macrosomia, and neonatal hypoglycemia.

Couples need to decide the risks they are willing to accept to have a child—specifically, the added maternal risks associated with ischemic heart disease, proliferative retinopathy, and hypertension. Preconception counseling helps women with renal insufficiency understand and cope with the possibility that more rapid deterioration of renal function may occur during pregnancy. A woman with vomiting or diarrhea associated with gastroenteropathy also should understand the added risk of wide glucose swings resulting from variable food intake and absorption.

The preconception assessment should include a history and physical examination with gynecologic evaluation. Women with diabetes for more than 5 yr should have a dilated eye exam by an ophthalmologist. Appropriate laboratory tests include a glycated hemoglobin level to evaluate the mean glucose levels over the previous two to three months, a urinalysis, serum creatinine, and 24-h urine albumin. A thyroid panel and EKG also may be indicated (Table 1).

Management before pregnancy focuses on achieving as close to normal glucose levels as possible. This involves nutritional counseling, instruction about an exercise program, and details regarding insulin administration. A dietician can help the patient devise meal plans to achieve or maintain ideal body weight and minimize high and low glucose levels. Regular exercise may also help normalize blood glucose levels in those with type 2 diabetes. As the patient is making significant changes for the sake of her future pregnancy, other health care issues, such as smoking cessation, avoidance of alcohol, and discontinuation of any unnecessary drugs, may also require attention *(21)*.

PSYCHOSOCIAL ISSUES

Diabetes invariably intensifies anxiety and other emotional responses already heightened by pregnancy. Most women fear that diabetes will harm their baby, and some worry about their own health. Glucose levels above the targeted range heighten a woman's fear, and hypoglycemic reactions intensify anxiety. Hope and discouragement rise and plummet with glucose levels.

During the first trimester, vomiting suppresses the desire to eat and upsets the regularity of meals. Hypoglycemic reactions that follow vomiting add to glucose variability and ambivalence about taking insulin. Heightened insulin sensitivity, particularly in the last weeks of the first trimester, increases swings in glucose levels, which accentuate the frequency of both hypoglycemic reactions and hyperglycemia. Frustration develops when glucose levels do not stay close to target goals. Conflicting emotions and increasing fear of hypoglycemic reactions create the anxiety surrounding elevated glucose levels. Financial worries may add to the distress and further influence diabetes management. Thus, emotions, physiologic changes, and financial concerns, which vary as widely as the personalities and coping styles of the women, influence the ability to follow medical recommendations.

Women seek emotional support from family, friends, and particularly from members of the health care team. Fortunately, intensified management does not adversely affect mood *(22)*, and women glean hope from normal glucose levels and even more from words of encouragement from physicians, nurses, and dieticians. Medical plans that lead to greater glucose stability provide education and support, particularly with regard to favorable outcomes of most pregnancies complicated by gestational diabetes, and provide reassurance.

In women with diabetes complications prior to pregnancy, fear of visual loss or worsening renal insufficiency saps energy and intensifies the anxiety normally accompanying pregnancy. This anxiety manifests differently in each individual. However, the psychological gains from near-normal glucose levels, plus constant support and encouragement,

Table 1
Management of Diabetes and Pregnancy

Preconception evaluation:	Recommend glucose self-monitoring before meals and at bedtime and near normal glycated hemoglobin levels.
	Perform history and physical.
	Order glycated hemoglobin, serum creatinine, 24 h urine albumin.
	Review glucose self-monitoring record.
	Discuss increased risk if any these present: ischemic heart disease, proliferative untreated retinopathy, serum creatinine > 2 mg/dL, proteinuria > 3 g/24 h or blood pressure increased despite treatment.
Screening:	Screen all women not previously known to have diabetes at 24–28 wk gestation with glucose level 1 h after a 50-g oral glucose solution.
GTT:	Indicated if screening glucose > 140 mg/dL, history stillbirth or fasting glycosuria present.
Diagnosis:	If fasting glucose >105 mg/dL two times or two values after 100-g GTT exceeds 105 mg/dL fasting, 190 mg/dL at 1 h, 165 mg/dL at 2 h, 145 mg/dL at 3 h.
Diet:	Recommend calories to promote weight gain (15–40 lbs) and prevent ketosis.
	Provide instruction regarding meal planning, regular timing of meals and snacks.
	Suggest avoidance of high concentrations of dietary sugar and fat.
Glucose goals:	Strive for as near normal glycemia as possible without severe hypoglycemia in type 1 diabetes.
	Recommend insulin for glucose > 105 mg/dL fasting or >120 mg/dL 2-h after meals in gestational diabetes.
	Suggest glucose goals of 70–90 mg/dL fasting and 90–120 mg/dL 2 h after meals; mutually agree on goals.
Monitoring:	Recommend glucose self monitoring fasting and 2 h after meals in gestational diabetes and if hypoglycemia occurs also before meals and periodically at 3 AM.
	Recommend monitoring urine for ketones if weight loss occurs.
Hypoglycemia:	Provide education about the signs/symptoms of hypoglycemia and advise women to eat for glucose <60 mg/dL.
	Recommend driving only when glucose rises to at least 70–90 mg/dL.
Fetal:	Assess fetal well-being, size, and growth by ultrasound.
Assessment:	Begin nonstress test twice weekly at 32 wk for uncomplicated diabetes.
	Start nonstress test weekly at 28 wk then twice weekly at 32 wk for high blood pressure, previous stillbirth, and other pregnancy complication.
Delivery:	Perform amniocentesis for fetal lung maturity if delivery planned before 39 wk.
	Monitor blood glucose every 1–2 h during labor.
Postpartum:	Anticipate decreased insulin need post-partum.
	Encourage breast feeding.

help buffer anxiety, though fear may resurface with each abnormal glucose check or hint of a complication.

Not all women are able to utilize the care given or conform to the rigorous schedule and multiple demands that a pregnancy complicated by diabetes demands. Each woman responds differently, so that guidelines and treatment regimens must be modified to take into account individual circumstances and limitations, as well as medical needs. Individualization of care becomes essential to achieve the best possible glucose levels and pregnancy outcome.

SCREENING FOR GESTATIONAL DIABETES

All pregnant women over age 25 and those under age 25 who are obese, have a family history of diabetes or are members of a high-risk ethnic population, such as African-American, Hispanic, and Native American, should undergo screening for glucose intolerance *(23)*. Screening, normally scheduled between 24–28 wk of gestation, involves the administration of a 50-g oral glucose solution with blood drawn for glucose measurement 1 h later. The test may be done at any time of the day, fasting or postprandial. When the plasma glucose equals or exceeds 140 mg/dL (7.8 mmol/L), the women should undergo a full 3-h glucose tolerance test *(9)*.

The American Diabetes Association (ADA) and the American College of Obstetricians endorse the two-step procedure previously described, in which a screening glucose determination precedes the glucose tolerance test. However, most countries outside North America use the World Health Organization (WHO) criteria, which recommends a single 75-g oral glucose-tolerance test for diagnosis of gestational diabetes *(24)*. This one-step procedure, which provides a direct comparison to the standard glucose-tolerance test used in nonpregnant adults, predicts adverse pregnancy outcomes as effectively as the two-step procedure *(25)*.

Glucose-Tolerance Test

The glucose-tolerance test, performed after an overnight fast, involves measurement of a fasting plasma glucose and glucose levels at 1, 2, and 3 h after a 100-g oral glucose solution. Two values that equal or exceed 105 mg/dL (5.8 mmol/L) fasting, 190 mg/dL (10.8 mmol/L) at 1 h, 165 mg/dL (9.2 mmol/L) at 2 h, and 145 mg/dL (8.1 mmol/L) at 3 h confirms the diagnosis of gestational diabetes *(9)*. These recommended criteria are the most widely used, though perinatal morbidity may be increased in patients with even lower values *(26)*.

Treatment Goals

Discussion of the risks and benefits of intensive diabetes management assists in setting treatment goals including glycemic targets. Recommended glycemic goals, set at 70–100 mg/dL (3.9–5.6 mmol/L) fasting and < 120 mg/dL (6.7 mmol/L) two hours postprandially, may require modification, depending on the risk of hypoglycemia *(20)*. Ideally, setting goals occurs prior to conception in women with type 1 or type 2 diabetes or immediately after diagnosis in those with gestational diabetes.

Glucose and Ketone Monitoring

The results of glucose self-monitoring provide a basis for determining the need for insulin therapy and for insulin-dose changes *(27)*. A diabetes educator or pharmacist can familiarize the woman with the meter used for monitoring. Some glucose meters cost less than $50, whereas those with memory capacity may cost $150 or more. The meters require periodic calibration using a reference solution. Similar readings between meters used for home monitoring and those in the physician's office further verify meter and operator accuracy. A discrepancy of more than 15% between meters should prompt comparison of the code on the glucose strips and the meters. Next, the meters should be cleaned, and a comparison test repeated. A continuing difference of more than 15% between meters necessitates replacement of the meter found inaccurate compared to a laboratory standard.

Urine dipstick evaluation also should be done at each office visit to check for urinary tract infection, protein, and ketones. Skipped meals and inadequate caloric intake lead to using fat for energy and ketonuria. Urine ketone testing, recommended for women with inadequate weight gain during pregnancy, provides a standard by which women can judge whether or not they have eaten enough. Trace urinary ketones usually do not require intervention. Moderate to large urinary ketones mean that the frequency and/or content of meals need modification. Ketonuria during gestation may vary inversely with the child's intelligence quotient *(28)*.

Diabetes Education

In addition to verbal instruction, women welcome written material covering the essentials of diabetes care, including meal planning, insulin administration, and ways to balance exercise with meals and insulin. The frequency and timing of self glucose monitoring require consideration of each woman's schedule, type of diabetes, and financial resources. Education regarding preventive care, such as the need for periodic ophthalmologic examination, also necessitates individualized counseling. Women with diabetic retinopathy may have acceleration of their retinopathy during pregnancy, whereas women with gestational diabetes and no previously existing eye disease do not need special ophthalmologic attention.

Insulin-treated women and their family members need to know the signs and symptoms of hypoglycemia and understand the importance of always keeping some source of sugar readily available. Women who take insulin should be instructed regarding the need to eat whenever glucose levels fall below 60 mg/dL, or when they sense a hypoglycemic reaction. Overtreatment of hypoglycemia causes rebound hyperglycemia and may contribute to poor glycemic control. Glucose tablets or gels work more quickly than milk or orange juice and result in a more consistent glycemic response without rebound hyperglycemia. Family members of women with type 1 diabetes need instruction regarding the use of glucagon for severe insulin reactions.

Nutritional Recommendations

Individualized nutritional assessment is central for devising a diet plan that meets maternal and fetal needs and optimizes glycemia *(29)*. Cultural, economic, and educational factors influence dietary recommendations. In addition to appetite and weight assessments, blood glucose levels, and the record of urinary ketones serve as guides to the individualized meal plan *(30)*.

Diabetes does not alter the general dietary recommendations for pregnancy, except that complex carbohydrates replace free sugars. Regular timing of meals and frequent snacks reduce the incidence of hypoglycemia. Women who use continuous subcutaneous insulin delivery by a pump have more flexibility with mealtimes and snacks than women who use injections. Day-to-day consistency and minimal intake of sucrose and other caloric sweeteners assist in attaining glycemic goals (9). The American Diabetes Association and the American Dietetic Association do not make specific recommendations for caloric intake or percent distribution of carbohydrate, protein, and fat for pregnant women.

Weight-gain recommendations, based on women's weight prior to pregnancy, vary from 15 pounds (7 kg) for obese women to 40 pounds (18 kg) for underweight women. Calories to promote an average weight gain of 25–30 pounds prevents ketonemia. A dietician and diabetes educator can help the woman with diabetes devise creative meal plans to suit her preferences.

The glycemic index defined as the percent increase in blood glucose after the ingestion of a food varies with both meal content and manner of preparation. Patients can develop their own "glycemic index" by monitoring blood glucose responses (21). Insulin must balance the quantity of food, especially carbohydrates. Three meals with three snacks are considered optimal and appropriate for nausea and vomiting associated with early pregnancy and also help avoid third trimester early satiety. Caffeine consumption should be decreased or avoided, although there is little direct evidence that caffeine alone adversely affects pregnancy (31).

Vitamin, mineral, and folate supplements help meet daily nutritional recommendations, as the typical American diet does not supply the 30 mg of iron recommended, and folate requirements more than double during pregnancy. Folate supplementation decreases the incidence of small-for-gestational-age births and neural-tube defects (21). The requirements for phosphorous, thiamine, and vitamin B6 increase by 33–50% with lesser increases in protein, zinc, and riboflavin requirements. Calcium requirement increases from 33% to as much as 400%/d during pregnancy. Vitamin B6, calcium, magnesium, iron, zinc, and copper are most likely to be present in 80% or less of the recommended daily requirements. Food sources rich in these nutrients—meats, poultry, fish, and dairy products—are all recommended in additional amounts during pregnancy (32).

Artificial sweeteners, though not essential, help reduce consumption of simple sugars. Aspartic acid, a metabolite of aspartame, does not readily cross the placenta, and methanol levels rise only minimally. Phenylalanine, the third breakdown product of aspartame, does cross the placenta with fetal levels consistently below toxic levels, even at twice acceptable daily intake. Acesulfame-K and saccharin do not appear harmful during pregnancy (32). Therefore, noncaloric sweeteners may be used in moderation (9).

Exercise

Weller reports up to a 90% success rate in maintaining women with gestational diabetes on diet therapy and exercise without the need for insulin therapy (33). However, exercise, as an adjunct in treating and maintaining normoglycemia, carries more potential risks during pregnancy than in nonpregnant adults. Physiologic changes during pregnancy influence these risks. Joints become more lax in pregnancy, the center of balance changes, and plasma volume expands. These changes make injury, dehydration, and hypovolemia more likely.

An exercise program must be individualized. Guidelines to avoid complications involve keeping the maternal heart rate below 150 beats/min at maximum exertion. The "talk test," meaning a woman should be able to talk at peak exercise, serves as a practical method to avoid over-exertion. Others recommendations include limiting exercise to levels that do not cause exhaustion, maintaining good hydration and ventilation, and stopping if any pain or bleeding occurs. Uterine activity may occur with exercise, but whether this causes pre-term deliveries remains unclear *(34)*. Medical contradictions to exercise include pre-term labor and hypertension, both of which may be increased in diabetes.

Insulin

Gestational diabetes often is managed by diet and exercise alone. However, insulin treatment is needed if diet and exercise do not consistently maintain the fasting plasma glucose < 105 mg/dL (5.8 mmol/dL) or the 2-h postprandial plasma glucose exceeds 120 mg/dL (6.7 mmol/L) two times within a 1–2 wk interval. About half the women with gestational diabetes will need insulin *(35)*. Oral hypoglycemic agents are not recommended during pregnancy, primarily because insulin more readily enables attainment of normoglycemia. Also, the safety of oral hypoglycemic agents remains questionable *(36)*.

Intensive insulin management enhances the ability to maintain glucose levels within the therapeutic goals of less than 90 mg/dL (5 mmol/L) fasting and less than 120 mg/dL (6.7 mmol/L) 2 h after meals *(21)*. As pregnancy progresses, increasing production of placental hormones causes insulin resistance and increasing insulin need, particularly between 20–24 wk gestation. Insulin resistance makes hypoglycemia an infrequent complication despite high insulin doses. Women with insulin-requiring gestational diabetes usually experience a continual increase in insulin requirements over the final weeks of pregnancy *(37)*.

Human insulin, the least immunogenic insulin, comes in several modifications that alter absorption and duration of action. Regular insulin, usually taken 30–45 min before meals, begins acting 30–60 min after injection. To obtain normal postprandial glucose levels and avoid preprandial hypoglycemia, sometimes as much as an hour needs to elapse between the injection of regular insulin and the meal. Also, because insulin absorption occurs more rapidly from the abdomen than from the legs or hips, using the abdomen for insulin injections before meals may help lower postprandial glucose concentrations.

Lispro insulin begins working in minutes and lasts about 2 h. Injection just prior to meals offers convenience and effectively lowers glucose levels 1 and 2 h postprandially without leading to preprandial hypoglycemia. Even when taken 15 min after meals, lispro effectively lowers postprandial glucose levels *(38)*. Because there are no clinical studies regarding the use of Lispro insulin during pregnancy, its use should be considered only if clearly indicated. A combination of NPH or Lente insulin with regular or Lispro insulin given before breakfast and supper usually maintains glucose levels within the therapeutic range throughout the day and night. Occasionally, high glucose levels after lunch necessitate a before-lunch insulin dose. An elevated fasting level may require NPH or Lente at bedtime (Table 2).

In women with gestational diabetes, adjustment of insulin therapy according to postprandial rather than preprandial blood glucose levels improves glucose levels and decreases the risk of neonatal hypoglycemia, macrosomia, and cesarean delivery *(39)*. When corticosteroids are used to enhance fetal-lung maturity, the insulin requirement may double the day after the steroid injection *(21)*. Insulin resistance ends abruptly with delivery. Therefore, insulin rarely is given following the onset of labor. The last injection normally occurs the night prior to planned induction.

Table 2
Insulin Dose Adjustments for Abnormal Glucose Levels[a]

Time	Glucose elevated	Glucose too low
Fasting	Increase PM NPH[b]	Decrease before supper/bedtime NPH
	Switch NPH from supper to bedtime	Increase bedtime snack
		Decrease AM NPH
After breakfast	Increase AM Regular	Decrease AM Regular
	Change breakfast content	Decrease AM NPH
	Give injection in abdomen[c]	
	Switch Regular to Lispro[d]	
	Increase time interval between insulin (Regular) injection and meal	
Before lunch	Increase AM Regular	Decrease AM Regular
		Decrease AM NPH
After lunch	Increase before lunch Regular	Decrease before lunch Regular/Lispro
	Switch Regular to Lispro	Change or increase lunch content
	Change or decrease lunch content	Decrease AM NPH
	Increase AM NPH	
Before supper	Increase before lunch Regular	Decrease before lunch Regular
	Increase AM NPH	Decrease AM NPH
	Increase before lunch Regular	
After supper	Increase before supper Regular	Decrease before supper Regular
	Change content of supper	Increase carbohydrates/calories at supper
	Give injection in the abdomen	
	Switch Regular to Lispro	
During night	Increase before supper/bedtime NPH	Decrease before dinner NPH or Regular
	Add bedtime snack	
	Move before supper NPH to HS	

[a]Change dose by 10%.
[b]Wherever NPH appears in table may substitute Lente.
[c]May apply to all after meal glucose elevations; abdominal injection decreases time for absorption.
[d]Lispro has not been studied specifically during pregnancy and thus should be used only when clearly indicated. It is more rapidly absorbed with shorter duration of action than Regular insulin.
Adapted from Pasui and McFarland (83).

Type 2 diabetes during pregnancy nearly always necessitates the use of insulin. A reduction in the insulin dose rarely occurs during the first trimester. A steady increase in insulin need begins during the second trimester and lasts until the last weeks of pregnancy. Usually, the insulin dose does not rise during the last 4 wk of gestation. Intensive management enhances the ability to maintain glucose levels within the therapeutic goals, though rigid glycemic control should not be maintained at the cost of symptomatic hypoglycemia.

Insulin requirements often double or triple by term. After delivery, the need for insulin declines dramatically. Exogenous insulin or oral hypoglycemic agents may not be needed for a variable period, sometimes up to several days or weeks. When glucose levels rise over 150 mg/dL, insulin may be restarted at the dose used before pregnancy. Women who do not nurse may restart oral hypoglycemic agents rather than continue to use insulin, particularly if the oral agents maintained normal glucose levels prior to pregnancy. Most women require a dose similar to that used prior to pregnancy within a few days post-partum.

Type 1 diabetes is difficult to manage during pregnancy, because extreme insulin sensitivity leads to wide swings in glucose levels. The sudden development of ketonuria without apparent reason may precede any other sign of pregnancy. During the first trimester, nausea and vomiting change food intake and accentuate glucose variability. Even close attention to detail, multiple glucose checks, regular timing of meals, and consistent insulin administration cannot completely eliminate periodic high and low glucose levels *(40)*. Frequent and severe hypoglycemic reactions occur most frequently between 10–15 wk gestation with recurrent hypoglycemic episodes causing rebound hyperglycemia. However, several mild reactions per week may need to be tolerated *(41)*.

In the second trimester, insulin need steadily increases with the greatest change occurring between 20–30 wk gestation. The average insulin dose increase found in more than 200 women with type 1 diabetes during pregnancy was 52 U/d. The degree of rise was positively related to initial maternal weight gain, particularly during the second trimester, and inversely related to diabetes duration. The dose was not related to level of glycemia, pregnancy complications, or pregnancy outcome. About 8% of women experience a fall in insulin requirement, which bears no relation to maternal characteristics or fetal outcome. A decreased insulin requirement after 36 wk gestation does not indicate an adverse prognosis *(42)*.

With delivery of the placenta, human placental lactogen, estrogen, and progesterone levels fall precipitously leading to decreased insulin resistance and decreased insulin need. Growth hormone and gonadotropins remain suppressed. The result is a relative state of "panhypopituitarism," another reason that insulin need decreases. In addition, high pre-partum insulin doses create stores of bound insulin that last for hours after the last injection.

Normally, women take an insulin dose the evening prior to elective delivery and no insulin the morning of induction. Glucose levels are measured every 1–2 h during labor and if the plasma glucose concentration rises to > 140 mg/dL (7.8 m*M*), 1–4 U of insulin may be given hourly. However, most women do not need any insulin during active labor. If glucose levels fall below 70 mg/dL, 5% dextrose in water given at a rate of 75 mL/h may replace the saline infusion *(21)*. Other protocols for insulin and intravenous fluid administration may assist in management *(43)*.

Following delivery, insulin need falls precipitously. In order to anticipate when to restart insulin therapy, glucose checks should be done before meals and at bedtime. A preprandial value of 150 mg/dL (8.3 mmol/L) or more signals the need to restart insulin *(21)*. The first dose should be slightly less than the prepregnancy dose. Subsequent dosage changes depend on glucose measurements done prior to meals and at bedtime.

The dose of insulin used prior to pregnancy most closely approximates the dose needed after delivery. When the dose prior to pregnancy is not known, 0.7 U/kg body weight provides a reasonable starting dose. This may be divided into two doses with 2/3 given before breakfast and 1/3 before supper. The morning dose may be divided into 2/3 intermediate acting insulin and 1/3 short-acting insulin and the PM dose 1/2 short-acting and 1/2 intermediate-acting insulin.

HYPOGLYCEMIA

The average glucose level obtained in intensively managed nonpregnant adults with type 1 diabetes is approx 155 mg/dL, compared to an average of 231 mg/dL in patients managed conventionally *(18)*. However, intensive therapy in nonpregnant adults also leads to three times the incidence of severe hypoglycemic reactions. Severe hypoglycemia occurs even more frequently during pregnancy, partly as a result of diminished epinephrine and growth-hormone responses to hypoglycemia *(11)*.

Clinically significant hypoglycemia that results in the requirement of assistance from another person occurs in nearly three quarters of pregnant women with type 1 diabetes. Fortunately, severe hypoglycemia during the early weeks of embryogenesis is not associated with increased embryopathy. However, in women with recurrent episodes of hypoglycemia, the clear benefits of strict glycemic control must be weighed against the hazards of hypoglycemia. Thus, hypoglycemia becomes the limiting factor in the management of insulin-dependent diabetes *(44)*. Education should include precautions about checking glucose levels before driving, postponing driving until glucose levels rise to 90 mg/dL *(21)*, and eating whenever glucose measurements register below 60 mg/dL. Table 2 outlines ways to adjust the insulin dose for low glucose levels.

FETAL SURVEILLANCE

Precise dating of the pregnancy, best established during the first two trimesters, assists in planning the time for delivery. A first trimester ultrasound examination allows accurate dating, and an ultrasound performed after 17 wk offers the opportunity to detect fetal anomalies *(45)*. Maternal alphafetoprotein screening enables detection of most neural tube defects, which are increased to 20–50/1000 pregnancies complicated by diabetes *(46)*. The screening test, offered between 16 and 20 wk gestation, uses a standard curve to enable data interpretation. Diabetes may alter the ranges of normal, requiring some adjustment of the standard curve *(47)*.

Serial ultrasonography, though not routinely required, may become necessary if fundal height measurements appear abnormal for dates. Ultrasonography may alert the practitioner to development of macrosomia, polyhydramnios, or intrauterine growth retardation, which occur with greater frequency in diabetes *(48)*. Adding fetal echocardiography to the ultrasound evaluation assists in detecting or excluding cardiac anomalies.

Fetal surveillance becomes especially important in the third trimester because intrauterine fetal demise occurs more commonly in pregnancies complicated by diabetes. Fetal surveillance consists of frequent physical examinations, maternal kick counts, nonstress tests, biophysical profiles, and contraction stress tests *(49,50)*. Nonstress testing often begins at 32 wk, though complications may lead to testing as early as 28 wk gestation. Conditions that prompt early testing include hyperglycemia, pyelonephritis, ketoacidosis, renal disease, hypertension, intrauterine growth retardation, and worsening retinopathy.

A negative contraction stress test done once weekly remains the gold standard for fetal surveillance, as the test gives almost no false-negative results. However, a positive test does not necessitate immediate delivery, as the false-positive rate is high *(50)*. The contraction stress test, a labor-intensive procedure, requires constant patient monitoring, and intravenous access, and may take hours to complete. For this reason, other, less invasive, forms of fetal surveillance predominate.

The nonstress test performed twice weekly requires only an external monitor and has a predictive value similar to that of a negative contraction stress test. A nonreactive nonstress test necessitates further evaluation of the fetus. The nonstress test should be performed at least twice weekly. Another noninvasive test, the biophysical profile, includes a nonstress test, estimation of amniotic fluid volume, and fetal movement parameters. A score of less that 7/10 may suggest fetal compromise *(50)*. A nonstress test and an estimate of amniotic fluid volume done twice weekly predict fetal outcomes, as well as the standard full biophysical profile *(51)*. Women with gestational diabetes who have normal glucose levels on diet alone and no obstetrical complications need not begin fetal testing until 40 wk gestation, as perinatal outcome approaches that of the nondiabetic population. Maternal assessment of fetal activity with daily kick counts may begin at 28 wk gestation.

DELIVERY AND POSTPARTUM CARE

Clinical factors including the type of diabetes influence timing of delivery. Delivery at 37 or 38 wk gestation, is the established pattern for women with diabetes antedating pregnancy who had no obstetrical or diabetes-associated complications and have near-normal glucose levels. Women with intensively managed gestational diabetes frequently deliver after spontaneously going into labor. Planned inductions usually occur at 39–40 wk for women with a favorable cervix. Those with an unfavorable cervix may be followed expectantly provided their glucose levels stay within the therapeutic range, and fetal assessment remains reassuring. Cervical ripening with prostaglandin agents at 40 wk may be necessary.

Although pre-term delivery decreases the incidence of intrauterine fetal demise, early delivery increases infant respiratory-distress syndrome and other complications, such as necrotizing enterocolitis. Elective delivery before 39 wk gestational age requires documentation of fetal lung maturity based on the amniotic fluid lecithin/sphingomyelin ratio and the presence of phosphatidylglycerol. The interpretation of the lecithin/sphingomyelin ratio differs by laboratory, though a lecithin/sphingomyelin ratio greater than two or three in the presence of phosphatidyl-glycerol suggests pulmonary maturity. When fetal testing does not prove reassuring, and lung maturity studies suggest pulmonary immaturity, the risks of delaying delivery must be weighed against the risk of infant developing respiratory distress. Corticosteroids widely used to promote lung maturity cause insulin resistance, which may produce significant hyperglycemia and may even precipitate diabetic ketoacidosis *(48)*.

The route of delivery requires consideration. Fetal tests which are not reassuring and an unfavorable cervix may necessitate cesarean delivery. Prostaglandins, used for cervical ripening, provide another alternative. If a fetus can tolerate the labor process, maternal morbidity may be reduced by vaginal delivery. However, vaginal delivery carries the risk of shoulder dystocia and cephalopelvic disproportion in macrosomic infants. Because of these risks, delivery should be contemplated after 38 wk gestation and if not pursued, careful monitoring of fetal growth performed. Cesarean delivery may be indicated if the estimated fetal weight exceeds 4500 g *(52)*.

RISK OF DEVELOPING DIABETES AFTER GESTATIONAL DIABETES

Women with gestational diabetes have a 33–50% chance of gestational diabetes recurrence in subsequent pregnancies *(53)*. The percentage of women with gestational diabetes who later develop type 2 or type 1 diabetes varies with the time of follow up, criteria used for initial diagnosis of gestational diabetes, and the criteria for diagnosis of type 2 diabetes. Studies show a wide variation in the incidence of diabetes following gestational diabetes with ranges varying between 6–62% (54,55). The 5-yr cumulative incidence of diabetes during follow-up after gestational diabetes mellitus is nearly 50% (56). An elevated fasting glucose level and the need for insulin therapy increase the risk of diabetes developing post-partum (12,57). Based on the prevalence of antibodies to glutamic acid decarboxylase in women with gestational diabetes, about 1.7% of women with gestational diabetes will develop type 1 diabetes (58).

As high as 20% of women with gestational diabetes tested in the early post-partum period have an abnormal oral glucose tolerance test (12). Abnormal glucose tolerance noted early postpartum occurs predominantly in women requiring insulin during pregnancy and in those diagnosed before the twenty-fourth week of gestation (59). Patients receiving at least 100 units/day of insulin have a 100% incidence of postpartum glucose intolerance (57).

Postpartum glucose screening is not needed for women managed by diet alone during pregnancy, because of the low incidence of postpartum glucose intolerance. Women requiring insulin during pregnancy may warrant a 2-h 75-g glucose tolerance test at the first post-partum visit (57). Another follow up method involves screening with a fasting plasma glucose, which should be below 110 mg/dL. The fasting plasma glucose is the preferred method of diagnosis of diabetes, because it is easier and faster to perform, more convenient and acceptable to patients, more reproducible, and less expensive (23). Long term follow up of women with previous gestational diabetes must be individualized. Every woman should have glucose measurement done if symptoms of hyperglycemia develop and periodically when asymptomatic (21). Measures to prevent glucose intolerance postpartum include exercise and a well-balanced dietary plan aimed at maintaining normal weight.

CONTRACEPTION

The risks associated with diabetes during pregnancy usually outweigh the risks associated with most types of contraceptive use. Current contraception options include sterilization, oral hormone regimens, injectable hormone treatments, the intrauterine device, barrier methods, spermicides and the rhythm method. Lifestyle, education, and a woman's ability to utilize a particular method influence the type of contraception recommended. In addition, medical complications associated with diabetes such as hypertension, cardiac disease, and renal disease and the effectiveness of specific contraceptive methods affect contraception choice (60).

Rhythm Method

The rhythm method, the least effective means of contraception, involves estimating from menstrual cycle lengths, examination of the cervical mucus, symptomatology, and records of basal body temperature the fertile period of the menstrual cycle. Based on a 28-d cycle, the time for abstinence falls from cycle d 10 though cycle d 19. Pregnancy rates with the rhythm method range from as low as 3.1% to over 80%/yr (61). Thus, this method is used when medical, moral or religious reasons preclude another more effective option. Use of an ovulation predictor kit for detection of the preovulatory luteinizing hormone surge increases accuracy of ovulation prediction. However, the added cost of the kit, often $20 or more, may limit repeated use (62).

Condoms

Latex condoms aid in prevention of pregnancy and sexually transmitted diseases. The added value of spermicides remains uncertain, whereas the use of lubricants decreases effectiveness and increases breakage. Water-based lubricants decrease this risk. The pregnancy rate for male condom use alone is 3.6/100 women-years *(61)*. The female condom has not gained popularity largely because of lack of availability and decreased sensation *(63)*.

Diaphragm

Consistent use of a diaphragm, another barrier method of conception, is associated with low failure rates when fitted by medical personnel to prevent slippage and urethral pressure. The diaphragm is filled with spermicidal jelly and left in place for at least eight hours after coitus. Additional spermicidal jelly must be placed intravaginally with each subsequent coitus.

Intrauterine Device

The intrauterine device (IUD) is a popular and effective method of contraception. The copper intrauterine device offers up to 10 years of contraception which relies on the slow metabolism of copper to prevent sperm capacitation and fertilization. Studies have revealed no increase in the infection rate in diabetic patients over the general population. Contraindications for insertion of the IUD include suspicion of any of the following: pregnancy, malignancy, infection, and behavior suggesting a high risk for contracting a sexually transmitted diseases *(64)*.

The contraceptive methods previously discussed do not involve systemic medication. The remaining reversible contraceptive methods use exogenous hormones to alter ovulation or the endometrial and cervical environment. Hormones may affect more than just reproductive function, and the metabolic effects need consideration, especially in women with diabetes *(65)*.

The Pill

Oral contraceptive pills contain various combinations of estrogen and progestational agents that alter ovulation and the endometrium, and have other metabolic effects. The "low dose" contraceptives contain 20–50 µg of estinyl estradiol. The most popular ones contain 35 µg or less of ethinyl estradiol combined with a progestin such as norethindrone, levonorgestrel, norgesterone, or ethynodiol diacetate, desogestrel, or norgestimate. The "mini-pill," or progestin-only pill, does not contain any ethinyl estradiol, only norethindrone or levonorgestrel.

The oral contraceptive pills contain monophasic, or triphasic progestin preparations, and some of the newer pills have phasic ethinyl estradiol doses also. The types of progestins used in oral contraceptives differ in their side-effect profiles. The androgenic side effects include alterations in lipid profiles, weight gain, and acne. Other side effects include nausea, breast tenderness, weight gain, increased blood pressure, menstrual irregularity, amenorrhea, and headache *(61)*. Failure rates with oral contraceptive use can range from 1/100 to 15/100 depending on compliance *(65)*.

Oral contraceptive use may impair glucose tolerance *(66)*. Reports vary regarding the extent and reason for the abnormal glucose tolerance, with no particular oral contraceptive identified as causing the least insulin resistance. Barrett reports an increased risk of myocardial infarction (MI) in oral contraceptive users who have diabetes *(67)*. However, the association of oral contraception use and cardiovascular disease remains to be clarified, because all adults with diabetes have an increased risk for cardiovascular disease *(68–70)*. Diabetes and oral contraceptive use may also increase the risk of Candida infections *(60,65)*.

Compared to the cardiovascular risk and insulin resistance state of pregnancy, the risks that may occur with oral contraceptive use are small. Therefore, in a young otherwise healthy diabetic woman, oral contraceptive use is a viable option for contraception. A monophasic low-dose oral contraceptive with low androgenic side effects makes a suitable choice.

Norplant

Norplant contains levonorgestrel designed for continuous subcutaneous release. The six silastic capsules placed under the skin administer 85 to 30 µg of the drug daily. Norplant provides five years of contraception with rates slightly better than oral contraceptions, averaging 8/100 users over 5 yr *(65)*. Norplant may raise fasting glucose levels and decrease total cholesterol.

Depo-Provera

Depo-medroxyprogesterone acetate, (or Depo-provera), the most widely used injectable contraceptive, has a failure rate of less than 32/100 users *(65)*. The injection is given every 12–13 wk, though hormone levels may not decrease enough to allow ovulation for 7–9 mo after injection The major side effects include disruption of the menstrual cycle, weight gain, and delayed fertility. Depo-provera does not significantly change glucose tolerance *(71)* or increase thromboembolic events. The drug provides an effective contraception choice for women who cannot take estrogens *(72)*.

Sterilization

Sterilization, considered a permanent method of contraception, has a risk equivalent to the risk of the surgical procedure performed. Diabetes does not alter the effectiveness of sterilization, but does increase surgical risks. Failure rates range from 7.5–36.5/1000 procedures. The highest failure rate occurs with a clip procedure and the lowest with unipolar cautery (73)

PROGRESSION OF DIABETIC COMPLICATIONS DURING PREGNANCY

Diabetic retinopathy may worsen significantly during pregnancy. Some of the untoward ophthalmologic changes occurring during pregnancy may be linked to the rapid normalization of glucose levels in women with previous chronic hyperglycemia. Also, hypertension is associated with progression of retinopathy during pregnancy *(74)*.

Diabetic nephropathy with reduced creatinine clearance increases pregnancy risks. When a reduction in renal function occurs during pregnancy, some women have continued deterioration of renal function postpartum *(75)*. Women with an initial serum creatinine exceeding 1.5 mg/dL and/or proteinuria of more than three grams in 24 h have an increased risk of early delivery, preeclampsia, cesarean delivery and lower birth weight infants. In one study by the third trimester 58% had greater than a 1 g/24 h increase in proteinuria and 36% demonstrated more than a 15% fall in creatinine clearance. Women with an initial creatinine clearance greater than 90 mL/min and less than 1 g of urine protein/24 h had less loss of renal function at follow-up *(76)*.

Fortunately, in a recent study there was a 100% perinatal survival in 46 pregnancies complicated by diabetic renal disease *(76)*. However, fetal deaths are more common in women with renal disease and increase with the degree of renal dysfunction and proteinuria *(77)*. Women with diabetes and hypertension are at particular high risk for a poor pregnancy outcome. These higher risks should be discussed when counseling women with renal disease who contemplate pregnancy.

About 10% of diabetic women who did not have renal disease during pregnancy will have diabetic nephropathy 10 years after delivery. Proteinuria appearing during pregnancy and elevated glucose levels during pregnancy are associated with the subsequent development of nephropathy. Pregnancy and increasing parity do no appear to increase the overall risk for diabetic nephropathy (44% after 27 yr of diabetes) *(78)*.

Kimmerle and coworkers studied the effect of diabetic nephropathy on the course of 36 pregnancies. From the first to the third trimester the percentage of women with proteinuria over 3 grams per day increased from 14–53% and those treated with antihypertensive medication from 53–97%. There were no intrauterine or perinatal deaths, but one child died suddenly four weeks postpartum. Of 36 newborns, 11 were born before wk 34 and had respiratory distress syndrome. Abnormal renal function in the first trimester, elevated diastolic blood pressure in the third trimester and an elevated glycated hemoglobin value were predictive of low birth weight *(79)*.

LACTATION

Breast feeding should be encouraged in women with diabetes managed by diet alone or with insulin. Insulin in breast milk is rendered inactive in the infant's gastrointestinal tract and thus, does not adversely affect the infant. For women taking insulin, blood glucose monitoring with appropriate insulin and diet adjustment needs to be continued to prevent maternal hypoglycemia. The maternal use of oral hypoglycemic agents usually is considered a relative contraindication to breast feeding, although the American Academy of Pediatrics considers tolbutamide compatible with breast feeding *(80)*.

Breast feeding, even for a short time, has a beneficial effect on the mother's glucose and lipid levels. Breast feeding results in higher high density cholesterol and decreased blood glucose levels *(81)*. Epidemiological studies suggest that exposure of genetically susceptible infants to cow's milk before the age of three months increases the risk of the child developing insulin dependent diabetes. This provides another reason to favor breast feeding *(82)*.

CONCLUSION

Diabetes mellitus commonly complicates pregnancy and increases risks for mother and infant. Universal screening at 24 to 28 wk gestation identifies women with gestational diabetes. Dietary measures are used initially, and insulin is added if fasting glucose levels exceed 105 mg/dL or 2-h postprandial glucose levels exceed 120 mg/dL. Results of glucose self-monitoring guide insulin modifications. Women with pre-existing diabetes require intensive glucose management before conception to ensure the lowest incidence of congenital anomalies. Because of the greater risk for stillbirth and macrosomia associated with diabetes during pregnancy, fetal surveillance begins in the third trimester with nonstress tests the most widely used. Ultrasound dating and determination of the lecithin/sphingomyelin ratio assist in timing delivery.

REFERENCES

1. Kitzmiller JL, Buchanan TA, Kjos S, Combs CA, Ratner RE. Pre–conception care of diabetes, congenital malformations, and spontaneous abortions. Diabetes Care 1996;19:514–541.
2. Persson B, Hanson U. Fetal size in relation to quality of blood glucose control in pregnancies complicated by pregestational diabetes mellitus. Br J Obstet Gynaecol 1996;103:427–33.
3. Hod M, Merlob P, Friedman S, Schoenfeld A, Ovadia J. Gestational diabetes mellitus: A survey of perinatal complications in the 1980's. Diabetes 1991;40(Suppl 2):74–78.
4. Thompson DM, Dansereau J, Creed M, Ridell L. Tight glucose control results in normal perinatal outcome in 150 patients with gestational diabetes. Obstet Gynecol 1994;83:362–366.
5. Langer O, Rodriguez DA, Xenakis EM, McFarland MB, Berkus MD, Arredondo F. Intensified versus conventional management of gestational diabetes. Am J Obstet Gynecol 1994;170:1036–47.
6. Demarini S, Mimouni F, Tsang RC, Khoury J, Hertzberg V. Impact of metabolic control of diabetes during pregnancy on neonatal hypocalcemia: a randomized study. Obstet Gynecol 1994;83: 918–922.
7. Engelgau MM, Herman WH, Smith PJ, German RR, Aubert RE. The epidemiology of diabetes and pregnancy in the U.S., 1988. Diabetes Care 1995;18:1029–1033.
8. Beischer NA, Oats JN, Henry OA, Sheedy MT, Walstab JE. Incidence and severity of gestational diabetes mellitus according to country of birth in women living in Australia. Diabetes 1991;40(Suppl 2):35–38.
9. American Diabetes Association: Clinical Practice Recommendations. Gestational diabetes mellitus diabetes. Diabetes Care 1997;20(Suppl 1):S44–S45.
10. Metzger BE, Phelps RL, Dooley SL. The mother in pregnancies complicated by diabetes mellitus. In: Porte D, Sherwin RS, eds. Ellenberg and Rifkin's Diabetes Mellitus, 5th ed. Appleton and Lange, Stamford, 1997, pp. 887–915.
11. Rosenn BM, Miodovnik M, Khoury JC, Siddiqi TA. Counterregulatory hormonal responses to hypoglycemia during pregnancy. Obstet Gynecol 1996;87:568–74.
12. Catalano PM, Vargo KM, Bernstein IM, Amini B. Incidence and risk factors associated with abnormal postpartum glucose tolerance in women with gestational diabetes. Am J Obstet Gynecol 1991;65:914–919.
13. Diabetes Control and Complications Trial Research Group. Pregnancy outcomes in the Diabetes Control and Complications Trial. Am J Obstet Gynecol 1996;174:1343–1353.
14. Rosenn B, Miodovnik M, Combs CA, Khoury J, Siddiqi T. Glycemic thresholds for spontaneous abortion and congenital malformation in insulin–dependent diabetes mellitus. Obstet Gynecol 1994;84:515–520.
15. Moses RG, Calvert D. Pregnancy outcomes in women without gestational diabetes mellitus related to the maternal glucose level. Diabetes Care 1995;18:1527–1533.
16. Sacks DA, Greenspoon JS, Abu-Fadil S, Henry HM, Wolde-Tsadik G, Yao JFF. Toward universal criteria for gestational diabetes: The 75-gram glucose tolerance test in pregnancy. Am J Obstet Gynecol 1995;172:607–614.
17. Elixhauser A, Weschler JM, Kitzmiller DR, et al. Cost-benefit analysis of preconception care of women with established diabetes mellitus. Diabetes Care 1993;16:1146–1157.
18. Diabetes Control and Complications Trial Research Group. The effect of intensive treatment of diabetes on the development and progression of long-term complications in insulin-dependent diabetes mellitus. N Engl J Med 1993;329:977–86.
19. Janz NK, Herman WH, Becker MP, et al. Diabetes and pregnancy: factors associated with seeking preconception care. Diabetes Care 1995;18:157–165.
20. American Diabetes Association: Clinical practice recommendations. Preconception care of women with diabetes. Diabetes Care 1997;20(Suppl 1):S40–S43.
21. American Diabetes Association: Clinical education series. Medical management of pregnancy complicated by diabetes. Alexandria, American Diabetes Association, 1993, pp. 2–107.
22. Langer N, Langer O. Emotional adjustment to diagnosis and intensified treatment of gestational diabetes. Obstet Gynecol 1994;84:329–334.
23. The Expert Committee on the Diagnosis and Classification of Diabetes Mellitus: Committee Report. Report of the Expert Committee on the Diagnosis and Classification of Diabetes Mellitus. Diabetes Care 1997;20:1183–1195.

24. Carpenter MW. Testing for gestational diabetes. In: Reece EA, Coustan DR, eds. Diabetes Mellitus in Pregnancy, 2nd ed. Churchill Livingstone, New York, 1995, pp. 261–275.
25. Pettitt DJ, Bennett PH, Hanson RL, Narayan KMV, Knowler WC. Comparison of World Health Organization and National Diabetes Data Group procedures to detect abnormalities of glucose tolerance during pregnancy. Diabetes Care 1994;17:1264–1268.
26. Berkus MD, Langer O, Piper JM, Luther MF. Efficiency of lower threshold criteria for the diagnosis of gestational diabetes. Obstet Gynecol 1995;86:892–896.
27. Laird J, McFarland KF. Fasting blood glucose levels and initiation of insulin therapy in gestational diabetes. Endocr Pract 1996;2:330–332.
28. Rizzo T, Metzger BE, Burns WJ, Burns K. Correlation between antepartum maternal metabolism and intelligence of offspring. N Engl J Med 1991;325:911–916.
29. Fagen C, King JD, Erick M. Nutrition management in women with gestational diabetes mellitus: A review by ADA's Diabetes Care and Education dietetic practice group. J Am Diet Assoc 1995;95:460–467.
30. American Diabetes Association: Clinical practice recommendations. Nutrition recommendations and principles for people with diabetes mellitus. Diabetes Care. 20 1997;(Suppl 1): S14–S17.
31. Infante-Rivard C, Fernandez A, Gauthier R, David M, Rivard GE. Fetal loss associated with caffeine intake before and during pregnancy. JAMA 1993;270:2940–2943.
32. Luke B, Murtaugh MA. Dietary management. In: Reece EA, Coustan DR, eds. Diabetes Mellitus in Pregnancy, 2nd ed. Churchill Livingstone, New York, 1995, pp 191–200.
33. Weller KA. Diagnosis and management of gestational diabetes. Am Fam Physician 1996;53:2053–2057;2061–2062.
34. Mulford MI, Jovanovic-Peterson, L, Peterson CM. Alternative therapies for the management of gestational diabetes. Clin Perinatol 1993;20:619–634.
35. Jovanovic-Peterson L, Peterson CM. Rationale for prevention and treatment of glucose–mediated macrosomia: A protocol for gestational diabetes. Endocr Pract 1996;2:118–129.
36. Piacquadio K, Hollingsworth DR, Murphy H. Effects of in-utero exposure to oral hypoglycaemic drugs. Lancet 1991;338:866–869.
37. McManus RM, Ryan EA. Insulin requirements in insulin-dependent and insulin-requiring GDM women during final month of pregnancy. Diabetes Care 1992;15:1323–27.
38. Bloomgarden ZT. The 32nd Annual Meeting of the European Association for the Study of Diabetes. Diabetes Care 1997;20:902–904.
39. DeVeciana M, Major CA, Morgan MA, et al. Postprandial versus preprandial blood glucose monitoring in women with gestational diabetes mellitus requiring insulin therapy. N Engl J Med 1995;333:1237–1241.
40. Rosenn BM, Miodovnik M, Holcberg G, Khoury JC, Siddiqi T. Hypoglycemia: the price of intensive insulin therapy for pregnant women with insulin-dependent diabetes mellitus. Obstet Gynecol 1995;85:417–422.
41. Kimmerle R, Heinemann L, Delecki A, Berger M. Severe hypoglycemia: incidence and predisposing factors in 85 pregnancies of type I diabetic women. Diabetes Care 1992;15:1034–1037.
42. Steel JM, Johnstone FD, Hume R, Mao JH. Insulin requirements during pregnancy in women with type I diabetes. Obstet Gynecol 1994;83:253–258.
43. Jovanovic-Peterson L, Peterson CM. The art and science of maintenance of normoglycemia in pregnancies complicated by insulin-dependent diabetes mellitus. Endocr Pract 1996;2:130–143.
44. Cryer PE. Hypoglycemia: The limiting factor in the management of IDDM. Diabetes 1994;43:1378–1389.
45. American College of Obstetricians and Gynecologists. Ultrasonography in pregnancy. ACOG Technical Bulletin 187. Washington, DC, 1993.
46. Becerra JE, Khoury MJ, Cordero JF, Erickson JD. Diabetes mellitus during pregnancy and the risks for specific birth defects: a population-based case-control study. Pediatrics 1990;85:1–9.
47. Martin AO, Dempsey LM, Minogue J, et al. Maternal serum a–fetoprotein levels in pregnancies complicated by diabetes: implications for screening programs. Am J Obstet Gynecol 1990;163:1209–1216.
48. American College of Obstetricians and Gynecologists. Diabetes and pregnancy. ACOG Technical Bulletin 200. Washington, DC, 1994.
49. Landon MB, Gabbe SG. Fetal surveillance in the pregnancy complicated by diabetes mellitus. Clin Perinatol 1993;20:549–560.
50. American College of Obstetrics and Gynecology. Antepartum surveillance. ACOG Technical Bulletin 188. Washington, DC, 1994.
51. Nageotte MP, Towers CV, Asrat T, Freeman RK. Perinatal outcome with the modified biophysical profile. Am J Obstet Gynecol 1994;170:1672–1676.

52. American College of Obstetricians and Gynecologists. Fetal macrosomia. ACOG Technical Bulletin 159. Washington, DC, 1991.

53. Moses RG. The recurrence rate of gestational diabetes in subsequent pregnancies. Diabetes Care 1996;19:1348–1350.

54. O'Sullivan JB. Diabetes mellitus after GDM. Diabetes 1991;40(Suppl 2):131–139.

55. Damm P, Kuhl C, Bertelsen A, Molsted-Pedersen L. Predictive factors for the development of diabetes in women with previous gestational diabetes mellitus. Am J Obstet Gynecol 1992;167:607–616.

56. Metzger BE, Cho NH, Roston SM, Radvany R. Prepregnancy weight and antepartum insulin secretion predicts glucose tolerance five years after gestational diabetes mellitus. Diabetes Care 1993;16:1598–1605.

57. Greenberg LR, Moore TR, Murphy H. Gestational diabetes mellitus: antenatal variables as predictors of postpartum glucose intolerance. Obstet Gynecol 1995;86:97–101.

58. Beischer NA, Wein P, Sheedy MT, Mackay IR, Rowley MJ, Zimmet P. Prevalence of antibodies to glutamic acid decarboxylase in women who have had gestational diabetes. Am J Obstet Gynecol 1995;173:1563–1569.

59. Dacus JV, Meyer NL, Muram D, Stilson R, Phipps P, Sibai BM. Gestational diabetes: Postpartum glucose tolerance testing. Am J Obstet Gynecol 1994;171:927–931.

60. Mestman JH, Schmidt–Sarosi C. Diabetes mellitus and fertility control: contraception management issues. Am J Obstet Gynecol 1993;168:2012–2020.

61. Stubblefield PG. Contraception. In: Copeland LJ, Jarrell JF, McGregor JA, eds. Textbook of Gynecology. Saunders, Philadelphia, 1993, pp.156–188.

62. Miller PB, Soules MR. The usefulness of a urinary LH kit for ovulation prediction during menstrual cycles of normal women. Obstet Gynecol 1996;87:13–17.

63. Sapire KE. The female condom (Femidom): a study of user acceptability. S Afr Med J 1995;85(Suppl 10):1081–1084.

64. American College of Obstetricians and Gynecologists. The Intrauterine Device. ACOG Technical Bulletin 164. Washington DC, 1992.

65. American College of Obstetrics and Gynecology. Hormonal Contraception. ACOG Technical Bulletin 198. Washington DC, 1994.

66. Peterson KR, Skouby SO, Jepsen PV, Haaber AB. Diabetes regulation and oral contraceptives. Lipoprotein metabolism in women with insulin dependent diabetes mellitus using oral contraceptives. Ugeskr Laeger 1996;158:2288–2292.

67. Barrett DH, Anda RF, Escobedo LG, Croft JB, Williamson DF, Marks JS. Trends in oral contraceptive use and cigarette smoking. Behavior Risk Factor Surveillance System, 1982 and 1988. Arch Fam Med 1994;3:438–443.

68. Poulter NR, Chang CL, Farley TM, Marmot MG. Reliability of data from proxy respondents in an international case–control study of cardiovascular disease and oral contraceptives. World Health Organization Collaborative Study in Cardiovascular Disease and Steroid Hormone Contraception. J Epidemiol Community Health 1996;50:674–680.

69. Petitti DB, Sidney S, Quesenberry CP Jr., Bernstein A. Incidence of stroke and myocardial infarction in women of reproductive age. Stroke 1997;28:280–283.

70. World Health Organization. A multinational case-control study of cardiovascular disease and steroid hormone contraceptives. Description and validation of methods. World Health Organization Collaborative Study of Cardiovascular Disease and Steroid Contraception. J Clin Epidemiol 1995;48:1513–1547.

71. Westhoff C. Depot medroxyprogesterone acetate contraception. Metabolic parameters and mood changes. J Reprod Med 1996;41(Suppl 5):401–406.

72. Frederiksen MC. Depot medroxyprogesterone acetate contraception in women with medical problems. J Reprod Med 1996;41(Suppl 5):414–418.

73. American College of Obstetrics and Gynecology. Sterilization. ACOG Technical Bulletin 222. Washington, DC, 1996.

74. Rosenn B, Miodovnik M, Kranias G, et al. Progression of diabetic retinopathy in pregnancy: association with hypertension in pregnancy. Am J Obstet Gynecol 1992;166:1214–1218.

75. Prudy LP, Hantsch C, Molitch ME, et al. Effect of pregnancy on renal function in patients with moderate-to-severe diabetic renal insufficiency. Diabetes Care 1996;1067–1074.

76. Gordon M, Landon MB, Samuels P, Hissrich S, Gabbe SG. Perinatal outcome and long-term follow-up associated with modern management of diabetic nephropathy. Obstet Gynecol 1996;87:401–9.

77. Holley JL, Bernardini J, Quadri KH, Greenberg A, Laifer SA. Pregnancy outcomes in a prospective matched control study of pregnancy and renal disease. Clin Nephrol 1996;45:77–82.

78. Miodovnik M, Rosenn BM, Khoury JC, Grigsby JL, Siddiqi TA. Does pregnancy increase the risk for development and progression of diabetic nephropathy? Am J Obstet Gynecol 1996;174:1180–1189.
79. Kimmerle R, Zass RP, Somville T, et al. Pregnancies in women with diabetic nephropathy: long-term outcome for mother and child. Diabetologia 1995;38:227–35.
80. Briggs GG, Freeman RK, Yaffe SJ, eds. Drugs in pregnancy and lactation, 4th ed. Williams & Wilkins, Baltimore, pp. 832–833.
81. Kjos SL, Henry O, Lee RM, Buchanan TA, Mishell DR. The effect of lactation on glucose and lipid metabolism in women with recent gestational diabetes. Obstet Gynecol 1993;82:451–455.
82. Hammond-McKibben D, Dosch HM. Cow's milk, bovine serum albumin, and IDDM: can we settle the controversies? Diabetes Care 1997;20:897–901.
83. Pausi K, McFarland KF. Management of diabetes in pregnancy. Am Fam Physician 1997;55:2731–2738.

11

An Algorithm for Diabetes Management During Glucocorticoid Therapy of Nonendocrine Disease

Susan S. Braithwaite, MD, Walter G. Barr, MD, Amer Rahman, MD, and Shaista Quddusi, MD

CONTENTS

INTRODUCTION

For the patient who has pre-existing type 1 or type 2 diabetes mellitus or the patient with new-onset of diabetes during glucocorticoid therapy ("steroid diabetes"), glucocorticoid therapy of nonendocrine disease poses dilemmas. Glucocorticoid therapy exacerbates hyperglycemia, and tapering of a glucocorticoid dose without adjustment of diabetes therapy may result in severe hypoglycemia.

To address the need for an operational guideline on how to prevent emergencies and meet standards of care with respect to glycemic control, an algorithm is suggested for monitoring and management of diabetes mellitus during glucocorticoid therapy of nonendocrine disease.

LITERATURE REVIEW

Methods

As an adaptation of heuristics concerning the general management of diabetes, an algorithm about diabetes management during glucocorticoid therapy evolved. In an effort to justify and modify the algorithm, Medline was searched from 1966 to August 1997 for human reports on glucocorticoids and [hyperglycemia or diabetes mellitus]. To uncover reports that might relate metabolic emergencies to specific glucocorticoid care plans, the retrieved articles were reviewed for additional and earlier citations. Original

From: *Contemporary Endocrinology: Hormone Replacement Therapy*
Edited by: A. W. Meikle © Humana Press Inc., Totowa, NJ

reports and studies *(1–58)* and English-language reviews *(59–65)* were selected according to the presence of information about pathophysiology, predictors, incidence, complications, and treatment of steroid diabetes in nonpregnant adults or adolescents. Additive effects, possibly attributable to cyclosporin or other immunosuppressive therapy, were not reviewed.

Cases of diabetic metabolic emergency were classified as ketoalkalosis, hypoglycemia, ketoacidosis, or hyperosmolar coma. Ketoacidosis was identified if either the diagnosis was stated by the authors, could be inferred from the case description or was documented by inclusion of chemistries. Reports of ketonuria without ketoacidosis were reviewed, but are not included here as cases of metabolic emergency. Because mixed pictures of ketoacidosis and diabetic hyperosmolar state were recognized, because classification varied among authors, and because biochemical data was incomplete in many of the reviewed cases, it was difficult to apply a consistent classification rule. Therefore, for the reader, case iteration is used as the method of clarifying classification according to type of metabolic emergency.

The retrieval did not recover any study designed to evaluate diabetes management plans during glucocorticoid therapy. Therefore recommendations on diagnosis and monitoring of diabetes and conventional insulin management of type 2 diabetes and type 1 diabetes were reviewed, as stated in current monographic publications and clinical practice guidelines of the American Diabetes Association (ADA) *(66–72)* and other authoritative literature about diabetes mellitus *(73–86)*. Some of these sources referred to the topics of patient eduction, glucose monitoring, or insulin management during glucocorticoid therapy *(60,66,78,87)*.

Occurrence of Steroid Diabetes

Steroid diabetes has been reported in several series to occur in 0–46.2% of glucocorticoid-treated adult patients *(4,7,11,15,21,30,32,33,37,39,42,50,53,57)*. Family history of diabetes, present in 33–80% of cases *(2,12,32,33,37,42)*, and glucocorticoid dose *(2,12,42,57)* have emerged as possible predictors of this complication. Steroid diabetes, if it is to occur, usually appears early, for example, within the first 1 to 3 mo after renal transplant *(32,33,37,39,42,55)*.

Occurrence of Diabetic Metabolic Emergency During Glucocorticoid Therapy

There are no prospective data about frequency or predictors of metabolic emergency during glucocorticoid therapy. Short-term therapy *(21,88)* and intra-articular injection *(89–93)* generally carry low risk to patient safety. In small retrospective series about glucocorticoid treatment, the complication of diabetic ketoacidosis is reported occasionally, and hyperosmolar coma is reported in 3–27% of diabetic patients (Table 1). Conversely, in a small retrospective series of 135 patients hospitalized for diabetic hyperosmolar state (some of whom also were acidotic), which included a 28% incidence of nursing-home residents, compared against 135 age-matched hospitalized controls, the use of glucocorticoids by hyperosmolar patients ($n = 10$) was not significantly different from use by controls ($n = 6$) *(51)*.

In the literature review, 62 cases of diabetic metabolic emergency during glucocorticoid therapy were identified, with 10 fatalities (Table 2). There was one example of "diabetic ketoalkalosis" *(94–96)*, in this instance probably promoted by antecedent vomiting and several months of ambulatory corticotropin and glucocorticoid treatment *(5)*.

Table 1
Frequency of Steroid Diabetes, Hyperosmolar States, and Diabetic Ketoacidosis in Retrospective Series Reporting These Complications

Cases/series	Medical condition	Steroid diabetes/ patients in series	Number of cases (Percent of diabetic patients)	
			Hyperosmolar Coma	Ketoacidosis
Ranney 1957 (4)	Leukemia, lymphoma	5/34 (14.7%)		2 (40%)
Smyllie 1968 (21)	Respiratory disease	9/550 (1.6%)		
Ruiz 1973 (32)	Renal transplant	15/253 (5.9%)	1 (7%)	1 (7%)
Hill 1974 (33)	Renal transplant	12/31 (39.7%)	1 (8%)	1 (8%)
Woods 1975 (37)	Renal transplant	11/202 (5.4%)	3 (27%)	
David 1980 (39)	Renal transplant	31/286 (10.8%)		
Arner 1983 (42)	Renal transplant	67/145 (46.2%)		
Thomas 1987 (50)	SLE and other connective tissue disease	8/	2 (25%)	
Shi 1989 (53)	SLE, pemphigus, chronic nephritis	28/286 (9.8%)	4 (14%)	

Table 2
Reported Cases of Metabolic Emergency During Glucocorticoid Therapy

Classification of cases	Diabetic ketoacidosis	Hyperosmolar coma
Total reviewed	17	43
Fatalities	1	8
Setting		
Ambulatory	10	18
Hospitalized	2	4
Not determinable	5	21
Duration of glucocorticoid therapy		
>2 wk	12	19
≤2 wk	1	8
Not determinable	4	16

There was 1 case of hypoglycemia, occurring in conjunction with sulfonylurea therapy of steroid diabetes following adrenalectomy and proving fatal (23). An unpublished case of insulin-induced hypoglycemia with seizure has been observed by one of the present authors during ambulatory tapering of glucocorticoid therapy initiated in the hospital for obstructive airway disease. During glucocorticoid treatment of nonendocrine disease, in the reviewed literature there were no cases of hypoglycemia. There were 17 cases of ketoacidosis (two cases on p. 411 of ref. 4, cases 1–2 [18], case 3 [24], cases 1–4 [25], case 1 [32], and the ketoacidosis cases in refs. 3,8,10,33,45,58). There were 43 cases identified as hyperosmolar coma (cases 1 and 2 of ref. 24, case 10 [32], cases 3, 5, and 11 [37], case W.H. and T.G. [50], and the hyperosmolar cases in refs. 8,9,13,14,17,19,20,26–29,33,43,46,51–53). One hyperosmolar case was precipitated by intra-articular injection of glucocorticoid *(52)* and one by alternate-day therapy in combination with hydrochlorothiazide *(46)*, and two were complicated by thrombotic events *(13,26)*.

Not all cases of metabolic emergency could be classified according to setting or duration of glucocorticoid treatment at onset. Some occurred during hospitalization, sometimes for massive-dose therapy. A majority of cases of ketoacidosis (60%) occurred in the ambulatory setting. A majority of cases of ketoacidosis and at least a plurality of cases hyperosmolar coma occurred during glucocorticoid treatment of greater than 2 wk duration (≥70% and ≥44%, respectively), sometimes during tapering of the glucocorticoid regimen *(26,50)*. However, at least three of the fatalities in the hyperosmolar coma group occurred during ambulatory glucocorticoid therapy that had been of less than 2 wk duration.

In summary, among reviewed diabetic metabolic emergencies occurring during glucocorticoid therapy, the number of each type was: severe hypoglycemia, 1; ketoalkalosis, 1; ketoacidosis, 17; and hyperosmolar coma, 43. The numbers of fatalities were one each in association with hypoglycemia and ketoacidosis and eight with hyperosmolar coma. Many of the foregoing cases occurred before monitoring of capillary blood glucose had gained widespread acceptance. Although this historical review may not provide an accurate impression of present-day risk, nevertheless the data underscore the importance of active preventive measures.

Occurrence of Chronic Complications of Diabetes During Glucocorticoid Therapy

There is a paucity of objective data on chronic complications of diabetes among glucocorticoid-treated patients, but there is abundant evidence on the importance of metabolic control to other diabetic populations *(80,97)*. Therefore during long-term glucocorticoid therapy the prevention of diabetic microvascular complications is an appropriate concern.

Authority for an Algorithm About Diabetes Management During Glucocorticoid Therapy

In the literature review there was a paucity of information about diabetes management during glucocorticoid therapy. From current monographic publications and clinical practice guidelines of the American Diabetes Association and other authoritative literature about diabetes, general recommendations are available on diagnosis, monitoring and conventional insulin management of type 2 diabetes and Type 1 diabetes. These citations are included as authority for the algorithm even though they are not based on data specific to the glucocorticoid-treated patient.

The principles of the algorithm with supporting references include: diagnosis of diabetes based upon venous plasma glucose concentrations *(69)*, avoidance of urine glucose monitoring for diagnosed diabetes *(71)*, self-monitoring of blood glucose by patients with diabetes (SMBG) *(72,87)*, tight glycemic control standards during relatively stable glucocorticoid therapy intended to be long-term *(70)*, modified glycemic control standards during periods of instability (target range premeal glucose having an upper bound of 200 mg/dL and during tapering a lower bound of 120 mg/dL) *(85)*, nonreliance upon glycosylated hemoglobin results during intervals of instability of control *(84)*, conservative dosing during initiation or adjustment of intermediate-acting insulin *(82,98)*, twice-daily injections of mixed intermediate- and short-acting insulin ("split-mixed" regimens) *(66,87)*, regular insulin supplementation for premeal hyperglycemia *(66)*, a rule for calculation of the supplement (an adaptation from sick-day management plans for type 1 diabetes) *(83)*, potential need for large supplemental doses *(78)*, the "two-thirds" rule for conversion from short-acting to intermediate-acting insulin management (adaptation of a venerable inpatient heuristic) *(73)*, specific ratios of morning to evening insulin and of intermediate- to short-acting insulin *(68,74)*, use of insulin infusion *(77,86)*, potential compensation for alternate-day variability of hyperglycemia during alternate-day glucocorticoid therapy *(49,87)*, gaining experience on insulin dosing through previous treatment courses with the same patient *(87)*, and need for individualization of therapy *(87)*.

For those patients who require revision or initiation of hypoglycemic treatment during glucocorticoid therapy, the only agent covered under the algorithm is insulin. The sulfonylureas currently marketed in the United States require gradual dosage adjustment and control steroid diabetes only infrequently or inconsistently *(12,42,53,55)*. There is insufficient evidence in glucocorticoid-treated patients to determine whether some who require evening insulin would be well served by daytime sulfonylurea therapy. The underlying disease may raise safety considerations that contraindicate metformin, and data on efficacy of metformin for steroid diabetes is limited *(12)*. Potential use of alpha-glucosidase inhibitors, meglitinides, or thiazolidinedione drugs *(99)* for steroid diabetes remains to be tested in man.

THE ALGORITHM

Patient Population

Unless otherwise specified the algorithm applies to ambulatory as well as hospitalized patients. Initiation of therapy refers to the first exposure of patients to glucocorticoid therapy in doses equivalent to at least 30–60 mg prednisone daily. Tapering refers to decrements from pharmacologic to physiologic doses of glucocorticoids, or rapid discontinuation of short-term therapy. For patients who under similar conditions of general health have received comparable courses of glucocorticoid therapy in the past, review of previous experience may permit management during glucocorticoid rechallenge that is simplified in comparison to what is described below.

The algorithm focuses on the needs of patients not yet treated with insulin or type 2 diabetes patients who use conventional insulin management plans. Patients having type 1 diabetes and patients who already are proficient at insulin self-management, including users of multiple daily injection plans or continuous subcutaneous insulin infusion, may benefit from algorithms more complex than what is described below. Use of the algorithm should be complemented by individualization of therapy when glycemic targets are not met.

Beneficial glucocorticoid therapy should not be denied to patients having diabetes. However, whenever possible, patients without known diabetes should be screened with a fasting venous plasma glucose, and diabetic patients should be rendered normoglycemic before starting glucocorticoids. Those who are poorly controlled when first starting glucocorticoids, who are extremely insulin resistant, who are at risk of dehydration, and/or who have any of the usual risk factors for hyperosmolar coma should be followed with special vigilance.

A Recommendation to Categorize Patients
Before Initiation of Glucocorticoid Therapy According
to Presence or Absence of Diabetes and by Glucocorticoid Treatment Plan

At initiation of glucocorticoid therapy patients should be classified as diabetic or nondiabetic. Diabetic patients should be further categorized according to glucocorticoid treatment plan to determine diabetes management strategies. Table 3 shows a proposed categorization, consisting of single injections of glucocorticoid or glucocorticoid therapy that will be rapidly tapered and discontinued over the short term (< 2 wk) (category 1); fixed-dose short-term therapy (< 2 wk) or intermediate-term therapy (2-4 wk) (category 2); and long-term therapy (> 4 wk) (category 3).

The categorization is used to establish target ranges for blood glucose, recommendations on preserving or adjusting the dose of intermediate acting insulin, and indications for newly starting insulin therapy, that differ according to glucocorticoid treatment plan. All of these high-dose glucocorticoid treatment plans place patients at potential risk *(57)*, and therefore the only potential candidates for observation without use of insulin in the face of hyperglycemia are those whose treatment is brief, i.e. patients receiving single-injections of glucocorticoid or rapidly-tapering regimens (category 1). Modified glycemic control targets are recommended for certain unstable glucocorticoid-treated patients (category 1 and 2). These targets differ from those appropriate to stable patients (category 3). They are derived from modified glycemic control targets that are applicable to hospitalized patients, under a similar rationale *(85)*.

Glucose Monitoring for All Patients Receiving Glucocorticoid Therapy

All ambulatory patients should perform glucose monitoring. For ambulatory patients without known diabetes, urine testing should be cost-effective and sufficient for detection of impending hyperglycemic crisis if performed twice daily at the initiation of therapy and three times weekly during long-term therapy. For all ambulatory patients in whom the diagnosis of diabetes is made, SMBG should be recommended. The physician conducting glucocorticoid therapy also should determine the fasting venous plasma glucose concentration before initiation of glucocorticoid therapy and at periodic intervals for hospitalized patients and, for ambulatory patients, initially at 1–2-wk intervals.

Glucocorticoid Therapy for Nondiabetic Patients

The patient should receive education on the possibility that diabetes mellitus will occur. Special educational emphasis is necessary for the elderly and their caregivers, for other patients at high risk for hyperosmolar coma, for patients having a family history of type 2 diabetes and for those receiving high-dose glucocorticoid therapy or intermediate-to-long term therapy (longer than 2–4 wk). The appearance of glycosuria or hyperglycemia requires confirmation of the diagnosis of diabetes by fasting venous plasma glucose criteria, education on SMBG, and treatment.

Target Blood Glucose Ranges for Patients
with Diabetes During Glucocorticoid Therapy

For patients who receive glucocorticoid therapy that will be long term (> 4 wk), the target blood glucose is 80–120 mg/dL before meals and 100–140 mg/dL at bedtime (category 3). For patients who receive fixed-dose short-term therapy (< 2 wk) or inter-

Table 3
**Target Blood Glucose Ranges and Indications for Newly Starting Insulin
for Patients with Known Diabetes, According to Glucocorticoid Treatment Plan**

Glucocorticoid Treatment Plan	Target Range Blood Glucose	Indications for Newly Starting Insulin Therapy
Category 1 Single injections of glucocorticoid Glucocorticoid therapy that will be rapidly tapered and discontinued over the short term (< 2 wk)	Premeal 120–200 mg/dL for those receiving insulin therapy	Individualization based on metabolic risk
Category 2 Fixed-dose, short-term therapy (< 2 wk) Intermediate-term therapy (2–4 wk)	Premeal 80–200 mg/dL	Premeal glucose over 140 mg/dL or current use of oral agents
Category 3 Long-term therapy (> 4 wk)	Premeal 80–120 mg/dL, bedtime 100-140 mg/dL	Premeal glucose over 140 mg/dL or current use of oral agents

mediate term glucocorticoid therapy (2–4 wk), the upper bound of the target range may be increased to 200 mg/dL (category 2).

For insulin-treated patients during rapid glucocorticoid tapering regimens that result in discontinuation or reduction from pharmacologic to physiologic doses of glucocorticoids within 2 wk, and for those who receive a single injection of glucocorticoid or glucocorticoid therapy that will be rapidly tapered and discontinued over the short-term (< 2 wk), the target range glucose is 120–200 mg/dL before meals (category 1). For slower glucocorticoid tapering regimens, the target range glucose is 80–120 mg/dL before meals and 100–140 mg/dL at bedtime.

Initiation of Glucocorticoid Therapy for Patients with Recognized Diabetes, Not Yet Taking Insulin

Patients with recognized diabetes not yet taking insulin should perform SMBG at least twice a day during initiation of glucocorticoid therapy. Not every patient with known diabetes will require revision of therapy with hypoglycemic drugs during glucocorticoid treatment *(35)*. For those who receive a single injection of glucocorticoid or short-term glucocorticoid therapy that will be rapidly tapered and discontinued within 2 wk (category 1), observation of hyperglycemia often is reasonable. Nevertheless, during short-term glucocorticoid therapy some patients become candidates for supplemental premeal regular insulin because they present special risk factors for hyperosmolar coma, because monitoring suggests impending metabolic emergency, or because they will require repeated courses of glucocorticoids. A starting dose might be 4 U for premeal blood glucose 141–240 and 8 U for blood glucose over 240 mg/dL.

For patients on oral agents for treatment of diabetes or any patients who have mean fasting blood glucose over 140 mg/dL prior to glucocorticoid treatment who will receive fixed-dose short-term, intermediate-term or long-term glucocorticoid therapy (categories 2 and 3), in general insulin should be prescribed. Oral agents, if any, may be discontinued. The physician may start with at least 8–10 U of premixed 70/30 NPH/ regular insulin before breakfast and 4–5 U of premixed 50/50 or 70/30 NPH/regular insulin before supper, or equivalent. Further compensatory supplementation and adjustment of the daily dose will be required, as described under the "rapid insulin adjustment sub-routine" below (Fig. 1).

Initiation of Glucocorticoid Therapy for Patients Already Taking Insulin

During initiation of glucocorticoid therapy, patients should perform SMBG at least QID. When the blood glucose exceeds 300 mg/dL, testing should be performed every 4 h until improvement is seen. Once the glucocorticoid dosage has stabilized, patients with type 2 diabetes may reduce testing to BID, or to QID three days weekly.

The needed adjustment of daily insulin requirement during glucocorticoid therapy is unpredictable but may exceed a 50% increase over the pretreatment requirement *(48)*. For insulin-taking patients who receive a single injection of glucocorticoid or short-term glucocorticoid therapy that will be rapidly tapered and discontinued within 2 wk (category 1), the daily insulin dose should be supplemented with regular insulin, but generally the dose of longer-acting insulin preparations should not be increased unless control prior to glucocorticoid therapy was unsatisfactory. A supplement of regular insulin, as a percent of the daily total dose of insulin, may consist of 20% for blood glucose over 240 mg/dL, or 8 U, whichever is larger, followed by a meal or snack. If the blood glucose exceeds 300 mg/dL, the dose with snack may be repeated every 4 h. Higher doses should be considered if the response is unsatisfactory. In treating hospitalized or experienced ambulatory patients, the physician may recommend more complex algorithms for premeal supplementation, including, for example, 10% supplements of regular insulin for intermediate blood glucose concentrations (141–240 mg/dL).

For insulin-taking patients who receive long-term glucocorticoid therapy (category 3), the daily insulin dose should be supplemented with regular insulin, but in addition the dose of longer-acting insulin should be increased. For some patients on fixed-dose short-term or intermediate-term glucocorticoid therapy (category 2), similar adjustments of daily insulin dose are appropriate; the likelihood of extending treatment duration should influence decisions to adjust longer-acting insulin doses. Normoglycemic patients should make an initial increase of the daily dose of insulin by 10%, and patients having mean fasting blood glucose over 140 mg/dL should increase by 20%. Management is simplified by converting to premixed insulin, giving 2/3 of the daily dose as premixed 70/30 NPH/ regular before breakfast and 1/3 of the daily dose as premixed 50/50 or 70/30 NPH/ regular before supper. For patients with preexisting diabetes who have shown propensity to hypoglycemia or whose daily dose exceeds 80 U, the split-mixed regimen may be converted temporarily to NPH, administered two-thirds before breakfast and one-third before bedtime, in daily amount equal to the total previously given as split-mixed insulin (Fig. 2). Further adjustment of the daily dose will be required, as described under the "rapid insulin adjustment sub-routine" below.

Rapid Insulin Adjustment Subroutine

The heart of the algorithm (Fig. 3) is a "rapid insulin adjustment" sub-routine having as its goal for appropriate patients a safe method of working up the daily dose of split-mixed insulin over several days.

Rapid Upward Insulin Adjustment

Starting daily doses of premixed insulin:

Premixed _70/30_ insulin before breakfast: ___8___ units.

Premixed _70/30_ insulin before supper: ___4___ units.

Supplements of regular insulin:

If premeal blood sugar is over 240 mg/dL before breakfast, lunch or supper, take

___8___ units of regular insulin.

Adjustment of daily doses of premixed insulin:

If yesterday's supplements of regular insulin added up to:	then please increase today's doses of premixed insulin by:
___8___ units	___4___ units before breakfast and
	___2___ units before supper.
___16___ units	___8___ units before breakfast and
	___4___ units before supper.
___24___ units	___12___ units before breakfast and
	___6___ units before supper.

- Test blood glucose before each meal and before the bedtime snack.
- If the premeal glucose exceeds 300 mg/dL twice in a row, call me.
- If you have a hypoglycemic insulin reaction or premeal glucose under 80 mg/dL, call me and do not make any upward adjustment of the premixed insulin.
- This is a **temporary** plan for rapid insulin adjustment.
- Call me every three days at (GET)FBS-GOOD.

Fig. 1. A typical plan is shown for a newly diabetic person or a person with known type 2 diabetes whose treatment is being converted from oral agents to insulin at the time of initiation of glucocorticoid therapy. For simplicity, the daily dose initially may consist of premixed insulin, administered 2/3 before breakfast and 1/3 before supper, using 70/30 NPH/regular insulin before breakfast and 50/50 or 70/30 NPH/regular insulin before supper. The pre-meal supplements initially are about 8 U, and later 8 U or 1/5 of the daily dose, whichever is greater, given as regular insulin for pre-meal glucose exceeding 240 mg/dL. Each day's daily dose may be increased by 2/3 the number of units given as regular insulin the day before. As control improves, supplementation with regular insulin will be discontinued, for pre-meal blood glucose levels consistently between 140–240 mg/dL upward adjustments of the split/mixed NPH/regular insulin doses will be made only every third day, and individualization of treatment plan will occur.

Rapid Upward Insulin Adjustment

New daily doses of NPH insulin:

NPH insulin before breakfast: _72_ units.

NPH insulin before bedtime snack: _36_ units.

Supplements of regular insulin:

If premeal blood sugar is over 240 mg/dL before breakfast, lunch or supper, take

_22_ units of regular insulin.

Adjustment of daily doses of NPH insulin:

If yesterday's supplements of regular insulin added up to:	then please increase today's doses of NPH insulin by:
_22_ units	_10_ units before breakfast and
	_5_ units before bedtime snack.
_44_ units	_20_ units before breakfast and
	_10_ units before bedtime snack.
_66_ units	_30_ units before breakfast and
	_15_ units before bedtime snack.

- Test blood glucose before each meal and before the bedtime snack.
- If the premeal glucose exceeds 300 mg/dL twice in a row, call me.
- If you have a hypoglycemic insulin reaction or premeal glucose under 80 mg/dL, call me and do not make any upward adjustment of the NPH insulin.
- This is a **temporary** plan for rapid insulin adjustment.
- Call me every three days at (GET)FBS-GOOD.

Fig. 2. A typical plan is shown for person with known type 2 diabetes who had satisfactory control on 108 U of split/mixed insulin at the time of initiation of long-term glucocorticoid therapy. The example demonstrates the option of temporary conversion of the daily dose to NPH insulin, administered before breakfast and bedtime, with 2/3 of the daily dose before breakfast and 1/3 before the bedtime snack. Supplementation with premeal regular insulin is calculated as in Fig. 1. As control improves, the total daily dose will be converted from NPH insulin to an individualized split/mixed NPH/regular regimen administered before breakfast and supper, and for premeal blood glucose levels consistently between 140-240 mg/dL upward adjustments of insulin dose will be made only every third day.

Concern about hypoglycemia may be raised by the physicians, nursing staff, or patients because the peak actions of supplements of regular insulin will overlap the peak actions of split-mixed insulin as recommended under the rapid insulin adjustment subroutine. In response to those concerns, it should be noted first that the risk of hypoglycemia is reduced during high-dose glucocorticoid therapy because of insulin resistance *(1,2,44,54)*, and adequacy of the total daily insulin dose may be a more important

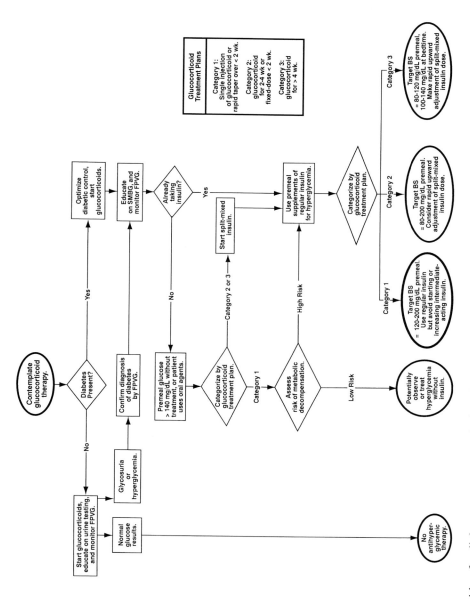

Fig. 3. An algorithm for diabetes management during glucocorticoid therapy of nonendocrine disease. FVPG, fasting venous plasma glucose. SMBG, self-monitoring of blood glucose.

consideration. Second, peak effects of insulin cannot be assumed to occur at the anticipated times when large doses are injected *(75)*; the actions of both regular and NPH insulin potentially are prolonged. Nevertheless, to address possible concerns about overlapping peak actions of insulin for patients requiring supplementation with regular insulin, an alternative plan is outlined under which the daily dose may be converted temporarily to split-dose NPH insulin rather than split-mixed NPH-regular insulin.

The daily dose is administered as either as split-mixed NPH-regular insulin before breakfast and supper or NPH insulin before breakfast and bedtime. In addition, premeal supplements of regular insulin should be taken before breakfast, lunch or supper. The next day, an increase of the daily dose of premixed or NPH insulin should be made in an amount equal to two-thirds of the number of units given as supplemental regular insulin the day before.

A premeal supplement, as number of units or percent of the daily total dose of insulin, whichever is higher, may consist of 8 units or 20% for blood glucose over 240 mg/dL before breakfast, lunch or supper (some experienced patients will also use 4 units or 10% for blood glucose 141–240 mg/dL). If the blood glucose exceeds 300 mg/dL, the dose with snack should be repeated every four hours, and if the response is unsatisfactory higher doses of supplemental regular insulin should be considered. For patients with severe fasting hyperglycemia increased hepatic glucose output contributes to the pathophysiology *(54)*. Patients like this may need insulin supplements in high dosage around the clock to gain initial control.

If hypoglycemia occurs the supplement of regular insulin should be reduced to perhaps 4 U or 10% for blood glucose over 240 mg/dL, and timing should be considered as a possible factor. The physician should be alert to the possibility of late snowballing of effect of large doses of subcutaneous insulin; hypoglycemia may occur after supplementation with regular insulin has been discontinued, necessitating a reduction of daily dosage.

For ambulatory patients premeal supplementation with regular insulin should be discontinued once premeal glucose readings are under 240 mg/dL, and at that point upward adjustments of daily dose should be made only every third day. Those who have been receiving the daily dose as NPH should be converted to a split-mixed regimen, administered two-thirds before breakfast as 70/30 premixed NPH/regular and one-third before supper as 50/50 or 70/30 NPH/regular insulin, in amount equal to the total previously given as a daily NPH dose. If premeal blood glucose levels have been under 240 mg/dL but have exceeded 140 mg/dL without episodes of hypoglycemia on the preceding 3 d, a 10% increase of the daily dose should be made.

Individualization of therapy is especially important as the patient begins to approach good control. Some patients taking a mixture of NPH/regular insulin at supper will have poor control at bedtime but hypoglycemia in the early morning. They are the ones who may fare better with a 50/50 than 70/30 mixture of NPH/regular insulin at supper or may do best without any intermediate acting insulin at night, taking only presupper regular insulin. Those patients using a small dose of glucocorticoid taken only in the morning sometimes may need no evening dose of insulin at all.

Some ambulatory patients are able implement their own insulin adjustments (Figs. 1 and 2), telephoning only every few days. The "rapid insulin adjustment" subroutine is also helpful to house officers. For patients not proficient at self-management, closer telephone surveillance is mandatory. If ambulatory therapy fails, for dehydration or impending hyperosmolar coma the patient may require hospitalization. In the dehydrated individual intravenous infusion is the best route to ensure absorption of insulin.

For already-hospitalized diabetic patients with poor control or perioperative patients having extreme insulin resistance due to high-dose glucocorticoid therapy, again insulin infusion may be the preferred therapy. The starting rate of insulin infusion for euglycemic patients with glucocorticoid-induced insulin resistance may be 2 U/h. To maintain glucose levels in the target range of 120–200 mg/dL the rate may have to be adjusted to 4 U/h or more. To correct greater degrees of hyperglycemia, higher rates of infusion are needed, following an initial priming bolus of intravenous insulin. About 2 h before the intravenous infusion is discontinued, subcutaneous split-mixed NPH-regular insulin should be administered. If all else is stable and if the insulin infusion rate has been consistent, it may be estimated that the needed amount of daily subcutaneous insulin is about 80% of the amount of intravenous insulin used during the preceding 24 h.

Tapering of Glucocorticoid Therapy for Patients Taking Insulin

During glucocorticoid tapering regimens, because severe hypoglycemia is judged a greater risk than moderate short-term hyperglycemia, there should be anticipatory reductions of the daily insulin dose. A special risk of hypoglycemia occurs when there is a change-over of care givers during glucocorticoid tapering, as may happen at the time of hospital discharge. The outpatient physician should be involved in discharge planning, but patient knowledgeability on self-adjustment is the best safety net.

It is expected that in most cases of new-onset steroid diabetes, resolution of the diabetic state will occur after discontinuation of glucocorticoid therapy (2,55,87). If insulin has been newly started because of the glucocorticoids, there is a good chance of insulin discontinuation by the time the glucocorticoid dosage reaches physiologic levels. If oral agents had been required for diabetic control prior to glucocorticoid therapy, they often might be resumed after discontinuation. Patients who required insulin prior to glucocorticoid therapy are likely to continue to require insulin. In order to anticipate the reduction of their daily insulin dose during glucocorticoid tapering, it is useful to review the augmentation of daily dose that occurred during glucocorticoid treatment.

Whenever a decrement in glucocorticoid dose is planned, if during the preceding three days the blood glucose has been less than 140 before meals or 160 mg/dL before bedtime, part of the anticipated reduction of the insulin dose should made, often by about 15–20% of the total daily insulin dose. When the daily insulin dose is less than 12–20 U, conversion to oral agents or insulin discontinuation may be considered.

Alternate-Day Glucocorticoid Treatment Plans

Some patients report greater daily variability of glycemic control than others. Since some patients require alternate-day insulin plans, individualization is necessary.

CONCLUSION

The suggested algorithm is merely a starting point for diabetes management during glucocorticoid therapy of nonendocrine disease. The algorithm addresses the need to prevent emergencies and meet standards of medical care for glycemic control. The physician must be prepared to modify the plan depending on patient characteristics and response. Further research on the pathogenesis and clinical behavior of steroid diabetes and outcomes research will be needed to determine the ideal treatment algorithm.

ACKNOWLEDGMENTS

The authors are indebted to Daniel Braithwaite, Sonya Chertkov, Mariko Inoue-King, Chen Yi Lin, Gene Michalik, and László Szilágyi for assistance in translation.

REFERENCES

1. Ingle DJ, Sheppard R, Evans JS, Kuizenga MH. A comparison of adrenal steroid diabetes and pancreatic diabetes in the rat. Endocrinology 1945;37:341–356.
2. Bookman JJ, Drachman SR, Schaefer LE, Adlersberg D. Steroid diabetes in man. Diabetes 1953;2:100–111.
3. Berg E-G. Nil nocere!: Über Schäden und Nebenwirkungen bei der therapeutischen Verwendung von Cortison and ähnlichen Steroidhormonen. Münchener Medizinische Wochenschrift 1956;98: 1614–1622.
4. Ranney HM, Gellhorn A. The effect of massive prednisone and prednisolone therapy on acute leukemia and malignant lymphomas. Am J Med 1957;22:405–413.
5. Simpson JR. Steroid diabetes: case report. Harper Hosp Bull 1957;15:43–51.
6. Grilliat JP, Kornig F, Vaillant G. Diabetes occurring during deltacortisone therapy of cirrhosis. Rev méd Nancy 1959;84:720–727.
7. Baldwin HS, Dworotzky M, Isaacs NJ. Evaluation of the steroid treatment of asthma since 1950. J Allergy 1961;32:109–118.
8. Gregory RL, Sayle BA. Steroid diabetes. Texas State J Med 1962;58:788–793.
9. Mach RS, DeSousa RC. Coma avec hyperosmolalité et déshydratation chez des malades hyper-glycémiques sans acidocétose. Schweizerische Medizinische Wochenschrift 1963;93:1256–1263.
10. Blereau RP, Weingarten CM. Diabetic acidosis secondary to steroid therapy. N Engl J Med 1964;271:836
11. Keeney EL. The condition of asthmatic patients after daily long-term corticosteroid treatment. Arizona Med 1964;21:463–469.
12. Miller SEP, Neilson JM. Clinical features of the diabetic syndrome appearing after steroid therapy. Postgrad Med J 1964;40:660–669.
13. Brocard H, Akoun G, Grand A. Diabéte stéroïde compliqué d'un coma de type hyperosmolaire. Bulletins et Memoires de la Société Médicale des Hôpitaux de Paris 1965;116:353–363.
14. Schwartz TB, Apfelbaum RI. Nonketotic diabetic coma. Yearbook Endocrinol 1965;1965–1966 series:165–181.
15. Walsh, Grant IWB. Corticosteroids in treatment of chronic asthma. Br Med J 1966;2:796–802.
16. Boyer MH. Hyperosmolar anacidotic coma in association with glucocorticoid therapy. JAMA 1967;202:95–97.
17. Plauchu M, Paliard P, Malluret J, Noel P, De Montgolfier R. Un nouveau cas d'état d'hyperosmolarité plasmatique ou de coma hyperosmolaire déclenché par les corticoïdes chez un diabétique latent, porteur d'une lymphose. Lyons M 1967;217:1921–1932.
18. Zangel V, Masszi J. Ketozisba átmenö steroid-diabetes három esete. Orvosi Hetilap 1967;108:395–396.
19. Kumar RS. Hyperosmolar non-ketotic coma. Lancet 1968;1:48–49.
20. Pyörälä K, Suhonen O, Pentikäinen P. Steroid therapy and hyperosmolar non-ketotic coma. Lancet 1968;1:596–597.
21. Smyllie HC, Connolly CK. Incidence of serious complications of corticosteroid therapy in respiratory disease: a retrospective survey of patients in the Brompton Hospital. Thorax 1968;23:571–581.
22. Williams ER. Systemic lupus erythematosus and diabetes mellitus. Br J Clin Practice 1968;22:461–463.
23. Arai J, Miyakawa Y, Kataoka K, Matsuki S, Asano S. Case of fatal hypoglycemic coma during sulfo-nylurea administration for the therapy of steroid diabetes following adrenalectomy. Saishin Igaku Recent Med 1969;24:2524–2529.
24. Spenney JG, Eure CA, Kreisberg RA. Hyperglycemic, hyperosmolar, nonketoacidotic diabetes: a com-plication of steroid and immunosuppressive therapy. Diabetes 1969;18:107–110.
25. Alavi IA, Sharma BK, Pillay VKG. Steroid-induced diabetic ketoacidosis. Am J Med Sci 1971; 262:(1)15–23.

26. Corcoran FH, Granatir RF, Schlang HA. Hyperglycemic hyperosmolar nonketotic coma associated with corticosteroid therapy. J Florida Med Assoc 1971;58:38–39.

27. Limas CJ, Samad A, Seff D. Hyperglycemic nonketotic coma as a complication of steroid therapy. NY State J Med 1971;71:1542–1543.

28. Szewczyk Z, Ratajczyk T, Rabczynski J. Hyperosmotic coma in steroid–induced diabetes complicating subacute glomerulonephritis in a 16-year-old boy. Polski Tygodnik Lekarski 1971;26:1988–1990.

29. Daouk AA, Malek GH, Kauffman HM, Kisken WA. Hyperosmolar non-ketotic coma in a kidney transplant recipient. J Urol 1972;108:524–525.

30. Lieberman P, Patterson R, Kunske R. Complications of long-term steroid therapy for asthma. J Allergy Clin Immunol 1972;49:329–336.

31. Owen OE, Cahill GF. Metabolic effects of exogenous glucocorticoids in fasted man. J Clin Invest 1973;52:2596–2605.

32. Ruiz JO, Simmons RL, Callender CO, Kjellstrand CM, Buselmeier TJ, Najarian JS. Steroid diabetes in renal transplant recipients: pathogenetic factors and prognosis. Surgery 1973;73:759–765.

33. Hill CM, Douglas JF, Rajkumar KV, McEvoy J, McGeown MG. Glycosuria and hyperglycaemia after kidney transplantation. Lancet 1974;2:490–492.

34. Kendall-Taylor P. Hyperosmolar coma in Cushing's disease. Lancet 1974;1:409.

35. Klein W. Treatment with glucocorticoids in diabetic patients. Zeitschrift fur Allgemeinmedizin 1974;50:1101–1106.

36. Simmons RL, Kjellstrand CM, Buselmeier TJ, Najarian JS. Glycosuria and hyperglycaemia after kidney transplantation. Lancet 1974;2 (letter):844.

37. Woods JE, Zincke H, Palumbo PJ, Johnson WJ, Anderson CF, Frohnert PP, et al. Hyperosmolar nonketotic syndrome and steroid diabetes: occurrence after renal transplantation. JAMA 1975;231:1261–1263.

38. Gunnarsson R, Arner P, Lundgren G, Magnusson G, Ostman J, Groth CG. Steroid diabetes after renal transplantation: a preliminary report. Scandinavian Journal of Urology and Nephrology 1977;42:191–194.

39. David DS, Cheigh JS, Braun DW, Fotino M, Stenzel KH, Rubin AL. HLA-A28 and steroid-induced diabetes in renal transplant patients. JAMA 1980;243:532–533.

40. Pagano G, Lombardi A, Ferraris GM, Imbimbo B, Cavallo-Perin P. Acute effect of prednisone and deflazacort on glucose tolerance in prediabetic subjects. Eur J Clin Pharmacol 1982;22:469–471.

41. Perlman K, Ehrlich RM. Steroid diabetes in childhood. Am J Dis Childhood 1982;136:64–68.

42. Arner P, Gunnarsson R, Blomdahl S, Groth C-G. Some characteristics of steroid diabetes: a study in renal-transplant recipients receiving high-dose corticosteroid therapy. Diabetes Care 1983;6:23–25.

43. Fujikawa LS, Meisler DM, Nozik RA. Hyperosmolar hyperglycemic nonketotic coma. A complication of short-term systemic corticosteroid use. Ophthalmology 1983;90:1239–1242.

44. Pagano G, Cavallo-Perin P, Cassader M, Bruno A, Ozzello A, Masciola P. An in vivo and in vitro study of the mechanism of prednisone-induced insulin resistance in healthy subjects. J Clin Invest 1983;72:1814–1820.

45. Ivanova II, Vasiutkova LA, Ivanov VA. Hyperglycemic coma after corticosteroid therapy. Sovetskaia Meditsina 1984;10:112–113.

46. Lohr R. Precipitation of hyperosmolar nonketotic diabetes on alternate-day corticosteroid therapy (letter). JAMA 1984;252:628.

47. Ferguson RP. A comparison of steroid and thiazide diabetes. Connecticut Medicine 1986;50:506–509.

48. Bruno A, Cavallo-Perin P, Cassader M, Pagano G. Deflazacort vs prednisone: effect on blood glucose control in insulin-treated diabetics. Arch Intern Med 1987;147:679–680.

49. Greenstone MA, Shaw AB. Alternate day corticosteroid causes alternate day hyperglycaemia. Postgrad Med J 1987;63:761–764.

50. Thomas JW, Vertkin A, Nell LJ. Antiinsulin antibodies and clinical characteristics of patients with systemic lupus erythematosus and other connective tissue diseases with steroid induced diabetes. J Rheumatol 1987;14:732–735.

51. Wachtel TJ SR, Lamberton P. Predisposing factors for the diabetic hyperosmolar state. Arch Intern Med 1987;147:499–501.

52. Black DM, Filak AT. Hyperglycemia with non-insulin-dependent diabetes following intraarticular steroid injection. J Family Practice 1989;28:(4)462–463.

53. Shi MZ, Zhang SF. Steroid diabetes: an analysis of 28 cases. Chinese J Intern Med 1989;28:139–141.

54. Ekstrand AV. Effect of steroid-therapy on insulin sensitivity in insulin-dependent diabetic patients after kidney transplantation. J Diabetic Complic 1991;5:(4)244–248.

55. Hricik DE, Bartucci MR, Moir EJ, Mayes JT, Shulak JA. Effects of steroid withdrawal on posttransplant diabetes mellitus in cyclosporine–treated renal transplant recipients. Transplantation 1991;51: 374–377.

56. Ogawa A, Johnson JH, Ohneda M, McAllister CT, Inman L, Alam T, et al. Roles of insulin resistance and ß–cell dysfunction in dexamethasone–induced diabetes. J Clin Investig 1992;90:497–504.

57. Gurwitz JH, Bohn RL, Glynn RJ, Monane M, Mogun H, Avorn J. Glucocorticoids and the risk for initiation of hypoglycemic therapy. Arch Int Med 1994;154:97–101.

58. Haggerty RD, Bergsman K, Edelson GW. Steroid-induced diabetic ketoacidosis. Practical Diabetology 1995;14:24–25.

59. McMahon M, Gerich J, Rizza R. Effects of glucocorticoids on carbohydrate metabolism. Diabetes Metab Rev 1988;4:17–30.

60. Genuth SM. Diabetes secondary to other endocrine dysfunctions. Clinical Diabetes 1990;8:74–79.

61. O'Byrne S FJ. Effects of drugs on glucose tolerance in non-insulin dependent diabetes (part I and II). Drugs 1990;40:203–219.

62. Caldwell JR, Furst DE. The efficacy and safety of low-dose corticosteroids for rheumatoid arthritis. Seminars in Arthritis and Rheumatism 1991;21:(1)1–11.

63. Pandit MK BJ, Gustafson AB. Drug-induced disorders of glucose tolerance. Ann Intern Med 1993;118:529–540.

64. Kirwan JR. Systemic corticosteroids in rheumatology. In: Klippel JH, Dieppe PA, eds. Rheumatology. Mosby, London, 1994:1–6.

65. Hetenyi G, Jr., Karsh J. Cortisone therapy: a challenge to academic medicine in 1959–1952. Perspect Biol Med 1997;40:426–439.

66. Kayne DM, Holvey SM. Drugs and hormones that increase blood glucose levels. In: Lebovitz HE, DeFronzo RA, Genuth S, Kreisberg RA, Pfeifer MA, Tamborlane WV, eds. Therapy for diabetes mellitus and related disorders, 2nd ed. American Diabetes Association, Alexandria, 1994, pp. 185–190.

67. Raskin P, Beebe CA, Davidson MB, Nathan D, Rizza RA, Sherwin R, eds. Pharmacologic intervention. In: Medical management of non-insulin-dependent (Type II) diabetes, 3rd ed. American Diabetes Association, Alexandria, 1994, pp. 40–49.

68. Santiago JV, Goldstein DE, Haymond M, Heins J, Schiffrin A, Simonson DC, et al., eds. Insulin treatment. In: Medical Management of Insulin–Dependent (Type I) Diabetes, 2nd ed. American Diabetes Association, Alexandria, 1994, pp. 35–51.

69. Expert Committee on the Diagnosis and Classification of Diabetes Mellitus AD. Report of the expert committee on the diagnosis and classification of diabetes mellitus. Diabetes Care 1997;20:1183–1197.

70. American Diabetes Association. Standards of medical care for patients with diabetes mellitus (position statement). Diabetes Care 1997;20:(Suppl 1)S5–S13.

71. American Diabetes Association. Urine glucose and ketone determinations (position statement). Diabetes Care 1996;19:(Suppl 1)S35.

72. American Diabetes Association. Self-monitoring of blood glucose (consensus statement). Diabetes Care 1996;19:S62–S66.

73. Metz R, Nice M, LaPlaca G. Evaluation of an eight-hour therapeutic regimen in uncontrolled diabetes. Diabetes 1967;16:341–345.

74. Skyler JS, Seigler DE, Reeves ML. A comparison of insulin regimens in insulin-dependent diabetes mellitus. Diabetes Care 1983;5:11–18.

75. Zinman B. The physiologic replacement of insulin: an elusive goal. N Engl J Med 1989;321:363–370.

76. Genuth S. Insulin use in NIDDM. Diabetes Care 1990;13:1240–1264.

77. Gavin LA. Perioperative management of the diabetic patient. Endocrinol Metab Clinics North Amer 1992;21:457–473.

78. Home PD, Alberti KGMM. Insulin therapy. In: Alberti KGMM, DeFronzo RA, Keen H, Zimmet P, eds. International Textbook of Diabetes Mellitus. John Wiley & Sons Ltd., Chichester, 1992:831–864.

79. Koivisto VA. Insulin therapy in type II diabetes. Diabetes Care 1993;16:29–39.

80. Lasker RD. The diabetes control and complication trial: implications for policy and practice. N Engl J Med 1993;329:1035–1036.

81. Zinman B. Insulin regimens and strategies for IDDM. Diabetes Care 1993;16:24–28.

82. Rosenzweig JL. Principles of insulin therapy. In: Kahn CR, Weir GC, eds. Joslin's Diabetes Mellitus, 13th ed. Lea & Febiger, Philadelphia, 1994, pp. 460–488.

83. Wolfsdorf JI, Anderson BJ, Pasquarello C. Treatment of the child with diabetes. In: Kahn CR, Weir GC, ed. Joslin's Diabetes Mellitus, 13th ed. Lea & Febiger, Philadelphia, 1994, pp. 530–551.

84. Goldstein DE, Little RR, Lorenz RA, Malone JI, Nathan D, Peterson CM. Tests of glycemia in diabetes. Diabetes Care 1995;18:896–909.
85. Hirsch IB, Paauw DS, Brunzell J. Inpatient management of adults with diabetes. Diabetes Care 1995;18:870–878.
86. Hawkins JB, Morales CM, Shipp JC. Insulin requirement in 242 patients with type II diabetes mellitus. Endocrine Practice 1996;1:385–389.
87. Siminerio LM, Carroll PB. Educating secondary diabetes patients. Diabetes Spectrum 1994;7:8–14.
88. Coles RS. Steroid therapy in uveitis. Int Ophthalmol Clin 1966;6:869–901.
89. Koehler BE, Urowitz MB, Killinger DW. The systemic effects of intra-articular corticosteroid. J Rheumatol 1974;1:(1)117–125.
90. Gottlieb NL, Riskin WG. Complications of local corticosteroid injections. JAMA 1980;243:(15)1547–1548.
91. Armstrong RD, English J, Gibson T, Chakroborty J, Marks V. Serum methylprednisolone levels following intra–articular injection of methylprednisolone acetate. Ann Rheum Diseases 1981;40:571–574.
92. Bertouch JV, Meffin PJ, Sallustio BC, Brooks PM. A comparison of plasma methylprednisolone concentrations following intra–articular injection in patients with rheumatoid arthritis and osteoarthritis. Aust NZ J Med 1983;13:583–586.
93. Weiss S, Kisch ES, Fischel B. Systemic effects of intraarticular administration of triamcinolone hexacetonide. Isr J Med Sci 1983;19:83–84.
94. Lim KC, Walsh CH. Diabetic ketoalkalosis: a readily misdiagnosed entity. Br Med J 1976;2:19.
95. Sanders G, Boyle G, Hunter S, Poffenbarger PL. Mixed acid-base abnormalities in diabetes. Diabetes Care 1978;1:362–364.
96. Pearson DW, Thomson JA, Kennedy AC, Toner PG, Ratcliffe JG. Diabetic ketoalkalosis due to ectopic ACTH production from an oat cell carcinoma. Postgrad Med J 1981;57:455–456.
97. The Diabetes Control and Complications Trial Research Group. The effect of intensive treatment of diabetes on the development and progression of long-term complications in insulin-dependent diabetes mellitus. N Engl J Med 1993;329:977–986.
98. Braithwaite SS, Barr WG, Thomas JD. Diabetes management during glucocorticoid therapy of nonendocrine disease. Endocr Prac 1996;2:320–325.
99. Weinstein SP, Holand A, O'Boyle F, Haber RS. Effects of thiazolidinediones on glucocorticoid-induced insulin resistance and GLUT4 glucose transporter expression in rat skeletal muscle. Metab Clin Exp 1993;42:1365–1369.

12

Management of the Exercising Diabetic

Robert E. Jones, MD

CONTENTS

INTRODUCTION

Diabetes mellitus is characterized by hyperglycemia resulting from either an absolute or relative insulin deficiency, and affects over 16 million people in the United States. Diabetes is classified into several types *(1)*, but the most frequently encountered categories are types 1 and 2 diabetes. Type 1 diabetes results from pancreatic-cell destruction, which causes in an absolute insulin deficiency. On the other hand, type 2 diabetes is characterized initially by insulin resistance followed by a progressive decline in insulin secretion *(2)*.

In addition to the use of hypoglycemic agents, the management of diabetes includes both dietary planning and suggestions for regular physical exercise. Whereas exercise has been shown to be beneficial in the treatment of diabetes through its effects on improving insulin sensitivity *(3)* and assisting with weight control, there are significant potential dangers associated with exercise in diabetics. For example, vigorous exercise in patients treated with insulin or sulfonylureas may be associated with hypoglycemia during or following the event, and, occasionally, the micro- or macrovasular complications associated with diabetes may be aggravated by participation in an exercise program. A variety of techniques may be implemented to reduce the risk of hypoglycemia in physically active diabetics and careful attention to the presence of existing complications should identify those individuals who are at risk for potential exacerbation due to exercise.

METABOLIC RESPONSES TO EXERCISE

The biochemical and hormonal responses to exercise are dependent on a variety of factors. For example, the degree of prior conditioning, the intensity of exercise, and the

From: *Contemporary Endocrinology: Hormone Replacement Therapy*
Edited by: A. W. Meikle © Humana Press Inc., Totowa, NJ

duration of the activity all play major roles in the adaptive responses and type of substrate fluxes noted during exercise.

Energy demands during exercise are met through the oxidation of fatty acids and glucose, and the synthesis and storage of these depot fuels, glycogen and triglycerides, is dependent on insulin. In addition, the glucose counterregulatory hormones, cortisol, growth hormone, catecholamines, and glucagon, either actively or permissively facilitate substrate mobilization by enhancing gluconeogenesis, lipolysis, or glycogenolysis. The concerted interplay between insulin and these counter-regulatory hormones allows for constancy of blood glucose levels and provides additional substrates for oxidation. During exercise in nondiabetic people, insulin levels fall, resulting in the mobilization of free fatty acids and the facilitation of gluconeogenesis from muscle-derived lactic acid and glycerol from adipocytes. Additionally, the decline in insulin concentration is also associated with cessation of glycogen synthesis in both muscle and liver, while permissively allowing glycogenolysis.

Exercise in Type 1 Diabetes

In contrast to normal individuals, insulin levels in type 1 diabetics are basically unregulated because of their reliance on injected insulin. If the type 1 patient is underinsulinized, substrate production and mobilization are unrestrained owing to the lack of opposition of the counterregulatory hormones. This may result in an exaggeration of preexisting hyperglycemia and may predispose to the development of ketoacidosis. If the patient is overinsulinized at the time of exercise, hypoglycemia will result owing to augmentation of tissue glucose uptake and suppression of hepatic gluconeogenesis. This insulin-induced stimulation of glucose uptake in muscle clearly augments noninsulin mediated glucose disposal that is already activated in exercising muscle *(4)*. Additionally, the suppression of lipolysis from elevated insulin levels also results in an impaired delivery of free fatty acids to myocytes and indirectly increases the oxidation of glucose because of the glucose-sparing actions of intracellular lipids.

Exercise in Type 2 Diabetes

The effects of exercise in type 2 diabetics are nearly identical but, because basal insulin secretion is generally maintained in these patients, the risk of developing ketoacidosis is nonexistent. However, if the patient is poorly controlled prior to exercise, a worsening of hyperglycemia may be observed. Similar to the risk seen with type 1 diabetics, type 2 patients treated with either insulin or a sulfonylurea may experience hypoglycemia during exercise. On the other hand, hypoglycemia is extremely rare in diabetics using metformin *(5)* and has not been described with the use of either glucosidase inhibitors or thiazolidinediones.

AVOIDANCE OF HYPOGLYCEMIA

Fatigue may be the only manifestation of a mild hypoglycemic reaction. As the degree of hypoglycemia increases, the sympathetic nervous system is activated, and, if corrective measures are not taken, neuroglycopenia may occur. The hypoglycemic effects of exercise may persist for many hours after completion of the event owing to delays in replenishment of hepatic or muscle glycogen and to the effect of exercise on enhancing insulin sensitivity. Post-exercise, late-onset hypoglycemia has been observed in young type 1 diabetics and may occur up to 24 h following strenuous exercise *(6)*.

Nutritional Supplements

Either adding nutritional supplements prior to exercise or reducing the insulin dosage are the mainstays of therapeutic approaches to prevent exercise-induced hypoglycemia *(7)*. Depending on specific circumstances, they can be used together or individually, but there can be no substitution for meticulous monitoring of capillary blood glucose before, during, and after exercise in order to assess the regimen or to prevent hypoglycemia. Ideally, exercise should be planned when blood glucose levels are highest, which is generally 1–3 h following a meal. Prior to exercise, blood glucose levels should be between 100 and 200 mg/dL (5.5–11.1 m*M*). If the patient is severely hyperglycemic (glucose in excess of 300 mg/dL or 16.7 m*M*), activity should be delayed in order to prevent an exacerbation of diabetic control. Relative pre-exercise hypoglycemia (glucose less than 80 mg/dL or 4.4 m*M*) should be treated by supplemental carbohydrate. Consumption of 15–20 g of readily absorbable carbohydrate is generally sufficient to prevent hypoglycemia during exercise.

Supplemental calories should be consumed immediately before and every 30–60 min during exercise. Simple carbohydrates, up to 40 g for adults and 25 g for children may be used, however, occasionally this approach is associated with an excessive glycemic excursion and may exacerbate fluid losses that normally occur during exercise. Dietary supplements containing a balanced mixture of complex carbohydrates, protein and fat such as whole milk *(8)* may provide a more prolonged, even absorption of glucose. This will provide longer protection against hypoglycemia without tending to dramatically elevate blood glucose levels. Usually, dietary supplementation is all that is required to prevent hypoglycemia during less strenuous exercise of modest duration (less than 45 min).

Alterations in Medical Regimen

Alterations in insulin dosage are usually necessary prior to more intense or extended periods of exercise. Lowering the amount of insulin projected to peak during the event by 15–25% is generally adequate to prevent exercise-induced hypoglycemia. Elite athletes may reduce their insulin dosage up to 40% prior to engaging in exhaustive competitions *(9)*. All adjustments in insulin dosage are dependent on the types of insulin employed, the schedule of injections and the time of day the exercise period is planned. For example, an exercise session that is planned prior to noon may necessitate a reduction in the dose of rapid-acting insulin administered in the morning. If a midafternoon event is scheduled, lowering the amount of intermediate-acting insulin may be needed. Patients who are managed with a single daily injection of intermediate-acting insulin may display a deterioration in control of fasting glucose levels if their dosage of insulin is decreased in order to accommodate an exercise session. In order to avoid this problem, the patient should be placed on twice-daily injections of insulin, and specific adjustments in dosage can be made on the timing of the exercise period. Patients managed using intensive, conventional insulin therapy based, on a regimen of ultralente and pre-prandial injections of a rapid-acting insulin such as regular or insulin lispro, frequently do not need any alteration in their dose of ultralente but should not use rapid-acting insulin prior to the event. A similar strategy can be taken for patients using an insulin pump that delivers a continuous supply of basal insulin. Generally, the basal rate does not need to be lowered, but boluses should be avoided prior to exercise. If the patient on an insulin pump is participating in either a water or contact sport, the pump should be disconnected and the tubing capped prior to the event. Once the insulin pump has been discontinued, which results in cessation of insulin delivery, the patient is at an increased risk for developing ketosis owing to the decline in insulin and the concurrent increase in counterregulatory hormones induced by exercise.

Therefore, the patient should be monitored closely, and the time off the pump should be kept to a minimum. Insulin lispro has gained in popularity for patients using a subcutaneous insulin-infusion device, and, because of its extremely short half-life, patients using this insulin in their pumps should be advised to limit their time off the pump to less than 3 h *(10)*. If the patient is using regular insulin in their pump, the time off the pump is longer and may be prolonged up to 4 h.

Other factors influencing the kinetics of insulin absorption must be considered while advising patients about avoiding exercise-related hypoglycemia. Local factors, such as increased blood flow can enhance the absorption of insulin from the injection site *(11)*, and patients should be advised to refrain from administering insulin into an extremity that will be exercised. Increased insulin sensitivity is one of the benefits derived from exercise, and physically active patients may develop lower insulin requirements as a consequence. Indeed, it is common to see reductions in insulin requirements ranging between 20–50% as patients improve their conditioning levels.

The phenomenon of post-exercise late-onset hypoglycemia can result in severe episodes of nocturnal neuroglycopenia and can be avoided by counseling the patient to increase their evening caloric intake and closely monitor capillary blood glucose levels. If the patient is just beginning an exercise program or is unaccustomed to an increased degree of physical activity, it may be prudent to prophylactically reduce the amount of insulin taken in the evening following exercise *(6)*.

There are a paucity of data concerning the use of oral hypoglycemics in patients participating in athletics. Sulfonylureas have been associated with prolonged or recurrent events of hypoglycemia, and it may be prudent to avoid the use of these agents in the management of diabetics who are participating in an intensive conditioning program or engaging in competitive sports. If the patient has failed diet therapy, these patients should be placed on insulin or changed to another oral agent not associated with hypoglycemia, such as troglitazone or acarbose. Using metformin in this circumstance may be inadvisable, owing to possible development of lactic acidosis secondary to exercise-induced hypoxemia or acidosis *(5)*.

Treatment and preventative measures against hypoglycemia are reviewed in Tables 1 and 2.

EFFECTS OF EXERCISE ON DIABETIC CONTROL AND COMPLICATIONS

It is clear that exercise has beneficial effects on both glucose homeostasis and insulin sensitivity, but several studies *(12–14)* have failed to document an improvement in long-term diabetic control in patients engaging in regular exercise or sports. However, short-term improvements in glycemic control have been noted *(15)*. The explanations underlying these observations are unclear, but may be related to pre-exercise carbohydrate loading *(9)*. This may result in hyperglycemia at the onset and during the event, or to overcorrection of hypoglycemia *(12)* either during or following exercise, or to physiologic barriers *(16)* described in type 2 diabetics. In addition to the immediate effects of

Table 1
Symptoms and Management of Hypoglycemia

Degree of hypoglycemia	Symptoms	Treatment	Return to activity
Mild	Fatigue, weakness, nausea, anxiety, tremor, palpitations	10–15g of readily absorbable carbohydrate	15 min following improvement in symptoms
Moderate	Tachycardia, diaphoresis, headache, mood, and personality changes	10–20 g of readily absorbable carbohydrate	15 min following improvement in symptoms
	Stupor, somulence, apathy	Observe patient closely following initial therapy; retreat for recurrent symptoms	Consider termination of activity
Severe	Loss of consciousness or seizures	Administer glucagon 1 mg IM or SC or give 50% dextrose IV	Medical reevaluation before exercising

Adapted with permission from ref. *25.*

Table 2
Recommendations for Pre-Exercise Planning

Schedule exercise 1–3 h after eating.
Pre-existing blood glucose should be between 100 and 200 mg/dL.
If glucose prior to exercise is <80 mg/dL, consume 15–20 g carbohydrate.
If glucose prior to exercise is >300 mg/dL or if urine ketones are positive, delay activity.
Consume carbohydrate immediately prior to and every 30–60 min during exercise.
Reduce insulin dose anticipated to peak during exercise by 15–25%.

Adapted with permission from ref. *7.*

exercise on diabetic control, it has been shown that the benefits of exercise in type 1 diabetics, at least, may persist long after participation in sports and are manifest as a reduction in the risk of macrovascular complications *(17)* without increasing the risk for microvascular complications, such as retinopathy *(18).*

ASSESSMENT GUIDELINES

The recommendations for evaluating a patient prior to participation in sports activities or a general conditioning program are based on the age of the patient, the type of diabetes and the length of time the patient has had diabetes. Because insulin resistance and asymptomatic hyperglycemia typically antedate the diagnosis of type 2 diabetes by several years, duration of illness is less critical in the assessment of type 2 diabetics.

General Assessment

The initial evaluation of the patient should include a general assessment of heath. Any symptoms suggesting vascular disease or pre-existing conditions which could be aggravated by participation in an exercise program should be investigated prior to granting medical clearance. Specific information crucial in assessing the patient with diabetes includes a review of the patient's short and long-term glycemic control, an evaluation of the frequency and duration of hypoglycemic episodes and a systematic investigation to diagnose any complications due to diabetes that could be aggravated by participation in sports.

Glycemic Control

Measuring a hemoglobin A_{1C} is indispensable in determining long-term metabolic control, and a careful review of the results of self-monitoring of capillary blood glucose will give an appraisal of short-term or day-to-day control. If the mean blood glucose is under 155 mg/dL (8.6 mM) and the hemoglobin A_{1C} is 7.2% or less, the patient is under good control *(19)*. On the other hand, a hemoglobin A_{1C} greater than 10% is consistent with poor control, and the patient should be counseled to avoid participation in competitive events, but enrollment in a conditioning program may benefit the overall control. In addition, symptoms of hyperglycemia or changes in weight should be obtained.

Hypoglycemia and Hypoglycemia Unawareness

A careful history of the frequency, duration, and presence of prodromal symptoms of hypoglycemia is also vital. The lack of an adrenergic prodrome to signal hypoglycemia is termed hypoglycemia unawareness and is typically manifest as recurrent, severe episodes of neuroglycopenia. Frequently, these patients also have difficulty in the effective counter-regulation of blood glucose, which results in prolonged episodes of hypoglycemia that generally require medical assistance to facilitate recovery. Obviously, these patients should be precluded from participation in sporting events, such as swimming, scuba diving, or climbing, where a sudden alteration in mental alertness could have drastic consequences. These patients should be encouraged to participate in activities where close supervision is possible. Because both alterations in the insulin regimen or supplemental feedings are used to prevent hypoglycemia during exercise, the history should also be directed to determine if the patient has unusual insulin-absorption kinetics or delayed gastric emptying.

Exercise-Induced Hypertension

Exercise-induced hypertension can be diagnosed by obtaining vital signs before and after moderate exercise *(20)*. This condition is defined as a peak systolic blood pressure greater than 210 mm Hg in men and 190 mm Hg in women *(21)*. If the response to exercise is normal, periodic re-evaluation to exclude exercise-induced hypertension should be undertaken. Although there is no consensus concerning management of these patients, it would be prudent to advise against participation in high-intensity events, and the patient should be directed to sports with low static demands.

Retinopathy

Diabetics with proliferative retinopathy should be excluded from contact sports or events like weightlifting because of the risk of vitreous hemorrhage or retinal detachment possibly resulting in blindness. Routine office funduscopy is usually inadequate to detect peripheral retinal lesions, and consultation with an ophthalmologist or retinal photographs are necessary to exclude retinopathy. It is not necessary to restrict activities of patients with mild background retinopathy or in the absence of retinal findings.

Nephopathy

The earliest manifestation of diabetic nephropathy is the presence of albuminuria or proteinuria *(22,23)*. The most sensitive screening test to detect this complication is the measurement of the microalbumin excretion rate. Although there is no evidence that exercise exacerbates fixed diabetic nephropathy, it may transiently increase the urinary excretion of albumin and protein. Exercising diabetics with incipient nephropathy should be monitored closely with periodic measurements of both creatinine clearance and protein excretion rates in order to ensure stability of renal function. Because of the close linkage between diabetic nephropathy and retinopathy (the renal-retinal syndrome *[24]*), patients with either component should be observed closely for the possible development of either complication.

Neuropathies

Peripheral sensory neuropathies are the most common neurologic complication of diabetes and can predispose to injury because of the risk of overusage owing to an increased pain threshold or because of joint laxity resulting from impaired proprioception. If a patient has normal vibratory and position sense on examination, it is very unlikely they have any significant sensory neuropathy. Dysfunction of the motor nerves is associated with weakness and atrophy, which serve to limit participation in a variety of different activities. Because these symptoms are owing to de-innervation, attempts to improve strength and bulk of the affected muscles are essentially fruitless.

The easiest diagnostic maneuvers to assess for the presence of autonomic neuropathy are determining the blood pressure and pulse response to orthostatic and Valsalva maneuvers. If these are normal, autonomic dysfunction is doubtful. The major clinical complications associated with autonomic neuropathies are diabetic gastroparesis with delayed gastric emptying and striking fluctuations in blood pressure.

Atherosclerosis

Monitored exercise tolerance testing should be considered in all type 2 diabetics over the age of 40 or those who have had the condition for over 10 yr. Type 1 diabetics with a greater than 15-yr history of diabetes should similarly be considered for screening. In addition to an increased risk for coronary-artery disease, diabetics have a several-fold higher chance of developing peripheral vascular disease. Diminished pulses, vascular bruits and delayed capillary refill times should prompt further evaluation of possible vascular insufficiency.

Conditions prompting limitations in sporting activities or conditioning programs are listed in Table 3.

CONCLUSIONS

If patients are carefully screened and counseled prior to participation in sports or a conditioning program, exercise appears beneficial in the management of diabetes and seems not to be associated with precipitating diabetic complications. The major exercise-related difficulty in diabetics is the occurrence of hypoglycemia, which can be immediate or may appear hours following exercise. The judicious use of nutritional supplements prior to and during exercise, coupled with carefully designed alterations in the patient's medical regimen, is generally adequate to avoid this problem. Periodic reassessment of

Table 3
Medical Conditions Potentially Limiting Strenuous Exercise

Hypoglycemia unawareness.
Proliferative diabetic retinopathy.
Persistent hyperglycemia.
Uncontrolled hypertension.
Significant peripheral sensory neuropathy.
Autonomic insufficiency.
Coronary artery disease.
Peripheral vascular disease.
Persistent albuminuria/proteinuria.
Nephropathy.
Noncompliance.

Adapted with permission from ref. *25*.

the patient and a critical review of both short- and long-term diabetic control are crucial in evaluating the efficacy of any therapeutic modifications made to accommodate an exercise program.

REFERENCES

1. Expert Committee on the Diagnosis and Classification of Diabetes Mellitus. Report of the expert committee on the diagnosis and classification of diabetes mellitus. Diabetes Care 1997;20:1183.
2. Seely BL, Olefsky JM. Potential cellular and genetic mechanisms for insulin resistance in the common disorders of diabetes and obesity. In: Moller DE, ed. Insulin Resistance. West Sussex, UK, Wiley, 1993:187–252.
3. Krotkiewski M, Lonnroth P, Mandroukas K, Wroblewski Z, Rebuffe-Svrive M, Holm G, et al. The effects of physical training on insulin secretion and effectiveness and on glucose metabolism in obesity and type 2 (non-insulin dependent) diabetes mellitus. Diabetologia 1985;28:881.
4. Ploug T, Galbo H, Richter EA. Increase muscle glucose uptake during contractions: no need for insulin. Am J Physiol 1984;247:E726.
5. Bailey CJ, Turner RC. Metformin. N Engl J Med 1996;334:574.
6. MacDonald MJ. Postexercise late-onset hypoglycemia in insulin dependent diabetic patients. Diabetes Care 1987;10:584.
7. Horton ES. Role and management of exercise in diabetes mellitus. Diabetes Care 1988;11:201.
8. Nathan DM, Madnek SF, Delahanty L. Programming pre-exercise snacks to prevent post- exercise hypoglycemia in intensively treated insulin dependent diabetics. Ann Int Med 1985;102:483.
9. Koivisto VA, Sane T, Ehyrquist F, Pelkonen R. Fuel and fluid homeostasis during long-term exercise in healthy subjects and type I diabetic patients. Diabetes Care 1992;15:1736.
10. HollemanF, Hoekstra JBL. Insulin lispro. N Engl J Med 1997;337:176.
11. Koivisto V, Felig P. Effects of acute exercise on insulin absorption in diabetic patients. N Engl J Med 1978;298:79.
12. Weiliczko MC, Gobert M, Mallet E. The participation in sports of diabetic children. A survey in the Rouen region. Ann Pediatr Paris 1991;38:84.
13. Selam JL, Casassus P, Bruzzo F, Leroy C, Slama G. Exercise is not associated with better diabetes control in type 1 and type 2 diabetic subjects. Acta Diabetol 1992;29:11.
14. Sackey AH, Jefferson IG. Physical activity and glycemic control in children with diabetes mellitus. Diabetes Med 1996;13:789.
15. Stratton R, Wilson DP, Endres RK, Goldstein DE. Improved glycemic control after a supervised eight week exercise program in insulin-dependent diabetic adolescents. Diabetes Care 1987;10:589.
16. Regensteiner JG, Sippel J, McFarling ET, Wolfel EE, Hiatt WR. Effects of non-insulin dependent diabetes on oxygen consumption during treadmill exercise. Med Sci Sports Exerc 1995;27:875.

17. LaPorte RE, Dorman JS, Tajima N, Cruickshanks KJ, Orchard TJ, Cavender DE, Becker DJ, Drash AL. Pittsburgh insulin-dependent diabetes mellitus morbidity and mortality study: physical activity and diabetic complications. Pediatrics 1986;78:1027.
18. Cruickshanks KJ, Moss SE, Klein R, Klein BE. Physical activity and proliferative retinopathy in people diagnosed with diabetes before age 30 years. Diabetes Care 1992;15:1267.
19. American Diabetes Association. Implications of the diabetes control and complications trial. Diabetes Care 1993;16:1517.
20. Blake GA, Levin SR, Koyal SN. Exercise-induced hypertension in normotensive patients with NIDDM. Diabetes Care 1990;7:799.
21. Lauer MS, Levy D, Anderson KM, Plehn JF. Is there a relationship between exercise systolic blood pressure and left ventricular mass? Ann Int Med 1992;116:203.
22. Mogensen CE, Christensen CK. Predicting diabetic nephropathy in insulin-dependent patients. N Engl J Med 1984;311:89.
23. Mogensen CE. Microalbuminuria predicts clinical proteinuria and early mortality in maturity-onset diabetes. N Engl J Med 1984;310:356.
24. Lloyd CE, Orchard TJ. Diabetes complications: the renal-retinal link. An epidemiological perspective. Diabetes Care 1995;18:1034.
25. Jones RE. The diabetic athlete. In: Lillegard W, Butcher JD, Rucker KS, eds. Handbook of Sports Medicine: A Symptom-Oriented Approach, 2nd ed. Butterworth Heinmann, Newton, MA, 1998.

V   ADRENAL

13 Glucocorticoids for Postnatal Treatment of Adrenal Insufficiency and for the Prenatal Treatment of Congenital Adrenal Hyperplasia

Lynnette K. Nieman, MD,
and Kristina I. Rother, MD

Contents

INTRODUCTION

Adrenal Insufficiency

Untreated, complete glucocorticoid insufficiency causes circulatory collapse and death. Although uncommon, the possibility of this endocrine emergency engenders vigilance, both for a new diagnosis of adrenal insufficiency as well as for exacerbation of a chronic known condition. Conversely, overtreatment of adrenal insufficiency with excessive glucocorticoid carries the morbidity associated with iatrogenic Cushing's syndrome. Thus, glucocorticoid insufficiency presents two major challenges for clinicians—timely diagnosis and appropriate treatment.

CAUSES OF ADRENAL INSUFFICIENCY

The causes of glucocorticoid insufficiency can be defined by the anatomic site of the defect. Primary adrenal insufficiency reflects an inability of the adrenal glands to synthesize steroids, whereas secondary adrenal insufficiency reflects an inability of the hypo-

From: *Contemporary Endocrinology: Hormone Replacement Therapy*
Edited by: A. W. Meikle © Humana Press Inc., Totowa, NJ

thalamic-pituitary unit to deliver corticotropin-releasing hormone (CRH) and/or adreno-corticotropin (ACTH), thus reducing trophic support to otherwise normal adrenal glands. This anatomic distinction results in an important clinical difference: patients with primary adrenal disease tend to have destruction of all layers of the adrenal cortex; as a result, mineralocorticoid, as well as glucocorticoid, function is lost. In contrast, the diminished ACTH levels in patients with secondary adrenal insufficiency markedly decrease cortisol production, but do not affect mineralocorticoid production, so that mineralocorticoid activity is intact.

Primary Adrenal Insufficiency

Primary adrenal insufficiency may be caused by a number of conditions. Autoimmune destruction of the glands is the most common etiology in the US (>80%), and may occur alone or in association with other endocrinopathies. These latter polyglandular failure syndromes tend to present either in childhood (type 1), in association with hypoparathyroidism and mucocutaneous candidiasis (1), or in adulthood (type 2), in association with insulin-dependent diabetes mellitus, autoimmune thyroid disease, alopecia areata, and vitiligo (2). Radiographically, these adrenal glands are small.

Infections cause about 15% of primary adrenal insufficiency, and typically include tuberculosis, systemic fungal diseases (histoplasmosis, coccidiomycosis, blastomycosis), and AIDS-associated opportunistic infections such as cytomegalovirus (CMV) (3). These adrenal glands tend to be large on CT scan.

Recently, there has been increased awareness that adrenal insufficiency may be the first presenting feature of adrenaleukodystrophy (4). This rare (1:25,000) X-linked condition is characterized by deficiency of peroxisomal very long-chain acyl CoA synthetase, the first step in oxidation in peroxisomes. This deficiency results in increased circulating amounts of very long-chained fatty acids (VLCFAs), which can be detected as an increase in plasma C26:0 fatty-acid levels. Incomplete penetrance of the genetic defect and variable accumulation of VLCFAs in adrenal gland, brain, testis, and liver account for the clinical phenotypes, which differ by age and presentation. Cerebral adrenaleukodystrophy, presenting in childhood, is characterized by cognitive and gait disturbances, whereas the adult form, adrenomyeloneuropathy, is characterized by spinal cord and peripheral nerve demyelination. In both forms, accumulation of VLCFAs in the adrenal cortex alter membrane function and inhibit signal transduction by ACTH. Because a substantial minority of patients in both groups present first with adrenal insufficiency, boys and young men with adrenal insufficiency should be screened for adrenaleukodystrophy.

Adrenal tissue may be replaced by bilateral metastases (most commonly primary carcinoma of the lung, breast, kidney, or gut, or primary lymphoma) (5), or by hemorrhage (6), leading to insufficient steroidogenesis. Bilateral adrenalectomy removes all steroidogenic tissue, leaving a life-long deficit.

Medications that inhibit specific enzymatic steps of steroidogenesis, including ketoconazole, mitotane, aminoglutethimide, trilostane, and metyrapone, can cause primary adrenal failure. These medications are usually prescribed in the setting of hypercortisolism to exploit this ability and reduce glucocorticoid production (7). However, this side effect of the imidazole derivatives may not be anticipated in patients treated for fungal disease.

The congenital adrenal hyperplasias (CAH) are a disparate group of genetic diseases that each reflect a deficiency of one of the enzymes needed for adrenal steroidogenesis (8). Patients with nearly complete deficiency of an enzyme required for cortisol synthesis present in childhood with adrenal insufficiency and salt-wasting crisis. This is most problematic in patients with mutation of the 21-hydroxylase (P450c21) or 11-β hydroxylase (P450c11) gene. The increase in ACTH levels caused by cortisol deficiency drives the intact steroidogenic pathways so that there is excessive production of the steroids just proximal to the enzymatic block, 17-hydroxyprogesterone and 11-deoxycortisol, respectively, in 21-hydroxylase and 11β-hydroxylase deficiency. Because of the increased levels of precursor steroids, adrenal androgen levels increase. As a result, severely affected girls may be virilized *in utero*, and less affected girls and women become hirsute after puberty.

The initial presentation of patients with primary adrenal insufficiency is either acute or chronic. The characteristic features of acute adrenal insufficiency include orthostatic hypotension, circulatory collapse, fever, hyperkalemia, hyponatremia, and hypoglycemia. These patients will often prove to have hemorrhage, metastasis, or acute infection and lack the typical history and clinical findings of patients with chronic primary adrenal insufficiency. The latter individuals present with a longer history of malaise, fatigue, anorexia, weight loss, joint and back pain, salt craving, and darkening of the skin. Although hyperpigmentation is dramatic in sun-exposed areas, it is present in other areas also and should be sought in the creases of the hands, extensor surfaces, recent scars, buccal and vaginal mucosa, and nipples. Associated biochemical features include hyponatremia, hypoglycemia, and hyperkalemia.

Secondary Adrenal Insufficiency

Suppression of the hypothalamic-pituitary-adrenal axis by exogenous or endogenous glucocorticoids is the most common cause of secondary adrenal insufficiency. It is important to recognize that this axis may not recover full function for up to 18 mo after cure of Cushing's syndrome *(9)* or discontinuation of medication *(10)*, during which time the patient should receive supplemental steroids in times of physiologic stress (*see* "Adjustment of Glucocorticoid Dose" section). Secondary adrenal insufficiency also may result from structural lesions of the hypothalamus or pituitary gland that interfere with CRH production or transport, or with corticotrope function. This includes tumors, destruction by infiltrating disorders, x-irradiation, and lymphocytic hypophysitis. Although the loss of ACTH function usually is accompanied by other pituitary deficiencies, isolated ACTH deficiency may occur, though rarely *(11)*.

DIAGNOSIS OF ADRENAL INSUFFICIENCY

The diagnosis of adrenal insufficiency rests on biochemical testing. If acute adrenal insufficiency is suspected in a patient without a known diagnosis, blood is obtained for measurement of cortisol when the intravenous line is inserted in preparation for immediate therapy. In patients with adrenal insufficiency, the cortisol value generally will return in the normal or subnormal range. Such a value is inappropriately low for the physiologic state of hypotension in which cortisol values are usually well above 18 μg/dL.

In a nonemergent presentation, the cortisol response to administration of ACTH is the gold standard test of adrenal steroidogenic ability *(12,13)*. In the classic test, 250 μg of ACTH (1-24, cosyntropin) is given either intravenously or intramuscularly at any time of the day. This supraphysiologic dose of ACTH delivers a maximal stimulus to the adrenal gland, so that the peak cortisol response measured 30–60 min later is greater than 18 μg/dL. The actual plasma cortisol value at 30 min is the most consistent measure, and does not change in relationship to the basal cortisol level. Although the absolute increase in cortisol is usually greater than 7 µg/dL, this criterion alone cannot be used to determine adequacy of the response. In particular, critically ill patients with a high basal cortisol level may not show a further increase after ACTH administration. The increased basal value in such patients reflects a normal adrenal response to the stressful condition. It is important to recognize that a normal response to ACTH, 250 µg, may occur in the setting of mild hypothalamic-pituitary disease, particularly of recent onset (14). In this setting, ACTH levels are reduced, but are adequate to sustain some adrenal steroidogenesis, so that cortisol secretion is apparently normal in response to a pharmacologic dose of ACTH.

Other tests, such as the metyrapone stimulation test, insulin-induced hypoglycemia, and lower doses of the ACTH stimulation test (15), may have value in specific circumstances but cannot be advocated as the appropriate initial screening test (13). Both insulin and metyrapone have significant morbidity in individuals who lack appropriate counterregulatory processes. The lower-dose ACTH tests have not yet been fully validated but hold promise.

Primary and secondary adrenal insufficiency may be distinguished by biochemical tests. The basal plasma ACTH in a sensitive RIA is generally above the normal range in primary adrenal insufficiency and may exceed the normal range before the cortisol response to ACTH stimulation is subnormal. Measurement of basal ACTH works as well as the CRH-stimulated ACTH value for discriminating primary and secondary adrenal insufficiency (16). Primary adrenal insufficiency may also be identified by failure of plasma aldosterone to reach 16 ng/dL at 30 min after cosyntropin, as normal individuals, and those with secondary adrenal insufficiency exceed this value (17).

Individuals suspected of having congenital adrenal hyperplasia should undergo additional measurement of steroids just before and after the enzymatic block to delineate the site of enzymatic deficiency, as detailed elsewhere (8). When a family has an affected infant, subsequent prenatal diagnosis for 21-hydroxylase deficiency using molecular probes of the 21-hydroxylase gene (8,18–21), or human leukocyte antigen (HLA) (22) genes, and material obtained from chorionic villous sampling at 8–10 wk gestation is now available, albeit primarily in the research setting. The 21-hydroxylase gene is closely linked to the HLA major histocompatibility complex on chromosome 6, so that affected siblings usually share the identical HLA type. A large number of different mutations have been reported in patients with 21-hydroxylase deficiency, so that molecular diagnosis is not a straightforward commercially available test. These molecular techniques have supplanted diagnostic measurement of 17-hydroxyprogesterone and testosterone in amniotic fluid at 16–18 wk, because they allow for earlier discontinuation of dexamethasone treatment of an unaffected fetus.

TREATMENT OF GLUCOCORTICOID INSUFFICIENCY

Chronic therapy of glucocorticoid insufficiency is designed to provide a physiologic amount of glucocorticoid. This is best done by administering 12–15 mg/M^2 of hydrocortisone daily in one or two oral doses. Ideally, the morning dose is given as soon after waking as possible; for individuals who feel extremely fatigued in the morning as blood levels are increasing, a strategy of taking the medication 30 min before arising may be helpful. Although many patients do well on a single morning dose, others complain of pronounced fatigue in the afternoon and evening. For these individuals, a split dose of hydrocortisone, in which about one third of the daily dose is given around 4 PM may be useful. Many adults complain of insomnia and overly vivid dreams if glucocorticoid is given later in the evening; this timing is best avoided.

Other glucocorticoids may be used for daily replacement therapy with regard to their relative potency to hydrocortisone (Table 1). Of these choices, hydrocortisone offers the advantage of a variety of dose tablets, which allows for fine adjustment and splitting of the daily dose.

Patients with primary adrenal insufficiency should also receive mineralocorticoid. When mineralocorticoid is not given as part of the chronic therapy of primary adrenal insufficiency, often the dose of hydrocortisone or other steroid with mineralocorticoid activity is increased to ameliorate hyperkalemia or salt craving. The problem with this approach is that the amount of administered glucocorticoid activity also increases—beyond the level of physiologic replacement—so that the patient becomes Cushingoid.

In suspected acute adrenal insufficiency, hydrocortisone is the treatment of choice, because it has both glucocorticoid and mineralocorticoid activity. Treatment with intravenous saline for volume expansion, glucose for hypoglycemia, and intravenous hydrocortisone, 100 mg, is started immediately after placement of an intravenous line and withdrawal of blood for documentation of the cortisol value. Patients with adrenal insufficiency will recover blood pressure and normalize symptoms rapidly, usually within an hour. Persistent symptoms should provoke evaluation of other causes.

Adjustment of Glucocorticoid Dose

All patients receiving chronic glucocorticoid replacement therapy should be instructed that they are "dependent" on taking glucocorticoids as prescribed and that failure to take or absorb the medication will lead to adrenal crisis and possibly death. They should also obtain a medical information bracelet or necklace that identifies this requirement (Medic Alert Foundation, 2323 Colorado Ave, Turlock, CA 95382; telephone 1-800-432-5378). Caregivers must educate these patients and their families about how to adjust their medication dosage for mild physiologic stress conditions and how to respond to more severe situations, including when to administer glucocorticoid.

Conventional wisdom recommends that the daily oral glucocorticoid dose be doubled for "stressful" physiologic conditions such as fever, nausea, and diarrhea. Apart from reduced absorption because of vomiting or diarrhea, there is relatively little data in the medical literature to support this requirement. Additionally, this practice may lead to chronic overmedication by the patient because of a liberal interpretation of what constitutes physical stress. Thus, education of when and how to change the dosage of steroid should be reinforced periodically—preferably with written material—and the dangers of excessive steroid use should be emphasized.

Supraphysiologic doses of glucocorticoid are given during maximally stressful situations—for example, in the setting of adrenal crisis, major surgery, trauma, or labor and delivery. (There are few data to support the need for 10-fold the physiologic replacement dose, as opposed to mere replacement, but the safety of not following this practice has not been established.) The patient or a family member should be taught how to administer intramuscular injections and should be given an emergency kit containing prefilled syringes with injectable steroid (dexamethasone 5 mg or hydrocortisone 100 mg). If the patient experiences trauma, vomiting, or is found unconscious, the medication should be

Table 1
Comparison of Commonly Used Glucocorticoids

Cortisone	8–12	25	0.8
Cortisol (hydrocortisone)	8–12	20	1
Prednisone	12–36	5	0.8
Dexamethasone	36–72	0.3	0
Fludrocortisone			250

administered, and the patient should be transported to the hospital. In the hospital, from 100–300 mg of hydrocortisone is given by vein each day, in a split dose every 6–8 h. These increases in oral or parenteral glucocorticoid doses should be continued only for a few days, until the acute event has resolved, and are then tapered by 50% each day until the usual oral dose may be resumed.

Glucocorticoid therapy may require adjustment when the metabolism of the agent might be altered. In particular, hyperthyroidism increases—and hypothyroidism decreases—the metabolism of glucocorticoids so that the administered dose of medication may need to be adjusted dramatically. Drugs such as rifampin, phenobarbital, and phenytoin, which induce hepatic microsomal enzymes that catabolize steroids, reduce the bioavailability of these agents.

Evaluation of Therapeutic Efficacy

In the setting of chronic adrenal insufficiency, clinical assessment is the best way to judge whether the glucocorticoid dose is correct. Symptoms of adrenal insufficiency such as nausea, anorexia, and diarrhea ameliorate quickly with the initiation of therapy, and the patient gains lost weight. Joint aches and pains may resolve more slowly. Salt craving decreases in patients with primary adrenal insufficiency when the mineralocorticoid replacement is appropriate.

Although biochemical abnormalities also normalize, these should not be used as an index of appropriate therapy. When glucocorticoid and mineralocorticoid replacement of patients with primary adrenal insufficiency is adequate, plasma ACTH levels decrease but still remain elevated in the range of 100–200 pg/mL. Plasma renin activity, however, normalizes completely and may be used to judge the adequacy of mineralocorticoid replacement. Increases in ACTH alone above 200 pg/mL suggest inadequate glucocorticoid replacement; if both ACTH and renin are increased, the mineralocorticoid dose should be increased before the glucocorticoid dose is adjusted to prevent iatrogenic Cushing's syndrome. Although hydrocortisone is metabolized to cortisol, plasma cortisol values should not be used to monitor therapy, because clearance from the bloodstream is rapid, and circulating values are low for most of the day. Other steroids, such as dexamethasone or prednisone, do not crossreact fully in the cortisol assays; thus, measurement of plasma cortisol does not provide a good measure of adequate replacement if these agents are used.

Clinical features are also the best way to monitor for glucocorticoid excess. The development of a Cushingoid habitus, weight gain, and in children, decreased linear growth, are worrisome, and suggest that the glucocorticoid dose should be decreased. The development of osteopenia is possible with more subtle overreplacement. If the patient is receiving hydrocortisone, increased urine free cortisol provides biochemical evidence that the dose is too high.

Pediatric patients receiving hydrocortisone for classical salt-wasting congenital adrenal insufficiency are monitored using these clinical criteria, and also measurement of the steroid immediately proximate to the enzymatic block *(8)*. Thus, in 21-hydroxylase deficiency, measurement of 17-hydroxyprogesterone provides an indirect index of the ability of administered glucocorticoid to inhibit ACTH secretion. With adequate treatment, morning levels of this index steroid are reduced but not fully normalized. The risk of over-treatment, ultimately leading to short stature from glucocorticoid excess, may be reduced by splitting the hydrocortisone dose into three evenly spaced intervals, and by adequate administration of fludrocortisone. Undertreatment is often signaled by continued excessive linear growth and the development of precocious puberty.

PRENATAL TREATMENT OF CONGENITAL ADRENAL HYPERPLASIA WITH DEXAMETHASONE

Prenatal treatment of a potentially affected fetus is used to prevent virilization of affected females. This approach, first advocated by David and Forest for treatment of 21-hydroxylase deficiency in 1984 *(23)*, is recommended for subsequent pregnancies after an affected child is born to a couple. In this setting, hormonal treatment of the fetus is begun—blind to its affected status and sex—by administering dexamethasone orally to the mother immediately after confirmation of pregnancy in a woman at risk for having affected offspring. This strategy is based on the fact that dexamethasone, when administered to a pregnant woman, is not bound to corticosteroid-binding globulin, crosses the placental barrier, and suppresses fetal ACTH levels, which stimulate adrenal androgen production. Dexamethasone is the agent of choice because as a synthetic fluorinated steroid it is not a ready substrate for 11β-hydroxysteroid dehydrogenase type 2 (11β-HSD-2). In contrast, only a small portion of maternally administered cortisol and prednisolone reaches the fetus in an active form because, at least during the last trimester, both placental and fetal 11β-HSD-2 rapidly convert these active 11-hydroxysteroids to inert 11-keto forms (cortisone, prednisone).

The recommended dexamethasone dose, 20 µg/kg/d in two or three divided doses *(8,19)*, should be started as early as 4–5 wk gestation to prevent virilization of an affected female fetus. Chorionic villous sampling (CVS) is performed at 8–10 wk; if the karyotype analysis reveals that the fetus is male, treatment is stopped. If the fetus is female, treatment is continued until the results of the DNA analysis of the affected gene or HLA type are available, when dexamethasone treatment is either discontinued, or, in the case of an affected female, continued to term.

Effectiveness of Treatment

Dexamethasone reduces genital masculinization in affected females substantially; about half of these infants require no genital surgery, and the rest require less surgical repair *(24–27)*. In keeping with the timing of genital development *in utero*, progression to virilization is reduced (Prader stage 2 or less) with treatment initiation before the 10th wk of gestation but is uniformly more severe (Prader stages 3 or 4) with later initiation of treatment *(26)*. Apart from the reduction in surgery, the additional psychological benefits of ameliorating the genital masculinization are difficult to quantitate in affected patients and their families but are likely to be substantial.

The relationship between increased fetal androgens and lower frequency of marriage and fewer children (28), an increased incidence of lesbian behavior (28,29) or less interest in sexual activity, and a more negative body image (30) reported in affected untreated females is not well understood. The contribution of fetal androgenization as opposed to the contributions of parental uncertainty about the sex assignment, and of the possible psychological trauma of genital surgery have not been distinguished. However, the potential contribution of fetal androgens to "masculinization" of the brain represented by these alterations from the female "norm" has been invoked as an additional reason to initiate early prenatal therapy.

Side Effects of Treatment

Few clear-cut adverse effects have been reported in neonates or children who received prenatal treatment with dexamethasone, but the number of studies and subjects is small. No teratogenic effects have been noted. Most treated newborns have normal weight and length; however, anecdotal reports have suggested an increased risk of fetal death after acute withdrawal of glucocorticoid therapy (in unaffected pregnancies) and possibly an increased incidence of adverse events in children born after short- or long-term prenatal treatment (18,25).

The potential for causing iatrogenic maternal Cushing's syndrome, with its known deleterious effects on fetal and maternal morbidity (31), is a concern. The incidence of significant maternal side effects is low in the first to early second trimester, but increases to between 10–50 % of treated mothers when dexamethasone is continued until term (24–27,32). These adverse effects include Cushingoid features, excessive weight gain, severe cutaneous striae, hypertension, abnormal glucose tolerance, proteinuria, acne, hirsutism, edema, and emotional irritability.

Seckl and Miller have recently summarized the most important current concerns regarding long-term fetal treatment (33). These include unnecessary treatment of unaffected fetuses, the known adverse effects on the mother, and potential adverse effects on the child. If a couple has a child with CAH, only one in four subsequent pregnancies will be affected, and only one in eight will be an affected female; thus, seven out of eight fetuses are treated unnecessarily during the early stages of pregnancy. Although the recommended treatment, 20 µg/kg/d of dexamethasone, is a supraphysiological dose for the mother, it does not consistently prevent virilization of an affected fetus. Other concerns, based in part on animal studies, include the possibility that prenatal glucocorticoid exposure may lead to an increased risk of later cardiovascular disease, to hippocampal damage (34), or to abnormalities in social play, reproductive behavior, avoidance and spatial learning. Regarding the latter point, increased avoidance, shyness, emotionality, and internalizing problems have been reported in children exposed to dexamethasone prenatally (35).

CONCLUSIONS

Prenatal treatment of affected females with 21-hydroxylase deficiency is effective in ameliorating the genital malformations caused by increased androgen concentrations. However, the effectiveness of treatment is unpredictable, and many questions regarding long-term consequences of this treatment remain unanswered. Therefore, we support the view that prenatal treatment with dexamethasone should be viewed as an experimental therapy, and patients should be closely supervised for long periods, optimally by inclusion in institutional review board-approved study protocols.

REFERENCES

1. Ahonen P, Myllarnieini S, Sipila I, Perheentupu J. Clinical variation of autoimmune polyendocrinopathy-candidiasis-ectodermal dystrophy (APECED) in a series of 68 patients. N Engl J Med 1990;322:1829–1836.
2. Betterle C, Volpato M, Greggio AN, Presotto F Type 2 polyglandular autoimmune disease (Schmidt's syndrome). J Pediatr Endocrinol Metab 1996;9 Suppl 1: 113–123.
3. Piedrola G, Casado JL, Lopez E, Moreno A, Perez-Elias MJ, Garcia-Robles R. Clinical features of adrenal insufficiency in patients with acquired immunodeficiency syndrome. Clin Endocrinol (Oxf)1996; 45:97–101.
4. Rizzo WB. X-linked adrenoleukodystrophy: A cause of primary adrenal insufficeincy in males. Endocrinologist 1992;2:177–183.
5. Ihde JK, Turnbull AD, Bajourunas DR. Adrenal insufficiency in the cancer patient: implications for the surgeon. Br J Surg 1990;77:1335–1337.
6. Rao RH, Vagnucci AH, Amico JA. Bilateral massive adrenal hemorrhage: early recognition and treatment. Ann Intern Med 1989;110:227–235.
7. Nieman LK. Cushing's Syndrome Treatment. In: Wayne Bardin C, ed. Current Therapy of Endocrinology and Metabolism. Saunders, Philadelphia, 1996, pp. 609–614.
8. New M.I. Minireview: 21-hydroxylase deficiency congenital adrenal hyperplasia. J Steroid Biochem Molec Biol 1994;48:15–22.
9. Avgerinos PC, Chrousos GP, Nieman LK, et al. The corticotropin-releasing hormone test in the postoperative evaluation of patients with Cushing's syndrome. J Clin Endocrinol Metab 1987;65:906–913.
10. Graber AL, Ney RL, Nicholson WE, et al. Natural history of pituitary-adrenal recovery following long-term suppression with corticosteroid. J Clin Endocrinol Metab 1965;25:11–16,.
11. Yamamoto T, Fukuyama J, Haasegawa K, Sugiura M. Isolated corticotropin deficiency in adults. Report of 10 cases and reveiw of the literature. Arch Intern Med 1992;152:1705–1712.
12. Oelkers H, Diederich S, Bahr V. Diagnosis and therapy surveillance in Addison's disease: rapid adrenocorticotropin (ACTH) test and measurement of plasma ACTH, renin activity, and aldosterone. J Clin Endocrinol Metab 1992;75:259–264.
13. Grinspoon SK, Biller BM. Clinical review 62: Laboratory assessment of adrenal insufficiency. J Clin Endocrinol Metab 1994;79:923–931.
14. Borst GC, Michenfelder HJ, O'Brian JT. Discordant cortisol responses to exogeneous ACTH and insulin-induced hypoglycemia in patients with pituitary diseases. N Engl J Med 1982;302:1462–464.
15. Dickstein G, Schechner C. Low dose ACTH test: a word of caution to the word of caution: when and how to use it. J Clin Endocrinol 1997;82:322.
16. Schulte HM, Chrousos GP, Avgerinos P, et al. The corticotropin-releasing hormone stimulation test: a possible aid in the evaluation of patients with adrenal insufficiency. J Clin Endocrinol Metab 1984;58:1064–1067.
17. Dluhy RG, Himathongkam T, Greenfield M. Rapid ACTH test with plasma aldosterone levels. Ann Intern Med 1974;80:693–696.
18. Miller WL. Genetics, diagnosis, and management of 21-hydroxylase deficiency. J Clin Endocrinol Metab 1994;78:241–246.
19. Barbat B, Bogyo A, Raux-Dermay MC, et al. Screening of CYP21 gene mutations in 120 French patients affected by steroid 21-hydroxylase deficiency. Hum Mutat 1995;5:126–130.
20. Speiser PW, New MI. Prenatal diagnosis and management of congenital adrenal hyperplasia. Clin Perinatol 1994;21:631–645.
21. Speiser PW, White PC, Dupont J, Zhu D, Mercado A, New MI. Molecular genetic prenatal diagnosis of congenital adrenal hyperplasia due to 21-hydroxylase deficiency by allele-specific hybridization. Recent Prog Horm Res 1994;49:367–371.
22. Couillin P, Nicolas H, Boue J, Boue A. HLA typing of amniotic-fluid cells applied to prenatal diagnosis of congenital adrenal hyperplasia. Lancet 1979;1:1076.
23. David MJ, Forest MG. Prenatal treatment of congenital adrenal hyperplasia resulting from 21-hydroxylase deficiency. J Pediatr 1984;105:799–803.

24. Forest MG, David M, Morel Y. Prenatal diagnosis and treatment of 21-hydroxylase deficiency. J Steroid Biochem Mol Biol 1993;45:75–82.

25. Lajic S, Wedell A, Ritzen EM, Knudzon J, Holst M. Scandinavian experience of prenatal treatment of congenital adrenal hyperplasia. Horm Res 1997;48(Suppl 2):22 (Abstr 87).

26. Mercado AB, Wilson RC, Cheng KC, Wei JQ, New MI. Prenatal treatment and diagnosis of congenital adrenal hyperplasia owing to 21-hydroxylase deficiency. J Clin Endocrinol Metab 1995;80:2014–2020.

27. Dorr HG, Sippell WG, Willig RP. Praenatale Diagnostik und Therapie des Adrenogenitalen Syndroms (AGS) mit 21-Hydroxylase Defekt. Monatsschr Kinderheilkd 1992;140:661–663.

28. Mulaikal RM, Migeon CJ, Rock JA. Fertility rates in female patients with congenital adrenal hyperplasia due to 21-hydroxylase deficiency. N Engl J Med 1987;316:178–188.

29. Dittmann RW, Kappes ME, Kappes MH. Sexual behavior in adolescent and adult females with congenital adrenal hyperplasia. Psychoneuroendocrinology 1992;17:153–170.

30. Kuhnle U, Bollinger M, Schwarz HP, Knorr D. Partnership and sexuality in adult female patients with congenital adrenal hyperplasia: first results of a cross-sectional qualtiy-of-life evaluation. J Steroid Biochem Mol Biol 1993;45:123–126.

31. Buescher MA, McClamrock HD, Adashi EY. Cushing's syndrome in pregnancy. Obstet Gynecol 1992;79:130–137.

32. Pang S, Clark AT, Freeman LC, et al. Maternal side-effects of prenatal dexamethasone therapy for fetal congenital adrenal hyperplasia. J Clin Endocrinol Metab 1992;75:249–253.

33. Seckl JR, Miller WL. Commentary: how safe is long-term prenatal glucocorticoid treatment? J Am Med Assoc 1997;277:1077–1079.

34. Uno H, Lohmiller L, Thieme C, Kemnitz JW, Engle MJ, Roecker EB, Farrell PM. Brain damage induced by prenatal exposure to dexamethasone in fetal rhesus macaques. I. Hippocampus. Brain Res Dev 1990;53:157–167.

35. Trautman PD, Meyer-Bahlburg HFL, Postelnek J, New MI. Effects of early prenatal dexamethasone on the cognitive and behavioral development of young children: results of a pilot study. Psychoneuroendocrinology 1995;20:439–449.

14

Mineralocorticoid Deficiency Syndromes

W. Reid Litchfield, MD, and Robert G. Dluhy, MD

CONTENTS

INTRODUCTION

Mineralocorticoid Physiology

Aldosterone, the most important mineralocorticoid in humans, is produced in the zona glomerulosa of the adrenal cortex. It acts on the principal cells of the distal convoluted tubule of the kidney, intestine, and salivary gland to stimulate sodium absorption and potassium excretion. The adrenocortical steroidogenic cells of the zona glomerulosa are unique in that they express aldosterone synthase activity, which converts corticosterone to aldosterone. On the other hand, these cells lack 17α-hydroxylase activity which is present in the cortisol-producing zona fasciculata.

Although the control of cortisol secretion is primarily regulated by adrenocorticotropin (ACTH), the control of aldosterone secretion is more complex. There are two major secretagogues of aldosterone secretion: potassium and angiotensin II. Minor regulators that either stimulate or inhibit aldosterone secretion include ACTH, vasopressin, dopamine, atrial natriuetic peptide, serotonin, somatostatin, and α-adrenergic agents.

Potassium depolarizes voltage-sensitive calcium channels on the plasma membrane of cells of the zona glomerulosa, resulting in an influx of calcium. This increase in cytosolic calcium activates a cascade of second messengers that result in aldosterone synthesis and release from the cell.

The renin-angiotensin system is the other major regulator of aldosterone secretion. The macula densa, a specialized group of cells located in the afferent arteriole and the distal convoluted tubule of the kidney, regulates renin release in response to baroreceptor stretch and the ion content of the luminal tubular fluid, respectively. The enzyme renin is the rate-limiting step in this cascade; an increase in the release of renin results in action

From: *Contemporary Endocrinology: Hormone Replacement Therapy*
Edited by: A. W. Meikle © Humana Press Inc., Totowa, NJ

Table 1
Etiologies of Aldosterone Deficiency/Resistance States

Secretagogue deficiency
    Hyporeninemia
        Diabetes mellitus
        Drugs (β-blockers, prostaglandin inhibitors)
    Ang II deficiency (ACE inhibitors) or blockade (AT1 receptor antagonists)
    Hypokalemia
Adrenocortical dysfunction
    Autoimmune destruction (idiopathic Addison's disease)
    Adrenal hemorrhage
    Infectious/infiltrative diseases (e.g., cytomegalovirus in AIDS patients)
    Steroidogenic defects (CMO deficiency)
    Drugs (heparin)
Intrinsic renal abnormalities
    Mineralocorticoid receptor antagonism (spironolactone, eplerenone)
    Epithelial sodium channel
        Mutation (pseudohypoaldosteronism type 1)
        Drugs (amiloride, trimethoprim, triamterene)

on angiotensinogen to produce the decapeptide angiotensin I (Ang I). Angiotensin-converting enzyme (ACE) converts this inactive peptide (Ang I) into the octapeptide Ang II, a potent vasoconstrictor as well as a secretagogue of aldosterone. Ang II can be further metabolized to angiotensin III (Ang III), which is equipotent in its effects on aldosterone secretion but lacks the vasoconstrictive properties of Ang II.

The renin-angiotensin system was previously viewed as a classic circulating hormonal system; recent studies have shown all components of this system in the kidney, heart, and peripheral vasculature allowing for the local regulation of function by generation of Ang II in these tissues.

ACTH can transiently increase aldosterone levels, particularly during stress. However, in ACTH-deficient patients, (e.g., steroid-suppressed subjects), aldosterone homeostasis is usually normal, because the zona glomerulosa is still normally regulated by potassium and the renin-angiotensin system.

ALDOSTERONE-DEFICIENCY SYNDROMES

Although the causes of aldosterone deficiency are numerous (Table 1), the clinical presentation is often similar and the severity of the syndrome related to the degree of the hormonal deficiency state. A general approach to organize the diagnosis of these conditions (Fig. 1) is based on the renin status of the patient; aldosterone deficiency can therefore be classified as hyporeninemic (secondary) or hyperreninemic (primary). Thus, hypoaldosteronism can arise from a deficiency of aldosterone secretagogues (primarily renin) or secondary to end-organ (adrenocortical) deficiency. In the latter circumstance, as well as in aldosterone-resistant states, the renin levels will be elevated. Drugs can produce mineralocorticoid deficiency by a variety of mechanisms, including renin/angiotensin lowering actions, direct effects on adrenocortical steroidogenesis, or by altering renal handling of potassium (Table 2; 1).

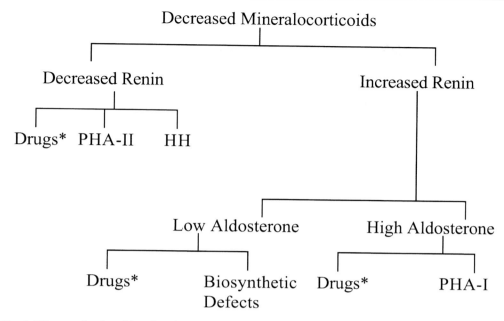

Fig. 1. Diagnostic algorithm for the mineralocorticoid-deficient patient.* *See* Table 2. Abbreviations: PHA, pseudohypoaldosteronism; HH, hyporeninemic hypoaldosteronism.

Hyporeninemic Hypoaldosteronism (HH)

Acquired

HH accounts for approx 10% of all cases of hyperkalemia and up to 50% of previously unexplained hyperkalemia *(1)*. It is a heterogeneous syndrome in which isolated aldosterone deficiency results from decreased renin release from the kidney. Acute provocative maneuvers, such as sodium restriction, volume depletion with diuretics and upright posture, fail to simulate renin release. Aldosterone responsiveness to Ang II and ACTH is variable, but patients fail to exhibit normal potassium-stimulated aldosterone production *(2)*.

This syndrome has multiple etiologies and occurs most commonly in the seventh decade of life. Many patients have interstitial renal disease and/or mild-to-moderate renal insufficiency. However, creatinine clearance remains above those levels that usually cause hyperkalemia (< 10 mL/min). Diabetes mellitus is the most common disease associated with HH, but other concurrent illnesses such as multiple myeloma, systemic lupus erythematosis, amyloidosis, cirrhosis, AIDS or sickle cell disease have also been reported. It has been hypothesized that autonomic insufficiency (e.g., diabetes mellitus) or prostaglandin deficiency (nonsteroidal anti-inflammatory medications) are alternative mechanisms that underlie the hyporeninemic state. Additionally, some patients with renal insufficiency are volume expanded, and this may contribute to the suppressed renin levels that are characteristic of HH.

The diagnosis of HH is established by demonstrating subnormal stimulation of renin and aldosterone levels following provocation with upright posture and a low sodium diet (or acute volume depletion with a diuretic, such as furosemide). Cortisol levels, by definition, are normal, and show physiologic responsiveness to cosyntropin. Serum

Table 2
Drug-Induced Hyperkalemia

Hypoaldosteronism
    Prostaglandin inhibitors (inhibit renin and aldosterone synthesis)
    β-blockers (inhibit renin release)
    ACE inhibitors (inhibit Ang II generation)
    Heparin (inhibits aldosterone synthesis)
    Ang II receptor blockers (inhibit Ang II action)
Decreased renal kaliuresis
    Potassium-sparing diuretics (spironolactone, amiloride, triamterene)
    Cyclosporine
    Lithium
    Digitalis
    Trimethoprim
    Pentamidine
Altered potassium distribution
    β-blockers
    α-blockers
    Hypertonic solutions (glucose, mannitol, saline)
    Digitalis
    Succinylcholine
    Insulin antogonists (somatostatin, diazoxide) or deficiency (diabetes mellitus)

Adapted with permission from ref. *1*.

potassium is consistently elevated, although symptomatic hyperkalemia is unusual. At least half of such patients also demonstrate hyperchloremic metabolic acidosis.

Treatment of HH is primarily mineralocorticoid replacement with fludrocortisone (Florinef®) in doses of 0.05–0.2 mg daily in conjunction with a high sodium (150–200 mmol/d) diet (*see* "Mineralcorticoid Replacement" section). However, patients with cardiovascular disease may not tolerate this regimen because of volume expansion. Potassium intake should also be restricted to 40–60 mmol/d. Potassium-binding resins (Kayexalate®) and loop diuretics (furosemide) can also be used to manage the hyperkalemia and/or permit usage of lower doses of fludrocortisone.

GENETIC–PSEUDOHYPOALDOSTERONISM TYPE II (PHA-II)

PHA-II, or Gordon's syndrome *(3)*, a genetic variant of HH, is seen in hypertensive adults and inherited in an autosomal dominant fashion *(4)*. This syndrome is sometimes referred to as familial hyperkalemia and hypertension. The kidney retains its ability to respond to the sodium-retaining effects of aldosterone, but does not show normal aldosterone-induced kaliuresis. Patients have normal renal function and usually no history of long-standing diabetes mellitus, which serves to distinguish them from patients with HH.

PHA-II is thought to arise from enhanced absorption of chloride ions in the early portions of the distal tubule, causing proximal sodium reabsorption and insufficient sodium delivery to the distal tubule for potassium exchange. This increased proximal absorption of sodium chloride causes volume expansion and suppression of the renin-angiotensin system. Low luminal sodium concentrations impairs distal tubular kaliuresis, results in hyperkalemia, and increases aldosterone levels to a variable degree through potassium-stimulated aldosterone production *(5)*. Treatment of the syndrome focuses on increasing sodium delivery to the distal tubule with thiazide or loop diuretics.

Hyperreninemic Hypoaldosteronism

PRIMARY ADRENAL FAILURE

Primary adrenal failure usually does not cause isolated mineralocorticoid deficiency but rather combined glucocorticoid and mineralocorticoid deficiencies *(6)*. Rarely, however, isolated mineralocorticoid deficiency may be seen *(7)*. Most cases result from autoimmune adrenal destruction but primary adrenal failure can also be seen as a result of bilateral adrenal hemorrhage *(8)*, tumor infiltration of the adrenal glands, some infections (AIDS *[7]*, histoplasmosis, mycobacterial infections, cytomegalovirus), or infiltrative diseases (amyloidosis *[9]*, hemochromatosis).

Treatment should focus on correcting the underlying illness, as many patients will have restoration of adrenocortical function after appropriate therapy. Usually combined glucocorticoid and mineralocorticoid replacement therapies are needed.

ACUTE, SEVERE ILLNESS

Critically ill patients can show selective hypoaldosteronism with elevated plasma renin activity (PRA) *(10)*, but these patients are not characteristically hyperkalemic. The fact that plasma cortisol levels are normal or high in these subjects indicates that there is selective adrenal deficiency of the zona glomerulosa. When ACTH is administered to these subjects cortisol responses are normal, but aldosterone shows a minimal response. There may be diminished aldosterone responsiveness to the infusion of Ang II in some of these patients as well *(10)*.

The etiology of this syndrome is not clearly defined. A number of possibilities for the selective hypoaldosteronism exist, but the most likely explanation relates to the chronic stress-related elevation of ACTH leading to altered steroidogenesis, favoring normal cortisol production but diminished production of mineralocorticoids such as aldosterone, corticosterone, and 18-hydroxycorticosterone *(11,12)*. Chronic hypoxia, as is seen with exposure to high altitudes, has been shown to result in hyperveninemic hypoaldosteronism with preserved cortisol biosynthesis *(13)*. Because many critically ill patients experience hypoxemia over the course of their illness, this may contribute to their hypoaldosteronism as well. Finally, hypokalemia, another common occurrence in the critically ill patient, may also contribute to the selective hypoaldosteronism.

BIOSYNTHETIC DEFECTS

Congenital hypoaldosteronism is a rare genetic disorder with an autosomal recessive pattern of inheritance. It is caused by deficiency of corticosterone 18-methyl oxidase (CMO, or P450c11Aldo), the enzyme that catalyzes the conversion of corticosterone to aldosterone (Fig. 2). Mutations in the gene coding for P450c11Aldo (CYP11B2) have been described that affect both CMO I *(14–16)* and CMO II *(17)* isoenzymes, but CMO I deficiency is less common. Patients present with signs of hypoaldosteronism, such as sodium wasting, hyponatremia, hyperkalemia, metabolic acidosis and hypotension. During infancy, CMO deficiency can also cause growth retardation. Hyperreninemia in infancy is marked but lacks diagnostic specificity, because elevated renin levels are

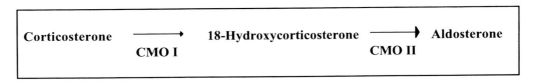

Fig. 2. Biosynthetic pathway of aldosterone production from its precursor corticosterone. Congenital hypoaldosteronism results from corticosterone 18-methyl oxidase (CMO) deficiency. CMO I and II deficiency have similar clinical presentations and are differentiated by the accumulation of 18-hydroxycorticosterone in CMO II deficiency but not in CMO I deficiency.

also seen in primary adrenal failure (Addison's disease), as well as in the aldosterone resistance syndromes (*see* "Pseudohypoaldosteronism Type 1" section). Symptoms are most pronounced early in life and tend to improve gradually as the child ages.

CMO I and CMO II deficiency can be difficult to differentiate clinically or in severity of symptoms *(18)*. However, the syndromes are easily differentiated biochemically. CMO II is characterized by extremely elevated 18-hydroxycorticosterone levels and a ratio of 18-hydroxycorticosterone to aldosterone exceeding 5. In contrast, 18-hydroxycorticosterone is lacking in CMO I deficiency. Treatment is similar for both syndromes and involves mineralocorticoid replacement with fludrocortisone *(19)*.

ALDOSTERONE-RESISTANCE SYNDROMES

Pseudohypoaldosteronism Type 1 (PHA-I)

This is rare, autosomal recessive disorder that was first described in 1958 and represents resistance of the renal tubule to the effects of aldosterone *(20)*. This syndrome arises from mutations of the amiloride-sensitive epithelial sodium channel (ENaC) resulting in loss of ENaC function *(21)*. Infants with this syndrome show biochemical signs of hypoaldosteronism including salt wasting, hypotension, hyperkalemia and hyperchloremic metabolic acidosis. This phenotype is the result of primary renal salt wasting and a secondary defect in potassium and hydrogen ion secretion. Affected individuals exhibit marked elevation of plasma renin activity and plasma aldosterone levels. Treatment with exogenous mineralocorticoids does not correct the hyperkalemia and formal testing of the hypothalamic-pituitary-adrenal axis is completely normal *(22)*. Treatment involves administration of potassium-binding resins, potassium-wasting diuretics and sodium chloride supplementation to maintain vascular volume. The syndrome is often self-limited, and salt supplementation can often be discontinued after several years.

Pseudohypoaldosteronism Type III (PHA-III)

PHA-III is most commonly diagnosed in normotensive adults with hyperkalemia. Plasma aldosterone are elevated, and there is impaired renal potassium excretory capacity that is refractory to exogenous mineralocorticoids. Most patients have tubulointerstitial renal disease (Fanconi syndrome, multiple myeloma, and so on). Treatment involves use of kaliuretic diuretics, potassium-binding resins, and sodium chloride supplementation to maintain intravascular volume.

DRUG-INDUCED HYPERKALEMIC STATES

Aldosterone Deficiency

INHIBITORS OF RENIN RELEASE

Inhibitors of the cyclooxygenase pathway of prostaglandin synthesis have been shown to reversibly inhibit renin release independent of the precipitation of renal insufficiency *(23,24)*. However, patients with underlying renal insufficiency (particularly diabetes mellitus—see HH) are at higher risk for clinically significant hypoaldosteronism and resultant hyperkalemia from these medications (Table 2). Because another important determinant of renin release is the sympathetic nervous system *(25,26)*, interruption of the adrenergic system with β-blockers can inhibit renin release, thereby secondarily decreasing the production of Ang II and aldosterone. However, precipitation of hyperkalemia with β-blockers alone is rare, usually occurring in patients with preexisting chronic renal insufficiency and/or diabetes mellitus.

INHIBITORS OF ANG II PRODUCTION OR ACTION

In normal subjects ACE inhibitors moderately reduce aldosterone levels by inhibiting Ang II formation. They can precipitate hyperkalemia, but usually this occurs only in the setting of underlying renal insufficiency or significant renovascular hypertension. This is particularly important in diabetic patients in which ACE inhibitors are the agents of choice to reduce protein excretion and preserve renal function. AT1 receptor agonists (losartan, valsartan) block the actions of Ang II resulting in 'functional' Ang II insufficiency. Hyperkalemia is not commonly seen with these agents, but would be expected in patients with renal insufficiency.

INHIBITORS OF ALDOSTERONE SECRETION

Heparin, even in low doses, has been shown to cause hypoaldosteronism and hyperkalemia *(27–29)*. A number of mechanisms have been proposed through which heparin may cause hypoaldosteronism. Chlorbutal, a preservative additive to commercial heparin preparations, has been shown to inhibit both the early and late biosynthetic phases of aldosterone production *(30)*. Heparin decreases Ang II-mediated aldosterone production by decreasing receptor number and binding affinity of Ang II receptors on adrenal glomerulosa cells *(31)*. Higher doses of heparin can also impair ACTH and potassium-stimulated aldosterone production *(30)*. These effects may be seen as early as four days after initiation of therapy. Although aldosterone levels may be reduced to some extent in all patients on heparin therapy, most subjects do not show overt hypoaldosteronism because they are able to compensate by increasing renin release from the kidney. Individuals with diabetes mellitus, renal insufficiency, or critical illness may exhibit impaired compensation and are therefore at higher risk of developing heparin-induced hypoaldosteronism. A high index of suspicion must be maintained when such patients are given heparin so that hypoaldosteronism can be recognized early, and appropriate therapy initiated.

In addition to inhibiting renin release, prostaglandin synthase inhibitors have also been shown to inhibit aldosterone secretion directly *(23)*. Spironolactone can cause 'functional' hypoaldosteronism by antagonizing the effects of aldosterone at the mineralocorticoid receptor. Amiloride, triamterene, trimethoprim therapy can all result in hyperkalemia; the mechanism of action is independent of aldosterone and involves a direct effect of the drug on blocking the aldosterone-regulated ENaC. This results in reduction of the transepithelial voltage in the renal tubule thus inhibiting kaliuresis *(32)*.

TREATMENT OF MINERALOCORTICOID DEFICIENCY

General Principles

There are several goals of therapy in mineralocorticoid deficient patients. The first is to assess the severity of the hyperkalemic state, and institute immediate treatment, if required.

Hyperkalemia may require emergency treatment if it is severe and especially if it occurs rapidly. Electrocardiographic features of life-threatening hyperkalemia (peaked T waves, shortening of QTc, and widening of QRS) mandate emergency treatment of the hyperkalemia *(33)*. Intravenous calcium gluconate (two to four ampules of 10% calcium gluconate) or calcium chloride (10 mL 10% calcium chloride over 2–5 min) will stabilize the myocardium by raising the threshold potential of the cell membranes and lowering excitability. Extracellular potassium can also be temporarily shifted into the intracellular compartment by intravenous administration of insulin (5 U/regular insulin with 50 mL 50% dextrose to prevent hypoglycemia) or sodium bicarbonate (50–150 mEq sodium bicarbonate) and also by nebulized albuterol. However, maneuvers to shift potassium into the intracellular compartment are only temporizing measures, lasting 20–30 min. Additional long-term therapies should be simultaneously initiated and directed at the etiology of the hyperkalemic state.

In the sodium and/or aldosterone-depleted subject, correction of the deficiencies will ultimately restore potassium homeostasis by promoting kaliuresis. Acidosis should be corrected with intravenous sodium bicarbonate administration. Hemodialysis can rapidly lower blood potassium levels and may be needed in some emergency cases. Additional therapies to lower potassium, such as potassium-binding resins (Kayexelate® 15–20 g po q2h; Resonium(50 g po/pr q4-6h) are useful in chronic hyperkalemic states, such as renal insufficiency (1 g of Kayexelate® has an in vitro exchange capacity of about 3 mEq of potassium). Potassium-binding resins should be complimented by a low potassium diet and, if needed, potassium-wasting diuretics (primarily furosemide). Some of these therapies, especially diuretics, are useful in treating elderly patients with hypoaldosteronism who are prone to volume overload as a result of renal insufficiency and/ or congestive heart failure. Finally, a careful history is necessary to identify possible medications that may have precipitated or worsened an underlying hyperkalemic state, such as hyporeninemic hypoaldosteronism (Table 2). Medications such as ACE inhibitors should be temporarily discontinued and judiciously reinstated later if they are felt to be absolutely necessary for the management of the patient.

A second major goal of therapy is to simultaneously correct the volume depletion and hypotension that occurs in many mineralocorticoid-deficient patients. Patients should be given intravenous isotonic saline or be maintained on a high salt diet; sodium chloride tablets (10–12 g/d) may be beneficial in some patients. Caution should be exercised not to hydrate those hyperkalemic patients who may also be concomitantly volume expanded (such as patients with renal insufficiency).

Mineralocorticoid Replacement

Along with a normal sodium intake (100–150 mmol/d), fludrocortisone (Florinef®), a synthetic mineralocorticoid, is the cornerstone of maintenance therapy of the aldosterone deficient patient. Most patients with aldosterone insufficiency require a daily dose of 0.1 mg/d (dose range 0.05–0.2 mg/d). Larger doses may be needed in selected patients, such as subjects with HH and PHA-III. Fludrocortisone can be administered in a single daily dose, although patients that require larger doses may benefit from twice-a-day dosing. Therapy should be initiated at very low doses in the elderly or patients with a history of congestive heart failure. When increasing the dose of fludrocortisone, patients should have their dosage increased gradually to prevent excessive sodium retention or rapid volume expansion. Ambulatory patients can monitor adequacy of treatment by recording accurate daily weights as a sensitive measure of salt and water retention.

Mineralocorticoid treatment is usually not necessary in the hospitalized acutely ill patient with primary adrenal insufficiency. In such patients, the pharmacological doses of parenteral glucocorticoids that are commonly used to prevent adrenal crisis (bolus hydrocortisone, 100 mg iv q8h or continuous hydrocortisone infusion, 10 mg/h) and exert sufficient mineralocorticoid action at the renal mineralocorticoid receptor to obviate the need for oral exogenous mineralocorticoid treatment. In addition, there are no parenteral mineralocorticoid formulations available to treat patients whose oral intake has been curtailed. Another cornerstone of management in acutely ill patients who are mineralocorticoid deficient is adequate sodium repletion, primarily with isotonic saline. It is emphasized that mineralocorticoid treatment alone never can replete extracellular volume in a mineralocorticoid and volume-depleted subject without providing adequate substrate (sodium). Careful attention should also be given to maintenance of blood pressure and renal function (such as the BUN/creatinine ratio and adequate urine output).

REFERENCES

1. Tan SY, Burton M. Hyporeninemic hypoaldosteronism. An overlooked cause of hyperkalemia. Arch Intern Med 1981;141:30–33.
2. Schambelan M, Stockigt JR, Biglieri EG. Isolated hypoaldosteronism in adults: a renin-deficiency syndrome. N Engl J Med 1972;287:573.
3. Gordon RD. Syndrome of hypertension and hyperkalemia with normal glomerular filtration rate. Hypertension 1986;8:93.
4. Mansfield TA, Simon DB, Farfel Z, Bia M, Tucci JR, Lebel M, et al. Multilocus linkage of familial hyperkalaemia and hypertension, pseudohypoaldosteronism type II, to chromosomes 1q31-42 and 7p11-q21. Nat Genet 1997;16:(2)202–205.
5. Schambelan M, et al. Mineralocorticoid-resistant renal hyperkalemia without salt-wasting (Type II pseudohypoaldosteronism): Role of increased renal chloride reabsorption. Kidney Int 1981;19:716.
6. Oelkers W. Adrenal insufficiency. N Engl J Med 1996;335:1206–1212.
7. Guy RJ, Turberg Y, Davidson RN, Finnerty G, MacGregor GA, Wise PH. Mineralocorticoid deficiency in HIV infection. BMJ 1989;298:496–497.
8. Dahlberg PJ, Goellner MH, Pehling GB. Adrenal insufficiency secondary to adrenal hemorrhage. Two case reports and a review of cases confirmed by computed tomography. Arch Intern Med 1990;150:905–909.
9. Agmon D, Green J, Platau E, Better OS. Isolated adrenal mineralocorticoid deficiency due to amyloidosis associated with familial Mediterranean fever. Am J Med Sci 1984;288:40–43.
10. Zipser RD, Davenport MW, Martin KL, Tuck ML, Warner NE, Swinney RR, et al. Hyperreninemic hypoaldosteronism in the critically ill: a new entity. J Clin Endocrinol Metab 1981;53:867–873.
11. Biglieri EG, Schambelan M, Slaton Jr. PE. Effect of adrenocorticotropin on desoxycorticosterone, corticosterone and aldosterone excretion. J Clin Endocrinol Metab 1969;29:1091
12. Kraiem Z, Rosenthal T, Rotzak R, Lunenfeld B. Angiotensin II and K challenge followed by prolonged ACTH administration in normal subjects. ACTA Endocrinol (Copenh) 1979;91:657
13. Slater JDH, Tuffley RE, Williams ES, Beresford CH, Sonksen PH, Edwards RHT, et al. Control of aldosterone secretion during acclimatization to hypoxia in man. Clin Sci 1969;37:237

14. Nomoto S, Massa G, Mitani F, Ishimura Y, Miyahara K, Toda K, et al. CMO I deficiency caused by a point mutation in exon 8 of the human CYP11B2 gene encoding steroid 18-hydroxylase (P450C18). Biochem Biophys Res Commun 1997;234:(2)382–385.

15. Mitsuuchi Y, Kawamoto T, Miyahara K, Ulick S, Morton DH, Naiki Y, et al. Congenitally defective aldosterone biosynthesis in humans: inactivation of the P-450C18 gene (CYP11B2) due to nucleotide deletion in CMO I deficient patients. Biochem Biophys Res Commun 1993;190:(3)864–869.

16. Peter M, Fawaz L, Drop SLS, Visser HKA, Sippel WG. A prismatic case. Hereditary defect in biosynthesis of aldosterone: aldosterone synthase deficiency 1964–1997. J Clin Endocrinol Metab 1997;82:(11)3525-3528.

17. Mitsuuchi Y, Kawamoto T, Naiki Y, Miyahara K, Toda K, Kuribayashi I, et al. Congenitally defective aldosterone biosynthesis in humans: the involvement of point mutations of the P-450C18 gene (CYP11B2) in CMO II deficient patients. Biochem Biophys Res Commun 1992;182:(2)974–979.

18. Peter M, Sippel WG. Congenital hypoaldosteronism: the Visser-Cost-Syndrome revisited. Pediatr Res 1996;39:554–560.

19. Yong AB, Montalto J, Pitt J, Oakes S, Preston T, Buchanan C. Corticosterone methyl oxidase type II (CMO II) deficiency: biochemical approach to diagnosis. Clin Biochem 1994;27:(6)491–494.

20. Cheek DB, Perry JW. A salt-wasting syndrome in infancy. Arch Dis Child 1958;33:252.

21. Chang SS, Grunder S, Hanukoglu A, Rosler A, Mathew PM, Hanukoglu I, et al. Mutations in subunits of the epithelial sodium channel cause salt wasting with hyperkalaemic acidosis, pseudohypoaldosteronism type 1. Nat Genet 1996;12:(3)248–253.

22. Oberfield SE, et al. Pseudohypoaldosteronism: multiple target organ unresponsiveness to mineralocorticoid hormones. J Clin Endocrinol Metab 1979;48:228.

23. Saruta T, Kaplan NM. Adrenocortical steroidogenesis: the effects of prostaglandins. J Clin Invest 1972;51:2246.

24. Franco-Saenz R, et al. Prostaglandins and renin production: a review. Prostaglandins 1980;20:1131.

25. Holdaas H, Dibona GF, Kiil F. Effect of low-level renal nerve stimulation on renin release from nonfiltering kidneys. Am J Physiol 1981;241:F156–F161.

26. Gross R, Hackenberg HM, Hackenthal E, Kirchheim H. Interaction between perfusion pressure and sympathetic nerves in renin release by carotid baroreflex in conscious dogs. J Physiol 1981;313:237–250.

27. Oster JR, Singer I, Fishman LM. Heparin-induced hypoaldosteronism and hyperkalemia. Am J Med 1995;98:(6)575–586.

28. Aull L, Chao H, Coy K. Heparin-induced hyperkalemia. DICP 1990;24:244–246.

29. Levesque H, Verdier S, Cailleux N, Elie-Legrand MC, Gancel A, Basuyau JP, et al. Low molecular weight heparins and hypoaldosteronism. BMJ 1990;300:1437–1438.

30. Sequeira SJ, McKenna TJ. Chlorbutal, a new inhibitor of aldosterone biosynthesis identified during examination of heparin effect on aldosterone production. J Clin Endocrinol Metab 1986;63:(6)780–784.

31. Azukizawa S, Iwasaki I, Kigoshi T, Uchida K, Morimoto S. Effects of heparin treatments in vivo and in vitro on adrenal angiotensin II receptors and angiotensin II-induced aldosterone production in rats. ACTA Endocrinol (Copenh) 1988;119:(3)367–372.

32. Velazquez H, Perazella MA, Wright FS, Ellison DH. Renal mechanism of trimethoprim-induced hyperkalemia. Ann Intern Med 1993;119:(4)296–301.

33. Clark BA, Brown RS. Potassium homeostasis and hyperkalemic syndromes. Endocrinol Clin North Am 1995;24:(3)573–591.

15

Dehydroepiandrosterone and Pregnenolone

Rakhmawati Sih, MD,
Hosam Kamel, MD, *Mohamad Horani,* MD,
and John E. Morley, MB, BCH

Contents

INTRODUCTION

Steroid hormones play a multifactorial role in human physiology. They facilitate coordinative processes that enable neural, endocrine, immune, and metabolic systems, separately or collectively, to operate in solving problems of survival and reproduction. Both pregnenolone and dehydroepiandrosterone (DHEA) are key hormones early in the pathway of steroid hormones biosynthesis (Fig. 1). Actually, pregnenolone is the precursor of all the known steroid hormones, and its formation from cholesterol via the action of cytochrome P450scc, is the rate limiting step in steroid hormone formation. DHEA and its sulfated conjugate, dehydroepiandrosterone sulfate (DHEAS), on the other hand, serve as precursors for both androgenic and estrogenic steroids, and are the most abundant steroid hormones in the human body. The plasma levels of both DHEA and pregnenolone have been shown to decline progressively with advancing age. Furthermore, based on multiple animal and human studies, there is now accumulating evidence to suggest a potential role for both these hormones in the prevention of multiple morbidities associated with the aging process. This chapter reviews the biological roles of DHEA and pregnenolone and draws implications for their possible role as antiaging agents.

DHEA

DHEA and its sulfated conjugate DHEAS are the most abundant steroid hormones in the human body *(1)*, despite that very little is known about their physiological role. For

From: *Contemporary Endocrinology: Hormone Replacement Therapy*
Edited by: A. W. Meikle © Humana Press Inc., Totowa, NJ

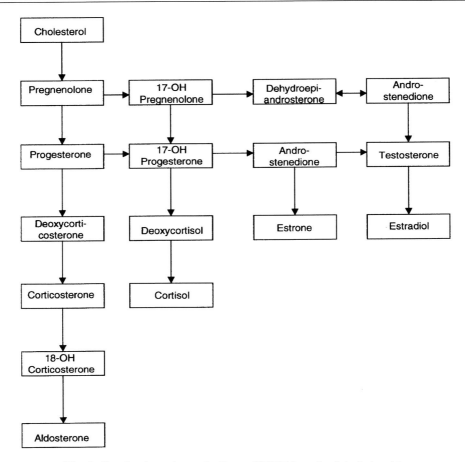

Fig. 1. Synthesis and metabolism of DHEA and related steroids.

many years, DHEA has enjoyed the reputation that it is the fountain of youth even though evidence for its beneficial effects in humans were virtually nonexistent. Over the past decade, however, this situation have changed. Two observations renewed interest among aging researchers in DHEA and DHEAS. The first of these is that circulating levels of these steroids decline markedly with aging. Second, animal studies have demonstrated the beneficial effects of DHEA administration in preventing obesity, diabetes, cancer, heart disease, and in enhancing the immune system. Collectively, these observations have led investigators to question whether DHEA administration can reverse some of the degenerative changes associated with human aging. This resulted in several human studies being conducted that tested the effects of DHEA administration on various organ systems. In this chapter, we discuss the biological role of DHEA and review its antiaging effects as demonstrated by both animal and human studies with special emphasis on the latter.

DHEA: Synthesis and Biological Role

DHEA is a C-19 steroid first isolated in 1934 from urine by Butenandt and Dannenbaum *(4)*. Most DHEA is produced in the adrenal cortex from cholesterol (Fig. 1) under the influence of the adrenocorticotrophic hormone (ACTH). The testes and ovaries contribute

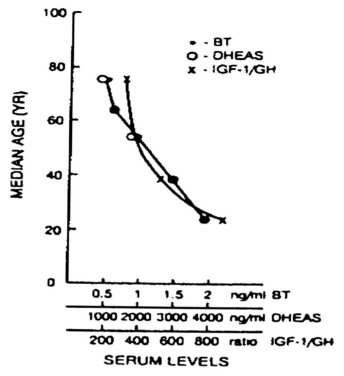

Fig. 2. Age-related decline in dehydroepiandrosterone sulfate blood levels in humans *(94)*.

5% of total DHEA production *(5)*. Ninety-nine percent of circulating DHEA is in the form of its water-soluble sulfate conjugate, DHEAS *(2)*. DHEAS function as an inactive reservoir and both DHEA and DHEAS are interconverted in peripheral and adrenal tissues *(5)*. DHEA(S) circulate in the blood in a free nonprotein-bound form as well as bound to albumin and sex hormone-binding globulin (SHBG) *(6)*.

How DHEA exerts its biologic actions remains a mystery. DHEA may act by influencing several key metabolic enzymes, such as glucose-6-phosphate dehydrogenase or glycerol-3-phosphate dehydrogenase, by altering physicochemical parameters via interpolation into cellular membranes, or by conversion to androgens, estrogens, or other metabolites. A putative binding site for DHEA has been demonstrated on hepatocytes and human leukocytes, but a specific DHEA receptor has not yet been characterized *(1)*.

DHEA and Aging

Both cross-sectional *(7)* and longitudinal studies *(8)* have demonstrated the decline of DHEA and DHEAS levels with advancing age (Fig. 2). It has been shown conclusively that with age, levels of DHEA and DHEAS in both sexes decrease at a relatively constant rate of 2%/yr. Hence, at age 80, levels are only about 20% of those at age 25 *(9)*. This decline has been attributed by some researchers to a decrease in number of functional zona reticularis cells, whereas others attributed it to intra-adrenal changes in 17-alpha hydroxylase activity *(10)*.

At all ages, the interindividual variability is very high and the normal range of serum DHEAS is therefore very wide. Most studies report 10–30% higher levels of DHEAS in men than women. This difference, however, largely disappears after age 50 *(9)*. Moreover, important genetic differences appear to exist, e.g., Japanese men have significantly lower levels than American white men *(11)*.

The decline in DHEA serum levels with age is parallel to the development of decreased immunity, physical frailty, decreased muscle mass, increased fat mass, decreased ability to cope, disrupted sleep patterns, and increased incidence of disease. Thus, DHEA can be viewed as a marker of aging in humans *(9)*. More importantly, low levels of DHEA and DHEAS are associated with a variety of morbidities and mortality. Low serum levels of DHEAS have been correlated with increased all-cause and cardiovascular mortality in men *(12)*, premenopausal breast cancer *(13)*, and gastric cancer *(14)*. Low DHEA levels may also be a risk factor for osteoporosis *(15,16)* although there are data that have not found any significant association of DHEAS levels with bone mineral density *(17)*.

DHEA: Antiaging Effects

Although numerous animal studies have demonstrated that DHEA has multiple antiaging effects, it should be kept in mind that most of these animal studies were conducted on rodents, which have little, if any, circulating DHEA. Hence, a major question is whether any of these beneficial consequences of DHEA administration demonstrated in animal models can be shown to be relevant in human beings. This led several investigators to administer DHEA to humans and monitor its biological effects. Table 1 summarizes these human studies. In the following section, we explore the various effects of DHEA as demonstrated by both animal and human studies.

DHEA and Cardiovascular Disease

Early studies conducted by Marmorston et al. *(18,19)* and Kask *(20)* indicated that levels of DHEA, DHEAS or their urinary metabolites, 17 ketosteroids were lower in men with arteriosclerotic disease, leading to the suggestion that DHEA and DHEAS might protect against cardiovascular disease *(21)*. Later on, in 1986, Barrett-Connor et al. examined this hypothesis in a large 12-yr longitudinal study *(22)* and reported that DHEAS levels were inversely related to the cardiovascular mortality in men. However, this inverse association between DHEAS levels and cardiovascular disease has not been consistently found in subsequent studies in women *(23)* or in other cohorts *(24–26)*.

A major concern in evaluating these epidemiological data are that the association between DHEA levels and cardiovascular disease may merely be epiphenomenon. That is, because the incidence of atherosclerosis is related to age, the decline in plasma DHEAS with aging may be coincidental and not casual *(27)*. This led investigators to conduct several animal studies to prospectively test the hypothesis that DHEA protects against atheroscleorosis. These studies showed that oral administration of DHEA has a great protective effect against ahterosclerosis in cholesterol-fed animals *(28–30)*.

Several factors may contribute to the protective effect of DHEA against cardiovascular disease. In human studies, oral administration of DHEA decreased the activity of glucose-6-phosphate dehydrogenase in erythrocytes *(31,32)*. These findings are important because glucose-6-phosphate dehydrogenase reduces NADPH, which is involved in cell proliferation and the synthesis of fatty acids and cholesterol. If the production of NADPH is blocked, fatty acid synthesis will be lowered, and the production of very low-density lipoproteins (VLDL) and their conversion to low-density lipoprotiens (LDL) will be greatly reduced. This will lead to less atheroma formation *(5)*.

Table 1
Overview of Human DHEA Studies

Researchers/ type of study	Dose and period of subjects	Age and number	Results
Yen et al. *(49)*;	50 mg cap oral/ sublingual	8 men/8 women, age:40–70	DHEA, A, T, DHT were similar in two routes, but there was rapid and marked elevation of DHEA for 2 h after sublingual than after oral route.
Yen et al. *(49)*; Randomized, placebo-controlled	50 mg oral cap for 6 mo	13 men/17 women, age: 40–70	Twofold increase of A, T, DHT in women with only slight increase in men. Small decrease in HDL in women, no change in other lipids No change in SHBG E1-E2 in both women and men No change in insulin sensitivity, body fat mass No change in libido Increase in perceived physical and psychological well-being (men, 67%; women, 84%)
Yen et al. *(49)*; Randomized, placebo-controlled	100 mg cap for 1 yr	8 men/8 women, age: 50–65	Increase in SHBG in women with no change in men Fivefold increase in A, T, DHT in women, but only twofold increase in men No change in gonadotropin in both groups Increase in lean body mass only in men Increased in IGF-I in both groups No change in: lipids profile, apolipoprotein, insulin, glucose, metabolic rate, and bone mineral density
Yen et al. *(49)*; Single-blind, placebo-controlled	50 mg cap: 2 wk placebo then 20	9 men	Stimulation of immune function Increase in NK cells and IL- 2
Buster et al. *(95)*; Open-label, noncontrolled trial	Placebo or 150 or 300 mg DHEA	8 postmenopausal women not on hormone replacement	Increase in DHEA, DHEAS, T No change in estradiol levels Increase in LET in one of subjects Direct assay of T overestimated it by 300%

(continued)

Table 1 (continued)

Researchers/ type of study	Dose and period of subjects	Age and number	Results
Vollenhoven et al. (96); Open noncontrolled trial	200 mg DHEA for 3–6 wk	10 women with SLE, average age 35.7 yr	Improved SLE activity Decrease requirement of prednisone Decrease in proteinuria Improvement in well being and energy Four subjects developed acneiform dermatitis Two subjects developed mild hirsutism who were also on prednisone
Arano et al. (97); Double-blind, randomized, placebo-controlled study	(1) 50 mg oral DHEA or placebo twice daily for 4 d beginning 2 d before tetanus vaccination	(1) 66 men, age > 65	(1) No difference between DHEAS group and placebo group, no detrimental effects of DHEAS on outcomes of tetanus vaccination
	(2) 50 mg oral DHEA or placebo for 2 d beginning with the day of influenza vaccination	(2) 67 elderly persons, age: ?	(2) 41.2% of DHEAS group have greater than fourfold increase in HAI titer, only 27% of placebo group have greater than fourfold increase in HAI titer Response to H1N1 antigen was 39.9% in placebo group and 47.1% in DHEAS group. Response to influenza B: Marked increase in titter in only three of placebo group and six of DHEAS group
Dyner et al. (98); Open-label uncontrolled trial	250–500–750 mg oral DHEA tid for 16 wk	31 homosexual men	No dose limiting side effects No sustained improvement in CD4 No change in P24 Ag or beta-macroglobulin Transient decrees in neopterin at 8 wk
Jakubowicz et al. (33); Double-blind placebo-controlled study	(1) Acute test: 300 mg of DHEA; 6 were given (L-NAME), a specific inhibitor of NO synthase. The rest of subjects were given intravenous saline.	(1) 14 men (out of 22)	(1) Increase in IGF-1 and C-GMP in saline group Increase in IGF-1 in DHEA-L-NAME group, which indicates that DHEA's effect is medicated via NO

Table 1 (continued)

Researchers/ type of study	Dose and period of subjects	Age and number	Results
	(2) 100 mg oral DHEA qd for 1 mo	(2) 22 men, mean	(2) Increase in plasma C-GMP and IGF-1 after 1 mo of DHEA replacement
Jesse and Loesser (27); Random-, ized double-, blind placebo-controlled trial	300 mg oral DHEA tid for 14 d	10 normal men	Platelet aggregation rates were prolonged in four out of five in DHEA group. No side effects reported
Beer et al. (34); Randomized, double-blind, and placebo-controlled trial	50 mg oral DHEA tid for 12 d	34 men, age: 47–75	Decrease in plasma plasminogen activator inhibitor type 1 (PAI-1) and tissue plasmin-ogen activator (tPA) Decrease in diastolic BP in DHEA group compared with slight increase in BP in placebo group. Two- to fivefold increase in serum DHEAS, no change in serum DHEA in DHEA group. 55% increase in A in DHEA group No change in systolic BP in both groups No change in body mass index in both groups
Heta et al. (99)	200 mg of intravenous injection of DHEAS in 20 mL of 5% dextrose	15 full pregnant women	20% increase in maternal cardiac output after 15 min, and increase 25% increase in stroke volume No change in heart rate or mean arterial pressure
Wolkowitz et al. (70)	30–90 mg of oral DHEA qd for 4 wk	3 men/3 women (major depression patients): age: 51–72	Increase in serum levels of DHEA, DHEAS Improvement in HDRS, global depression, SCL90, BDI, improvement in automatic memory functions Return of behavioral and cognitive measures to baseline after DHEA withdrawal

(continued)

Table 1 (continued)

Researchers/ type of study	Dose and period of subjects	Age and number	Results
Friess et al., (100); placebo-controlled study	Single 500 mg oral dose	Ten young healthy men, mean age: 24.9	Significant increase in REM sleep, with no change in other sleep variables DHEA may play a role of GABAa-agonist/antagonist
Buffington et al. (101); case report	0.25 mg dexametha-zone for 1 mo, then 0.25 mg + DHEA (150 bid)	One woman (NIDDM, primary amenorrhea), age: 15	No change in body weight, and percent of body fat Dex treatment caused eightfold increase in serum cortisol, 28-fold decrease in DHEAS, and fivefold decrease in testosterone DHEA administration did not affect cortisol levels, but caused increase in DHEAS and testosterone DHEA caused increase in the disappearance rate of glucose in response to intravenous insulin, suggesting enhanced peripheral tissue insulin sensitivity DHEA caused threefold increase in the hypoglycemic response to intravenous insulin, and 30% increase insulin binding
Bates et al. (60); Randomized, double-blind placebo controlled trial	50 mg oral DHEA qd for 3 wk	15 patients	Insulin sensitive index increased in the DHEA group No change in weight body mass index
Casson et al. (102); Placebo-controlled randomized trial	50 mg oral DHEA qd for 3 wk	11 postmeno-pausal women	Increase in DHEA, DHEAS, T, free T Decrease in fasting triglycerides with no change in other lipid profile Increase in insulin sensitivity Increase in SHBG
Usiskin et al. (103)	1,600 mg DHEA/d for 28 d	6 obese men	No change in total body weight, body fat mass, tissue insulin sensitivity, serum lipids, or fat distribution.

Table 1 (continued)

Researchers/ type of study	Dose and period of subjects	Age and number	Results
Jones, et al. (104); case report	Oral DHEA	Patient with advanced prostate cancer	Symptoms improved Cancer flared Previously hormonally unresponsive cancer responded transiently to third-line hormonal therapy with diethylstilbesterol.
Labri et al. (105); noncontrolled trial	10% DHEA cream for 12 mo	Fourteen 60–70-yr-old post-menopausal women	Stimulation of vaginal epithelium maturation No estrogenic effect observed on endometrium Bone mineral density at the hip significantly increased Decreased alkaline phosphatase, and urinary/hydroxyproline/creatinine ratio Increase in serum osteocalcin, a marker of bone formation
Danenberg et al. (106); Prospective ran-, domized, double-blind study	Either DHEA (50 mg qd po) for 4 d or a placebo. Antibody response to the influenza vaccine was measured before and 28 d after vaccination.	71 volunteers, age 61–89 yr	Increased DHEAS in the DHEA group No enhancement in established immunity Decrease in attainment of protective antibody titter against A/Texas strain in subjects with nonprotenctive baseline antibody titer following DHEA treatment compared with placebo.
Wolf et al. (92); double-blind, placebo-controlled trial	DHEA 50 mg for 2 wk daily, then 2-wk wash-out period and a 2-wk placebo period	40 healthy men and women (mean age 69 yr)	DHEA, androstenedione, and testosterone increased in both groups No strong beneficial effects in psychological or cognitive parameter
Evans et al. (107); Randomized, double-blind trial	DHEAS 50 mg po bid for 4 d, or a placebo. Tetanus vaccine given before the fifth dose	66 individuals, age 65 yr or older	No difference noted between groups

(continued)

Table 1 (continued)

Researchers/ type of study	Dose and period of subjects	Age and number	Results
Evans et al. *(107)*; Randomized, double-blind trial	DHEAS 50 mg po immediately before and 24 h after vaccination	67 individuals	Number of individuals who developed influenza protective titer was not different in the two groups. The mean log increase in the antibody response was greater in the DHEAS group.
Diamond et al. *(108)*	Single daily percutaneous application of a 10% DHEA cream	15 postmeno-pausal women, age 60–70 yr	9.8% decrease in subcutaneous skinfold thickness 12 mo. 11% decrease in fasting plasma glucose levels and a 17% decrease in fasting insulin levels. Overall trend towards a decrease in total cholesterol and its lipoprotein fractions. Plasma triglycerides were not affected. HDL cholesterol decreased by 8%

A, androstenedione; T, testosterone; DHT, dihydroeiandrosterone; SHBG, sex hormone binding globulin; HDL, High density lipoprotein; E1, estrone; E2, estradiol; LFT, liver function test; nk, natural-killer cells; IL, interleukin; SLE, systemic lupus erythromatosis; C-GMP, cyclic guanosine monophosphate; IGF, insulin growth factor-1; REM, rapid eye movement; HDRS, Hamilton Depression Rating Scale;, BDI, Beck Depression Inventory; SCL, symptom check list; NIDDM, noninsulin-dependent diabetes mellitus.

Both in vitro and in vivo studies showed that DHEA and DHEAS have inhibitory effect on platelet activation. When DHEAS was added to pooled platelet-rich plasma before the addition of the agonist arachidonate the platelet aggregation was inhibited. Inhibition of platelet aggregation by DHEA was both dose- and time-dependent. Inhibition of platelet aggregation by DHEA was accompanied by reduced platelet thromboxane B2 production. The effect of DHEA on platelet function was also tested in vivo. In Jesse et al. *(27)* in a randomized, double-blind study, 10 normal men received either DHEA 300 mg ($n = 5$) or placebo capsule ($n = 5$) orally three times/d for 14 d. Platelet aggregation was either slowed or completely inhibited in the DHEA group.

DHEA administration has also been shown in human studies to enhance nitric oxide activity, a potent vasodilator, a mechanism that may be involved in the protective action of DHEA against coronary artery disease *(33)*. Finally, Beer et al. in a double-blind, placebo controlled study demonstrated that the administration of DHEA to human subjects caused a decrease in both plasma plasminogen activator inhibitor type 1 (PAI-1) and tissue plasminogen activator (tPA) antigens *(34)*. Both PAI-1 and tPA antigens are circulating markers of fibrinolytic potential, and their elevation is a risk factor for heart disease in men.

DHEA AND CANCER

Animal studies have repeatedly shown that DHEA supplementation slows the development of several cancers such as testicular cancer *(35)*, skin cancer *(36)*, pancreatic cancer *(37)*, and colorectal cancer *(38)*. Epidemiological studies have shown low DHEA levels to be associated with premenopausal breast cancer *(13)*, gastric cancer *(14)*, lung cancer *(39)*, bladder cancer *(40)*, and hairy cell leukemia *(41)*. In vitro, DHEA has been shown to have paradoxical effects, slowing the growth of human breast cancer cells in some studies *(42,43)*, but not in others *(44)*. This was attributed to the activation of androgen receptors in a human breast cancer cell line *(43)*. Prospective human studies are required before definitive statements can be made concerning the role of DHEA supplementation in cancer prevention in humans.

DHEA AND IMMUNOMODUALTION

Although DHEA and DHEAS levels decline significantly with age, cortisol levels do not, creating the potential for greater suppression of cellular immunity *(5)*. This is correlated with increased incidence and severity of infectious diseases and cancers in the elderly; and higher circulating levels of interlukin (IL)-6 and autoantibodies *(45)*. Multiple studies have suggested that DHEA has a role in enhancing immunity. DHEAS supplementation reverses the age associated dysregulation of IL-6 production in mice *(46)*, and enhances immune responses in aged mice to pnemococcal *(47)*, and hepatitis B vaccinations *(48)*. Yen et al. *(49)* conducted a placebo-controlled trial in which he administered DHEA 50 mg/d to nine healthy older men for 5 mo duration. DHEA resulted in enhanced T-cell mitogenesis and natural killer-cell activity, as well as increased production of growth factors.

Recently there have been growing interest in DHEA in relation to the acquired immune deficiency syndrome (AIDS). Changes in cytokine production in patients with AIDS are very similar to those seen in aging, but less dramatic. Chatteron et al. in an 11-yr longitudinal study *(50)* demonstrated that in patients infected with the HIV virus, there is a progressive decline in serum DHEA levels which in some cases preceded a precipitous fall in CD4 cell count. In another study by Dyner et al. DHEA supplementation to patients with AIDS resulted in a 40% reduction in serum neopterine, one of the markers of HIV infection progression, but did not have any effect on CD4 cell count *(33)*. Although the role of DHEA in the treatment of AIDS has not yet been determined, the drug appears to show potential for clinical benefit that warrant evaluation in large, randomized, controlled trials.

DHEA AND DIABETES MELLITUS

Several lines of evidence indicate that insulin influences DHEA metabolism. Both insulin receptors and insulin-like growth factor I receptors have been identified on human adrenal glands *(51)*, suggesting a possible role for insulin in the regulation of adrenal function. Moreover, eidemiologic studies report that serum DHEA in men is reduced in conditions characterized by insulin resistance and hyperinsulinemia, such as obesity *(52)*, hypertension *(53)*, and untreated type II diabetes mellitus *(54)*. In addition in a series of elegant studies Nestler et al. was able to demonstrate that in men: 1-insulin infusion acutely lowers serum DHEA levels *(55)*, 2-amelioration of insulin resistance and hyperinsulinemia is associated with a rise is serum DHEA over a broad range of ages *(56)*, 3-insulin acutely increases the metabolic clearance rate of DHEA *(57)*, and 4-insulin inhibits adrenal androgen production *(58)*.

These observations led investigators to suggest that reduced serum DHEA may be an indicator of insulin sensitivity problems and that insulin resistance may be ameliorated by DHEA administration *(59)*. Bates et al. in a placebo-controlled trial, administered 50 mg of DHEA daily to 15 postmenopausal women for three weeks period and was able to demonstrate a significant enhancement in insulin sensitivity index *(60)*. A similar effect of DHEA on insulin sensitivity was demonstrated by Casson et al. who administered 50 mg of DHEA to 11 postmenopausal women for a period of three weeks *(61)*. Larger placebo-controlled trials, however, are needed in different sex and age groups before making definitive conclusions regarding the biological effect of DHEA in patients with diabetes mellitus.

DHEA AND OSTEOPOROSIS

Low serum levels of DHEA were postulated as a possible risk factor for the development of osteoporosis *(62)*. A positive correlation between serum levels of DHEAS and bone mineral density in the lumbar spine, femoral neck, and radius mid-shaft has been demonstrated in women aged 45–69 yr *(63)*. However, the mechanism(s) by which DHEA may offer protection against osteoporosis remain an enigma. DHEA may have a non-estrogenic effect on bone as there were no significant differences in estrogen levels among women with different bone densities *(63)*. However, DHEA may be converted by bone osteocytes to estrogen resulting in slowing down of bone resorption. Furthermore, a metabolite of DHEA and DHEAS, 4-androstene-3 beta,17 beta-diol, has an affinity for estrogen receptors *(64)* and may act as an antiresortptive agent. Prospective placebo-controlled trials are needed, however, to confirm the protective effect of DHEA against osteoporosis and to define recommendations for therapeutic interventions.

DHEA AND THE CENTRAL NERVOUS SYSTEM

DHEAS has been shown to improve memory in young and old mice *(90)*. The administration of a steroid sulfatase inhibitor enhances memory and acetylcholine levels while increasing DHEA levels *(91)*. These animal studies have suggested a role for DHEAS in memory consolidation, whereas increasing DHEA levels DHEAS levels in the human brain were found to be higher (3.0 ng/g) than the levels in the adrenal gland (2.9 ng/g), which in turn are three to four times higher than plasma levels *(65)*. This suggests that DHEAS could be a neuroreactive steroidal hormone *(5)*. Patients with Alzheimer's disease were found to have lower levels of DHEA and DHEAS *(66,67)*. However, the weight of evidence from recent studies does not strongly support a role in Alzheimer's disease *(5)*. In male nursing home patients, plasma DHEAS levels were inversely related to the presence of organic brain syndrome and to the degree of dependence in activities of daily living *(68)*.

Pilot studies of DHEA administration to medical or psychiatric patients noted improvement in mood, energy, libido, and in some cases memory *(69)*. DHEA when administered to depressed patients resulted in improvement in their depressive symptoms *(70)*. Also, length and quality of sleep were found to have improved as did well-being, in aged men and women treated with DHEA 50 mg/d for 3 mo *(49,71)*. Thus, it appears form the initial pilot studies that DHEA is involved in behavior. Larger scale double-blind trials addressing this issue are currently underway. A recent carefully controlled study failed to demonstrate an effect of DHEA on mood *(92)*.

Current DHEA Status

Although the results from initial human studies appear promising, they still need to be confirmed by large-scale controlled studies. At the present time, a beneficial effect of DHEA administration in humans has not yet been firmly established, and the side effects of chronic DHEA administration are virtually not known. Thus, it does not seem reasonable at the present time to dispense DHEA. This status, however, is expected to change in the near future given the magnitude of current human DHEA-related research. It is expected that a therapeutic role for DHEA will be established which could take the form of hormone replacement therapy or as pharmacologic therapy for specific pathologic conditions (1).

PREGNENOLONE

Pregnenolone is the precursor of all of the known steroid hormones (Fig. 1), and as such posses several typical steroid hormonal effects (72,73). The formation of pregnenolone, by the conversion from cholesterol via the action of cytochrome P450scc (side-chain cleavage), is the rate limiting step in steroid hormone formation. Like DHEA, its secretion from the adrenal also declines with age showing a 60% reduction at 75 yrcompared to the mean values observed at 35 yr.

Effects of Pregnenolone on Physical Decline

Similar to its derivatives, pregnenolone may be involved in the modulation of muscle strength, osteoporosis and immune function which may be achieved directly or from its conversion to other steroid hormones. In a recent animal study, injection of pregnenolone prior to administration of a lysozyme antigen, increased titers of antilysozyme IgG compared with controls suggesting its role in the regulation of body's immune response (87).

In the 1940s and 1950s, pregnenolone was safely used as a treatment for rheumatoid arthritis and other inflammatory conditions. Outcomes in the treatment of rheumatoid arthritis were variable, improving symptoms in majority of patients in most studies, but having few effects in other studies (74,75). From anecdotal evidence volunteered by our subjects in preliminary studies, pregnenolone administration mitigated "aches and pains" attributed to arthritis. The mechanism of the anti-inflammatory effects of pregnenolone is unclear, and its impact on aspects of frailty in humans has not been explored.

Pregnenolone and the Central Nervous System

In addition to serving as a precursor for the formation of different steroids, pregnenolone also appears to directly affect both GABAA (gamma amino butyric acid)A and NMDA (N methyl D aspartate) receptors in the central nervous system (CNS) (76,77). As a neurosteroid, pregnenolone may have a role in the regulation of behavior, mood, anxiety, learning, and sleep. Within animal brains, regional alterations in the concentration of pregnenolone sulfate have been associated with different physiological states, i.e., stress, diurnal cycles, or sexual activities (78).

During the mid 1940s, several experiments were performed examining the effects of pregnenolone on psychomotor performance in humans. In a study of nearly 300 factory workers who were given up to 70 mg of pregnenolone for up to 3 months, pregnenolone improved production efficiency in groups deemed to be working under more stressful conditions, those being paid per piece rather than paid per hour *(79,80)*. Effects of pregnenolone administration on psychomotor performance in pilots included a decrease in fatigue and an improvement in targeting scores *(81)*. In a recent study in humans, 1 mg doses of pregnenolone affected EEG patterns during sleep, improved sleep efficiency and decreased intermittent wakefulness *(82)*.

Pregnenolone and Memory

In animal studies of steroid hormones and memory, intracerebro-ventricular infusion of pregnenolone in mice showed a direct dose-response relationship with memory retention in foot shock active avoidance training. When infused into the nucleus basalis magnocellularis, a part of the brain observed to undergo marked cell loss in patients with Alzheimer's dementia *(83)*, pregnenolone sulfate enhanced memory performance in rats *(84)*. Our group also demonstrated that pregnenolone when injected in mice brains enhances posttraining memory processes *(88,89)*. The effect of pregnenolone on memory in humans has not been established.

Pregnenolone in Humans

In our preliminary study, 22 healthy men and women aged 20–88 yr were given 500 mg pregnenolone each day for a period of 12 wk. This study found no effects on strength, balance, or memory *(93)*. Early studies had suggested that pregnenolone may improve attention span and performance in humans *(94)*.

Pregnenolone: Side Effects Profile

Problems often arise that preclude prolonged hormonal replacement. For example, in men prostatic hypertrophy and polycythemia are risks of long term testosterone replacement. Multiple studies in humans and animals have demonstrated no significant untoward effects owing to pregnenolone even with long-term administration. Specifically, there have been no reported effects on glucose, weight, heart rate, blood pressure, gastrointestinal symptoms, or menstrual cycles *(74,75,85)*. One case of mild rash was reported to occur with oral pregnenolone *(86)*. The minimum of side effects noted with pregnenolone may be attributed to the maintenance of normal steroid patterns, minimizing the disruption of feedback mechanisms in steroid formation and competition of steroid for receptor binding sites. Pregnenolone alone or with small amounts of androgens, estrogens or DHEA may avoid the side effects of large doses of these derivatives. Pregnenolone could serve as a precursor of indigenous synthesis of these hormones and may facilitate their actions through allosteric effects exerted by binding at different loci of the same receptors.

CONCLUSIONS

Because there are many tantalizing clues suggesting salutary effects of DHEA and pregnenolone on the aging process, so far controlled studies have failed to demonstrate these benefits in a convincing manner. There is a clear need for further long term controlled studies. Our preliminary studies have questioned whether commercially available DHEA always contains the amounts of DHEA stated on the bottle. This further confuses an already complex field.

REFERENCES

1. Nestler JE. DHEA: a Coming of age. Ann NY Acad Sci 1995;774:ix–xi.
2. Horani MH, Morley JE. The viability of the use of DHEA. Clin Geriatr 1997;5(4):34–48.
3. Longcope C. Adrenal and gonadal androgen secretion in normal females. Clin Endocrinol Metab 1986;15:213–228.
4. Butenandt A, Danenbaum H. Isolierung neuen, physiologisch unwirksamen Sterindervates aus Mannerharn, Seine Verknupfung mit Dehdro-androsterone und Androsteron. Z Physiol Chem 1934;229:192–195.
5. Watson RR, Huls A, Araghinikuam M, Chung S. Dehydroepiandrosterone and diseases of aging. Drugs Aging 1996;9(4):274–291.
6. Dunn JF, Nisula BC, Rodbard D. Transport of steroid hormones:Binding of 21 endogenous steroid to both testosterone-binding globulin and corticosteroid-binding globulin in human plasma. J Clin Endocrinol Metab 1965;53:58:68.
7. Vermeulen A. Adrenal Androgens. Raven Press, New York, 1980, pp. 207–217.
8. Orentreich N, Brind JL, Vogelman JH, Andres R, Baldwin H. Long-term longitudinal measurements of plasma dehydroepiandrosterone sulfate in normal men. J Clin Endocrinol Metab 1992;75:1002–1004.
9. Vermeulen A. dehydroepiandrosterone sulfate and aging. Ann NY Acad Sci 1995, 774:121–127.
10. Liu CH, Laughlin GA, Fischer UG, Yen SS. Marked attenuation of ultradian and circadian rhythms of dehydroepiandrosterone in postmenopausal women:evidence for a reduced 17,20-desmolase enzymatic activity. J Clin End Metab 1990;71(4):900–906.
11. Rotter JI, Wong L, Lifrank ET, Parker LM. A genetic component of the variation of dehydroepiandrosterone sulfate, Metabolism 1985;34:731–736.
12. Barrett-Connor E, Khaw KT, Yen SS. A prospective study of dehydroepandrosterone sulfate, mortality, and cardiovascular disease. N Engl J Med 1986;315:1519–1524.
13. Helzouer KJ, Gordon GB, Alberg AJ, Bush TL, Comstock GW. Relationship of prediagnostic serum levels of dehydroepiiaandrosterone and dehydroepiandrosterone sulfate to the risk of developing premenopausal breast cancer. Cancer Res 1992;52:1–4.
14. Gordon GB, Helzouer KJ, Alberg AJ, Comstock GW. Serum levels of dehydroepiandrosterone and dehydroepiandrosterone sulfate and the risk of developing gastric cancer. Cancer Epid Biomark Prevent 1993;2:33–35.
15. Szathmari M, Szucs J, Feher T, Hollo I. Dehydroepiandrosterone sulfate and bone mineral density. Osteoporosis Intl 1994;4:84–88.
16. Nordin BE, Robeertson A, Seamark RF, Bridges A, Philcox JC, Need AG, Horowitz M, Morris HA, Deam S. The relation between calcium absorption , serum dehydroepiandrosterone and vertebral mineral density in postmentopausal women. J Clin Endocrinol Metab 1985;60:651–657.
17. Barrett-Connor E. Kiltz-Silverstein D, Edelstein SL. A prospective study of dehydroepiandrosterone sulfate (DHEAS) and bone mineral density in older men and women. Am J Epidemiol 1993;137:201–206.
18. Marmorston J, Lewis JJ, Bernesetein JL, Sobel H, Kuzna O, Alexander R, Magidson O, Moore FJ. Excretion of urinary steroids by men and women with myocardial infarction. Geriatrics 1957;12:297–300.
19. Marmorston J, Griffith CC, Geller PJ, Fishman EL, Welsch F, Weiner JM. Urinary steroids in the measurement of aging and of . JAGS 1975;23:481–492.
20. Kask E. Ketosteroids and arteriosclerosis. Angiology 1959;10:358–368.
21. Khaw KT. Dehydroepiandrosterone, dehydroepiandrosterone sulphate and cardiovascular disease. J Endocrinol 1996;150:S149–S153.
22. Barrett-Connor E, Khaw K-T, Yen SSC. A prospective study of dehydroepiandrosterone sulfate, mortality, and cardiovascular disease. N Engl J Med 1986;315:1519–1524.
23. Barrett-Connor E., Edelstein SL. A prospective study of dehydroepiandrosterone sulfate and cognitive function in an older population: the Rancho Bernardo Study. JAGS 1994;42:420–423.
24. LaCroix AZ, Yano K, Reed DM. Dehydroepiandrosterone sulfate, incidence of myocardial infarction and extent of atherosclerosis in men. Circulation 1992;86:1529–1535.
25. Hautanen A, Mnttari M, Manninen V, Tenkanen L, Huttunen JK, Frick MH, Adlercreutz H. Adrenal androgens and testosterone as coronary risk factors in the Helsinki Heart Study. Atherosclerosis 1994;105:191–200.
26. Newcornewr LM, Manson JE, Barbieri RL, Hennekens CH, Stampfer MJ. Dehdroepiandrosterone sulfate and the risk of myocardial infarction in US male physicians: a prospective study. Am J Epidemiol 1994;140:870–875.

27. Jesse RL, Loesser K, Eich DM, Zhen Y, Hess M, Nestleer JE. Dehydroepiandrosterone Inhibits Human Platelet Aggregation in vitro and in vivo. Ann NY Acad Sci 1995;774:281–290.
28. Gordon GB, Bush DE, Weisiman HF. Reduction of atherosclerosis by administration of dehydroepiandrosterone. A study in the hypercholesterolemic New Zealand white rabbit with aortic intimal injury. J Clin Invest 1988;82:712–720.
29. Arad Y, Badimon JO, Badimon L, Hemmberec W, Ginsberg HN. Dehydroepiandrosterone feeding prevents aortic fatty streak formation and cholesterol accumulation in cholesterol-fed rabbit. Atherosclerosis 1989;9:159–166.
30. Eich DM, Nestler JE, Johnson DE, Doworkin GH, KO D, Wechsler, Hess ML. Inhibition of accelerated coronary atherosclerosis with dehydroepiandrosterone in the heterotopic rabbit model of cardiac transplantation. Circulation 1993;87:261–269.
31. Kawai S, Yahata N, Nishida S, et al. Dehydroepiandrosterone inhibits B 16 mouse melanoma cell growth by induction of differentiation. Anticancer Res 1995;15:427–431.
32. Ivanovic S, Agbaba D, Zivanov-Stakle D, et al. The urinary dehydroepiandrosterone, androsterone and eticholanolone excretion of healthy women and women with benign and malignant breast disease. J Clin Pharm Ther 1990;15:213–219.
33. Jakubowicz D, Beer N, Rengifo R. Effect of dehydroepoandrosterone on cyclic-guanosine monophophate in men of advancing age. Ann NY Acad Sci 1995;774:312–315.
34. Beer NA, Jakubowicz DJ, Matt DW, Beer RM, Nestler JE. Dehydroepiandrosterone reduces plasma plasminogen activator inhibitor type 1 and tissue plasminogen activator antigen in men. Am J Med Sci 1996;311(5):205–210.
35. Rao MS. Subbarao V, Yeldandi AV, et al. Inhibition of spontaneous testicular leydig cell tumor development in F-344 rats by dehydroepiandrosterone. Cancer Lett 1992;65:123–126.
36. Schwartz AG, Pashko LL. Cancer chemoprevention with the adrenocortical steroid dehydroepiandrosterone and structural analogs. J Cell Biochem 1993;17G (Suppl):73–79.
37. Schwrtz AG, Pashko LL. Cancer prevention with dehydroepiandrosterone and no-androgenic structural analogs. J Cell Biochem 1995;22 (Suppl):210–217.
38. Klamm RC, Holbrooke CT, Nyce JW. Chemotherapy of murine colorectal carcinoma with cisplatin plus 3'-deoxy'3'-azidothymidine. Anticancer Res 1992;12:781–787.
39. Bhatavdekar JM, Patel DD, Chikhikaar RR, et al. Levels of circulating peptide and steroid hormones in men with lung cancer. Neoplasma 1994;41:101–103.
40. Gordon GB, Helzlsouer KJ, Comstock GW. Serum levels of dehydroepiandrosterone and its sulfate and the risk of developing bladder cancer. Cancer Res 1991;51:1366–369.
41. Magee JM, Mckenzie S, Filippa DA, et al. Hairy cell leukemia:durability of response to splenectomy in 26 patients and treatment of relapse with androgens in six patients. Cancer 1985;56:2557–2562.
42. Liberto MH, Sonohara S, Brentant MM. Effects of androgens on proliferation and progesterone receptor levels in T47D human breast cancer cells. Tumour Biol 1993;14:38–45.
43. Boccuzzi G, DiMonaco M, Brignardello E, et al. Dehydroepiandrosterone antiestrogenic action through androgen receptor MCF-7 human breast cancer cell line. Anticancer Res 1993;13:2267–2272.
44. Boccuzzi G, DiMonaco M, Brignardello E, et al. Influence of dehydroepiandrosterone and 5-en-androstene-3 beta, 17 beta-diol on the growth of MCF-7 human breast cancer cells induced by 17 beta-estradiol. Anticancer Res 1992;12:799–803.
45. Daynes RA, Araneo BA, Ershler WB, et al. Altered regulation of IL-6 production with normal aging:possible linkage to the age-associated decline in dehydroepiandrosterone and its sulfated derivatives. J Immunol 1993;150:5219–5230.
46. Daynes RA, Araneo BA. Prevention and reversal of some age-associated changes in immunologic responses by supplemental dehydroepiandrosterone sulfate therapy. Aging Immun Infect Dis 1992;3:135–154.
47. Garg M, Bondada S. reversal of age associated decline in immune response to Pnu-immune vaccine by supplementation with the steroid hormone dehydroepiandrosterone. Infection Immun 1993;61:2238–2241.
48. Araneo BA, Woods ML, II, Dynes RA. Reversal of the immunosenescent phenotype by dehydroepiandrosterone: hormone treatment provides an adjutant effect on the immunization of aged mice with recombinant hepatitis B surface antigen. J Infect Dis 1993;167:830–840.
49. Yen SSC, Morales AJ, Khorram O. Replacement of DHEA in aging men and women: potential remedial effects. Ann NY Acad Sci 1995;774:128–142.
50. Chatterton RT Jr, Green D, Harris S, Grossman A, Hechter O. Longitudinal study of adrenal steroids in a cohort of HIV-infected patients with hemophilia. J Lab Clin Med 1996;127(6):545–552.

51. Kamio T, Shigematsu K, Kawai K, Tsuchiyama H. Immunoreactivity and receptor expression of insulin-like growth factor I and insulin in human adrenal tumors. An immunohistochemical study of 94 cases. Am J Pathol 1991;138:83–91.

52. Sonka J. Dehydroepiandrosterone. Metabolic effects. In: Charvat J, ed. Acta Universitais Carolinae, Universita Krlova Praha, Prague, 1976, pp. 1–171.

53. Nafziger An, Herrington DM, Bush TL. Dehydroepiandrosterone and dehydroepiandrosterone sulfate: Their relation to cardiovascular disease. Epidemiol Res 1991;13:267–293.

54. Barrett-Conor E. Lower endogenous androgen levels and dylipidemia in men with non-insulin-dependent diabetes mellitus. Ann Intern Med 1992;117:807–811.

55. Nestler JE, Usiskin KS, Barlascini CO, Welty D, Clore JN, Blackard WG. Suppression of serum dehydroepiandrosterone sulfate levels by insulin:An evaluation of possible mechanisms. J Clin Endocrinol Metab 1989;69:1040–1046.

56. Nestler JE, Beer NA, Jakubowicz DJ, Beer RM. Effects of a reduction in circulating insulin by metformin on serum dehydroepiandrosterone sulfate in nondiabetic men. J Clin Endocrinol Metab 1994;78:549–554.

57. Nestler JE, Kahwaash Z. Sex-specific action of insulin to acutely increase the metabolic clearance rate of dehydroepiandrosterone in humans. J Clin Invest 1994;94:1484–1489.

58. Nestler JE, McClanahan MA, Clore JN, Blackard WG. Insulin inhibits adrenal 17, 20-lyase activity in man. J Clin Endocrinol Metab 1992;74:362–367.

59. Nestler JE. Regulation of human dehydroepiandrosterone metabolism by insulin. Ann NY Acad Sci 1995;774:73–81.

60. Bates GW Jr, Egerman RS, Umstor ES, Buster JE, Casson PR. Dehydroepiandrosterone attenuates study-induced declines in insulin sensitivity in postmentopausal women. Ann NY Acad Sci 1995;774:291–293.

61. Casson PR, Faquin LC, Stenz FB, Straugh AB, Anderson RN, Abraham GE, Buster JE. Replacement of dehydroepiandrosterone enhances T-lymphocyte insulin binding in postmentopausal women. Fertil Steril 1995;63(5):1027–1031.

62. Nordin BE, Robertson A, Seamark RF, Bridges A, et al. The relation between calcium absorption, serum dehydroepiandrosterone, and vertebral mineral density in postmenopausal women. J Clin Endocrinol Metab 1985;60(4):651–657.

63. Szathmari M, Szucs J, Feher T, Hollo I. Dehydroepiandrosterone sulphate and bone mineral density. Osteoporosis Int. 1994;4(2):84–88.

64. Rozenberg S, Ham H, Bosson D, Peretz A, Robyn C. Age, steroids and bone mineral content. Maturitas 1990;12(2):137–143.

65. Maewska MD. Neuronal actions of DHEAS: possible roles in brain development, aging, memory and affect. Ann NY Acad Sci 1995;774:111–121.

66. Nasman B, Olsson T, Backstrom T, et al. Serum dehydorepiandrosterone sulfate in Alzheimer's disease and in multi-infarct dementia. Biol Psychiatry 1991;30:684–690.

67. Dodt C, Dittman J, Hruby J, et al. Different regulation of adrenocorticotropin and cortisol secretion in young mentally healthy elderly and patients with senile dementia of Alzheimer's type. J Clin Endocrinol Metabol 1991d;72:272–276.

68. Rudman D, Shetty KR, Mattson DE. Plasma deydroepiandrosterone sulfate in nursing home men. J Am Geriatr Soc 1990;38:421–427.

69. Kalimi M, Reglson W (Eds). 1990. The Biologic Role of Dehydroepiandrosterone. Walter de Gruyter, Berlin.

70. Wolkowitz OM, Reus VI, Roberts E, et al. Antidepressant and cognition-enhancing effects of DHEA in major depression. Ann NY Acad Sci 1995;774:337–339.

71. Morales AJ, Nolan JJ, Nelson JC, et al. effects of replacement dose of dehydroepiandroosterone in men and women of advancing age. J Clin Endocrinol Metab 1994;78:1360–1367.

72. Seley H. correlations between the chemical structure and pharmacological actions of the steroids. Endocrinology 1942;30:437–453.

73. Seley H. The pharmacology of steroid hormones and their derivatives. Rev Can Bio 1942;1:573–632.

74. McGavack TH, Chevalley J, Weissberg J. the use of Δ5 pregnenolone in various clinical disorders. J Clin Endocrinol 1951;11:559–577.

75. Brugsh HG, Manning RA. A comprehensive study of pregnenolone, 21 acetoxypregnenolone and ACTH. N Eng J Med 1951;d244:628–632.

76. Wu FS, Gibbs TT, Farb DH. Pregnenonolone sulfate: a positive allosteric modulator at N-Methyl-D-aspartate receptor. Mol Pharmacol 1991;40:333–336.

77. Irwin RP, NJ, Rogawski MA, et al. Pregnenolone sulfate augments NMDA receptor mediated increases in intracellular Ca 2+ in cultured rat hippocampal neurons. Neurosci Lett 1992;141:30–34.

78. Akwa Y, Young J, Kabbadj K, Sancho MJ, et al. Neurosteroid:biosynthesis, metabolism and function of pregnenolone and dehydroepiandrosterone in the brain. J Steroid Biochem Mol Biol 1991;40(1–3):71–81.

79. Pincus G, Hoagland H. Effects on industrial production of the administration of 5 pregnenolone to factor workers, I. Psychosom Med 1945;7:342–346.

80. Pincus G, Hoagland H, Wilson CH, Fay NJ. Effects on industrial production of the administration of 5 pregnenolone to factory workers, II. Psychosom Med 1945;7:347–352.

81. Pincus G, Hoagland H. effects of administered pregnenolone on fatiguing psychomotor performance. J Aviat Med 1944;15:98–115,135.

82. Stiger A, Trachsel L, Guldner J, et al. Neurosteroid pregnenolone induces sleep-EEG changes in man compatible with inverse agonistic GABAA-receptor modulation. Brain Res 1993;615:267–274.

83. Saper CB, German DC, White CL. Neuronal pathology in the nucleus basalis and associated cell groups in senile dementia of the Alzheimer's type:possible role in cell loss. Neurology 1985;35:1089–1095.

84. Mayo W, Dellu F, Robel P, et al. Infusion of neurosteroids into the nucleus basalis magnocellularis affects cognitive processes in the rat. Brain Res 1993;607:324–328.

85. Henderson E, Weinberg M, Wright WA. Pregnenolone. Endocr Rev 1950;10:455–474.

86. Tyler ET, Payne S, Kirsch. Pregnenolone in male infertility. West J Surg 1943;56:459–463.

87. Morfin R. Courchy G. Pregnenolone and dehydroepiandrosterone as a precursors of native 7-hydroxylated metabolites which increases the immune response in mice. J Steroid Biochem Molec Biol 1994;50:91–100.

88. Flood JF, Morley JE, Roberts E. Memory-enhancing effects in male mice of pregnenolone and steroids metabolically derived from it. Proc Natl Acad Sci USA 1992;89(5):1567–1571.

89. Flood JF, Morley JE, Roberts E. Pregnenolone sulfate enhances post-training memory processes when injected in very low doses into limbic system structures:the amygdala is by far the most sensitive. Proc Natl Acad Sci USA 1995;92(23):10,806–10,810.

90. Flood JF, Morley JE, Roberts E. Memory-enhancing effects in male mice of pregnenolone and steroids metabolically derived from it. Proc Natl Acad Sci USA 1992;89(5):1567–1571.

91. Li PK, Rhodes ME, Burke ME, Johnson DA. Memory enhancement mediated by the steroid sulfatase inhibitor (p-O-sulfamoyl)-N-tetradecanoyl tyramine. Life Sci 1997;60(3):PL45–51.

92. Wolf OT, Neumann O, Hellammer DH, Geiben AC, Strasburger CJ, et al. Effects of a two-week physiological dehydroepiandrosterone substitution on cognitive performance and well-being in healthy elderly women and men. J Clin Endocrinol Metab 1997;82(7):2363–2367.

93. Sih R. Morley JE, Kaiser FE, Herning M. Effects of pregnenolone on aging. J Investig Med 1997;45(7):348A [Abstract].

94. Morley JE, Kaiser F, Raum WJ, Perry HM, III, Flood JF, et al. Potentially predictive and manipulable blood serum correlates of aging in the healthy human male:progressive decreases in bioavailalable testosterone, dehydroepiandrosterone sulfate. Proc Natl Acad Sci USA 1997;94(14):7537–7542.

95. Buster JE, Casson PR, Straughan AB, et al. Postmenopausal steroid replacement with micronized dehydroepiandrosterone:preliminary oral bioavailability and dose proportionality studies. Am J Obstet Gynecol 1992;166(4):1163–1168.

96. Vollenhoven RF, Engelman EG, McGuire JL. Dehydroepiandrosterone in systemic lupus erythromaotosus. Results of a double-blind, placebo-controlled, randomized clinical trial. Arthritis Rheum 1995;38(12):1826–1831.

97. Araneo B, Dowell T, Woods ML, et al. DHEAS as an effective vaccine adjuvant in elderly humans. Proof-of-principal studies. Ann NY Acad Sci 1995;774:23248.

98. Dyner TS, Lang W, Geaga J, et al. An open-label dose-escalation trial of oral dehydroepiandrosteronee tolerance and pharmackinetics in patients with HIV disease. J AIDS 1993;6:459–465.

99. Friss E, Trachse L, Guldner J, et al. DHE administration increases rapid eye movement sleep and EEG power in the sigma frequency range. Am J Physiol 1995;268:E107–113.

100. Buffington CK, Pourmotabbed G, Kitabchi AE. Case report:amelioration of insulin resistance in diabetes with dehydroepiandrosterone. Am J Med Sci 1993;306(5):320–324.

101. Casson PR, Faquin LC, Stenz FB, Straughn AB, Anderson RN, et al. Replacement of dehydroepiandrosterone enhances T-lymphocyte insulin binding in postmentopausal women. Fertil Steril 1995;63(5):1027–1031.

102. Usiskin KS, Butterworth S, Clore JN, Arad Y, et al. Lack of effect of dehydroepiandrosterone in obese men. Int J Obese;14(5):457–463.

103. Jones JA, Nguyen A, Straub M, et al. Use of DHEA in a patient with advanced prostate cancer: a case report and review. Urology 1997;50(5):784–4788.

104. Labrie F, Diamond P, Cusan L, et al. Effect of 12-month dehydroepiandrosterone replacement therapy on bone, vagina, and endometrium in postmentopausal women. J Clin Endo Metabol 1997;82(10):3498–3505.

105. Danenberg HD, Benyehuda A, Zakayrones Z, et al. Dehydroepiandrosterone treatment is not beneficial to the immune response to influenza in elderly subjects. J Clin Endo Metab 1997, 82:2911–2914.

106. Evans TG, Judd ME, Dowel T, et al. The use of oral dehydroepiandrosterone sulfate as an adjuvant in tetanus and influenza vaccination of the elderly. Vaccine 1996;14(16):1531–1537.

107. Diamond P, Cusan L, Gomez JL, et al. Metabolic effects of 12-month percutaneous dehydroepiandrosterone replacement therapy in postmentopausal women. J Endocrin 1996;150 (Suppl S):S43–50.

VI GONADAL

16 Androgen Replacement Therapy of Male Hypogonadism

A. Wayne Meikle, MD

INTRODUCTION

Male hypogonadism is a relatively common disorder in clinical practice and has significant effects on the fertility, sexual function and general health of patients *(1–8)*. Disorders of sperm and testosterone production may be caused by primary, secondary, or tertiary hypogonadism. Some are relatively common and others are rare. Klinefelter's syndrome is a primary testicular disorder occurring in about 1 in 500 men and resulting in both androgen deficiency and infertility *(9–11)*. In men with clinical manifestations of primary or secondary hypogonadism, deficiency of testosterone usually can be treated effectively. Fertility in some men with primary testicular disease, such as Klinefelter's syndrome, is irreversible, but those with gonadotropin deficiency resulting in infertility can often be treated successfully *(12–14)*. Both testosterone deficiency and infertility can be corrected using gonadotropin or gonadotropin-releasing hormone (GnRH) therapy in men with hypogonadotropic hypogonadism. Understanding the pathophysiology of hypogonadism is needed to plan and use appropriate hormonal replacement therapy in men with deficiency of testosterone and sperm production.

OVERVIEW OF PHYSIOLOGY OF THE TESTES

GnRH made by the hypothalamus and secreted in a pulsatile pattern stimulates the release of gonadotropins (luteinizing [LH] and follicle stimulating hormone [FSH]) *(1,8)*.

From: *Contemporary Endocrinology: Hormone Replacement Therapy*
Edited by: A. W. Meikle © Humana Press Inc., Totowa, NJ

In the testis, Leydig cells comprise a small proportion of the mass of the testes and synthesize and secrete testosterone in response to LH, which is regulated by feedback effects of testosterone and its metabolites. The seminiferous tubule compartment comprises about 85% of the mass of the testes and contains Sertoli cells surrounding developing germ cells that produces mature spermatozoa. FSH binds to receptors and stimulates the Sertoli cells to produce an androgen-binding protein enabling the testes to concentrate testosterone many-fold above the serum levels. Sertoli cells also make inhibin, which has feedback influence on FSH secretion (14–18).

Testosterone and its potent 5-alpha metabolite, dihydrotestosterone (DHT), have important physiologic influences during embryogenesis, puberty and adulthood (8). During fetal development, testosterone and DHT result in normal differentiation of male internal and external genitalia (19,20).

During puberty, testosterone and DHT are required for the development and maintenance of male secondary sexual characteristics. DHT results in growth of the prostate and masculinization of the skin (8,21). The remaining androgen effects are from the actions of testosterone and include growth of the seminal vesicles, phallus and scrotum; growth of skeletal muscle; lowering of body fat; stimulation of long bone growth and mass, and closure of epiphyses; growth of normal male hair pattern; enlargement of the larynx resulting in deepening of the voice; enhancement of sexual behavior and function (libido and potency); and initiation of sperm formation. In adults, testosterone and DHT are required for the maintenance of libido and potency, muscle mass and strength, fat distribution, bone mass, erythropoiesis, prostate growth, male pattern hair growth, and spermatogenesis.

Pathophysiology

Hypogonadism is caused by disorders of the testes (primary, as listed in Table 1), pituitary (secondary), or hypothalamus (tertiary) (1,8). Testosterone deficiency may occur as the result of Leydig cell dysfunction from primary disease of the testes, inadequate LH secretion from diseases of the pituitary, or impaired GnRH secretion by the hypothalamus. Infertility may be observed in men with testosterone deficiency, seminiferous tubules disease, or hypogonadotropic hypogonadism.

Pinpointing the cause of hypogonadism makes it possible to tailor successful replacement therapy Table 2. Men with primary gonadal failure usually have either isolated azoospermia or oligospermia or combined with testosterone deficiency. In most of these men with impaired spermatogenesis, infertility is not reversible but special techniques for isolation of sperm from the testes make fertility possible in some cases with any sperm formation. In contrast, hormonal therapy in men with hypogonadotropic hypogonadism may stimulate spermatogenesis adequate for fertility. Testosterone therapy is offered to men with androgen deficiency when successful fertility is improbable or not desired. When fertility is desired in men with potentially correctable infertility, hormonal therapy with gonadotropins may be used in those with a secondary or tertiary disorder and GnRH in those with tertiary disease.

General Manifestations

CLINICAL PRESENTATION

The clinical presentation of male hypogonadism depends on the stage of sexual development (1,8). If androgen deficiency occurs during fetal development from defects in

Table 1
Causes of Hypogonadism

Gonadal defects
    Genetic Defect; Klinefelter's Syndrome, myotonic dystrophy, Prader-Willi Syndrome
    Polyglandular autoimmune failure syndromes (eg. Schmidt Syndrome)
    Anatomic Defects
    Toxins; cytotoxic agents, spironolactone, alcohol
    Radiation
    Orchitis; usually a result of mumps
Hormone Resistance
    Androgen insensitivity
    Luteinizing hormone insensitivity
Hypopituitarism
    Idiopathic
    Tumor
    Other causes
Hyperprolactinemia
    Usually owing to pituitary adenoma
    Idiopathic increased prolactin production
Gonadotropin deficiency
    Hypogonadotropic Hypogonadism
    Isolated congenital idiopathic GnRH deficiency
        GnRH deficiency with anosmia - Kallman Syndrome
        Acquired GnRH deficiency is very uncommon
    Respond to pulsatile GnRH administration
    Hypothalamic Insufficiency
    LH or FSH Deficiency
Systemic diseases
    Chronic Diseases
    Malnutrition / Starvation
    Massive Obesity
    AIDS/HIV

Table 2
Laboratory Testing of Hypogonadism

Hypothalmic	*Primary hypogonadism*	*Seminiferous Tubule disease*	*Leydig cell failure*	*Pituitary disease*	*Hypothalmic disease*
Testosterone	Low	Normal	Low	Low	Low
LH	High	Normal	High	Low	Low
FSH	High	High	Normal	Low	Low
Sperm count	Low	Low	Low	Low	Low
LH and FSH response to GnRH	Normal	Not done	Not done	Low	Normal

Review: Interpreting the results: 1. Testosterone low, LH and FSH elevated; primary hypogonadism; order karyotype. 2. Testosterone low, LH and FSH normal or low; secondary hypogonadism, obtain PRL and CT scan of head to screen for mass lesion; remaining pituitary hormones must be tested for deficiency. 3. Testosterone and LH normal, FSH high; abnormal seminiferous tubule compartment; order semen analysis. 4. Testosterone, LH and FSH high; androgen resistance syndrome.

Table 3
Clinical Presentation of Peripubertal Hypogonadism

Small testes, phallus, and prostate (prepubertal testes are between 3 and 4 mL in volume and less
  than 3 cm long by 2 cm wide; peripubertal testes are between 4 and 15 mL in volume and from
  3–4 cm long by 2–3 cm wide)
Lack of male-pattern hair growth
Scant pubic and axillary hair, if adrenal androgens are also deficient
Disproportionately long arms and legs (from delayed epiphyseal closure, eunuchoidism; with the
  crown-to-pubis ratio < 1 and an arm span more than 6 cm greater than height)
No pubertal growth spurt
No increase in libido or potency
Reduced male musculature
Gynecomastia
Persistently high-pitched voice

androgen synthesis, metabolism, or androgen responsiveness, various manifestations of male pseudohermaphroditism may be observed.

Prepubertal. In boys with prepuberal hypogonadism, expression of the androgen deficit is seldom recognized before the age for onset of puberty unless associated growth retardation or other anatomic and endocrine abnormalities are found. Failure of puberty is well characterized by several clinical features as shown in Table 3.

Postpubertal. Postpubertal loss of testicular function may be manifested by infertility and androgen deficiency, and the clinical symptoms and signs may evolve slowly, making them relatively difficult to detect. These symptoms and signs in aging men may be mistaken for symptoms of aging and go unrecognized. The growth of male pattern body hair usually slows, but the voice and the size of the phallus, testes and prostate change little. In younger men, a delay in temporal hair recession and balding may go unnoticed as a manifestation of hypogonadism. Patients with postpubertal hypogonadism may have some or all of these clinical findings as summarized in Table 4.

GOAL OF ANDROGEN THERAPY

In testosterone replacement therapy, a safe general principle is to mimic the normal concentrations of testosterone (350–1050 ng/dL) and its active metabolites (22–26) and thereby avoiding unphysiologically high testosterone serum concentrations to prevent possible side-effects or low concentrations to prevent androgen deficiency. Although it is known that patients experience symptoms with androgen deficiency, it is not known whether unphysiologically high concentrations carry health risks. Until that is known, the safe course would be to duplicate normal physiology as closely as possible. When these goals are met, physiological responses to androgen replacement therapy can be achieved and allow virilization in prepuberal males and restoration or preservation of virilization in postpuberal men. The therapy should not have untoward effects on the prostate, serum lipids, and cardiovascular, liver, and lung function. Therapy should allow self-administration, be convenient, and cause minimal discomfort. Pharmacokinetic preparations should be reproducibility responses from day to day. Cost of treatment is also a consideration for each patient. None of the currently available androgen replacement therapies achieves the ideal, but the relative merits of each will be discussed. A review will be made

Table 4
Clinical Presentation of Postpubertal Hypogonadism

Progressive decrease in muscle mass
Loss of libido
Impotence
Infertility with oligospermia or azoospermia
Hot flashes (with acute onset of hypogonadism)
Osteoporosis
Anemia
Adult testes are usually between 15 and 30 mL and 4.5–5.5 cm long by 2.8–3.3 cm wide
Mild depression
Reduced energy

comparing the pharmacokinetics of different androgen preparations widely used for substitution therapy.

PHARMACOLOGY OF ANDROGENS

Historical Aspects

The first evidence that the testes produced virilizing substances came from Berthold *(27)* who transplanted testes from roosters into the abdomen of capons, which made them behave like normal roosters. Butenandt *(28)* was the first to obtain testosterone from urine and David *(29)* crystallized it from the urine of bulls. Testosterone was then chemically synthesized by Butenandt and Hanisch *(30)* and Ruzick and Wettstein *(31)*. After its synthesis, testosterone was introduced for treatment of hypogonadism. Since oral testosterone was ineffective, pellets were implanted subcutaneously or the methyl derivative (methyltestosterone) was administered orally. In the 1950s, testosterone ester injections gained widespread acceptance *(32)*. Other derivatives were prepared in an attempt to prepare steroids with anabolic properties. In the 1970s testosterone undecanoate, an oral preparation, became available for clinical use in some countries. Since derivatives of testosterone have hepatic toxicity, emphasis in recent years has been on delivering pure testosterone preparations, including long-acting testosterone esters, injection of testosterone microspheres, oral testosterone cyclodextrines and scrotal and nonscrotal patch systems and topical dihydrotestosterone. Although testosterone is metabolized to potent metabolites by steroid 5-alpha-reductase to form dihydrotestosterone and aromatase to form estradiol, chemical modification of testosterone results in compounds that are poor substrates for these enzymes. In contrast, testosterone esters release pure testosterone into the circulation.

Oral Testosterone Preparations

PURE TESTOSTERONE

Unesterified pure testosterone administered orally may be well absorbed by the gut, but it is largely metabolized by the liver to inactive products. Oral doses of 200 mg, compared to normal mean production of about 5 mg/d, are needed to exceed the liver's capacity to metabolize testosterone in normal men *(33–36)*. Further, 400–600 mg of pure testosterone administered orally are required to achieve replacement therapy. For these reasons, oral testosterone has not been used for replacement therapy.

Table 5
Structure of Testosterone and Its Derivatives

Generic name	R	X	Other modifications
Natural androgens			
Testosterone	H	H	
5α-Dihydrotestosterone	H	H	4,5-ane
Unmodified 17β esters			
Testosterone propionate	COCH2CH3	H	
Testosterone enanthate	$CO(CH_2)_5CH_3$	H	
Testosterone cypionate		H	
Testosterone undecanoate	$CO(CH_2)_8CH_2 = CH_2$	H	
Modified 17β esters			
Methanolone acetate	$COCH_3$	H	$1\text{-}CH_3$; 1,2-ene; 4,5-ane
Nandrolone phenylpropionate		H	19-nor CH_3
Nandrolone decanoate	$CO(CH_2)_6CH_3$	H	19-nor CH_3
17α-alkylation			
Methyltestosterone	H	CH_3	
Fluoxymesterone	H	CH_3	9-F; 11-OH
Methandroestenolone	H	CH_3	1,2-ene
Oxandrolone	H	CH_3	C_2 replaced by O; 4,5-ane
Oxymethelone	H	CH_3	2 = CHOH; 4,5-ane
Stanozole	H	CH_3	4,5-ane; [3,2-c]pyrazole
Danazole	H	$CH^{\underline{o}}C$ H	[2,3-d]isozazole
Norethandrolone	H	CH_2C H_3	19-nor CH_3
Ethylestrenole	H	CH_2C H_3	19-nor CH_3; 3-H
Modified androgen			
Mesterolone	H	H	$1\text{-}CH_3$; 4,5-ane

17-ALPHA-METHYLTESTOSTERONE

17-alpha-methyltestosterone was the first synthesized derivative of testosterone and is effective orally (Table 5). Peak blood levels are achieved between 1.5 and 2 h after ingestion, and it is cleared with a half-life of about 150 min, suggesting that several doses daily would be required to maintain a therapeutic level of the steroid (37). In men treated with the steroid, many articles have confirmed hepatic toxicity, including cholestasis, peliosis, elevation of liver enzymes and reduction of HDL-cholesterol (38–41). It has been withdrawn from the market in some countries and is not currently recommended for use. In addition, measurement of the steroid in the blood to monitor adequate dosing is not possible in most clinical laboratories.

FLUOXYMESTERONE

This steroid is a 17-alpha-methyltestosterone steroid with a fluorine in the 9 position. It has a longer half-time in serum than the parent steroid, but it has the risk of hepatoxicity and is not recommended for clinical use (38,42–44).

MESTEROLONE

Mesterolone is a derivative of 5-alpha-dihydrotestosterone with a methyl group in the one position. Liver toxicity has not been reported with its use. It is not metabolized to estrogen and is weak in suppression of gonadotropins *(45–50)*. Dosing for treatment of hypogonadism cannot be monitored and is considered unsatisfactory for replacement therapy for hypogonadism *(32)*.

TESTOSTERONE UNDECENOATE

This is a 17-beta-long aliphatic side-chain ester of testosterone. When given orally, it is absorbed well by the gut and much of it enters the lymphatics rather than the hepatic portal system. Consequently, it enters the systemic circulation (63%) without substantial hepatic transformation *(51)*. This preparation is not available in the US.

Testosterone undecanoate is effective when administered orally and on average maximum levels could be observed 5 h after its administration *(52–59)*. However, the serum testosterone profiles have shown a high interindividual variability of the time when maximum concentrations were reached, and the maximal concentrations achieved, and ranged from 17–96 nmol/L. Even with administration of 40 mg of testosterone undecanoate three times a day only short-lived peaks of testosterone have been observed indicating that the fluctuations with this preparation are considerable *(26,60,61)*. Investigators have also reported considerable intra-individual as well as inter-individual variability and disproportionately high DHT levels. For these reasons testosterone undecanoate has not been considered a satisfactory preparation for androgen replacement therapy of hypogonadal men.

Sublingual

Sublingual administration of testosterone complexed with hydroxypropyl-beta-cyclodextrin results in a rapid rise in serum testosterone but subnormal concentrations occur within 2 h of use *(62–65)*. The short half-life and its bitter taste limit its practical use for long-term replacement therapy.

TESTOSTERONE CYCLODEXTRIN

A recently studied sublingual preparation has more promise as an oral mucosa absorbed preparation for treatment of testosterone deficiency in hypogonadal men than testosterone undecanoate *(62–65)*. Testosterone cyclodextrin contains natural testosterone, which is surrounded by a carbohydrate ring (2-hydroxypropyl-beta cyclodextrin), a facilitator of absorption of testosterone through the oral mucosa *(66)*. A preliminary study on a small number of hypogonadal men for 7 d established that 2, 5, or 5.0 mg tid, appeared to be the appropriate dosages for androgen replacement *(63)*. Studies in hypogonadal men (age range 22–60 yr) with basal serum T levels of less than 250 ng/dL have demonstrated that the 5 mg dose produces peak testosterone concentrations of about 1400 ng/dL within 60 min after administration and the nadir is reached at 360 min on average 67 (Fig. 1). The calculated half life was about 68 min, and the profile of estradiol and DHT paralleled those for testosterone. When 5 mg was administered three times/d, a reduction in serum FSH but not LH was observed and a small reduction in serum HDL without adverse profiles for liver function tests, changes of hematocrit, blood pressure, or gynecomastia. Sexual activity was benefitted. The pharmacokinetic studies indicate no accumulation of testosterone between doses. Thus, with this preparation, serum testosterone

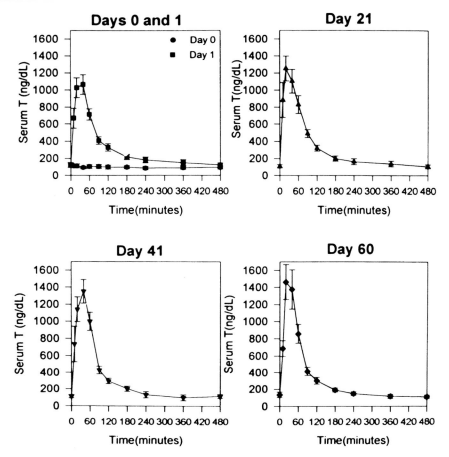

Fig. 1. Mean (± SEM) serum T levels before (D 0) and after administration of SLT 5.0 mg at time 0 min on d 1, 21, 41, and 60 in hypogonadal men (*n* = 18) *(64)*.

concentrations would be expected to be subnormal during the night and within approx 3 h following administration of a dose. This preparation has not been marketed as yet, but it is presumed to be in the near future.

Intramuscular Preparations

Testosterone Esters Overview

Testosterone propionate has a short release phase of only 2–3 d and should not be used for long-term replacement therapy *(68)*. Testosterone enanthate, cypionate, and cyclohexane carboxylate have similar steroid release profiles when injected intramuscularly, and injections of about 200 mg every 2 wk provides concentrations of testosterone above or in the normal range for about 2 wk *(68–70)*. There are also preparations of combinations of the short and long-acting esters available in Europe. They produce even higher initial peaks than the longer acting esters. The longest acting testosterone ester preparation is testosterone-trans-4-n-butylcyclohexyl-carboxylate. Blood levels are sustained for about 12 wk after a large injection of 600 mg in a volume of 2.4 mL *(71)*.

Esterification of the testosterone at the 17 position with propionic or enanthic acid prolongs the intramuscular retention and duration of activity of testosterone in proportion to the length of the fatty acid. When administered intramuscularly *(72)*, the androgen ester is slowly absorbed into the circulation where it is then rapidly metabolized to active unesterified testosterone *(73)*. Intrinsic potency, bioavailability and rate of clearance from the circulation are determinants of the biological actions of androgens.

In hypogonadal patients the baseline untreated serum concentration is low, so the profile following androgen administration is a reflection of the pharmacokinetics of the exogenously administered testosterone alone. Most of the data reviewed following androgen therapy has been based on the increases of testosterone serum concentrations over basal levels in hypogonadal patients.

NANDROLONE PHENYLPROPIONATE AND DECANOATE

Nandrolone phenylpropionate and decanoate are 17-beta-hydroxyl esters of 19-nortestosterone *(74,75)*, which have prolonged action when injected, are used to treat refractory anemias rather than for androgen replacement therapy.

TESTOSTERONE PROPIONATE

Single Dose Pharmacokinetics. Nieschlag et al. *(68)* showed that a single dose of 50 mg of testosterone propionate injected at 1800 h in hypogonadal men results in supraphysiologic peak concentrations. Two days after the injections concentrations are subnormal. These pharmacokinetics indicate that testosterone propionate would have to be administered every two days to maintain therapeutic concentrations of testosterone. This illustrates why testosterone propionate is impractical for routine long-term androgen replacement therapy.

TESTOSTERONE ENANTHATE AND CYPIONATE COMPARISONS

Following intramuscular injections of testosterone enanthate (194 mg) and cypionate (cyclopentylpropionate, 200 mg) in hypogonadal men, comparable pharmacokinetics have been observed over a 10-d interval, as shown in Fig. 2. This provides evidence for the recommendation that these two preparations are interchangeable for androgen replacement therapy *(69,70)*. However, both preparations result in supraphysiologic concentrations of testosterone from day one to four after the injection. In other studies, the pharmacokinetics of testosterone cyclohexane carboxylate and testosterone enanthate gave similar profiles for the peak concentrations, but the cyclohexane carboxylate had slightly lower values on subsequent days despite comparable effects on suppression of LH. Based on these and other studies, a satisfactory regimen is to administer 200 mg of one of these ester preparations once every two weeks intramuscularly *(76,77)*.

Multiple-Dose Pharmacokinetics. Based on simulation pharmacokinetics, 250 mg of testosterone enanthate injected at weekly intervals would result in supraphysiological maximal testosterone serum concentrations up to 78 nmol/L shortly after the injection and supraphysiological minimal testosterone serum concentrations up to 40 nmol/L just before the next injection is given *(77)*. Injecting 250 mg of testosterone enanthate every 2 wk results in maximal supraphysiological testosterone serum concentrations up to 51 nmol/L shortly after injection and testosterone serum levels at the lower range for normal testosterone serum concentration (12 nmol/L) before 2 wk. If the injection interval is extended to 3 or 4 wk, 14 d after the injection of testosterone, serum concentrations would be below the normal range.

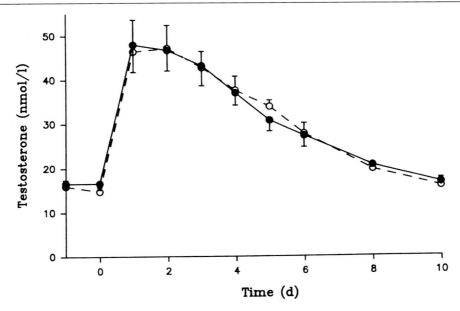

Fig. 2. Comparative pharmacokinetics of 194 mg of testosterone enanthate and 200 mg of testosterone cypioate after intramuscular injection to 6 normal volunteers. Closed circles, mean + or – SEM of testosterone enanthate kinetics; open circles, mean ± SEM of testosterone cypionate kinetics *(77)*.

Snyder and Lawrence *(78)* used a different approach and administered 100 mg/wk (*n* = 12), 200 mg/2 wk (*n* = 10), 300 mg/3 wk (*n* = 9) and 400 mg/4 wk (*n* = 6) of testosterone enanthate to hypogonadal patients during a study period of 3 mo (Fig. 3). The conclusions from their studies are comparable to those cited above with the 250 mg dose administered at intervals of 1–4 wk. If a 100 mg dose is used, the injection interval should be about seven days to maintain physiologic levels of testosterone. If 200–250 mg are used, the interval should be no more than 2 wk to provide testosterone levels within physiologic range by the end of the injection interval *(78)*. If the interval is extended to three weeks, the supraphysiologic concentrations will be even greater shortly after an injection of 300 mg and levels may or may not be sustained in the normal range for 3 wk.

Demisch and Nickelsen *(79)* concluded from their studies that 250 mg of testosterone enanthate given once every three weeks would provide adequate concentrations of both, total and "free" testosterone during the first and second week. However, by the third week, total testosterone concentrations were subnormal and and erectile disturbances were reported by the patients. Thus, whether 200–250 mg of testosterone enanthate or a comparable preparation is used, the interval should be no more than every two weeks to maintain testosterone concentrations within the physiologic range for adult normal younger men.

TESTOSTERONE ESTER COMBINATIONS

Testosterone mixtures of short acting and intermediate acting esters of testosterone *(77)* have been advocated by some and used widely in some parts of the world for substitution therapy of male hypogonadism. These combinations have been used based on the rationale that the short acting preparation would produce normal concentrations

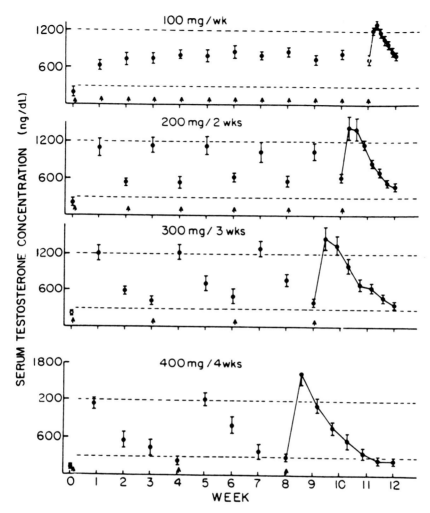

Fig. 3. Serum testosterone concentrations during testosterone replacement therapy in adult primary hypogonadal men. Testosterone enanthate was administered by intramuscular injection (arrows) for 12 wk in four dosage regimens: 100 mg weekly; 200 mg every 2 wk; 300 mg every 3 wk; and 4000 mg every 4 wk. Blood was sampled weekly until the last dose and more frequently thereafter *(78)*.

shortly after the injection and the intermediate acting preparation subsequently. As shown from the pharmacokinetic studies above (*see* Table 6), it is unnecessary to combine the short and intermediate acting preparation because the intermediate acting preparations provide high concentrations of testosterone within hours after their administration. No advantage has been shown either from pharmacokinetic or therapeutic studies to favor combination preparation over intermediate preparations alone.

Testosterone Buciclate

Administration of 600 mg of testosterone buciclate injected intramuscularly to hypogonadal men produced serum testosterone concentrations within the normal range

Table 6
Pharmacokinetics and Safety of Androgens

Preparation	Peak	Trough	T monitoring	DHT	Estradiol	Lower dysfunction	HDL Chol	Skin irritation
T propionate	1 d	2–3 d	None	Dose dep	Dose dep	None	Dose dep	None
T enanthate	1–2 d	10–14 d	1 wk	Dose dep	Dose dep	None	Dose dep	None
T cypionate	1–2 d	10–14 d	1 wk	Dose dep	Dose dep	None	Dose dep	None
T buccilate	2–4 wk	12–14 wk	4–6 wk	Dose dep	Dose dep	None	Dose dep	None
T pellets	1 mo	6 mo	3–4 mo	Dose dep	Dose dep	None	Dose dep	None
T undeconate	2–6 h	2–6 h		Increased	Normal	None	Dose dep	None
T cyclodextrin	1 h	6 h	2–4 h	Normal	Normal	None	Dose dep	None
Methyl T	1.5–2 h	4–5 h	None	Low	Low	Yes	30% dec.	None
Fluroxymesterone				Low	Low	Yes		None
Mesterolone				Low	Low	None		None
T scrotal	3–5 h	20–24 h	12 h	Elevated	Normal	None	Modest	Minimal
T Nonscrotal	6–8 h	24 h	12 h	Normal	Normal	None	Modest	Yes
DHT topical	4–8 h	20–24 h	DHT 12 h	Elevated	Low	None	Modest	Minimal

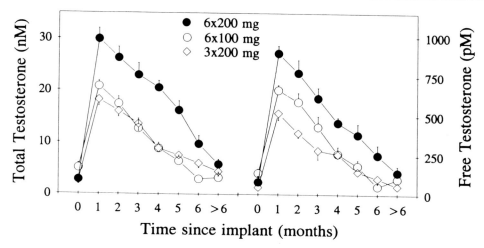

Fig. 4. Plasma total (left) and free (right) testosterone following a single implantation in 43 hypogonadal men *(174).*

for about 8 wk. Pharmacokinetic analysis showed a terminal elimination half-life of 29.5 d *(71).* Serum DHT concentrations were not elevated above normal, and gonadotropins were significantly suppressed with the 600 mg dose but not with the 200 mg dose. No adverse biochemical or prostate responses were reported, and SHBG did not change and serum estradiol increased only slightly. It is unknown if this preparation will find use for male contraceptive therapy or replacement for hypogonadism.

Testosterone Microspheres

Testosterone microspheres are made by preparing testosterone with microencapsulated, biodegradable 85:15 molar lactide:glycolide copolymer *(80).* This preparation is then injected intramuscularly and results in therapeutic levels of testosterone for about 10 wk. The injection of 2.5 mL is painful, and serum testosterone concentrations are inconsistent.

Subcutaneous Testosterone Implants

Fused pellets or silastic capsules of pure testosterone implanted subcutaneously release testosterone in sufficient quantities to maintain physiologic concentrations of testosterone for 4–6 mo *(81,82).*

Subdermal Testosterone Pellets

Bioavailability. The bioavailability of testosterone from subdermal pellet implants approaches 100% by 6 mo (Fig. 4) and is proportional to the dose administered, so that a 6×200 mg dose regimen gives twice that of either 6×100 mg or 3×200 mg regimen.

The pharmacokinetics of testosterone pellet implanted in 43 hypogonadal men (6×100 mg, 3×200 mg, 6×200 mg; total of 111 implants) indicated that testosterone concentrations remained in the normal range for 4–6 mo depending on the dose and were reproducible (Fig. 4) *(81,82).* An initial peak was observed during the first day and a subsequent peak testosterone levels were achieved 2–4 wk after implantation. By 6 mo, plasma testosterone levels returned to the baseline after the 600 mg dose, whereas elevations were sustained beyond 6 mo following the 1200 mg dose. Plasma-free testosterone and total testosterone correlated well ($r = 0.90$), except during the first 3 mo following insertion of the implant when free testosterone levels were significantly higher after the 600 mg regimen with a greater surface area.

The pharmacodynamics of testosterone pellet implants indicated the expected biological effects of implantation on clinical state (well-being, sexual function), gonadotropin suppression (in men with hypergonadotropic hypogonadism), SHBG levels, and biochemistry (81,82). A good relationship was observed between suppression of elevated gonadotropins in men with primary hypogonadism and maintenance of physiological testosterone levels. These results suggest that monitoring of testosterone and gonadotropin levels are useful in monitoring responses to the therapy. Thus, clinical monitoring is readily augmented by blood testosterone levels, as well as gonadotropin suppression in men with hypergonadotropic hypogonadism.

Topical Androgen Preparations

Topical creams containing testosterone have been used in the treatment of microphallus in children (83). The applications probably are effective because of systemic absorption rather than local absorption in the penis.

Percutaneous DHT in Hypogonadal Men

Dihydrotestosterone (DHT) applied to the skin in a hydroalcoholic gel twice daily can produce sustained concentrations of DHT (84,85).

The topical application of a single daily dose of 125 mg of DHT to the abdominal skin of hypogonadal patients rapidly increased the plasma concentrations of DHT from 0.41 ± 0.20 nmol/L before treatment to 8.66 ± 1.12 nmol/L on d 4. Two applications of a dose of 125 mg twice daily at 0800 hand 2000 h increased the plasma level of DHT to 15.25 ± 1.94 nmol/L on d 4 of treatment (86) (Fig. 5). DHT concentrations between 0800 h to 200 h demonstrated values between approx 3–5 nmol/L. Percutaneous DHT therapy for up to 3 mo maintained stable serum DHT concentrations. Best results were obtained when the gel was applied to a large area of the thorax, shoulders, and arms to an area larger than 20×20 cm.

With the percutaneous DHT treatment, the increased ratio of DHT/testosterone ratio to around 5, whereas in normal men the DHT/testosterone ratio ranges between 0.1–0.2. Plasma testosterone and estradiol concentrations did not rise with DHT therapy, but 3 alpha-androstanediol glucuronide rose, SHBG did not increase, and no change in gonadotropins was observed (86).

Clinically, improvement in virilization and sexual function were reported after the daily topical application of 250 mg of DHT. Vermeulen and Deslypere (87) reported that long-term transdermal DHT therapy in elderly males resulted in a moderate decrease in plasma LDL and HDL cholesterol levels, but this was not confirmed by other studies. DHT therapy did not result in enlargement of the prostate as determined by ultrasound study (86,88).

Transdermal Testosterone

Trans-Scrotal Testosterone

As shown in Fig. 6, a 60 cm^2 and 40 cm^2 Testoderm applied to the scrotum of hypogonadal men resulted in peak concentrations of testosterone with either dose

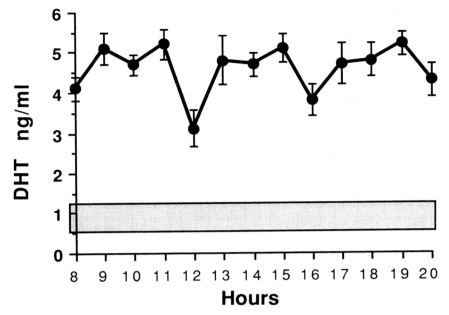

Fig. 5. Plasma DHT levels from 0800 h to 2000 h on d 4 of DHT administration 125 mg twice daily. (The shaded area represents the range for normal men) *(86)*.

between 3–5 h and the peak concentrations of testosterone were 12 and 17 nmol/L, respectively. In a 12-wk study of 54 hypogonadal men, 44 of them used the 40 cm² patch for 4 wk followed by the 60 cm² patch for the next 8 wk; and blood levels of testosterone were obtained at 3–5 h after patch application (Fig. 7) *(89)*. Peak testosterone concentrations increased progressively during the first 3 wk and then remained stable. An earlier preparation delivered 2.4 mg and 3.6 mg/d, respectively; and later systems delivered 4 and 6 mg/d.

With these systems 61.5% achieved normal concentrations of testosterone and 80% had normal levels when the combined concentrations of testosterone plus DHT were made *(89)*. During chronic Testoderm therapy, estradiol levels were in the normal range and DHT concentrations remained elevated *(25,89–95)*.

NONSCROTAL TESTOSTERONE PATCH THERAPY (ANDRODERM)

Pharmacokinetics. After two 2.5 mg Androderm systems were applied to non scrotal skin at about 10 PM, testosterone was continuously absorbed during the 24-h dosing period and the serum testosterone concentration profile mimicked the normal circadian variation observed in healthy young men (Fig. 8) *(23,96,97)*. Peak testosterone concentrations occurred in the early morning hours with minimum concentrations in the evening. In addition, bioavailable testosterone, DHT, and estradiol serum testosterone concentrations (BT) measured during Androderm treatment paralleled the serum testosterone profile (Fig. 8) and remained within the normal reference range.

Clinical Studies. In clinical studies of the 2.5 mg Androderm, 93% of patients were treated with two systems daily, 6% used three systems daily, and 1% used one system daily *(23,96,97)*.

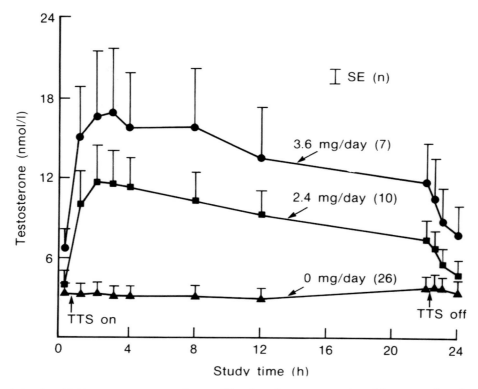

Fig. 6. Study of 24 h serum concentration profile of total testosterone in subjects wearing placebo (*n* = 26), Testoderm-TTS 2.4 mg (*n* = 10) or Testoderm-TTS 3.6 mg (*n* = 7). The Testoderm systems where applied to the scrotum immediately after the experimental zero hour blood sample was taken and were then worn continuously for 22 h at which time they were removed. The data represent means + or – SE for each sampling time. (Reproduced with permission from ref. *89*.)

In those clinical trials of men between the ages of 15 and 65 yr, the 2.5 mg Androderm systems produced mean morning serum concentrations of testosterone within the normal reference range in 92% of patients.

Suppression of gonadotropins to normal in men occurred in about one-half of men with primary hypogonadism treated with Androderm for 6–12 mo *(23,96–98)*. Androderm therapy had positive effects on fatigue, mood, and sexual function as determined from questionnaires and nocturnal penile tumescence *(23,96–98)*.

Comparison with Intramuscular Testosterone. In a study of 66 patients previously treated with testosterone injections, subjects were randomized to receive either Androderm or intramuscular testosterone enanthate (200 mg every 2 wk) treatment for 6 mo *(96)*. The percent of serum concentrations of testosterone, bioavailable testosterone, DHT and estradiol that were within the normal range was 92, 89, 85, and 77%, respectively. Sexual function assessment and lipid profiles were comparable between groups.

Effect on Plasma Lipids. In another study of 29 hypogonadal men withdrawn from androgen therapy for 8 wk of androgen, Androderm treatment for one year decreased cholesterol 1.2% and HDL 8% but increased the ratio of Cholesterol/HDL 9% *(96)*. However, these results were not significantly different from their baseline hypogonadal state.

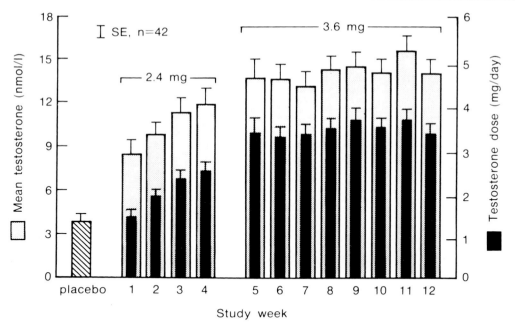

Fig. 7. Weekly serum Cmax levels of total testosterone obtained 3–5 after application (tmax) of a Testoderm-TTS (left ordinate). In the figure the time periods labeled 2.4 mg and 3.6 mg refer to the weeks during which subjects wearing Testoderm-TTS delivering 2.4 mg/d or Testoderm-TTS delivering 3.6 mg/d. The dose of testosterone delivered over the 22 h of wearing on the day of measurement was estimated from residual hormone in used systems compared with the contents of unused systems (right ordinate). (Reproduced with permission from ref. *89*).

Management of Skin Irritation. Contact dermatitis occurs in approx 10% of men following several weeks of use of Androderm. Pretreatment of the skin site where the active area of the patch will applied with 0.1% triamcinolone acetonide cream has been shown to greatly reduce contact dermatitis and itching *(99,100)*. These glucocorticoid cream preparations do not significantly affect testosterone absorption and the quantity of glucocorticoid applied and absorbed is insufficient to produce significant alteration of the hypothalamic-pituitary-adrenal axis. Hydrocortisone is less effective, and ointments should be avoided because they will diminish testosterone delivery.

TESTODERM® TTS

Recently, a nonscrotal testosterone delivery system (Testoderm® TTS) was approved for replacement testosterone therapy in testosterone-deficient men. It restores physiologic levels of testosterone and DHT following daily use and has a favorable side-effect profile with less than 1% discontinuing therapy because of adverse skin reactions.

Human Chorionic Gonadotropin

Human chorionic gonadotropin (hCG), binds to the LH receptors on Leydig cells and like LH stimulates endogenous testosterone production from the testes. Thus, hCG is an alternative to testosterone therapy in inducing pubertal development in boys and treating

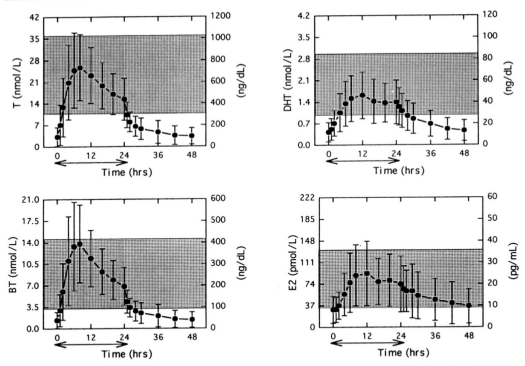

Fig. 8. Serum concentration profiles of T, BT, DHT, and E2 during and after the nighttime application of two TTD systems to the back of 34 hypogonadal men (mean± SD). The shaded areas represent 95% confidence intervals for morning hormone levels in normal men between the ages of 20–65 yr. The arrow denotes the 24-h duration of TTD system application. (Reproduced with permission from ref. *23.*)

androgen deficiency in men with gonadotropin deficiency. In young prepubertal boys (e.g., 13–14 yr of age) presenting with hypogonadotropic hypogonadism and delayed puberty, hCG may be begun at a dosage of 1000–2000 international units (IU) IM or subcutaneously (SC) weekly *(101)* and then slowly increased during the next 1–2 yr to the adult dosages of 1000–2000 IU, IM, or SC, two to three times weekly *(see* Table 7). Some men with gonadotropin deficiency require either higher or lower dosages of hCG. Both subcutaneous and IM administration are equally effective, but the subcutaneous route is more acceptable for self administration.

Therapy can be monitored by assessing the clinical response to treatment, such as the progression of virilization and growth in prepubertal boys and by measuring the serum testosterone concentration, which should be maintained within the normal range *(102)*.

hCG therapy has two major advantages over testosterone replacement therapy. First, it stimulates growth of the testes, which may be important to boys who have never gone through puberty *(102)*. Second, it may stimulate sufficient intratesticular testosterone production prior to the initiation of spermatogenesis,

There are several disadvantages of hCG treatment. hCG treatment requires frequent injections, is expensive, elevates estradiol relative to testosterone and may cause gynecomastia. Development of neutralizing antibodies to hCG may reduce the efficacy of hCG or make it completely ineffective *(1,8)*.

Table 7
Treatment of Male Hypogondism

Group	Goal of therapy	Plasma testosterone	Preparation	Usual dose
Delayed adolescence	Short-term maintenance, initial	100–300 ng/dL	hCG	500 IU IM 1–2/wk
			Androderm	2.5 mg patch; 12 h at night
			TE or TC	50–100 mg q 3–4 wk
	Subsequent	300–400 ng/dL	Androderm	2.5 mg/daily
			TE or TC	100 q 2/wk
Adult	Long-term maintenance	400–1000 ng/dL		
Hypogonadotrophic hypogonadism			GnRH[a]	5–30 µg SC q 2 h
Hypogonadism	Subreplacement		hCG	1000–4000 IU IM 1–3×/wk
			Androderm	5 mg/d
			Testoderm	4 or 6 mg/d
			TE or TC	200 mg q 2wk or q 1 wk IM
			Fluroxymesterone	5–10 mg/d p.o.
			Methyltestosterone	5–25 mg daily
			Testosterone undecanoate[b]	200 p.o. qid

[a]Experimental, requires programmed pump.
[b]Not available in US.
hCG, human chorionic gonadotropin; GnRH, gonadotropin-releasing hormone; TE, testosterone enanthate; TC, testosterone cypionate.

Summary of Therapy

The available testosterone esters for intramuscular injection (testosterone propionate, testosterone enanthate, testosterone cypionate, testosterone cyclohexane carboxylate) do not achieve satisfactory serum testosterone profiles for the treatment of male hypogonadism (Table 7). Doses and injection intervals frequently prescribed in the clinic result in initial supraphysiologic androgen levels and subnormal levels prior to the next injection. Injections of 100 mg of testosterone enanthate or cypionate IM at weekly intervals would more closely approximate normal physiology than 200–250 mg every 2–3 wk. However, an injection frequency more often than 2 wk may be unacceptable to many patients. Further, there is no advantage in combining short-acting testosterone esters (i.e., testosterone propionate) and longer-acting esters (i.e., testosterone enanthate) for testosterone replacement therapy. Since both the short-acting and intermediate-acting esters show maximal serum concentrations shortly after injection.

Of the clinically available injectable androgen esters, 19-nortestosterone hexoxyphenyipropionate shows the best pharmacokinetics. However, as a derivative of the naturally occurring testosterone, 19-nortestosterone might not possess its full pharmacodynamic spectrum and therefore is not an ideal drug for treatment of male hypogonadism *(74,75)*.

Oral administration of testosterone undecanoate results in undesirably high interindividual and intraindividual variability of concentrations of testosterone. Multiple daily doses are required. The submucosal preparation testosterone cyclodextrin has a more reproducible profile; but as with the testosterone undeconoate preparation, the testosterone elevations are only short-lived, resulting in wide fluctuations of serum concentrations.

The most favorable pharmacokinetic profile of testosterone is observed when using either the trans-scrotal or nonscrotal testosterone patch systems. The scrotal system has the disadvantage of supraphysiologic DHT concentrations. Daily administration of Androderm in the evening results in serum testosterone concentrations in the normal range, mimicking the regular circadian rhythm. The nontranscrotal system has the disadvantage of local skin reactions, which can often be successfully managed with topical glucocorticoid administration. The scrotal system has the disadvantage of requiring shaving of the scrotum and adequate scrotal size and adherence. Currently, several satisfactory options for testosterone replacement therapy are available to clinicians in various countries. Of course, the treatment must be tailored for each patient, and important considerations include ease of use, physiologic replacement, side effects and cost. All of these should be discussed with the patient before making the selection. Although testosterone esters, testosterone enanthate and cypionate, are effective, safe, and the least expensive androgen preparations available (particularly if self-administered), they require administration by injection into a large muscle. These two preparations are considered equally effective and have been popular in the past for treatment of hypogonadal men (Table 7).

ADULTS

In adults with hypogonadism, androgen replacement therapy is begun by administering either testosterone enanthate or cypionate 200 mg, intramuscularly (IM), every 2 wk. Figures 2 and 3 display the fluctuations of serum testosterone concentrations after intramuscular injection of 200 mg of either ester. They result in testosterone levels at or above the normal range 1–4 d after administration and then gradually fall over the subsequent

2 wk and may be below the normal range before the next injection. Administering 100 mg weekly produce a better pattern of testosterone levels, but higher doses at less frequent intervals produce greater fluctuations *(77,78)*. Patients, family members or friends can be taught to give deep intramuscular injections of testosterone esters; otherwise, injections by nursing personnel in the clinic are needed.

The therapeutic efficacy of androgen replacement is assessed by monitoring the patient's clinical and serum testosterone responses *(1,8)*. There is considerable variability in response to testosterone therapy in hypogonadal men and include improvement in libido, potency, sexual activity, feeling of well-being, motivation, energy level, aggressiveness, stamina, and hematocrit may occur during the first few weeks to months of androgen replacement therapy. Body hair, muscle mass and strength, and bone mass increase over months to years. In sexually immature, eunuchoidal men, androgen replacement also stimulates development of secondary sexual characteristics, which requires many months to years to achieve adult status and, if epiphyses are unfused, long bone growth will occur.

If injectable forms of testosterone are used, testosterone levels during therapy should be in the mid-normal range 1 wk after an injection and above the lower limit of the normal range preceding the next injection. In some hypogonadal men treated with testosterone esters, disturbing fluctuations in sexual function, energy level, and mood are associated with fluctuations in serum testosterone concentrations between injections. Thus some patients may complain of reduced energy level and sexual function a few days before their next testosterone injection and have serum testosterone levels below the eugonadal range at that time. Shortening the dosing interval of testosterone ester administration from every 2 wk to every 10 d is recommended in these patients.

Men who have been hypogonadal for prolonged intervals may experience alarming changes in sexual desire and function, which may be a stress to their relationship with a spouse *(1,8)*. Counseling of patients and their partners before beginning androgen replacement is recommended to help reduce or alleviate these adjustment problems. Beginning with lower replacement doses may be wise, particularly in elderly hypogonadal men.

Prepubertal

Androgen replacement therapy in prepubertal hypogonadism is usually started at about 14 yr of age. The earliest sign of puberty in boys is enlargement of the testes and an increase in testis size to more than 8–10 mL is usually the first clinical indication of spontaneous puberty. Increases in serum LH and testosterone levels (initially at night) are the hormonal signals that also indicate the onset of puberty *(1,8)*. Growth, virilization, and psychological adjustment are evaluated clinically during androgen replacement therapy. Severe emotional and psychological distress in affected boys and their families makes earlier institution of androgen replacement therapy a prudent choice. It is often difficult to accurately distinguish between simple delayed puberty and hypogonadism. Therefore, only transient androgen therapy is used until it is determined that permanent hypogonadism is established and dictates continuous treatment to induce puberty and maintain sexual function *(1,8)*. Also, in young boys with delayed puberty and also markedly retarded bone age and short stature, excessive androgen treatment causes rapid virilization and increase in long bone growth, and may lead to premature closure of epiphyses, resulting in compromised adult height *(1,8)*. However, this does not affect the ultimate height in those with simple delayed puberty.

In boys with simple delayed puberty, gradual replacement therapy with testosterone (is indicated and) is usually begun using a 50 or 100 mg of testosterone enanthate or cypionate IM monthly *(1,8)*. The design of the regimen in boys is to duplicate the changes in testosterone that occur with puberty in normal boys and thus, gradual virilization and progression of secondary sexual development. This regimen will stimulate long bone growth and initiate virilization without interfering with the onset of spontaneous puberty. If simple delayed puberty or hypogonadism is diagnosed, dosage of testosterone ester is increased to 50–100 mg every 2 wk. These higher dosages are continued for approx 6 mo and then stopped for 3–6 mo for assessment of the spontaneous onset and progression of puberty. If spontaneous pubertal development and growth do not occur, androgen therapy is reinstituted for another 6 mo. This will produce further virilization, but full virilization can be achieved over the next few years with full adult replacement doses. Full adult replacement dosages are seldom needed in those with simple delayed puberty.

POTENTIAL BENEFITS OF ANDROGEN THERAPY

Testosterone Replacement Therapy in Aging Men

Most studies have confirmed an age related decline in testosterone beginning in the fourth decade of life and about 20% of men by age 60 have serum testosterone concentrations of less than 300–350 ng/dL *(2–5,24,25,103–107)*. Because SHBG rises in aging men, bioavailable testosterone (non-SHBG-bound), or free testosterone concentrations may better reflect the deficiency of testosterone than the total testosterone concentration. Thus, these measurements are recommended when the testosterone concentration is between 350 and 450 ng/dL.

Testosterone Effects on Body Composition

Studies in older men treated with testosterone replacement have generally confirmed that body fat mass declines and lean body mass increase. In addition, some aspects of muscle strength improve; when visceral fat was measured by CT scan, a reduction in fat was also reported. These studies were relatively short and ranged in length from 3–18 mo. Several forms of therapy have been used and include testosterone esters, the scrotal patch and a gel preparation. The studies are too small and of inadequate length to make it possible to compare one treatment modality to another.

Katznelson et al. *(108)* studied the effects of testosterone enanthate 100 mg/wk at intervals of 6 mo for 18 mo on bone density and lean body mass. Before treatment hypogonadal men had higher than normal percent body fat (26.4 vs 19.2% in age matched controls). During testosterone enanthate therapy, the percent body fat decreased 14% on average, subcutaneous fat 13%, and lean body mass increased 7%. Spinal BMD and trabecular BMD increased by 5 and 14%, respectively, but radial BMD did not change. Markers of bone formation and resorption decreased significantly.

Bhasin and associates *(109)* treated younger hypogonadal men for only 10 wk and reported a mean weight gain of 4.5 kg, a 5 kg increase in fat-free mass without a change in percent fat. Sih et al. *(110)* reported that older men treated with testosterone cypionate for 12 mo had significantly lower 1,25 dihydroxyvitamin D levels, but testosterone cypionate had no demonstrable influence on osteocalcin, calcium, phosphate, alkaline phosphatase, 25 hydroxyvitamin D, or PTH concentrations.

Muscle Performance and Wasting

In addition, the measurement of the triceps and quadriceps increased significantly as did muscle strength measured by one repetition maximum of weight lifting. These results are in agreement with cross-sectional studies in men with the AIDS wasting syndrome *(111)*. Testosterone therapy is being considered and used for management of weight loss and wasting associated with AIDS *(112–114)*. Free testosterone concentrations correlated significantly with total body potassium ($r = 0.45$) and muscle mass ($r = 0.45$) and total testosterone levels were correlated with exercise functional capacity ($r = 0.64$). Sih et al 110 reported improvement of bilateral grip strength in older hypgonadal treated with testosterone at 3, 6, 9, and 12 mo of therapy.

Mood

In elderly men, the effects of testosterone therapy on mood and sexual behavior have not been studied extensively *(65,115–118)*. But some studies have suggested that testosterone improves spatial cognition, sense of well-being, and libido. Impotence in older men may be corrected if the cause is androgen deficiency. Some men have androgen deficiency and impotence caused by other factors; testosterone therapy will not correct their impotence.

Wang et al. *(65)* studied the effect of testosterone enanthate *(18)* and sublingual testosterone *(33)* in 51 hypogonadal men treated for 60 d. When compared with the baseline period, T replacement led to a significant decrease in anger, irritability, sadness, tiredness and nervousness with an improvement in energy level, friendliness and sense of well-being in all subjects as a group. These results suggest that T replacement therapy enhances mood parameters and reduces anger, irritability, and nervousness. Sih et al. *(110)* did not report on effects of testosterone replacement on mood, but did assess memory and observed no influence.

Leptin

Testosterone cypionate therapy significantly reduced leptin concentrations in elderly men *(110)*. Although they did not report a reduction in BMI with testosterone therapy, they did observe a significant correlation between BMI, body fat, and triglyceride levels.

OSTEOPOROSIS

ANDROGEN DEFICIENCY AND OSTEOPOROSIS

Effects of Androgens in Normal Men. Androgens affect both by the peak bone mass achieved during development and the subsequent amount of bone loss. The dramatic increase in both cortical and trabecular bone density during puberty in boys *(119,120)* is attributed to the pubertal rise in testosterone or one of its metabolites. During the puberty an increase in serum alkaline phosphatase heralds a rise in osteoblast activity, and subsequent bone density increases. In normal boys, peak trabecular bone density is usually achieved by the age of 18 yr *(120)* is and peak cortical bone density is often reached a few years later. Bone density remains relatively stable in young adult males and then declines slowly after age 35 yr *(121)*, and the bone loss is regulated by genetic, endocrine, mechanical, and nutritional factors. In about 55% of men with vertebral crush fractures, secondary causes of osteoporosis may be detected, and the most common causes are glucocorticosteroid therapy, hypogonadism, skeletal metastases, multiple myeloma, gastric surgery, and anticonvulsant and neuroleptic treatment *(122–125)*.

Although hypogonadism is found in up to 20% of men with vertebral crush fractures or osteoporosis, the clinical features of testosterone deficiency may not always be present. There is little published information on the treatment of primary osteoporosis in men, although calcitonin, bisphosphonates and testosterone have been recommended in the management of osteoporosis in men *(126)*.

AGING AND OSTEOPOROSIS

Osteoporosis is one of the leading causes of morbidity and mortality in the elderly. Bone is lost with advancing age in both men and women, leading to an increased incidence of osteoporotic fractures of the fore-arm, vertebral body, and femoral neck. Although aging women lose more bone than aging men, men still lose 30% of their trabecular bone and 20% of their cortical bone *(121)*.

By the ninth decade of life, 4% of men will have sustained a fore-arm fracture, 7% a vertebral fracture, and 5% a femoral neck fracture. The absolute number of osteoporotic fractures is rising in men, because of an aging population with an increase in the age-specific incidence of fractures. Even if the age-specific incidence of fractures stabilizes, demographic trends suggest that a further increase in the number of men with osteoporotic fractures is inevitable. Thus, despite lower rates of osteoporosis in men than in women, one-fifth of all hip fractures occur in men and hypogonadism is one of the most common underlying causes *(127,128)*.

It is clear that hypogonadism during and after the teenage years can affect bone mineral density (BMD). It is less clear whether the decline in testosterone with aging accounts for the loss of bone mass. Further, study is needed to clarify this association, but androgen replacement in aging hypogondal men does improve BMD.

GLUCOCORTICOIDS, ANDROGENS, AND OSTEOPOROSIS

Osteoporosis is associated with both hypogonadism and corticosteroid therapy. Testosterone levels are reduced about 33% by long-term oral prednisolone treatment, but are minimally affected by therapeutic doses of inhaled corticosteroids *(129–132)*. In addition, glucocorticoid therapy may cause a variety of adverse systemic effects including adrenal suppression, dermal thinning and a reduction in total bone calcium.

Praet et al. *(133)* concluded that patients with chronic bronchitics treated with corticosteroids, even at low doses, are at risk for osteoporosis and hypogonadism might contribute to their low BMD and low osteocalcin levels.

BONE DENSITY IN HYPOGONADAL MEN

Studies in Men with Primary Hypogonadism. Stepan et al. *(134)* measured BMD of the lumbar spine in 12 men castrated for sex offenses up to 11 yr previously (mean 5.6 yr) and repeated the measurement in 9 at intervals of 1–3 yr. As shown in Fig. 9, BMD decreased progressively in the following years and biochemical markers of bone resorption and bone formation were increased compared to age-matched normal men. These findings suggest that gonadal steroid deficiency is associated with increased bone turnover and loss.

Medically induced secondary hypogonadism following daily administration of a long-acting GnRH analog to men with benign prostatic hyperplasia has also been reported to reduce bone mass and increase bone turnover *(135)*. The GnRH analog therapy produced

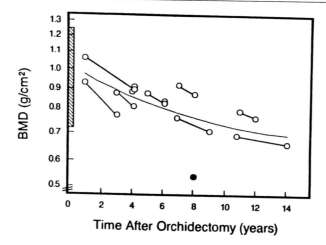

Fig. 9. Scattergram of lumbar spinal bone mineral density (BMD) as a function of time after orchidectomy in 12 men. In 8 patients the measurement was repeated after 1-3 years. The hatched bar indicates the normal range for 20 men matched for age. The solid circle represents the value for one man who developed a hip fracture. (Reproduced with permission from ref. *134.*)

severe testosterone deficiency in all men and reduced BMD in 10 of 17 men over a period of 6–12 mo). The rise in serum alkaline phosphatase and osteocalcin levels corroborated an elevation of bone turnover without an alteration of serum concentrations of calcium, vitamin D metabolites, and parathyroid hormone.

HYPERPROLACTINEMIC HYPOGONADISM AND OSTEOPOROSIS

Greenspan et al. *(136)* measured cortical and trabecular bone density in 18 men between the ages of 30 and 79 with secondary hypogonadism caused by prolactin-secreting tumors. They reported that both cortical and trabecular bone mineral density were significantly decreased in the hyperprolactinemic men compared to age-matched controls. Although their findings suggest that hypogonadism in hyperprolactinemic men leads to osteopenia, other hormone deficiencies, such as growth hormone, also may have an adverse influence on BMD.

Following medical, surgical or radiation therapy of the prolactin-secreting tumors, the effects of restoration of gonadal steroid secretion on bone density in 20 men was performed serially for 6–48 mo by Greenspan et al. *(137)*. In men whose serum testosterone levels normalized (Group I), there was a significant correlation between the change in serum testosterone levels and the change in cortical bone density. In contrast, men who remained hypogonadal (Group II) had no improvement in cortical bone density. However, neither trabecular nor cortical bone density changed significantly in either group.

Constitutionally Delayed Puberty and Bone Density

Finkelstein et al. have assessed BMD in men with a history of delayed puberty to further investigate if there may be a critical period in development that affects achievement of a normal peak bone mineral density. Trabecular and cortical BMD in 23 adult men with histories of constitutionally delayed puberty were compared to a matched group of normal men *(138)*. Both radial and spinal bone mineral density were significantly lower in men with histories of delayed puberty than in normal controls (Fig. 10a,b). These findings indicate that men with histories of constitutionally delayed puberty have

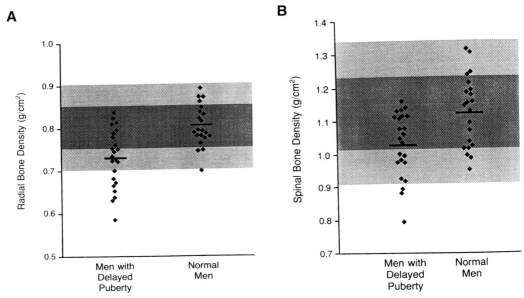

Fig. 10. Radial bone density (panel a) and spinal bone density panel b) in 23 men with histories of delayed puberty and 21 normal controls. The horizontal lines indicate the group means, and the shaded areas the mean ± 1 SD and ± 2 SD. for the normal men. (Reproduced with permission ref. *138*).

decreased radial and spinal bone mineral density and may be at increased risk for osteoporosis. Finkelstein et al. also suggest that the timing of puberty is an important determinant of peak bone mass and that studies should be conducted to determine the benefits of androgen replacement therapy in these men.

Testosterone Therapy in Men with Idiopathic Hypogonadotropic Hypogonadism and Bone Density

Men with idiopathic hypogonadotropic hypogonadism (IHH) are hypogonadal due to an isolated absence of hypothalamic gonadotropin-releasing hormone (GnRH) secretion and have no other anterior pituitary hormonal deficiencies. Finkelstein et al. measured cortical and trabecular bone density in 23 young men with IHH *(139)*. These men, regardless of whether the epiphyses are open or fused, have severe osteopenia of both cortical and trabecular bone. They concluded that the osteopenia of IHH men is a result of inadequate pubertal bone accretion rather than post-maturity adult bone loss.

To assess the effects of androgen replacement on bone mass in IHH men, they made longitudinal measurements of cortical and trabecular bone density in 21 of these 23 men during normalization of serum testosterone levels with either pulsatile GnRH, human chorionic gonadotropin, or intramuscular testosterone therapy for an average of 2 yr Finkelstein et al. *(140)*. In the men with fused epiphyses (Group I), a small but significant increase in cortical bone density was observed without a change in trabecular bone density. These responses are similar to those described above for adult men with hyperprolactinemic hypogonadism. In contrast, men with skeletal immaturity initially showed increases in (Group II) both cortical and trabecular bone density in response to normalization of testosterone and the increase in cortical bone density increased more in

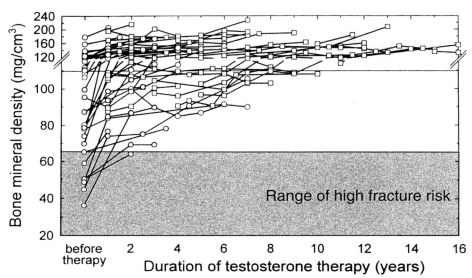

Fig. 11. Increase in BMD during long term testosterone substitution therapy up to 16 yr in 72 hypogonadal patients. Circles indicate hypogonadal patients with first QCT measurement before initiation of testosterone substitution therapy, squares show those patients already receiving testosterone therapy at the first QCT. The dark shaded areas indicates the range of high fracture risk, the unshaded area shows the range without significant fracture risk, and the light shaded area indicates the intermediate range where fractures may occur. (Reproduced with permission from ref. *126*.)

the skeletally immature than in the mature men. However, even after therapy, bone density remained subnormal. The explanation for the failure of testosterone normalization to correct the osteopenia may suggest that other factors are involved or deficiency of gonadal steroids at a critical time in bone maturation has irreversible consequences on achieving peak bone mass.

TESTOSTERONE THERAPY IN ACQUIRED HYPOGONADISM AND BONE DENSITY

Recently, Behre et al. *(126)* reported on the long-term effects of androgen replacement therapy on BMD in hypogonadal men. During the first year of therapy BMD increased 26% (Figs. 11,12). In 72 hypogonadal men long-term therapy maintained BMD in the age-dependent reference range independent of the whether the patients had primary or secondary hypogonadism. This suggests that older men will have benefit in BMD following treatment with androgen replacement therapy for hypogonadism. Katznelson et al. *(141)* also investigated bone density and the effects of androgen replacement therapy in 29 men with acquired primary or secondary hypogonadism, Spinal bone density was significantly lower than that of age-matched normal men and increased significantly (5% by DXA and 13% by QCT) during 12–18 mo of androgen replacement therapy.

MECHANISM OF ACTION OF ANDROGENS ON BONE

The mechanism(s) whereby androgens affect bone density is still unclear. Data suggest that androgens may stimulate bone formation directly, and several observations are consistent with this notion. First, androgen receptors have been found on osteoblasts. Second, both aromatizable and non-aromatizable androgens stimulate proliferation of

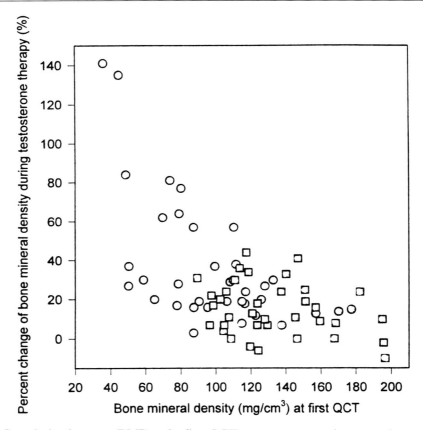

Fig. 12. Correlation between BMD at the first QCT measurement and percent change in BMD during testosterone substitution therapy. Circles indicate hypogonadal patients with first QCT measurement before initiation of testosterone substitution therapy; squares show those patients already receiving testosterone therapy at the first QCT. (Reproduced with permission from ref. *126*.)

human osteoblasts in vitro. However, it is still unclear whether the ability of testosterone to stimulate bone formation and inhibit bone resorption is due to testosterone itself or one of its metabolites such as estradiol or dihydrotestosterone.

It is known that testosterone can be converted to dihydrotestosterone by human bone in vitro. However, inhibition of dihydrotestosterone formation by administration of an inhibitor of 5-α-reductase has no effect on bone mass in humans *(142)* or rats. The aromatization of testosterone into estrogens may be important for many of the effects of testosterone on bone:

1. Estrogen receptors are present in human osteoblasts *(143–150)*.
2. Estrogens appear to maintain bone mass in castrated male-to-female transsexuals.
3. A man with complete estrogen resistance owing to a genetic defect in the estrogen receptor had severe osteopenia despite normal testosterone levels and complete virilization *(151)*.

This finding provides compelling evidence that estrogens are required for a normal peak bone mass in men. However, in men cortical bone mineral density is higher than in women *(120)*; whether this is secondary to the larger muscle mass in men than in women is unknown.

THERAPY OF ANDROGEN-DEFICIENCY BONE LOSS

Androgen replacement therapy has been shown to increase in BMD in hypogonadal men and particularly, those with skeletal immaturity *(136,138)*. However, what serum concentration of testosterone and the duration of the deficiency needed to cause osteoporosis is unknown. In men with modest decreases of serum testosterone concentrations, osteoporosis is observed. It is important to know if testosterone therapy will prevent osteoporosis without causing undue risks. Studies comparing various forms of androgen replacement therapy on management and prevention of osteoporosis should be conducted. For some men, androgens are contraindicated, and designer estrogens or bisphosphonates may provide benefits in preventing bone loss after induction of hypogonadism with medical or surgical therapy.

Furthermore, no data comparing different modes of androgen replacement (e.g., parenteral vs topical) on bone density are available. The use of nonandrogenic agents to prevent bone loss in hypogonadal men with contraindications to testosterone therapy (e.g., men with prostate cancer receiving GnRH analog therapy or after surgical castration) has not been investigated. However, since bone resorption is increased in them, antiresorptive therapy would seem to be logical.

PRECAUTIONS OF ANDROGEN THERAPY IN AGING MEN

Several complications of androgen replacement therapy have been reported. With testosterone preparations, the risk of adverse influences on water retention, polycythemia, hepatotoxicity, sleep apnea, prostate enlargement, and cardiovascular appear small.

Water Retention

Although some increase in body weight thought to be due to water retention has been reported with androgen therapy, the risk of peripheral edema, hypertension and congestive heart failure is uncommon. In studies involving 120 older men treated for 3–9 mo, exacerbation of peripheral edema or congestive heart failure was not reported. A small percentage of men had some rise in blood pressure during androgen replacement therapy compared to the control interval *(152)*.

Polycythemia

Androgens stimulate erythropoiesis, which accounts for higher hematocrits in normal men compared to hypogonadal men. Since older men tend to have lower hematocrits than younger men (unless they have underlying diseases that raise hematocrits), the risk of polycythemia is small *(152)*. The mean rise in hematocrit has been between 0 and 7.0%. Although Sih et al. *(110)* reported that 24% of older men treated with injections of testosterone cypionate (200 mg every 2 wk) had hematocrits above 52%. Testosterone patch therapy appears to have a lower risk for hematocrit elevation than injections of 200 mg of testosterone esters given every 2 wk *(153)*. However, testosterone replacement therapy may cause polycythemia so that men with a history of polycythemia should be followed closely and men in general should have periodic screening of hematocrit for the development of polycythemia.

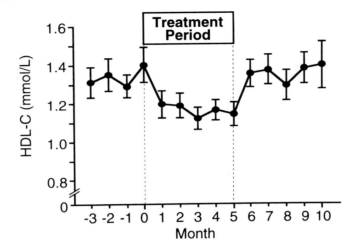

Fig. 13. Mean ± SE plasma HDL cholesterol levels in the subjects during the course of the study (*n* = 19 until month 7, *n* = 8–15 thereafter). All data points during the treatment period (testosterone enanthate, 200 mg IM/wk) were significantly decreased (*p* < 0.05) compared with the baseline and posttreatment values. Reprinted with permission from ref. *157*.

Sleep Apnea

Recent studies of testosterone therapy in older men have not reported sleep apnea as a complication. However, men with a history of sleep apnea were generally excluded from participation *(152)*.

Serum Lipids

An elevation of total cholesterol and a suppression of HDL are known risk factors for cardiovascular disease. Many studies have shown a reduction in total cholesterol and LDL-cholesterol in response to androgen replacement therapy without an adverse profile for HDL-cholesterol. Higher than usual replacement doses of testosterone have been associated with adverse lipid profiles.

ANDROGEN EFFECTS ON PLASMA LIPIDS

In hypogonadal men following medical castration using GnRH agonists, alpha lipoproteins are higher and beta-lipoproteins are lower. Moorjani et al. *(154)* reported that GnRH and antiandrogen administration to older men with prostate cancer had significant elevations of HDL-cholesterol without a change in VLDL or LDL-cholesterol. In contrast, surgical castration resulted in no rise in HDL cholesterol, but apoprotein B levels rose.

In other studies in healthy younger men Golderberg *(155)* reported that men treated with a GnRH agonist had elevation of HDL-cholesterol, apo AI and apo B levels and no change in triglycerides. If androgen replacement is done along with GnRH therapy, the rise is HDL cholesterol can be aborted *(156–160)*. Mean HDL cholesterol rose 26% during treatment with GnRH alone and the mean levels of HDL2 rose 63%; HDL3 17%; and apo AI 17%. GnRH plus 100 mg/week of TE produced only a slight decrease in HDL cholesterol without a significant change in HDL2 or 3 and apo AI (Figs. 13,14). Bagatell et al. *(158)* showed that estradiol was important in preventing the drop in HDL2 in men treated with testosterone. When estrogen synthesis was inhibited with testolactone, HDL2

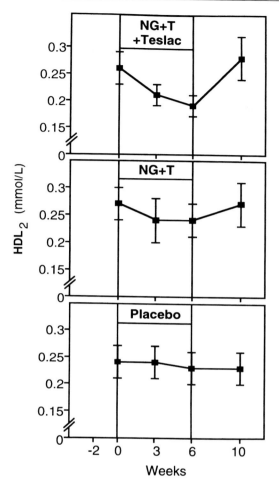

Fig. 14. Mean (± SE) high-density lipoprotein-2 cholesterol levels during the study in men receiving Nal-Glu (NG) plus T plus Teslac (top panel; *n* = 10), Nal-Glu plus T (middle panel; *n* = 10), or placebo (bottom panel; *nn* = 9). Reprinted with permission from ref. *158.*

was suppressed significantly. Whether the effects of androgen on lipids accounts for the differences in rates of CAD reported in epidemiology studies is uncertain.

Androgen Therapy in Delayed Puberty. Kirkland et al. *(161)* injected TE for 3 mo to 14 boys with delayed puberty who were between 13 and 16 yr of age. The dose was 100 mg/mo for the first month and 200 mg for the second and third month. Serum testosterone was in the normal range for adults, and plasma HDL levels decreased by a mean of 7.4 mg/dL after the 100 mg injection and 13.7 mg/dL after the 200 mg injections. While there appears to be a cause and effect relationship between androgen therapy and plasma lipid changes, the relationship is complex because androgens also are associated with changes in body composition and metabolic variables *(162).*

Relationship of Dose and Lipids. Higher than normal replacement doses of androgen (Testosterone enanthate, 200 mg/wk) used for medical birth control therapy have been associated with a 13% suppression of HDL and suppression of apo AI and HDL2 and 3 subfractions *(156–159).* The magnitude of effects of androgen replacement has varied somewhat from study to study. Smaller effects on lipids have been found by other investigators who also administered esters of testosterone. In older men treated with Testosterone cypionate, no effects of therapy were reported for cholesterol, LDL, HDL, or triglycerides.

Anabolic Steroids and Lipids. Anabolic steroids derivatives of testosterone administered orally have profound influences on lipid profiles in contrast with the more modest effects of testosterone esters or transdermal testosterone administration. Although oral methyltestosterone therapy, HDL decreases by more than 30% with striking changes in the HDL2 subfraction and apo AI and AII. LDL cholesterol rises about 30–40% with a decrease of 65–80% in Lp(a) levels (at least in women) (163,164). The more profound influence of anabolic androgens compared with testosterone preparations appears to be related to the metabolism of testosterone to estradiol. Synthetic androgens are not efficiently converted to estrogen. Thus, estrogens may reverse some of the adverse effects of testosterone on lipid profiles (165,166). In addition, testosterone administered parenterally avoids the excessive androgen influence on the liver during first pass clearance. Thus, oral nonaromatizable androgens have a greater suppression of HDL-cholesterol than do aromatizable androgens, such as testosterone.

Prostate Disease

BENIGN PROSTATE ENLARGEMENT

Progressive growth of the prostate occurs in both the transition and peripheral zones of the prostate as men age (167–170). In both normal and hypogonadal aging men, androgen withdrawal results in a significant reduction in prostate volume of both zones (Fig. 15) (169). In our studies, the reduction appears to be proportional to the volume of the prostate. We found a high correlation with the volume of the prostate and age in men receiving Testosterone enanthate, during androgen withdrawal and during androgen therapy with Androderm. Following 8 wk of androgen withdrawal, Androderm treatment resulted in growth of the prostate to the size observed during testosterone enanthate therapy. Over the next 9 mo further enlargement was not observed. In a cross-sectional study, Behre and Niesclag (171) reported that in untreated hypogonadal men, no significant correlation existed between prostate volume and age. In contrast, testosterone-treated men and normal men showed a positive correlation with prostate volume and age, and no significant age-adjusted differences were observed between the testosterone-treated men and normal controls (Fig. 16). Serum concentrations of PSA were not elevated above those expected in men of comparable age, which is consistent with results reported recently by Sih et al. (110) who observed no change in PSA in older hypogonadal men treated with injections of a testosterone ester. Although there are limitations in study design, these observations do not suggest that androgen replacement therapy will cause growth of the prostate beyond what will occur in men with normal gonadal function.

PROSTATE CANCER

Prostate cancer is an androgen responsive cancer, but evidence that testosterone therapy causes prostate cancer is lacking (172,173). An undiagnosed prostate cancer may grow in response to testosterone therapy. A PSA and digital rectal examination is recommended in men age 40 or over before initiation of androgen replacement therapy for hypogonadism. Further, screening for prostate cancer in men on testosterone therapy should follow the usual guidelines for normal men of comparable age.

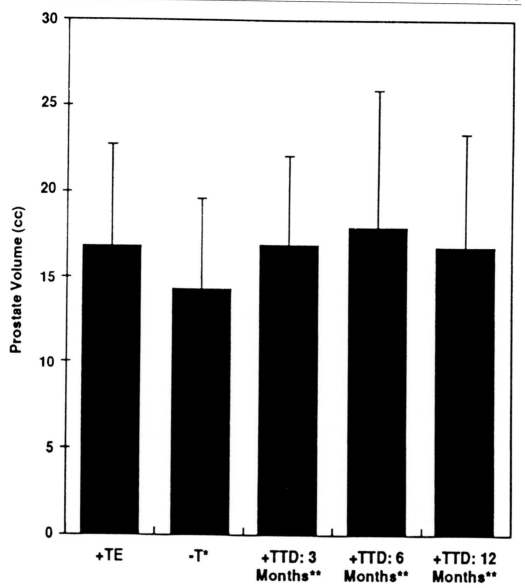

Fig. 15. Prostate volume measured by TRUS. (T, testosterone; TE, testosterone enanthate; TTD, testosterone transdermal system.) (Reproduced with permission from ref. *169.*)

OTHER CONSIDERATIONS OF
TREATMENT OF ANDROGEN DEFICIENCY

The main use of androgen replacement therapy is in the management of men with hypogonadism. The cause of the hypogonadism should be established to determine if it might be reversible. If so, therapy should be directed at correction of the underlying cause. For example, hyperprolactinemia from a pituitary tumor can be treated with bromocryptine, which will often correct the testosterone deficiency. Some tumors of the

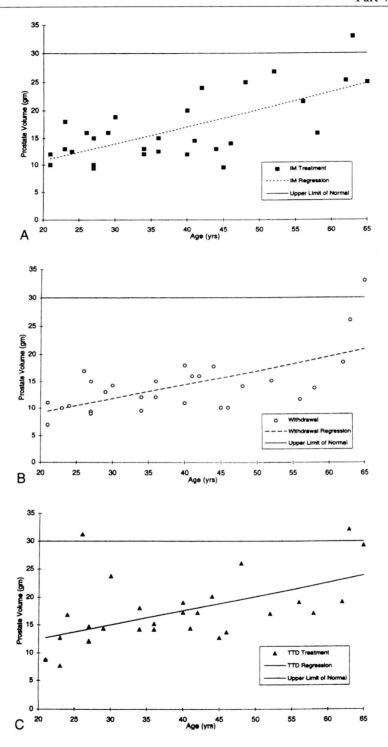

Fig. 16. Linear regression of prostate volume with age. **(A)** Prostate volume correlated signifi-cantly with age during therapy with testosterone enanthate ($r = 0.69, p < 0.01$). **(B)** Prostate volume correlated significantly with age after an 8-wk testosterone withdrawal interval ($r = 0.64, p < 0.01$).

pituitary or hypothalamus may require surgical or irradiation therapy. Thus, in addition to secondary or tertiary hypogonadism, other deficiencies, such as ACTH, growth hormone, and TSH may exist and require management. Systemic illness and glucocorticoid therapy will cause hypogonadism and depending on the clinical situation, androgen replacement therapy may be considered in such patients. In aging men, androgen replacement therapy requires the usual monitoring for diseases incident to age, but may offer benefits in bone preservation, lean body mass, mood, and sexual function.

For men who desire fertility at some time in their life, hormonal therapy directed at enhancing spermatogenesis may offer them that opportunity. After fertility therapy is deemed a success or a failure, resumption of conventional testosterone therapy is then indicated.

Severe gynecomastia or small testes may contribute to psychological problems or social embarrassment for some hypogonadal boys and men. Gynecomastia usually does not regress and may worsen during hormonal replacement therapy of hypogonadism, and plastic surgery (reductive mammoplasty) is a reasonable alternative. Some patients with secondary hypogonadism may have enlargement of the testes in response to gonadotropin therapy, but such therapy is not indicated in men with primary hypogonadism, such as those with Klinefelter's syndrome who have extremely small testes. Surgical implantation of testicular prostheses is an option for some men.

SUMMARY OF ANDROGEN REPLACEMENT THERAPY

The hormone replacement goals for management of male hypogonadism depend upon both the cause and the stage of sexual development in which gonadal failure occurs. Androgen replacement therapy is indicated to stimulate and sustain normal secondary sexual characteristics, sexual function, and behavior in prepubertal boys and men with either primary or secondary hypogonadism. Several options for replacement therapy are available in various countries and the availability of those preparations should be taken into consideration by the clinician before therapy is instituted. The goal is to normalize physiology as closely as possible and at the lowest cost. All of these factors influence the decision, which is shared with the physician and patient. Parenteral testosterone esters, testosterone enanthate or cypionate, are the effective, safe, and relatively inexpensive androgen preparations widely available for this purpose. They produce early supraphysiologic concentrations of testosterone, may be more prone to cause gynecomastia and polycythemia. Transdermal testosterone results in more physiologic testosterone and estradiol concentrations with a circadian variation, but they are more expensive than testosterone ester preparation that require an intramuscular injection. They allow monitoring of therapeutic response by assessing testosterone concentrations. The scrotal patch has fewer skin reactions than the nonscrotal patch, but it results in supraphysiologic concentrations of DHT. Newer preparations include a sublingual form that appears to have widely fluctuating testosterone concentrations. A DHT dermal preparation is available in some parts of the world but does not produce normal concentrations of testosterone or estradiol. The oral testosterone undecanoate results in unpredictable concentrations

(C) Prostate volume correlated significantly with age during 1 yr of testosterone transdermal system treatment ($r = 0.55$, $p < 0.01$). (IM = intramuscular; TTD = testosterone transdermal system.) (Reproduced with permission from ref. *169*.)

of testosterone and high DHT levels and is not recommend widely in countries where it is available. In boys or men with secondary hypogonadism, gonadotropin therapy may be used instead of testosterone therapy to stimulate endogenous testosterone production. Because of their greater expense and complexity, however, these modalities are usually reserved for men with gonadotropin deficiency who desire fertility and in whom spermatogenesis must be initiated and maintained. In some patients gonadotropin therapy may be begun with hCG alone. In men with partial or previously treated gonadotropin deficiency, or in men with postpubertal hypogonadotropic hypogonadism, hCG treatment alone may be sufficient to stimulate spermatogenesis and fertility. As discussed in detail elsewhere, men with prepubertal hypogonadotropic hypogonadism require the combined treatment with hCG plus human menopausal gonadotropins to initiate sperm production and fertility. In those with a selective deficiency of GnRH, such as Kallmann's syndrome, pulsatile GnRH therapy has been shown to stimulate testosterone production and spermatogenesis.

REFERENCES

1. Santen RJ. Male Hypogonadism. In: Yen SSC, Jaffe RB, eds. Reproductive Endocrinology, 3rd ed. Saunders, Philadelphia, 1991, pp. 739-794.
2. Korenman SG. Androgen function after age 50 years and treatment of hypogonadism. Curr Ther Endocrinol Metab 1994;5:585-7.
3. Korenman S, Morley J, Mooradian A, et al. Secondary hypogonadism in older men: its relation to impotence. J Clin Endocrinol Metab 1990;71:963-9.
4. Mastrogiacomo I, Feghali G, Foresta C, Ruzza G. Andropause: incidence and pathogenesis. Arch Androl 1982;9:293-6.
5. Vermeulen A, Kaufman JM. Ageing of the hypothalamo-pituitary-testicular axis in men. Horm Res 1995;43:25-8.
6. Ou Y, Hwang T, Yang C, et al. Hormonal screening in impotent patients. J Formos Med Assoc 1991;90:560-4.
7. Wortsman J, Rosner W, Dufau M. Abnormal testicular function in men with primary hypothyroidism. Am J Med 1987;82:207-12.
8. Griffin JE, Wilson JD. Disorders of the Testes and Male Reproductive Tract. In: Wilson JD, Foster DW, eds. William's Textbook of Endocrinology, 8th ed. Saunders, Philadelphia, 1992:799-852.
9. Nielsen J, Wohlert M. Chromosome abnormalities found among 34,910 newborn children: results from a 13-year incidence study in Arhus, Denmark. Hum Genet 1991;87:81-3.
10. Tunte W, Niermann H. Incidence of Klinefelter's syndrome and seasonal variation. Lancet 1968;1:641.
11. Luciani J, Guichaoua M. Chromosome abnormalities in male infertility. Ann Biol Clin (Paris) 1985;43:71-4.
12. McClure RD. Endocrine investigation and therapy. Urol Clin North Am 1987;14:471-88.
13. Huang CC, Huang HS. Successful treatment of male infertility due to hypogonadotropic hypogonadism—report of three cases. Chang Keng I Hsueh 1994;17:78-84.
14. Nachtigall LB, Boepple PA, Pralong FP, Crowley WF, Jr. Adult-onset idiopathic hypogonadotropic hypogonadism—a treatable form of male infertility. N Engl J Med 1997;336:410-5.
15. Nachtigall LB, Boepple PA, Seminara SB, et al. Inhibin B secretion in males with gonadotropin-releasing hormone (GnRH) deficiency before and during long-term GnRH replacement: relationship to spontaneous puberty, testicular volume, and prior treatment—a clinical research center study. J Clin Endocrinol Metab 1996;81:3520-5.
16. Seminara SB, Boepple PA, Nachtigall LB, et al. Inhibin B in males with gonadotropin-releasing hormone (GnRH) deficiency: changes in serum concentration after short-term physiologic GnRH replacement: a clinical research center study. J Clin Endocrinol Metab 1996;81:3692-6.
17. Anawalt BD, Bebb RA, Matsumoto AM, et al. Serum inhibin B levels reflect Sertoli cell function in normal men and men with testicular dysfunction. J Clin Endocrinol Metab 1996;81:3341-5.
18. McLachlan RI, Finkel DM, Bremner WJ, Snyder PJ. Serum inhibin concentrations before and during gonadotropin treatment in men with hypogonadotropic hypogonadism: physiological and clinical implications. J Clin Endocrinol Metab 1990;70:1414-9.

19. MacDonald PC, Wilson JD. Familial incomplete male pseudohermaphroditism, Type 2. N Engl J Med 1974;291:944-949.
20. Walsh PC, Harrod MJ, Goldstein JL, MacDonald PC, Wilson JD. Familial incomplete male pseudohermaphroditism, type 2, decreased dihydrotestosterone formation in pseudovaginal perineoscrotal hypospadias. N Engl J Med 1974;291:944-949.
21. Imperato-McGinley J, Peterson RE, Gantier T, et al. Hormonal evaluation of a large kindred with complete androgen insensitivity: evidence of a secondary 5 alpha-reductase deficiency. J Clin Endocrinol Metab 1982;54:931-941.
22. Meikle AW, Mazer NA, Moellmer JF, et al. Enhanced transdermal delivery of testosterone across nonscrotal skin produces physiological concentrations of testosterone and its metabolites in hypogonadal men. J Clin Endocrinol Metab 1992;74:623-8.
23. Meikle AW, Arver S, Dobs AS, Sanders SW, Rajaram L, Mazer NA. Pharmacokinetics and metabolism of a permeation-enhanced testosterone transdermal system in hypogonadal men: influence of application site- -a clinical research center study. J Clin Endocrinol Metab 1996;81:1832-40.
24. Matsumoto A. Clinical use and abuse of androgens and antiandrogens. In: Becker K, ed. Priniciples and Practice of Endocrinology and Metabolism. 2nd ed. J.B. Lippincott, Philadelphia, 1995:1110-1122.
25. Matsumoto AM. Hormonal therapy of male hypogonadism. Endocrinol Metab Clin North Am 1994;23:857-75.
26. Cantrill J, Dewis P, Large D, Newman M, Anderson D. Which testosterone replacement therapy? Clin Endocrinol (Oxf) 1984;21:97-107.
27. Berthold A. Transplantation der Hoed. Archiv fur Anatomie, Physiologie und wissenschaftliche Medicin, Berlin. 1849:42-46.
28. Butenandt A. Uber die chemische Untersuchung des Sexualhomons. A angew Chem 1931;44:905-908.
29. David k, Dingermanse E, Freud J, Laqure E. Uber krystallinisches mannliches Hormon aus Hoden (Testosteron), wirksamer als aus Harn oder aus Cholesterin bereitetes Androsteron. Hoppe-Seyler's Z physiol Chem 1935;233:281-282.
30. Butenandt A, Hanisch G. Uber Testosteron, Umwandlung des Dehydro-androsterons in Androstendiol und Testosteron; ein Weg zur Darstellung des Testosterons aus Cholesterin. Hoppe- seyler's Z Physiol Chem 1935;237:89-98.
31. Ruzick L, Wettstein A. synthetische Darstellung des Testishormons, Testosteron (androsten 3-on-17ol). Helv chim Acta 1935;18:1264-1275.
32. Nieschlag E, Behre H. Pharmacology and clinical uses of testosterone. In: Nieschlag E, Behre H, eds. Testosterone: action, deficiency, substitution. Berlin, Heidelberg, New York: Springer-Verlag; 1990:92-108.
33. Daggett P, Wheeler M, Nabarro J. Oral testosterone: a reappraisal. Horm Res 1978;9:121-9.
34. Johnsen S, Bennett E, Jensen V. Therapeutic effectiveness of oral testosterone. Lancet 1974;2:1473-5.
35. Nieschlag E, Hoogen H, Bolk M, Schuster H, Wickings E. Clinical trial with testosterone undecanoate for male fertility control. Contraception 1978;18:607-14.
36. Nieschlag E, Cuppers H, Wickings E. Influence of sex, testicular development and liver function on the bioavailability of oral testosterone. Eur J Clin Invest 1977;7:145-7.
37. Alkalay D, Khemani L, Wagner WE J, Bartlett M. Sublingual and oral administration of methyltestosterone. A comparison of drug bioavailability. J Clin Pharmacol New Drugs 1973;13:142-51.
38. Lie J. Pulmonary peliosis. Arch Pathol Lab Med 1985;109:878-9.
39. Westaby D, Ogle S, Paradinas F, Randell J, Murray-Lyon I. Liver damage from long-term methyltestosterone. Lancet 1977;2:262-3.
40. Paradinas F, Bull T, Westaby D, Murray-Lyon I. Hyperplasia and prolapse of hepatocytes into hepatic veins during longterm methyltestosterone therapy: possible relationships of these changes to the developement of peliosis hepatis and liver tumours. Histopathology 1977;1:225-46.
41. Pezold F. Anabolic hormones in chronic hepatitis. Oral therapy with 1 alpha, 17 alpha-bis(acetylthio)-17 alpha-methyltestosterone. Munch Med Wochenschr 1968;110:2663-8.
42. Doerr P, Pirke K. Regulation of plasma oestrogens in normal adult males. I. Response of oestradiol, oestrone and testosterone to HCG and fluoxymesterone administration. Acta Endocrinol (Copenh) 1974;75:617-24.
43. Jones TM, Fang VS, Landau rL, Rosenfield RL. The effects of fluoxymesterone administration on testicular function. Clin Endocrinol Metab 1977;43:121-129.
44. Nadell J, Kosek J. Peliosis hepatis. Twelve cases associated with oral androgen therapy. Arch Pathol Lab Med 1977;101:405-10.

45. Kovary P, Lenau H, Niermann H, Zierden E, Wagner H. Testosterone levels and gonadotrophins in Klinefelter's patients treated with injections of mesterolone cipionate. Arch Dermatol Res 1977;258:289-94.

46. Wang C, Chan C, Wong K, Yeung K. Comparison of the effectiveness of placebo, clomiphene citrate, mesterolone, pentoxifylline, and testosterone rebound therapy for the treatment of idiopathic oligospermia. Fertil Steril 1983;40:358-65.

47. Ros A. Our experience with mesterolone therapy. Evaluation of 22 hormonal steroids constituting the gas chromatographic picture in the total neutral urinary fraction. The effectiveness of mesterolone in the therapy of oligoastenospermias. Attual Ostet Ginecol 1969;15:37-53.

48. Gerhards E, Nieuweboer B, Richter E. On the alkyl-substituted steroids. V. Testosterone excretion in man after oral administration of 1alpha-methyl-5alpha-androstane-17beta ol-3-one(mesterolone) and 17-alpha-methyl-androst-4-en-17beta-ol-3-one (17 alpha-methyltestosterone). Arzneimittelforschung 1969;19:765-6.

49. Komatsu Y, Tomoyoshi T, Okada K. Clinical experiences with mesterolone, an orally administered androgen, in male urology. Hinyokika Kiyo 1969;15:663-9.

50. Aakvaag A, Stromme S. The effect of mesterolone administration to normal men on the pituitary-testicular function. Acta Endocrinol (Copenh) 1974;77:380-6.

51. Schurmeyer T, Wickings E, Freischem C, Nieschlag E. Saliva and serum testosterone following oral testosterone undecanoate administration in normal and hypogonadal men. Acta Endocrinol (Copenh) 1983;102:456-62.

52. Tauber U, Schroder K, Dusterberg B, Matthes H. Absolute bioavailability of testosterone after oral administration of testosterone-undecanoate and testosterone. Eur J Drug Metab Pharmacokinet 1986;11:145-9.

53. Luisi M, Franchi F. Double-blind group comparative study of testosterone undecanoate and mesterolone in hypogonadal male patients. J Endocrinol Invest 1980;3:305-8.

54. Maisey N, Bingham J, Marks V, English J, Chakraborty J. Clinical efficacy of testosterone undecanoate in male hypogonadism. Clin Endocrinol (Oxf) 1981;14:625-9.

55. Tax L. Absolute bioavailability of testosterone after oral administration of testosterone- undecanoate and testosterone [letter]. Eur J Drug Metab Pharmacokinet 1987;12:225-6.

56. Gooren L. Long-term safety of the oral androgen testosterone undecanoate. Int J Androl 1986;9:21-6.

57. Frey H, Aakvaag A, Saanum D, Falch J. Bioavailability of oral testosterone in males. Eur J Clin Pharmacol 1979;16:345-9.

58. Coert A, Geelen J, de Visser J, van der Vies J. The pharmacology and metabolism of testosterone undecanoate (TU), a new orally active androgen. Acta Endocrinol (Copenh) 1975;79:789-800.

59. Nieschlag E, Mauss J, Coert A, Kicovic P. Plasma androgen levels in men after oral administration of testosterone or testosterone undecanoate. Acta Endocrinol (Copenh) 1975;79:366-74.

60. Skakkebaek N, Bancroft J, Davidson D, Warner P. Androgen replacement with oral testosterone undecanoate in hypogonadal men: a double blind controlled study. Clin Endocrinol (Oxf) 1981;14:49- 61.

61. Conway A, Boylan L, Howe C, Ross G, Handelsman D. Randomized clinical trial of testosterone replacement therapy in hypogonadal men. Int J Androl 1988;11:247-64.

62. Salehian B, Wang C, Alexander G, et al. Pharmacokinetics, bioefficacy, and safety of sublingual testosterone cyclodextrin in hypogonadal men: comparison to testosterone enanthate: a clinical research center study. J Clin Endocrinol Metab 1995;80:3567-75.

63. Stuenkel CA, Dudley RE, Yen SS. Sublingual administration of testosterone-hydroxypropyl-beta-cyclodextrin inclusion complex simulates episodic androgen release in hypogonadal men. J Clin Endocrinol Metab 1991;72:1054-9.

64. Wang C, Eyre DR, Clark R, et al. Sublingual testosterone replacement improves muscle mass and strength, decreases bone resorption, and increases bone formation markers in hypogonadal men: a clinical research center study. J Clin Endocrinol Metab 1996;81:3654-62.

65. Wang C, Alexander G, Berman N, et al. Testosterone replacement therapy improves mood in hypogonadal men: a clinical research center study. J Clin Endocrinol Metab 1996;81:3578-83.

66. Pitha J, Anaissie E, Uekama K. gamma-Cyclodextrin:testosterone complex suitable for sublingual administration. J Pharm Sci 1987;76:788-90.

67. Salehian B, Wang C, Alexander G, et al. Pharmacokinetics, bioefficacy, and safety of sublingual testosterone cyclodextrin in hypogonadal men: comparison to testosterone enanthate: a clinical research center study. J Clin Endocrinol Metab 1995;80:3567-75.

68. Nieschlag E, Cuppers H, Wiegelmann W, Wickings E. Bioavailability and LH-suppressing effect of different testosterone preparations in normal and hypogonadal men. Horm Res 1976;7:138-45.

69. Schulte-Beerbuhl M, Nieschlag E. Comparison of testosterone, dihydrotestosterone, luteinizing hormone, and follicle-stimulating hormone in serum after injection of testosterone enanthate of testosterone cypionate. Fertil Steril 1980;33:201-3.

70. Schurmeyer T, Nieschlag E. Comparative pharmacokinetics of testosterone enanthate and testosterone cyclohexanecarboxylate as assessed by serum and salivary testosterone levels in normal men. Int J Androl 1984;7:181-7.

71. Behre HM, Nieschlag E. Testosterone buciclate (20 Aet-1) in hypogonadal men: pharmacokinetics and pharmacodynamics of the new long-acting androgen ester. J Clin Endocrinol Metab 1992;75:1204-10.

72. Junkmann K. Long-acting steroids in reproduction. Recent Prog Horm Res 1957;13:389-419.

73. Fujioka M, Shinohara Y, Baba S, Irie M, Inoue K. Pharmacokinetic properties of testosterone propionate in normal men. J Clin Endocrinol Metab 1986;63:1361-4.

74. Knuth U, Behre H, Belkien L, Bents H, Nieschlag E. Clinical trial of 19-nortestosterone-hexoxyphenylpropionate (Anadur) for male fertility regulation. Fertil Steril 1985;44:814-21.

75. Belkien L, Schurmeyer T, Hano R, Gunnarsson P, Nieschlag E. Pharmacokinetics of 19-nortestosterone esters in normal men. J Steroid Biochem 1985;22:623-9.

76. Nankin H. Hormone kinetics after intramuscular testosterone cypionate. Fertil Steril 1987;47:1004-9.

77. Behre H, Oberpenning F, Nieschlag E. Comparative pharmacokinetics of testosterone preparations: application of computer analysis and simulation. In: Nieschlag E, Behre H, eds. Testosterone-action, deficiency, substitution. Springer-Verlag, Berlin, Heidelberg, New York, 1990, pp. 115-134.

78. Snyder PJ, Lawrence DA. Treatment of male hypogonadism with testosterone enanthate. J Clin Endocrinol Metab 1980;51:1335-9.

79. Demisch K, Nickelsen T. Distribution of testosterone in plasma proteins during replacement therapy with testosterone enanthate in patients suffering from hypogonadism. Andrologia 1983;15 Spec No:536-41.

80. Bhasin S, Swerdloff RS, Steiner B, et al. A biodegradable testosterone microcapsule formulation provides uniform eugonadal levels of testosterone for 10–11 weeks in hypogonadal men. J Clin Endocrinol Metab 1992;74:75-83.

81. Handelsman D, Conway A, Boylan L. Suppression of human spermatogenesis by testosterone implants. J Clin Endocrinol Metab 1992;75:1326-32.

82. Handelsman D, Conway A, Boylan L. Pharmacokinetics and pharmacodynamics of testosterone pellets in man. J Clin Endocrinol Metab 1990;71:216-22.

83. Choi S, Kim D, de Lingnieres B. Transdermal dihydrotestosterone therapy and its effects on patients with microphallus. J Urol 1993;150:657-660.

84. Chemana D, Morville R, Fiet J, et al. Percutaneous absorption of 5 alpha-dihydrotestosterone in man. II. Percutaneous administration of 5 alpha-dihydrotestosterone in hypogonadal men with idiopathic haemochromatosis; clinical, metabolic and hormonal effectiveness. Int J Androl 1982;5:595-606.

85. Kuhn J, Laudat M, Roca R, Dugue M, Luton J, Bricaire H. Gynecomastia: effect of prolonged treatment with dihydrotestosterone by the percutaneous route. Presse Med 1983;12:21-5.

86. Schaison G, Nahoul, K, Couzinet, B. Percutaneous dihydrotestosterone (DHT) treatment. In: Nieschlag E, Behre HM, ed. Testosterone-action, deficiency, substitution. Springer-Verlag, Berlin, Heidelberg, New York, 1990, pp. 155-164.

87. Vermeulen A, Deslypere J. Long-term transdermal dihydrotestosterone therapy: effects on pituitary gonadal axis and plasma lipoproteins. Maturitas 1985;7:281-7.

88. De Lignieres B. Transdermal dihydrotestosterone treatment of 'andropause.' Annals Med 1993;25:235-241.

89. Place V, Atkinson, L, Prather, DA, Trunell, N, Yates, FE. Transdermal testosterone replacement through genital skin. In: Nieschlag E, HM Behre, ed. Testosterone: action, deficiency, substitution. Springer-Verlag, Berlin, Heidelberg, New York, 1990, pp. 165-180.

90. Ahmed SR, Boucher AE, Manni A, Santen RJ, Bartholomew M, Demers LM. Transdermal testosterone therapy in the treatment of male hypogonadism. J Clin Endocrinol Metab 1988;66:546-51.

91. Bals-Pratsch M, Knuth UA, Yoon YD, Nieschlag E. Transdermal testosterone substitution therapy for male hypogonadism. Lancet 1986;2:943-6.

92. Cunningham GR, Cordero E, Thornby JI. Testosterone replacement with transdermal therapeutic systems. Physiological serum testosterone and elevated dihydrotestosterone levels. JAMA 1989;261:2525-30.

93. Findlay JC, Place V, Snyder PJ. Treatment of primary hypogonadism in men by the transdermal administration of testosterone. J Clin Endocrinol Metab 1989;68:369-373.

94. Carey PO, Howards SS, Vance ML. Transdermal testosterone treatment of hypogonadal men. J Urol 1988;140:76-79.

95. Findlay JC, Place VA, Snyder PJ. Transdermal delivery of testosterone. J Clin Endocrinol Metab 1987;64:266-8.

96. Meikle AW, CardosaDeSousa JC, Dacosta N, Bishop DK, Samlowski WE. Direct and indirect effects of Murine Interleukin-2, Gamma interferon, and tumor necrosis factor on Testosterone synthesis in mouse leydig cells. J Androl 1992;13:1-7.

97. Meikle A, Arver, S, Dobs, AS, Sanders, SW, Mazer, NA. Androderm: a permeation enhanced non-scrotal testosterone transdermal system for the treatment of male hypogonadism. In: Bhasin S, Gabelnick HL, Spieler JM, Swerdloff RS, Wang C, eds. Pharmacol, Biol Clin Appli Androgens. Wiley-Liss, Inc, New York, 1996.

98. Arver S, Dobs AS, Meikle AW, Allen RP, Sanders SW, Mazer NA. Improvement of sexual function in testosterone deficient men treated for 1 year with a permeation enhanced testosterone transdermal system. J Urol 1996;155:1604-8.

99. Meikle A, Annand D, Hunter C, et al. Pre-treatment with topical corticosteroid cream improves local tolerability and does not significantly alter the pharmacokinetics of the androderm testosterone transdermal system in hypogonadal men. Endocrine Soc 1997;79th:P01-322.

100. Wilson D, Kaidbey K, Boike S, Jorkasky D. Use of topical corticosteroid cream in the pretreatment of skin reactions associated with Androderm testosterone transdermal system. Endocrine Soc 1997;79th:P01-323.

101. Balducci R, Toscano V, Casilli D, Maroder M, Sciarra F, Boscherini B. Testicular responsiveness following chronic administration of hCG (1500 IU every six days) in untreated hypogonadotropic hypogonadism. Horm Metab Res 1987;19:216-21.

102. Finkel D, Phillips J, Snyder P. Stimulation of spermatogenesis by gonadotropins in men with hypogonadotropic hypogonadism. N Engl J Med 1985;313:651-5.

103. Baker HW, Hudson B. Changes in the pituitary-testicular axis with age. Monogr Endocrinol 1983;25:71-83.

104. Carter HB, Pearson JD, Metter EJ, et al. Longitudinal evaluation of serum androgen levels in men with and without prostate cancer. Prostate 1995;27:25-31.

105. Tenover JS, Matsumoto AM, Plymate SR, Bremner WJ. The effects of aging in normal men on bioavailable testosterone and luteinizing hormone secretion: response to clomiphene citrate. J Clin Endocrinol Metab 1987;65:1118-1126.

106. Nankin HR, Calkins JH. Decreased bioavailable testosterone in aging normal and impotent men. J Clin Endocrinol Metab 1986;63:1418-1420.

107. Bremner WJ, Vitiello MV, Prinz PN. Loss of circadianrhythmicity in blood testosterone levels with aging in normal men. J Clin Endocrinol Metab 1983;56:1278-1281.

108. Katznelson L, Finkelstein JS, Schoenfeld DA, Rosenthal DI, Anderson EJ, Klibanski A. Increase in bone density and lean body mass during testosterone administration in men with acquired hypogonadism. J Clin Endocrinol Metab 1996;81:4358-65.

109. Bhasin S, Storer TW, Berman N, et al. Testosterone replacement increases fat-free mass and muscle size in hypogonadal men. J Clin Endocrinol Metab 1997;82:407-13.

110. Sih R, Morley J, Kaiser F, Perry HM, Patrick P, Ross C. Testosterone replacement in older hypogonadal men: a 12-month randomized controlled trial. J Clin Endocrinol Metab 1997;82:1661-7.

111. Grinspoon S, Corcoran C, Lee K, et al. Loss of lean body and muscle mass correlates with androgen levels in hypogonadal men with acquired immunodeficiency syndrome and wasting. J Clin Endocrinol Metab 1996;81:4051-8.

112. Klein SA, Klauke S, Dobmeyer JM, et al. Substitution of testosterone in a HIV-1 positive patient with hypogonadism and Wasting-syndrome led to a reduced rate of apoptosis. Eur J Med Res 1997;2:30-2.

113. Rabkin JG, Rabkin R, Wagner GJ. Testosterone treatment of clinical hypogonadism in patients with HIV/AIDS [In Process Citation]. Int J STD AIDS 1997;8:537-45.

114. Holzman D. Testosterone wasting and AIDS [news]. Mol Med Today 1996;2:93.

115. Morales A, Johnston B, Heaton J, Clark A. Oral androgens in the treatment of hypogonadal impotent men. J Urol 1994;152:1115-8.

116. Burris AS, Banks SM, Carter CS, Davidson JM, Sherins RJ. A long-term, prospective study of the physiologic and behavioral effects of hormone replacement in untreated hypogonadal men. J Androl 1992;13:297-304.

117. O. Carroll R, Shapiro C, Bancroft J. Androgens, behaviour and nocturnal erection in hypogonadal men: the effects of varying the replacement dose. Clin Endocrinol 1985;23:527-38.

118. Hubert W. Psychotropic effects of testosterone. In: Nieschlag E, Behre HM, ed. Testosterone: action, deficiency, substitution. Springer-Verlag, Berlin, Heidelberg, New York, 1990, pp. 51-65.

119. Krabbe S, Christiansen C. Longitudinal study of calcium metabolism in male puberty. I. Bone mineral content, and serum levels of alkaline phosphatase, phosphate and calcium. Acta Paediatr Scand 1984;73:745-9.

120. Bonjour J, Theintz G, Buchs B, Slosman D, Rizzoli R. Critical years and stages of puberty for spinal and femoral bone mass accumulation during adolescence. J Clin Endocrinol Metab 1991;73:555- 63.

121. Scane AC, Sutcliffe AM, Francis RM. Osteoporosis in men. Baillieres Clin Rheumatol 1993;7:589-601.

122. Baillie S, Davison C, Johnson F, Francis R. Pathogenesis of vertebral crush fractures in men. Age Ageing 1992;21:139-41.

123. Halbreich U, Palter S. Accelerated osteoporosis in psychiatric patients: possible pathophysiological processes. Schizophr Bull 1996;22:447-54.

124. Halbreich U, Rojansky N, Palter S, et al. Decreased bone mineral density in medicated psychiatric patients. Psychosom Med 1995;57:485-91.

125. Keely E, Reiss J, Drinkwater D, Faiman C. Bone mineral density, sex hormones, and long-term use of neuroleptic agents in mem. Endocr Pract 1997;3:209-213.

126. Behre H, Kliesch S, Leifke E, Link T, Nieschlag E. Long-term effect of testosterone therapy on bone mineral density in hypogonadal men. J Clin Endocrinol Metab 1997;82:2386-2390.

127. Seeman E, Melton LJd, WM OF, Riggs BL. Risk factors for spinal osteoporosis in men. Am J Med 1983;75:977-83.

128. Seeman E. The dilemma of osteoporosis in men. Am J Med 1995;98:76s-88s.

129. Kuhn JM, Gay D, Lemercier JP, Pugeat M, Legrand A, Wolf LM. Testicular function during prolonged corticotherapy. Presse Med 1986;15:559-62.

130. Lukert BP. Glucocorticoid-induced osteoporosis. South Med J 1992;85:2s48-51.

131. Reid IR, Veale AG, France JT. Glucocorticoid osteoporosis. J Asthma 1994;31:7-18.

132. MacAdams MR, White RH, Chipps BE. Reduction of serum testosterone levels during chronic glucocorticoid therapy. Ann Intern Med 1986;104:648-651.

133. Praet JP, Peretz A, Rozenberg S, Famaey JP, Bourdoux P. Risk of osteoporosis in men with chronic bronchitis. Osteoporos Int 1992;2:257-61.

134. Stepan JJ, Lachman M, Zverina J, Pacovsky V, Baylink DJ. Castrated men exhibit bone loss: effect of calcitonin treatment on biochemical indices of bone remodeling. J Clin Endocrinol Metab 1989;69:523-7.

135. Goldray D, Weisman Y, Jaccard N, Merdler C, Chen J, Matzkin H. Decreased bone density in elderly men treated with the gonadotropin-releasing hormone agonist decapeptyl (D-Trp6-GnRH). J Clin Endocrinol Metab 1993;76:288-90.

136. Greenspan SL, Neer RM, Ridgeway EC, Klibanski A. Osteoporosis in men with hyperprolactinemic hypogonadism. Ann Intern Med 1986;104:777-782.

137. Greenspan SL, Oppenheim DS, Klibanski A. Importance of gonadal steroids to bone mass in men with hyperprolactinemic hypogonadism. Ann Intern Med 1989;110:526-31.

138. Finkelstein JS, Neer RM, Biller BM, Crawford JD, Klibanski A. Osteopenia in men with a history of delayed puberty. N Engl J Med 1992;326:600-4.

139. Finkelstein JS, Klibanski A, Neer RM, Greenspan SL, Rosenthal DI, Crowley WF, Jr. Osteoporosis in men with idiopathic hypogonadotropic hypogonadism. Ann Intern Med 1987;106:354- 61.

140. Finkelstein JS, Klibanski A, Neer RM, et al. Increases in bone density during treatment of men with idiopathic hypogonadotropic hypogonadism. J Clin Endocrinol Metab 1989;69:776-83.

141. Katznelson L, Finkelstein J, Baressi C, Klibanski A. Increase in trabecular bone density and altered body composition in androgen replaced hypogonadal men. Endocrine Soc 1994;75th:1524A.

142. Matzkin H, Chen J, Weisman Y, et al. Prolonged treatment with finasteride (a 5 alpha-reductase inhibitor) does not affect bone density and metabolism. Clin Endocrinol (Oxf.) 1992;37:432-436.

143. Pederson L, Kremer M, Foged N, et al. Evidence of a correlation of estrogen receptor level and avian osteoclast estrogen responsiveness. J Bone Miner Res 1997;12:742-52.

144. McDonnell D, Norris J. Analysis of the molecular pharmacology of estrogen receptor agonists and antagonists provides insights into the mechanism of action of estrogen in bone. Osteoporos Int 1997;7 Suppl 1:S29-34.

145. Hoyland J, Mee A, Baird P, Braidman I, Mawer E, Freemont A. Demonstration of estrogen receptor mRNA in bone using in situ reverse-transcriptase polymerase chain reaction. Bone 1997;20:87- 92.

146. Grese T, Cho S, Finley D, et al. Structure-activity relationships of selective estrogen receptor modulators: modifications to the 2-arylbenzothiophene core of raloxifene. J Med Chem 1997;40:146-67.

147. Fiorelli G, Gori F, Frediani U, et al. Membrane binding sites and non-genomic effects of estrogen in cultured human pre-osteoclastic cells. J Steroid Biochem Mol Biol 1996;59:233-40.

148. Kobayashi S, Inoue S, Hosoi T, Ouchi Y, Shiraki M, Orimo H. Association of bone mineral density with polymorphism of the estrogen receptor gene. J Bone Miner Res 1996;11:306-11.

149. Frolik C, Bryant H, Black E, Magee D, Chandrasekhar S. Time-dependent changes in biochemical bone markers and serum cholesterol in ovariectomized rats: effects of raloxifene HCl, tamoxifen, estrogen, and alendronate. Bone 1996;18:621-7.

150. Mano H, Yuasa T, Kameda T, et al. Mammalian mature osteoclasts as estrogen target cells. Biochem Biophys Res Commun 1996;223:637-42.

151. Smith EP, Boyd J, Frank GR, et al. Estrogen resistance caused by a mutation in the estrogen- receptor gene in a man [see comments] [published erratum appears in N Engl J Med 1995 Jan 12;332(2):131]. N Engl J Med 1994;331:1056-61.

152. Tenover J. Androgen therapy in aging men. In: Bhasin S, Galelnick H, Spieler J, Swerdloff R, Wang C, eds. Pharmacology, biology, and clinical applications of androgens. Wiley-Liss, Inc, New York, 1996, pp. 309-318.

153. Arver S, Meikle A, Dobs A, Sanders S, Mazer N. Hypogonadal men treated with the Androderm testosterone transdermal system had fewer abnormal hematocrit elevations than those treated with testosterone enanthate injections. Endocrine Soc 1997;79th:P01-327.

154. Moorjani S, Dupont A, Labrie F, et al. Changes in plasma lipoproteins during various androgen suppression therapies in men with prostatic carcinoma: effects of orchiectomyy, estrogen, and combination treatment with luteinizing hormone-releasing hormone agonist and flutamide. J Clin Endocrinol Metab 1988;66:314-322.

155. Goldberg RB, Rabin D, Alexander AN, Doelle GC, Getz GS. Suppression of plasma testosterone leads to an increase in serum total and high density lipoprotein cholesterol and apoproteins A-1 and B. J Clin Endocrinol Metab 1985;60:203-207.

156. Bagatell C, Bremner W. Androgen and progestagen effects on plasma lipids. Prog Cardiovasc Dis 1995;38:255-71.

157. Bagatell C, Heiman J, Matsumoto A, Rivier J, Bremner W. Metabolic and behavioral effects of high-dose, exogenous testosterone in healthy men. J Clin Endocrinol Metab 1994;79:561-7.

158. Bagatell C, Knopp R, Rivier J, Bremner W. Physiological levels of estradiol stimulate plasma high density lipoprotein2 cholesterol levels in normal men. J Clin Endocrinol Metab 1994;78:855-61.

159. Bagatell C, Knopp R, Vale W, Rivier J, Bremner W. Physiologic testosterone levels in normal men suppress high-density lipoprotein cholesterol levels [see comments]. Ann Intern Med 1992;116:967-73.

160. Byerley L, Lee WN, Swerdloff RS, et al. Effect of modulating serum testosterone levels in the normal male range on protein, carbohydrate, and lipid metabolism in men: implications for testosterone replacement therapy. Endocrine J 1993;1:253-262.

161. Kirkland R, Keenan B, Probstfield J, et al. Decrease in plasma high-density lipoprotein cholesterol levels at puberty in boys with delayed adolescence. Correlation with plasma testosterone levels. JAMA 1987;257:502-7.

162. Mooradian AD, Morley JE, Korenman SG. Biological actions of androgens. Endocr Rev 1987;8:1-28.

163. Hromadova M, Hacik T, Malatinsky E, Sklovsky A, Cervenakov I. Some measures of lipid metabolism in young sterile males before and after testosterone treatment. Endocrinol Exp 1989;23:205- 11.

164. Friedl K, Hannan CJ J, Jones R, Plymate S. High-density lipoprotein cholesterol is not decreased if an aromatizable androgen is administered. Metabolism 1990;39:69-74.

165. Watts N, Notelovitz M, Timmons M, Addison W, Wiita B, Downey L. Comparison of oral estrogens and estrogens plus androgen on bone mineral density, menopausal symptoms, and lipid-lipoprotein profiles in surgical menopause [published erratum appears in Obstet Gynecol 1995 May;85(5 Pt 1):668]. Obstet Gynecol 1995;85:529-37.

166. Hickok L, Toomey C, Speroff L. A comparison of esterified estrogens with and without methyltestosterone: effects on endometrial histology and serum lipoproteins in postmenopausal women. Obstet Gynecol 1993;82:919-24.

167. Meikle AW, Stephenson RA, McWhorter WP, Skolnick MH, Middleton RG. Effects of age, sex steroids, and family relationships on volumes of prostate zones in men with and without prostate cancer. Prostate 1995;26:253-259.

168. Meikle AW. Endocrinology of the prostate and of benign prostate prostatic hyperplasia. In: Degroot LJ, ed. Endocrinology, 3rd ed. W.B. Saunders, Philadelphia, 1995, pp. 2459-2473.

169. Meikle AW, Arver S, Dobs AS, et al. Prostate size in hypogonadal men treated with a nonscrotal permeation-enhanced testosterone transdermal system. Urology 1997;49:191-6.
170. Meikle AW, Stephenson RA, Lewis CM, Middleton RG. Effects of age and sex hormones on transition and peripheral zone volumes of prostate and benign prostatic hyperplasia in twins. J Clin Endocrinol Metab 1997;82:571-575.
171. Behre HM, Bohmeyer J, Nieschlag E. Prostate volume in testosterone-treated and untreated hypogonadal men in comparison to age-matched normal controls. Clin Endocrinol (Oxf) 1994;40:341-9.
172. McWhorter WP, Hernandez AD, Meikle AW, et al. A screening study of prostate cancer in high risk families. J Urol 1992;148:826-828.
173. Meikle AW, Smith J. Epidemiology of prostate cancer. Urol Clin North Am 1990;17:709-718.
174. Handelsman D. Androgen delivery systems: testosterone pellet implants. In: Bhasin S, Gabelnick HL, Spieler JM, Swerdloff RS, Wang C, eds. Pharmacology, Biology and Clinical Applications of Androgens. Wiley-Liss, Inc, New York, 1996, pp. 459-469.

17 Androgen Replacement
Sexual Behavior, Affect, and Cognition

Max Hirshkowitz, PhD, Claudia Orengo, MD, PhD, and Glenn R. Cunningham, MD

CONTENTS

INTRODUCTION

An awareness of the relationship between erectile function and testicular integrity has existed since antiquity *(1)*. However, some castrated men retain potency and erectile function for many years *(2)*. Most authors attribute this to the complexity of human sexual function, the importance of learned behavior, or both. Clinicians began using testosterone to restore libido and erectile function in the late 1930s, when a synthetic form became available. It was not until 1979 that testosterone's ability to restore libido was more rigorously demonstrated. Subsequently, investigators have examined if a "threshold" for androgen's effects on erectile function exists and whether there is a progressive beneficial effect, even when levels are in the "normal" range. Another issue concerns the possibility that some components of sexual behavior are androgen-dependent, whereas others are not. Even today the literature contains relatively few randomized placebo-controlled double-blind studies comparing more than one delivery system. Nonetheless, much progress has been made in the last 20 years. We review here the effects of testosterone deficiency on sexual behavior and function and the beneficial effects of testosterone replacement in testosterone deficient men.

Findings from animal studies have linked androgen and aggressive behavior in our minds. Male sexuality, even in humans, apparently involves aggressive behavioral features, thereby perpetuating this notion. Decreased aggressiveness reported in sex offenders after

From: *Contemporary Endocrinology: Hormone Replacement Therapy*
Edited by: A. W. Meikle © Humana Press Inc., Totowa, NJ

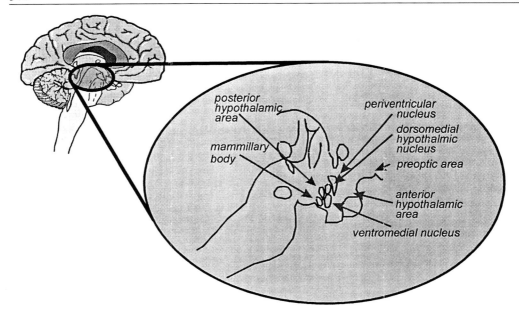

Fig. 1. Brain areas associated with sexual activity. Human brain with an inserted parasagittal section of rhesus monkey brain. Electrical stimulation and lesion sites shown to affect sexual behavior include dorsomedial hypothalamic nucleus, preoptic, anterior hypothalamic, and posterior hypothalamic areas. In nonhuman primates, androgen receptors are found in the amygdala, lateral septum, and premammillary bodies.

castration is taken by many as supporting evidence. However, controlled studies in normal men typically do not confirm the association between testosterone and aggression. A model is evolving that considers such aggressive behavior as an interaction between androgen and an impulse-control deficit. Finally, recent data indicate possible relationships between androgen, mood, and cognition. Testosterone's potential beneficial effects on mood and cognitive function have attracted clinical interest and are explored in a number of studies.

NEUROPHYSIOLOGY

Research from a variety of mammalian species has suggested that the steroid hormones testosterone and 17-estradiol may play a variety of regulatory roles in the central nervous system (CNS). During brain development, sex steroids appear to play a fine-tuning function in certain regions of the brain, modifying events related to neuronal survival and synapse formation *(3)*. In adult brain, sex steroids are capable of modulating synaptic transmission or neurosecretion in numerous hypothalamic and extrahypothalamic brain areas by interacting with specific receptors *(4)*. Therefore, it is reasonable to expect that these brain-related events have some functional or behavioral consequences. Figure 1 illustrates CNS areas implicated in sexual behavior and androgen receptor localization.

CNS Androgen Receptor Localization

Androgen receptors (ARs) are found in the hypothalamus, pituitary, and preoptic areas. Using ^{3}H-testosterone, Michael and colleagues *(5)* identified ARs in the amygdala, lateral septum, and premammillary bodies of nonhuman primates. Studies in intact, adult rats using double-label immunocytochemistry indicate the distribution of AR immuno-reactivity is similar in males and females (6). The vast majority of AR$^+$ cells in ventral tegmental area and substantia nigra (SN) pars compacta were tyrosine hydroxylase immunopositive, approximately half in the SN pars lateralis, and one third in the lateral retrorubral fields. The authors argue that receptor alignments are consistent with "estrogen influence over motor behaviors and androgen involvement in motivational functions." In rams, ARs have been found in many ventromedial somatostatin(+) neurones; however, the neurochemical phenotype of most AR+ cells in the arcuate nucleus remains unknown (7).

An antiandrogen can inhibit male copulatory activity in rats when injected systemically (8). Medial preoptic area (MPOA) implanted hydroxyflutamide (OHF) prevented restoration of sexual behavior by systemically administered testosterone. The greatest effect occurred at the ventromedial nucleus of the hypothalamus, a partial effect was found at the medial amygdala, and no effect at the lateral septum. Upon discontinuation of OHF, sexual activity was restored in most animals. Thus, male sexual behavior is affected by blockade of specific androgen-containing brain sites.

Apomorphine (APO) increases erectile behavior in intact adult rats (9). Castration prevents this response, and testosterone replacement (testosterone propionate >60 µg/kg) restores it within 24 h. Yawning, which is a centrally mediated behavior that accompanies erections in the rat, also is reduced by castration and restored by testosterone replacement. These responses are known as the penile erection/stretching/yawning phenomena. The effects of APO on penile erection/stretching/yawning are thought to be mediated by the CNS. They probably involve dopaminergic receptors (10). Dopamine antagonists that cross the blood–brain barrier antagonize these effects of APO; whereas, dopamine antagonists with only peripheral effects, such as domperidone, do not block APO-induced erections (11). Lesions of the paraventricular nucleus in the hypothalamus prevent APO-induced erections (12), and applying APO to this nucleus increases erectile responses (13).

CNS Lesion and Electrical Stimulation Studies

In general, studies using electrical brain stimulation and brain lesions to localize areas mediating sexual activity correlate well with AR mapping. Stimulation of forebrain, dorsomedial, and lateral hypothalamic nuclei produce penile erections, mating behavior, or both in laboratory animals (14–18). Similar activities are evoked by anterior cingulate gyrus and tegmental stimulation. Lesioning the medial preoptic areas is associated with cessation of male mating activity (19). Implantation of crystalline testosterone in the anterior hypothalamic preoptic areas restored sexual behavior that ceased after rats were castrated; however, implants in other areas had significantly less or no effect (20).

PERIPHERAL PHYSIOLOGY

Reflexes

The importance of lower motor neurons and of neurons in the major pelvic ganglion (MPG) in erections is illustrated by midthoracic transection of the spinal cord in castrated rats. Rats were castrated at age 120 d. Five days later the spinal cord was completely transected at the midthoracic level. Penile erections and penile flips were markedly influenced by testosterone treatment (21). When rats were castrated and the spinal cord

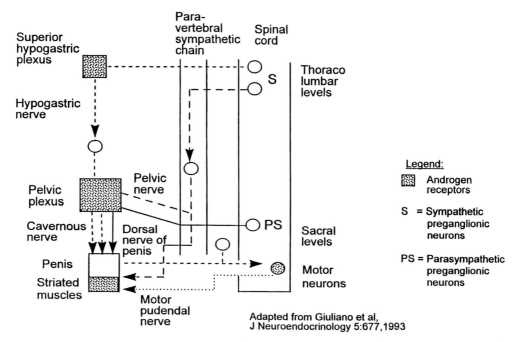

Fig. 2. Neural innervation of rat penile erections. Neurons and skeletal muscle demonstrated to possess androgen receptors are identified. Since little specific binding of androgen is observed in the corpora cavernosa of adults, the penis is not labeled to have androgen receptors; however, androgen receptors are present and responsive during development of the penis.

was transected at age 30 d, animals that survived had autonomic bladders, but remained healthy *(22)*. Capsules containing testosterone were implanted at 90 d of age. Penile reflexes were observed when rats were 100–110 d of age. Removal of the testosterone capsules caused a reduction in penile erections ($p < 0.05$) and penile flips ($p < 0.01$), and these parameters increased ($p < 0.025$) within 12 h of initiating testosterone treatment. In a second experiment, the investigators demonstrated that these reflexes were testosterone-dose dependent. Subsequently other investigators demonstrated that enzymes required for synthesis of neurotransmitters in both the sympathetic hypogastric ganglion *(23)* and the parasympathetic MPG are regulated by androgen *(24)*. Figure 2 provides a schematic representation of neural circuits and ARs involved in rat penile erections.

Autonomic nervous system enervation of the corpora cavernosa is considered the major affector of penile erections. Electrical stimulation of the MPG evokes erection. Preganglionic neurons of the parasympathetic pathway are located in the intermediolateral column of the sacral spinal cord. Their axons are in the pelvic nerves, synapsing with neurons in the MPG. Castration of adult rats reduces intracavernosal pressure, reversible with androgen replacement *(25)*. Interestingly, pelvic nerves axotomy does not impair the response; however, the response is reduced by concurrent castration and is restored by androgen replacement *(26)*. Furthermore, sectioning pelvic nerves in castrated rats further reduces intracavernosal pressure during MPG stimulation. ARs and nitric oxide synthase I (NOS I; neuronal nitric oxide synthase) co-localize to these neurons *(27)*. Castration reduces NOS I mRNA levels in these neurons and NADPH-diaphorase, which is linked to NOS *(28)*.

Nitric Oxide Synthase

Nonadrenergic, noncholinergic nerves whose neurons are located in the MPG release nitric oxide (NO), vasoactive polypeptide (VIP), and calcitonin gene-regulated peptide (CGRP) in the corpora cavernosa. These agents relax smooth-muscle cells in arterioles and in the trabeculae of the corpora cavernosa. NO is the most important smooth-muscle relaxer but under some circumstances, as demonstrated by the n-NOS knockout rat, other mediators may maintain erectile function. NO works via a cGMP mechanism to lower intracellular calcium concentrations and cause smooth-muscle relaxation.

NOS in the corpora cavernosa is partially androgen regulated. Castration reduces intracavernosal pressure and NOS activity. Both are restored by testosterone replacement (29,30). Castration reduces mRNA and nNOS protein in the cavernosa (31,32). Finasteride, a 5α-reductase inhibitor, reduces the effect of testosterone on NOS activity; thus, DHT may be more important than testosterone. Castration also decreases NOS positive nerve fibers density (33). Interestingly, castration-induced NOS activity reduction can be reversed by MPG stimulation when NOS activity is measured during an erection. This indicates that NOS activity can respond acutely to neural stimulation (34). Reduced intracavernosal pressure observed in castrated rats is not limited by substrate; it can be increased by combining sodium nitroprusside infusion (a NO donar) and MPG stimulation (31). Not all penile NOS activity is androgen dependent given that infusing a NOS inhibitor into corpora cavernosa of castrate rats further reduces intracavernosal pressure.

Androgen-stimulated increases in intracavernosal NOS and androgen potentiation of electrical MPG stimulation may be mediated by ARs in neurons of the MPG or by ARs in the corpora cavernosa. However, penile ARs decline during development and are very sparse in the adult rat (35,36) and other species (37). ARs in cultured smooth muscle cells from rat corpora cavernosa appear to be down regulated by estrogen (38). AR presence in MPG neurons argues for the androgen's major effect being at this level.

Penile erections depend on both increasing arterial inflow and decreasing venous outflow. Castration-related increases in penile outflow indicate that androgen may have additional effects (29). Venous outflow normally declines when sinusoids of the corpora cavernosa become engorged; therefore, the increased outflow may result from changes in tissue compliance of the corpora or the tunica albuginea.

The fifth and sixth lumbar segments of the rat spinal cord contain motor neurons that innervate bulbospongiosus and ischiocavernosus muscles (39). To identify the motor neurons, investigators stained the axons by injecting these muscles with horseradish peroxidase. These neurons are not developed in androgen resistant rats or in females; however, they concentrate radioactive testosterone or DHT (but not estradiol) in normal males. Bulbospongiousus muscles in rats augment intracavernosal pressure during penile erection (40) and androgen may directly affect bulbospongiousus and ischiocavernosus-striated muscle (41).

In summary, rat models provide data concerning androgen-related mechanisms underlying male sexual behavior. Androgen plays a role at many levels, including: hypothalamus, spinal cord (L5-L6) motor neurons to the bulbocavernosus muscles, hypogastric sympathetic ganglion, MPG, bulbospongiousus and ischiocavernosus muscles, and possibly corpora cavernosa receptors.

ANDROGEN AND MALE SEXUALITY

Most clinical testosterone deficiency studies examine adult men with congenital or acquired hypogonadism. Other than Klinefelter's syndrome and myotonic dystrophy, most hypogonadal men age 20–50 yr have secondary hypogonadism. However, the majority of hypogonadal men are age 50 yr, or older. Except in cases of surgical or chemical castration for stage D prostate cancer, testosterone deficiency typically is partial. Some testicular testosterone production usually remains and this can obscure effects of testosterone deficiency. Recently, a few studies have experimentally induced testosterone deficiency in young healthy men by using GnRH agonists or antagonists. This paradigm provides an unparalleled opportunity for observing acute effects of complete deficiency of testicular androgens.

Methods

SELF-REPORT

Self-report is a simple and direct approach to assessing sexual function. Quantitative indices can be derived from data collected during interviews, rating scales, diaries, and questionnaires. Information from the sexual partner also is useful. Validated questionnaires have appeared in the literature *(42–44)*. Some are inventories designed for single time administration to assess sexual dysfunction. Others assess sexual practices, preferences, and satisfaction. Salient inquiries include the frequency and intensity of sexual thoughts, interest, activity, and enjoyment.

Data concerning sexuality obtained in this manner, however, suffers from problems common to all self-reported information. The circumstances—sometimes called demand characteristics—can influence the response. Potential secondary gains and hidden agendas must be considered carefully. Some individuals minimize disclosure of their sexuality because of mistrust, embarrassment, or repression; whereas, others eagerly report intimate details of their sex life. Thus, differences in personality and personal style can influence self-report and obscure differences by inflating variance. Nonetheless, proper sampling and experimental design can avoid systematic errors in results.

ERECTILE RESPONSE TO VISUAL SEXUAL STIMULATION OR SEXUAL FANTASY

Visual sexual stimulation (VSS) is a technique used to objectively assess erectile responsiveness. VSS typically involves continuously measuring penile circumference increase when a subject views filmed or videotaped explicit material depicting nudity and sexual activities performed by adults. Sometimes, penile rigidity is measured. Variations on this approach include having subjects engage in sexual fantasy (SF) or listen to sexually arousing audiotaped material while monitoring erection.

Applying this technique overcomes some limitations of self-reported data; however, personality factors and individual differences still may influence results. In some individuals, sexual response may be inhibited by the laboratory setting and the presence of monitoring equipment on the penis. In repeated measure designs, order effects are critical. Initial embarrassment or sympathetic nervous system activity (via peripheral vasoconstrictive response) may decline in subsequent trials as a subject becomes more comfortable with procedures. The subject's sexual orientation and activity preference, compared to that depicted in the material presented should be considered. Aging studies must consider this carefully because attitudes, mores, and practices have changed considerably in the past six decades. Notwithstanding these factors, VSS provides an objective physiologic index of sexual responsiveness.

SLEEP-RELATED ERECTIONS (SREs)

Erectile capability can be indexed by evaluating sleep-related penile erections (sometimes referred to as nocturnal penile tumescence [NPT]). Nonvolitional, naturally occurring, SREs are found in all sexually potent, healthy men (45,46). These erections are tightly coupled with rapid eye movement (REM) sleep and appear unaffected by behavioral factors. Sexual abstention, viewing sexually explicit material, masturbation, and increased sexual activity all fail to alter SREs (47). Consequently, SRE testing provides objective, quantitative indices of erectile function. Therefore, failure to attain full erections during consolidated REM sleep is taken to indicate erectile pathology.

Strain gauges placed around the penis are used to record SREs by continuously measuring penile circumference. Concurrently, sleep-state assessment is preferred to determine coupling between SREs and REM sleep. Because circumference increase can occur without penile rigidity, penile resistance to buckling is a critical parameter for judging erectile quality. SREs are most commonly summarized according to frequency, magnitude, duration, and quality (rigidity).

Karacan and associates (48) studied SREs in young boys, young adults, middle-aged men, and the elderly. Their results have subsequently been replicated (42,49). Except for a sharp increase during adolescence, SREs in men age 3–80 yr are fairly consistent. With advancing age, small statistically reliable total tumescence time (duration) decline is found, accounting for approx 15% of variance (49a). Frequency and magnitude measures show little or no decline with age in healthy potent seniors.

At puberty, the ratio of SREs to REM sleep increases dramatically (see Fig. 3). This rise in spontaneous erectile activity paralleling increased circulating androgen suggests testosterone may potentiate erectile activity. In a study investigating SRE association with aging and endocrine function, bioavailable testosterone (but not total testosterone) was found to decline with age (50), and SRE frequency and duration correlated with bioavailable testosterone. Overall, age appeared to be the controlling factor; however, SRE duration was related to bioavailable testosterone within the 55–64 yr age group but not in younger or older groups. These authors suggest that age alters a central SRE activation threshold to account for the age-related testosterone association with SREs. Finally, another link between SREs and testosterone is the finding that peak levels occur near REM sleep transitions.

Testosterone levels are low early during the sleep period and gradually increase toward morning. Sleep-cycle disorganization is marked by testosterone alterations, and day sleep is associated with testosterone elevation (51,52). In healthy men, 3–5 rapid REM episodes occur each night. Testosterone peaks were first reported occurring proximal to shifts from NREM to REM sleep by Evans and colleagues (52). This finding was not confirmed by another research group (53) who instead found LH rises preceded testosterone peaks (lag time 20–140 min). Miyatake and colleagues (54) also found no sleep-stage association with testosterone level; however, mean level rather than peaks were analyzed. Subsequently, the REM-testosterone relationship was quantitatively demonstrated (54). Pulsatile peak testosterone levels were concentrated within a 20 min temporal window surrounding transitions from NREM to REM sleep. Interestingly, the CNS organizational state transition to REM sleep also marks the activation of spontaneous SREs.

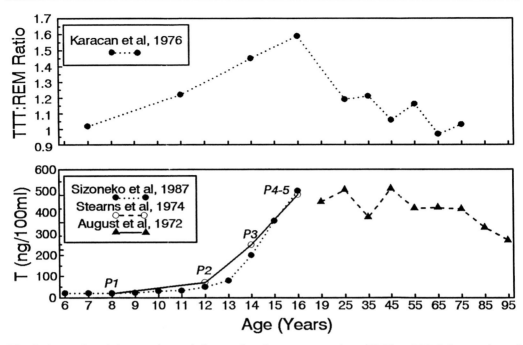

Fig. 3. Age-related changes in total sleep-related tumescence time (TTT) to REM sleep ratio and testosterone levels. Puberty stages (P) 1–5 are shown on the bottom panel. As puberty approaches, TTT:REM sleep ratio increases to a peak at age 16 yr. The ratio stabilizes slightly higher than 1:1 by age 25 yr. Testosterone rises dramatically during puberty, stabilizing at adult levels by age 16 yr.

If SREs are androgen-dependent, prepubescent SRE poses an interesting question. The presence of adrenal androgen during the first 2 yr of life may partially explain SREs in the very young; however, androgen remains low for half a decade or more. The dramatic SRE increase during puberty and its rapid decline by the end of the next decade to normal adult levels may reflect initial receptor supersensitivity and subsequent down-regulation. This model is supported by the finding that spontaneous erectile activation compared to REM sleep declines after puberty while testosterone levels remain high. Another theoretical perspective posits SREs having a very low, discrete, step-like androgen threshold for occurrence followed by a more continuous correlated association, once threshold is met. Finally, SRE may be influenced by both REM sleep and androgen, with one subserving a permissive role and the other a modulating one.

Androgen Deficiency and Replacement in Hypogonadal Men

SELF-REPORT

Davidson and colleagues *(56)* provided the initial scientific evidence for androgen's effects in hypogonadal men. They studied six men between the ages of 32 and 65. Subjects received placebo, 100, or 400 mg of testosterone enanthate (TE) IM every 4 wk for 5 mo. Treatments were varied at random within and among the subjects; subjects maintained daily logs of sexual activity. Paired t tests comparing placebo and 400 mg TE revealed significant differences for total erections ($p < 0.001$), nocturnal erections

Table 1
Self-Reported Effects of Androgen Deficiency

Investigators	n	Study design	Treatment	Findings
Davidson et al. (56)	6	On and off treatment	Placebo, Testosterone enanthate 100 or 400 mg/4 wk	**TE 400 mg vs Placebo:** TE → ↑ total erections ↑ nocturnal erections ↑ coital frequency
Luisi and Franci (112)	26	Double-blind, random	Testosterone undecanoate (40 mg tid) Mesterolone (50 mg tid)	**TU vs Baseline or Mesterolone:** TU → ↑ libido ↑ erections ↑ ejaculations
Skakkebaek et al. (113)	12	Double-blind, crossover	Placebo or testosterone undecanoate (40 mg qid)	**TU vs Placebo:** TU → ↑ sexual thoughts ↑ sexual excitement ↑ sexual acts ↑ ejaculations
Clopper et al. (61)	9	Single-blind, crossover	Placebo, hCG 2000 + hMG 75 tiw or testosterone enanthate (200 mg/2 wk)	**Tx vs Placebo:** Tx → ↑ libido ↑ ejaculations **TE vs hCG + hMG:** ↑ TE ejaculations

TE, testosterone enanthate; TU, testosterone undecanoate; Tx, treatment.

($p < 0.02$), coital frequency ($p < 0.05$), and erections culminating in orgasm ($p < 0.001$). Subsequent reports using different delivery systems confirm these findings (see Table 1).

ERECTILE RESPONSE TO VSS AND SF

Bancroft and Wu (57) studied eight hypogonadal men with testosterone levels <270 ng/dL during VSS. Subjects were studied while hypogonadal and during treatment with TU (160 or 240 mg/d). They reported no VSS maximal circumference change or latency to achieving erection difference between normal men, hypogonadal men, or testosterone treated hypogonadal men. Similar observations were made in a double-blind, crossover study involving six hypogonadal men (58). Subjects were treated with placebo, 200 mg or 400 mg of TE IM at monthly intervals. The total duration of erections and the time with maximal circumference were similar in hypogonadal and normal men and were not affected by testosterone treatment. The hypogonadal men had a slower loss of tumescence than the normal controls. A third study evaluated 9 hypogonadal males and 12 eugonadal controls (59). VSS-related penile magnitude and duration did not differ between hypogonadal men and eugonadal controls. Although testosterone replacement failed to alter magnitude or duration, it was associated with increased ($p < 0.01$) penile rigidity. These authors concluded that erectile responses to VSS predominantly involves an androgen independent system but may be influenced by androgen sensitive mechanisms.

Subjects also have undergone erection monitoring while fantasizing about "the most sexually exciting scene." Eight hypogonadal males were studied before and during treatment with TU (160 mg/d) (57). Maximum penile circumference increase was less in the hypogonadal men than in the age matched normal controls and was not improved by treatment. However, testosterone replacement improved the latency to achieve an erection. Other studies of six *(58)* and nine hypogonadal men *(59)* yielded less consistent results *(58)*. One investigation found no significant differences in erectile magnitude or duration; however, penile rigidity in hypogonadal men during SF improved ($p < 0.02$) with testosterone replacement *(59)*.

SLEEP-RELATED ERECTIONS

Androgen deficiency and androgen replacement alter SREs (*see* Table 2). Men with severe and previously untreated hypogonadism demonstrate little or no SRE *(60)*. All parameters of SRE increased over a year in which serum testosterone levels were normalized. Nine gonadotropin deficient males (age 16–20 yr) were evaluated in a cross-over designed study comparing gonadotropin (2000 units of hCG + 75 IU of hMG tiw) treatment, TE (200 mg/2 wk), and placebo *(61)*. Similar testosterone levels were achieved with both therapies. Total tumescence time ($p < 0.001$), duration of erections >80% of maximal tumescence ($p < 0.004$), and maximal circumference ($p < 0.001$) improved with both treatments.

Techniques used to monitor SREs and penile rigidity have varied across studies. Researchers employ different study designs and a variety of androgen replacement regimens; however, all studies indicate androgen-related SREs changes. Androgen deficiency is associated with fewer spontaneous SREs, reduced maximum increase in penile circumference (magnitude), shorter duration of erections, and poorer rigidity of the penis (quality) during erections *(114)*. Adequate testosterone replacement in the absence of comorbid disease increases and sometimes normalizes SREs.

The effects of testosterone on libido in hypogonadal men are best explained by an effect on the CNS. A CNS effect of androgen also could explain the differences in the frequency of SREs and perhaps the duration of SREs observed during androgen replacement. A local effect of testosterone at the level of the spinal cord, pelvic ganglia and/or corpora cavernosa would help to explain differences in penile circumference and rigidity that have been observed during hypogonadal and androgen replaced states.

Manipulating Testosterone Levels in Eugonadal Men

The effect on sexual behavior of varying serum testosterone levels within the normal or supernormal range interests clinical investigators. At one time, indescriminant treatment with testosterone was common; however, this practice is much less frequent today. If administering exogenous testosterone produces beneficial effects, one could justify such therapy under specific conditions. It also could help answer the question concerning whether testosterone exerts an effect when levels exceed a threshold or whether there is a continuous effect even when levels are within or exceed the normal range. Bhasin and colleagues *(62)* have convincingly demonstrated anabolic effects of supraphysiological doses of testosterone in young men. Is there a similar effect on sexual behavior?

Buna and coworkers *(63)* administered leuprolide to reduce gonadotropin and testosterone secretion and two doses of testosterone microspheres to restore serum levels of testosterone to low or high normal ranges. Daily logs of sexual activity and SRE studies in a sleep laboratory were conducted before and after 9 wk of treatment. Pretreatment testosterone levels in the two groups were similar (15.5 ± 2.1 and 16.6 ± 2.5 nmol/L). Treatment levels were 10.5 ± 1.7 and 26.5 ± 3.4 nmol/L ($p < 0.05$). No differences in

Table 2
Sleep-Related Erections in Androgen-Deficient Males

Investigators	n	Study design	Treatment	Findings
Kwan et al. *(56)*	6	Double-blind, placebo, crossover	Placebo, Testosterone enanthate 200 or 400 mg IM/mo	**TE vs Placebo:** TE → ↑ change in penile circumference ↑ SRE duration
O'Carroll et al. *(86)*	4	Off and on treatment	Testosterone undecanoate (160 mg/d)	**TU vs no treatment:** TU → ↑ change in penile circumference ↑ SRE duration
Cunningham & Hirshkowitz *(114)*	6	On and off treatment	Testosterone cypionate (200 mg/2 wk)	**TC (1–4 d) vs (7–8 wk):** TC (1–4 d) → ↑ number of SREs ↑ max circumference increase ↑ SRE duration ↑ penile rigidity
Burris and Sherins *(60)*	6	Off and on treatment	Testosterone enanthate 200 mg IM/ 2 wk or hCG 2000 + hMG 75 tiw	**No Tx vs Tx:** TX → ↑ number of SREs ↑ max circumference increase ↑ SRE duration ↑ penile rigidity
Arver et al. *(115)*	20	On TE, off Tx, on transdermal	Testosterone enanthate (200 mg/2 wk) or transdermal (7.5 mg/d)	**No Tx vs Tx:** No Tx → ↑ number of SREs ↑ SRE duration ↑ penile rigidity **TE vs Transdermal:** no differences
Clopper et al. *(61)*	9	Single-blind, crossover	Placebo, hCG 2000 + hMG 75 tiw or testosterone enanthate (200 mg IM/2 wk)	**Tx vs Placebo:** Tx → ↑ SRE duration ↑ change in penile circumference ↑ max circumference increase **TE vs hCG + hMG:** no differences
Carani et al. *(59)*	8	Off and on treatment	Multiple treatments	**Tx vs no Tx:** Tx → ↑ number of maximum SREs ($p < 0.07$) ↑ rigidity ($p < 0.07$)

TE, testosterone enanthate; TU, testosterone undecanoate; Tx, treatment; IM, intramuscular.

sexual behavior were observed when comparing parameters prior to and during treatment or during the two treatments. Similarly, no SRE differences were noted in the number, the magnitude, or duration of nocturnal erections.

The effects of TE (150 mg IM) versus placebo on SRE in normal men has been examined (64). Subjects were studied in a sleep laboratory two days after the injection, a time when testosterone levels would be supernormal or high normal. There were no significant differences in the number, magnitude or duration of sleep related erections. However, penile rigidity and the duration of maximal rigidity were increased by testosterone injections ($p < 0.0025$ and $p < 0.025$, respectively).

To explore possible benefits of testosterone therapy in men with normal serum levels of testosterone but who complained of sexual dysfunction, O'Carroll and Bancroft (65) conducted a double-blind, cross-over study using placebo or Sustanon, 250 mg IM/wk (testosterone-proprionate 30 mg; testosterone phenylproprionate 60 mg; testosterone isocaproate 60 mg; testosterone decanoate 100 mg). There was a 4 wk baseline period followed by 6 wk of placebo and 6 wk of testosterone therapy or 6 wk of testosterone therapy and 6 wk of placebo. Patients were divided into two groups, those complaining principally of loss of sexual interest or those complaining primarily of erectile failure. Treatment increased testosterone levels ($p < 0.01$). The frequency of sexual thoughts was increased ($p < 0.02$) by testosterone treatment in the group with low sexual interest; however, there was no increase in sexual activity or in mood. Testosterone therapy provided no benefit to the group of men complaining of erectile dysfunction.

These studies support the concept that a testosterone threshold exists for sexual behaviors. The threshold seems to be somewhat below the normal serum testosterone level range for young adult men. One cannot justify testosterone treatment of erectile dysfunction when serum testosterone levels are normal. Whether testosterone treatment improves libido within the normal serum testosterone range will require further studies.

Sexuality and 5α-Reductase Deficiency and Inhibition

Associations between testosterone level and sexual function could be mediated directly by testosterone or indirectly by its metabolites (DHT and estradiol). There are at least two 5α-reductase enzymes; therefore, inhibiting both would be necessary to ascertain if DHT is necessary for sexual function. The effects of a 5α-reductase inhibitor or an aromatase inhibitor on CNS would depend on it crossing the blood brain barrier. Many of these inhibitors are steroids; therefore, they likely cross this barrier in sufficient quantities to influence CNS activity.

Males with an inherited defect in type 2 5α-reductase reportedly develop normal libido and have normal penile erections. Penile development in these individuals is delayed but occurs at puberty (66). These men have rudimentary prostates; consequently, pharmaceutical type-1 and type-2 5α-reductase activity inhibitors have been developed in an effort to treat or prevent benign prostatic hyperplasia, male pattern baldness, and possibly prostate cancer. Three to four percent of men treated with finasteride (67), a type-2 inhibitor, or with GI198745 (unpublished data), an inhibitor of both the type-1 and type-2 enzymes, report reduced libido or potency. In a double-blind, placebo-controlled trial conducted at our laboratory we gave 20 sexually active men (age 41–64 yr) finasteride 5 mg or placebo for 12 wk (68). A sexual function questionnaire was administered weekly and no loss of libido or erectile dysfunction was found. We also studied these men for four nights in the sleep laboratory, twice during baseline and twice at the end of the treatment period. No consistent SRE frequency, magnitude, duration, or quality differences were observed with finasteride treatment compared to placebo. Thus, it appears that either testosterone or DHT can provide normal men with androgenic stimulation required for normal libido and erectile function. However, the possibility that a longer treatment period could adversely affect sexual function in some men remains. Finasteride is a type 2 inhibitor; therefore, it also is possible that type 1 5α-reductase activity in the brain could be responsible for maintaining libido and erectile function. Studies with GI198745 (unpublished) indicate a comparable incidence of erectile problems, making it likely that some men have a pre-existing condition that in conjunction with 5α-reductase inhibition causes the problem. As noted early, animal studies suggests DHT is more potent than testosterone with respect to potentiating neural stimulation of erections.

Whereas estrogen is thought to be the major steroid required by the CNS for sexual behavior in the rat, estrogen treatment of men usually reduces libido and potency *(69)*. No consistent changes in libido or in sexual function have been noted in men treated with either an aromatase inhibitor *(70,71)* or with an anti-estrogen. At this time, the clinical observations in males having either an aromatase deficiency or estrogen insensitivity are too few to provide definitive insights.

Surgical and Chemical Castration

In Men with Normal Sexuality

Surgical or medical (GnRH agonist treatment) castration for stage D prostate cancer reportedly reduces libido. Of 11 men studied, post-treatment libido was absent in five, poor in three, and fair in three *(72)*. All reported satisfactory erectile function before treatment; however, after five or more months no patient reported spontaneous erections and none had attempted intercourse following treatment. Four subjects had VSS-induced erections with a 10 mm or more circumference increase.

A double-blind study of the GnRH antagonist, Nal-Glu, randomized 50 men, age 20–40 yr into 5 groups: Nal-Glu alone, Nal-Glu + TE 50 mg IM/week, Nal-Glu + TE 100 mg IM/week, Nal-Glu + TE 100 mg IM/week + testolactone (an aromatase inhibitor) 250 mg po qid, and placebo *(71)*. After a 4 wk pretreatment phase, there were six treatment weeks and four recovery weeks. Men receiving Nal-Glu alone experienced less frequent sexual desire ($p < 0.05$), fewer sexual fantasies, less sexual intercourse, fewer spontaneous erections ($p < 0.55$ compared to baseline and $p < 0.05$ compared to posttreatment) and less frequent masturbation ($p < 0.05$). These parameters normalized within 3 wk of treatment cessation. Other groups did not differ from baseline on these parameters. Mean nadir testosterone levels in subjects receiving 50 mg of TE/wk were in the borderline low range (8.9 ± 0.6 nmol/L). Since testolactone blocks the conversion of testosterone to estradiol at least in peripheral tissues, it did not appear that estrogen is required for normal sexual function in the adult male.

The GnRH agonist leuprolide, initially stimulates and subsequently decreases gonadotropin secretion. Usually testosterone levels are suppressed within 3 wk. In a double blind, placebo controlled study involving 10 normal men ages 21–35, Hirshkowitz and colleagues *(73)* treated five men with leuprolide and five men with placebo injections. Subjects were studied for two successive nights in a sleep laboratory during a control period, and after 4, 8, and 12 wk of treatment. Second night data were used for the analysis. REM sleep measures and sleep efficiency were similar in the two groups. Significant ($p < 0.05$) reduction in total tumescence was observed at 8 and 12 wk. There was a trend for the number of SREs to decrease ($p < 0.14$) and a tendency toward reduced maximal penile circumference at 8 wk.

IN SEX OFFENDERS

Surgical castration of sex offenders was common practice in some European countries after the second World War II *(74)*. A survey of 39 sex offenders (mean age, 49.3 yr) revealed that although sexual activity declined after castration, 31% still reported ability to engage in sexual intercourse *(75)*. The strongest diminution of sexuality occurred when castration was performed later in life (age 46–59 yr). Heim compared these data to previously published work and found less cessation of coitus (69%) than previously reported by Cornu (90%) or Langeluddeke (82%).

Antiandrogens that suppress LH and testosterone secretion and/or antagonize testosterone action have been used to treat sex offenders. In one study *(76)*, 19 paraphilic men were administered cyproterone acetate. Significantly decreased sexual fantasies and masturbation were found; however, no decline occurred in self-reported libido, potency, or coitus. A placebo-controlled study of cyproterone acetate (CPA) on hypersexual men found it reduced sexual drive and arousal *(77)*. Medroxyprogesterone acetate (MPA), a synthetic progestin with gonadatropin-suppressing and anti-androgen properties, and CPA blunted a variety of sexual behaviors in seven pedophiles *(78)*. Both drugs reduced self-reported sexual thoughts, sexual fantasies, number of early morning erections, frequency of masturbation, pleasure derived from masturbation, and level of sexual frustration. MPA also was found to dramatically reduce SREs in three sex offenders *(79)*.

ANDROGEN AND AGGRESSIVE BEHAVIOR

In many species, androgens appear to increase aggressive behavior. Attempts to find analogous androgen-related increases in man have yielded mixed results. In a case report, MPA reduced aggressive sexual behavior and sexual acting out in a male schizophrenic *(80)*. Interestingly, it also suppressed SREs. Sex hormone administration is part of sex change protocols. Fifteen male-to-female transexuals treated with estrogen and antiandrogens were less prone to aggression and anger *(81)*. By contrast, androgens given to 35 female-to-male transsexuals increased aggression and sexual arousability.

Anabolic steroids abuse is anecdotally implicated in aggressive behavior and violent crime. A prospective double-blind, placebo-controlled study examined whether testosterone would increase aggressive tendencies in normal men *(82)*. After excluding competitive athletes and men with psychiatric disturbances, 600 mg TE or placebo were administered weekly for 6 wk to 43 eugonadal men. Subgroups with and without strength-training exercise regimens also were formed. No treatment-related changes were found on any subscales of the Multi-Dimensional Anger Inventory, the Mood Inventory, or the subjects significant-others' rating of mood or behavior on the Observer Mood Inventory. By contrast, double-blind, placebo-controlled, testosterone injection in 35 hypogonadal adolescents increased aggression scores on the Olweus Multifaceted Aggression Inventory *(83)*. Elevation was found for self-reported physical aggressive behaviors and aggressive impulses; however, verbal aggression did not increase.

These apparently discrepant findings can be explained by the androgen-disinhibition model. Some theorist believe that testosterone-related aggressive behavior manifests when impulse control problems occur. Thus, under normal circumstances, aggression is inhibited; however, when disinhibition occurs, it is unmasked. As such, the data showing no relationship between substantial testosterone supplementation and aggression in normal men does not rule out exacerbation of aggression among individuals prone to violence. The androgen-disinhibition model is supported by studies in squirrel monkeys *(84)*. Dominant males testosterone level rose to 202.9 ng/mL during mating season compared to 28 ng/mL in subordinates. Although alcohol (0.1–1.0 g/kg, PO) reduced testosterone in a dose-response manner in dominant males, low doses (0.1 and 0.3 g/kg) also increased aggressive behaviors. At time periods other than mating season, alcohol had no effect on aggressive behavior or testosterone.

ANDROGEN AND AFFECT

Data concerning the relationship between androgen and affect derive from three sources: 1) Studies involving testosterone-supplementation in eugonadal men, 2) Mood assessment during androgen replacement therapy in hypogonadal men, and 3) Crossectional and intervention research on men with depression.

TE administered to healthy eugonadal men appears not to alter mood. No significant change from placebo-baseline was found in 31 men, age 21–41 yr, given TE for 4 wk *(85)*. Ratings were made on scales for cheerfulness, lethargy, relaxation, tension, energy, unhappiness, irritability, readiness to fight, and easiness to anger. Similarly, no mood difference was found in 43 men administered 600 mg TE IM or placebo for 6 wk, regardless of whether they were in an exercise or nonexercise subgroup *(82)*.

In an early study, six men with hypogonadism, age 32–65 years, received two doses of TE (100 and 400 mg/mo) for 5 mo *(56)*. Subjects completed the Profile of Mood States (POMS) test at weekly intervals throughout most of the study and were seen by a psychologist once each month. No significant androgen-related changes were found in mood. By contrast, TU administered double-blind in four successive, 1-month periods (40, 80, 120, 160 mg/d in crossover design) reportedly improved mood *(86)*. Eight subjects recorded their mood states daily in diary format and completed visual analog scales rating 10 separate mood states. Significant testosterone-related improvements were found for several scales, including: cheerful-happy, tense-anxious, and relaxed. More recently, 51 hypogonadal men rated their moods before and on days 21, 41, and 60 of testosterone replacement (TE 200 mg q 20 d or sublingual testosterone cyclodextrin [2.5 or 5.0 mg tid]) *(87)*. Compared to baseline, testosterone replacement led to significantly decreased anger, irritability, sadness, tiredness, and nervousness. Increases occurred for energy level, friendliness, and sense of well being scales. Similarly, mood and energy improved with transdermal testosterone administration using scrotal patches *(88)*.

Androgen replacement also has been applied to men with low testosterone levels associated with Klinefelter's syndrome. No reported mood or energy differences were reported for four men given 160 mg TU or placebo in a double-blind, crossover study *(89)*. In a larger trial, 30 men with Klinefelter's syndrome were given testosterone *(90)*. Follow-up telephone interviews revealed improved mood, less irritability, more energy, and drive, less tiredness, more endurance and strength, less need for sleep, better concentration, and better relations with others during testosterone treatment.

The interrelationship between hypogonadism, fertility, and depression was psychometrically explored using the POMS *(60)*. Untreated hypogonadal men had higher depression, anger, fatigue and confusion scores than infertile men and eugonadal controls. During treatment, scores improved; however, hypogonadal men continued to score higher in depression than the other subjects.

Studies often find lower testosterone levels in depressed men than non-depressed men
(91–94). However, other studies report no difference related to depression *(95–98)*. Other
studies have found a negative correlation between testosterone levels and severity of
depression *(91,98,99)*.

Notwithstanding mixed results in correlational studies; testosterone administration
has been used experimentally to treat patients with depression. In the older literature,
testosterone reportedly alleviates depressive symptoms *(100)*. More recently, the antidepressant effect of a synthetic weak androgen, mesterolone was compared to amitriptyline
in men with depression *(101)*. Mesterolone relieved depression as effectively as amitriptyline. Additionally, a double-blind, placebo controlled study claimed mood enhancement with the weak androgen, dehydroepiandrosterone *(102)*.

In summary, testosterone supplementation may improve mood in patients with depression, hypogonadism, or both. The lack of change in normal eugonadal men may represent
a "ceiling effect" inherent in mood assessment tools or a threshold effect for testosterone.
Alternatively, testosterone may reduce an inhibitory depressogenic factor and have no
effect when such is not present. Additional work focused on testosterone supplementation and depressive disorder type and depth will likely elucidate the apparent interaction.

ANDROGEN AND COGNITION

Well established sex differences exist for verbal fluency and visual-spatial tasks.
Although the nature vs nurture issue remains unresolved, some evidence implicates a role
of androgen in certain cognitive abilities. The classic sex difference literature concerning
cognition derives from IQ tests.

Snow and Weinstock *(103)* reviewed the Wechsler Adult Intelligence Scale (WAIS)
literature to compare non-brain injured males and females on specific subtests. Women tend
to outperform men by 0.33 of the standard deviation on the Digit Symbol subtest. By
contrast, men outperform women, to the same extent or more, on the Arithmetic and
Information subtests. Several studies also found male superiority on Block Design and
Comprehension subtests. Notwithstanding subtest differences, overall IQ scores do not
differ. Hormonal differences between men and women have been suggested as one of many
possible underlying biological mechanisms to account for differential cognitive abilities.

Correlational approaches provide some evidence for a relationship between androgen,
visuo-spatial abilities, and verbal abilities. In 117 healthy young men, serum testosterone
correlated positively with measures of spatial ability and field dependence-independence
(104). By contrast, a significant negative correlation was found between testosterone and
measures of verbal production. Cognitive function was determined by five spatial and six
verbal ipsative test scores. Another study examined the relationship between serum
testosterone, estradiol and ACTH levels, and spatial, verbal, and musical abilities *(105)*.
For the 26 men (mean age 19 yr) and 25 women (mean age 18.7 yr) testosterone and
estradiol levels were not significantly related to any of the cognitive or musical tests;
however, the testosterone/estradiol ratio was significantly negatively correlated with
spatial tests, and ACTH was significantly positively correlated with spatial and musical
tests. Correlations were stronger for women than men. Other cognitive abilities assessed
in 59 men also reportedly correlate with bioavailable testosterone, including: the Folstein
Mini Mental Status Examination, animal naming, Rey visual design learning test and Rey
auditory verbal learning test *(106)*.

Although some researchers report simple correlations, others find a more complex relationship. For example, cognitive performance was explored in normal men and women grouped according to relatively high or low salivary testosterone concentrations *(107)*. Men with lower salivary testosterone performed better than other groups on spatial-mathematical tasks. Women with higher testosterone scored higher than low-testosterone women on these same measures. Testosterone concentration did not significantly relate to scores on tests that usually favor women. The authors suggest a nonlinear relationship exists between testosterone and spatial ability. Other data support possible nonlinearity. In two studies, moderate levels of androgens were associated with better spatial performance *(108,109)*.

Beyond crossectional descriptive and correlational investigations, several reports describe cognitive changes associated with testosterone administration. Eight treated hypogonadal men tended to have better picture identification ability than 12 untreated hypogonadal men *(110)*. Superior verbal fluency and verbal memory occurred when patients were hypogonadal compared to when they were treated.

In the study of transsexuals previously mentioned with reference to aggression *(81)*, the contribution of sex hormones to cognitive functioning also was assessed. Administering androgens to females was associated with increased spatial ability performance and a deterioration in verbal fluency. Male to female hormone therapy improved verbal fluency, suggesting that sex hormones quickly and directly influence sex-specific cognitive abilities. Finally, in a placebo-controlled study, WAIS block design subtest scores in elderly men (not selected for hypogonadism) improved after testosterone administration compared to placebo *(111)*.

These data, when considered together, suggest a CNS role of testosterone facilitating visual-spatial abilities and decreasing verbal abilities. Although an oversimplification, the results provides a fascinating clue about central actions of testosterone. It also establishes a basis for exploring testosterone replacement as a means to improve cognitive function, as well as mood, in men with primary or secondary hypogonadism.

CONCLUSIONS

As our knowledge base expands, it is becoming apparent that testosterone influences both central and peripheral nervous system mechanisms. Although a role for testosterone in sexual behavior has long been known, its relationship with aggression, mood, and cognition are being uncovered. Some simple notions require modification based on systematic experimentation (for example, testosterone's role in aggression). The availability of clinical paradigms, most notably androgen replacement in hypogonadal men, provide an opportunity to observe and measure changes as the hormonal levels are therapeutically normalized. We see not only self-reported increases in the level of sexual desire but also objective improvements in erectile capability indexed using SREs. Emotion and learned behavior have long been known to modulate human sexual response. Correlational and some experimental studies find mood and specific cognitive abilities affected by testosterone. Experimental models involving surgical castration in animals and androgen blockade in humans open additional avenues to explore how changes in testosterone alter sexual function, mood, and intellect. Finally, AR localization and its relationship with other neurotransmitter systems add important pieces to the complex puzzle of androgenic influence on human sexuality.

REFERENCES

1. Newerla GJ. The history of the discovery and isolation of the male hormone. NEJM 1943;228(2):39–47.
2. Hammond TE. The function of the testes after puberty. Br J Urol 1993;6:128–141.
3. Breedlove SM. Sexual dimorphism in the vertebrate nervous system. J Neurosci 1992;12:4133–4142.
4. McEwen BS. Our changing ideas about steroid effects on an ever-changing brain. Sem Neurosci 1991;3:497–507.
5. Michael RP, Rees HD, Gonsall RW. Sites in the male primate brain at which testosterone acts as an androgen. Brain Res 1989;502:11–20.
6. Kritzer MF. Selective colocalization of immunoreactivity for intracellular gonadal hormone receptors and tyrosine hydroxylase in the ventral tegmental area, substantia nigra, and retrorubral fields in the rat. J Comp Neurol 1997;379 (2):247–260.
7. Herbison AE. Neurochemical identity of neurones expressing oestrogen and androgen receptors in sheep hypothalamus. J Reprod Fertil (Supp) 1995;49:271–283.
8. McGinnis MY, Williams GW, Lumia AR. Inhibition of male sex behavior by androgen receptor blockade in preoptic area or hypothalamus, but not amygdala or septum. Physiol Behav 1996;60(3):783–789.
9. Heaton JPW, Varrin SJ. Effects of castration and exogenous testosterone supplementation in an animal model of penile erection. J Urol 1994;151:797–800.
10. Yamada K, Furukawa T. Direct evidence for involvement of dopaminergic inhibition and cholinergic activation in yawning. Psychopharmacology 1980;67:39.
11. Pehek E, Thompson J, Eaton R, Bazzett T, Hull E. Apomorphine and haloperidol, but not domeridone, affect penile reflexes in rats. Pharmacol Biochem Behav 1988;31:201.
12. Argiolas A, Melis MR, Mauri A, Gessa GL. Paraventricular nucleus lesion prevents yawning and penile erection induced by apomorphine and oxytocin but not by ACTH in rats. Brain Res 1987;421 (1-2):349–352.
13. Melis MR, Argiolas A, Gessa GL. Apomorphine-induced penile erection and yawning: site of action in brain. Brain Res 1987;415(1):98–104.
14. MacLean PD, Ploog DW. Cerebral representation of penile erections. J Neurophysiol 1962;25:29–55.
15. MacLean PD, Denniston RH, Dua S. Further studies on cerebral representation of penile erection: caudal thalamus, midbrain, and pons. J Neurophysiol 1963.26:274–293.
16. Malsbury CW. Facilitation of male rat copulatory behaviour by electrical stimulation of the medial preoptic area. Physiol Behav 1971;7:707–805.
17. Perachio AA, Marr LD, Alexander M. Sexual behavior in male rhesus monkeys elicited by electrical stimulation of preoptic and hypothalamic areas. Brain Res 1979;177:127–44.
18. Robinson BW, Mishkin M. Penile erections evoked by forebrain structures in macaca mulatta. Arch Neurol 1968;19:184–189.
19. Slimp JC, Hart BL, Goy RW. Heterosexual, autosexual and social behavior of adult male rhesus monkeys with medial preoptic-anterior hypothalamic lesions. Brain Res 1978;142:105–122.
20. Davidson JM. Hormones and sexual behavior in the male. Hospital Practice, 1975, pp. 126.
21. Hart BL. Testosterone regulation of sexual reflexes in spinal male rats. Science 1967;155:1283,1284.
22. Hart BL, Wallach SJR, Melese-D'Hospital PY. Differences in responsiveness to testosterone of penile reflexes and copulatory behavior of male rats. Hormones Behav 1983;17:274–283.
23. Melvin JE, Hamil RW. Gonadal hormone regulation of neurotransmitter synthesizing enzymes in the developing hypogastric ganglion. Brain Res 1986;383:38.
24. Melvin JE, Hamill RW. The major pelvic ganglion: androgen control of postnatal development. J Neurosci 1987;7(6):1607–1612.
25. Mills TM, Wiedmeier VT, Stopper VS. Androgen maintenance of erectile function in the rat penis. Biol Reprod 1992;46:342–348.
26. Giuliano F, Rampin O, Schirart A, Jardin A, Rousseau J-P. Autonomic control of penile erection: modulation by testosterone in the rat. J Neuroendocrinol 19935:677–683.
27. Schirar A, Bonnefond C, Meusnier C, Devinoy E. Androgens modulate nitric oxide synthase messenger ribonucleic acid expression in neurons of the major pelvic ganglion in the rat. Endocrinol 1997; 138(8):3093–3102.
28. Schirar A, Chang C, Rousseau JP. Localization of androgen receptor in nitric oxide synthase- and vasoactive intestinal peptide- containing neurons of the major pelvic ganglion innervating the rat penis. J Neuroendocrinol 1997;5:677.
29. Mills TM, Stopper VS, Wiedmeier VT. Effects of castration and androgen replacement on the hemodynamics of penile erection in the rat. Biol Reproduction 1994;51:234–238.

30. Lugg JA, Rajfer J, Gonzalez-Cadavid NF. Dihydrotestosterone is the active androgen in the maintenance of nitric oxide-mediated penile erection in the rat. Endocrinol 1995;36(4):1495–1501.

31. Reilly CM, Zamorano P, Stopper VS, Mills TM. Androgenic regulation of NO availability in rat penile erection. J Androl 1997;18(2):110–115.

32. Chamness SL, Ricker DD, Crone JK, Dembeck CL, Maguire MP, Burnett AL, Chang TSK. The effect of androgen on nitric oxide synthase in male reproductive tract of the rat. Fertil Steril 1995;63:1101–1107.

33. Zvara P, Sioufi R, Schipper HM, Begin LR, Brock GB. Nitric oxide mediated erectile activity is a testosterone dependent event: a rat erection model. Int J Impotence Res 1995;7:209–219.

34. Lugg J, Ng C, Rajfer J, Gonzalez-Cadavid NF. Cavernosal nerve stimulation in the rat reverses castration-induced decrease in penile NOS activity. Am J Physiol 1996;271:E354–61.

35. Rajfer J, Namkung PC, Petra PH. Identification, partial characterization and age-related changes of a cytoplasmic androgen receptor in the rat penis. J Steroid Biochem 1980;13:1489.

36. Takane KK, George FW, Wilson JD. Androgen receptor of rat penis is downregulated by androgen. Am J Physiol 1990;258:E46–E50.

37. Nonomura K, Sakakibara N, Demura T, Mori T, Koyanagi T. Androgen binding activity in the spongy tissue of mammalian penis. J Urol 1990;144:152.

38. Lin M-C, Rajfer J, Swerdloff RS, Gonzalez-Cadavid NF. Testosterone down-regulates the levels of androgen receptor mRNA in smooth muscle cells from the rat corpora cavernosa via aromatization to estrogens. J Steroid Biochem Molec Biol 1993;45(5):333–343.

39. Breedlove SM, Arnold AP. Hormone accumulation in a sexually dimorphic motor nucleus of the rat spinal cord. Science 1980;210:564–566.

40. Leipheimer RE, Sachs BD. Relative androgen sensitivity of the vascular and striated-muscle systems regulating penile erection in rats. Physiol Behav 1993;54:1085–1090.

41. Max SR, Toop J. Androgens enhance in vivo 2-deoxyglucose uptake by rat striated muscle. Endocrinol 1983;113(1):119–126.

42. Reynolds CF, Frank E, Thase ME, Houck PR, Jennings R, Howell JR, Lilienfeld SO, Kupfer DJ. Assessment of sexual functioning in depressed, impotent, and healthy men: factor analysis of a brief sexual function questionnaire for men. Psychiatry Res 1988;24:231–250.

43. Derogatis LR, Melisanatos N. The DSFI: a multidimensional measure of sexual functioning. J Sex Marital Therapy 1979;5:244.

44. Geisser ME, Jefferson TW, Spevak M, Boaz T, Thomas RG, Murray FT. Reliability and validity of the Florida Sexual History Questionnaire. J Clin Psychology 1991;47(4):519–528.

45. Hirshkowitz M, Moore CA, Karacan I. NPT/Rigidometry. In: Kirby RS, Carson C, Webster GD, eds. Impotence: Diagnosis and Management of Male Erectile Dysfunction. Oxford, UK. Butterworth-Heinemann, 1991, pp. 62–71.

46. Ware JC, Hirshkowitz M. Monitoring penile erections during sleep. In: Kryger MH, Roth T, Dement WC, eds. Principles and Practice of Sleep Medicine. W. B. Saunders, Philadelphia, 1994, pp. 967–977.

47. Ware JC, Hirshkowitz M, Thornby J, Salis P, Karacan I. Sleep-related erections: absence of change following presleep sexual arousal. J Psychosom Res 1997;42:547–553.

48. Karacan I, Williams RL, Thornby JI, et al. Sleep-related penile tumescence as a function of age. Am J Psychiatry 1975;132:932–937.

49. Ware JC, Hirshkowitz M. Characteristics of penile erections during sleep recorded from normal subjects. J Clin Neurophysiol 1992;9:78–87.

49a. Reynolds CF, Thase ME, Jennings JR, et al. Nocturnal penile tumescence in healthy 20- to 59-year olds: a revisit. Sleep 1989;12:368–73.

50. Schiavi RC, White D, Mandeli J, Schreiner-Engel P. Hormones and nocturnal penile tumescence in healthy aging men. Arch Sex Behav 1993;22:207–215.

51. Takahashi Y, Kipnis DM, Daughaday WH. Growth hormone secretion during sleep. J Clin Invest 1968;47:2079.

52. Evans JI, MacLean AW, Ismail AAA, Love D. Concentration of plasma testosterone in normal men during sleep. Nature 1971;229:261–262.

53. Judd HL, Parker DC, Rakoff JS, Hopper BR, Yen SSC. Elucidation of mechanism(s) of the nocturnal rise of testosterone in men. J Clin Endocrinol Metab 1973;38:134.

54. Miyatake A, Morimoto Y, Oishi T, Hanasaki N, Sugita Y, Iijima S, Teshima Y, Hishikawa Y, Yamamura Y. Circadian rhythm of serum tesosterone and its relation to sleep: comparison with the variation in serum luteinizing hormone, prolactin, and cortisol in normal men. J Clin Endocrinol 1980;51:1365–1371.

55. Roffwarg HP, Sachar EJ, Halpern F, Hellman L. Plasma testosterone and sleep: relationship to sleep stage variables. Psychosom Med 1982;44:73–84.

56. Davidson JM, Camargo CA, Smith ER. Effects of androgen on sexual behavior in hypogonadal men. J Clin Endocrinol Metab 1979;48:955.

57. Bancroft J, Wu FCW. Changes in erectile responsiveness during androgen replacement therapy. Arch Sex Behav 1983;12(1):59–663.

58. Kwan M, Greenleaf WJ, Mann J, Crapo L, Davidson JM. The nature of androgen action on male sexuality: A combined laboratory-self-report study on hypogonadal men. Clin Endocrinol Metab 1983;57(3):557–562.

59. Carani C, Granata J, Bancroft P, Marrama R. The effects of testosterone replacement on nocturnal penile tumescence and rigidity and erectile response to visual erotic stimuli in hypogonadal men. Psychoneuroendocrinology 1995;20(7):743–753.

60. Burris AS, Banks SM, Carter CS, Davidson JM, Sherins RJ. A long-term, prospective study of the physiologic and behavioral effects of hormone replacement in untreated hypogonadal men. J Androl 1992;13(4):297–304.

61. Clopper RR, Voorhess ML, MacGillivray MH, Lee PA, Mills B. Psychosexual behavior in hypopituitary men: a controlled comparison of gonadotropin and testosterone replacement. Psychoneuroendocrinol 1993;18(2):149–161.

62. Bhasin S, Storer TW, Berman N, Callegari C, Clevenger B, Phillips J, Bunnell TJ, Tricker R, Shirazi A, Casaburi R. The effects of suprophysiologic doses of testosterone on muscle size and strength in normal men. New Engl J Med 1996;335:1.

63. Buena F, Swerdloff RS, Steiner BS, Lutchmansingh P, Peterson MA, Pandian MR, Galmarini M, Bhasin S. Sexual function does not change when serum testosterone levels are pharmacologically varied within the normal male range. Fertil Steril 1993;59:1118–1123.

64. Carani C, Scuteri A, Marrama R, Bancroft J. Brief Report: The effects of testosterone administration and visual erotic stimuli on nocturnal penile tumescence in normal men. Hormones Behav 1990;24:435–441.

65. O'Carroll R, Bancroft J. Testosterone therapy for low sexual interest and erectile dysfunction in men: a controlled study. Br J Psychiatry 1984;145:146–151.

66. Imperato-McGinley J, Peterson RE, Gautier T, Sturla E. Androgens and the evolution of male-gender identity among male pseudohermaphrodites with 5α-reductase deficiency. N Engl J Med 1979;300:1233–1237.

67. Gormley GJ, Stoner E, Bruskewitz RC, Imperato-McGinley J, Walsh PC, McConnell JD, Andriole GL, Geller J, Bracken BR, Tenover JS, et al. The effect of finasteride in men with benign prostatic hyperplasia. The Finasteride Study Group. New Engl J Med 1992;327:1185–1191.

68. Cunningham GR, Hirshkowitz M. Inhibition of steroid 5α-reductase with finasteride:sleep-related erections, potency, and libido in healthy men. J Clin Endocrinol Metab 1995;80(6):1934–1940.

69. Bergman B, Damber JE, Littbrand B. Sexual function in prostatic cancer patients treated with radiotherapy, orchiectomy or oestrogens. Br J Urol 1984;56(1):64–69.

70. Radlmaier A, Eickenberg HU, Fletcher MS, Fourcade RO, Reis Santos JM, van Aubel Olg JM, Bono AV. Estrogen reduction by aromatase inhibition for benign prostatic hyperplasia: results of a double-blind, placebo-controlled, randomized clinical trial using two doses of the aromatase-inhibitor atamestane. Prostate 1996;29:199–208.

71. Bagatell CJ, Heiman JR, Rivier JE, Bremner WJ. Effects of endogenous testosterone and estradiol on sexual behavior in normal young men. J Clin Endocrinol Metab 1994;7:711–716.

72. Greenstein A, Plymate SR, Katz PG. Visually stimulated erection in castrated men. J Urol 1995;153:650–652.

73. Hirshkowitz M, Moore, CA, O'Connor S, Bellamy M, Cunningham GR. Androgen and sleep-related erections. J Psychosom Res 1997;42:541–546.

74. Heim N, Hursch CJ. Castration for sex offenders: treatment or punishment? A review and critique of recent European literature. Arch Sex Beh 1979;8(3):281–304.

75. Heim N. Sexual behavior of castrated sex offenders. Arch Sex Behav 1981;10(1):11–19.

76. Bradford JMW, Pawlak A. Double-blind crossover study of cyproterone acetate in the treatment of the paraphilias. Arch Sex Behav 1993;22:383–402.

77. Cooper AJ. A placebo controlled trial of the antiandrogen cyproterone acetate in deviant hypersexuality. Comp Psychiatr 1981;22:458.

78. Cooper AJ, Sandhu S, Losztyn S, Cernovsky Z. A double-blind placebo controlled trial of medroxyprogesterone acetate and cyproterone acetate with seven pedophiles. Can J Psychiatr 1992;37:687–693.

79. Wincze JP, Bansal S, Malamud M. Effects of medroxyprogesterone on subjective arousal, arousal to erotic stimulation, and nocturnal penile tumescence in male sex offenders. Arch Sex Behav 1986;15:293–305.

80. Cooper AJ, Losztyn S, Russell NC, Cernovsky Z. Medroxyprogesterone acetate, nocturnal penile tumescence, laboratory arousal, and sexual acting out in a male with schizophrenia. Arch Sex Behav 1990;19:361.

81. Van Goozen SH, Cohen-Kettenis PT, Gooren LJ, Frijda NH, Van de Poll, NE. Gender differences in behaviour: activating effects of cross-sex hormones. Psychoneuroendocrinology 1995;20(4):343–363.

82. Tricker R, Casaburi R, Storer TW, Clevenger B, Berman N, Shirazi A, Bhasin S. The effects of supraphysiological doses of testosterone on angry behavior in healthy eugonadal men: a clinical research center study. J Clin Endocrinol Metab 1996;81(10):3754–3758.

83. Finkelstein JW, Susman EJ, Chinchilli VM, Kunselman SJ, D'Arcangelo MR, Schwab J, Demers LM, Liben LS, Lookingbill G, Kulin HE. Estrogen or testosterone increases self-reported aggressive behaviors in hypogonadal adolescents. J Clin Endocrinol Metab 1997;82:2433–2438.

84. Winslow JT, Miczek KA. Androgen dependency of alcohol effects on aggressive behavior: a seasonal rhythm in high-ranking squirrel monkeys. Psycholpharmacol 1988;95:92–98.

85. Anderson RA, Bancroft J, Wu FCW. The effects of exogenous testosterone on sexuality and mood of normal men. J Clin Endocrinol Metab 1992;75:1503–1507.

86. O'Carroll R, Shapiro C, Bancroft J. Androgens, behavior and nocturnal erection in hypogonadal men: the effects of varying the replacement dose. Clini Endocrinol 1985;23:527–538.

87. Wang C, Alexander G, Berman N, Salehian B, Davidson T, McDonald V, Steiner B, Hull L, Callegari C, Swerdloff RS. Testosterone replacement therapy improves mood in hypogonadal men: a clinical research center study. J Clin Endocrinol Metab 1996;81(10):3578–3583.

88. Cunningham GR, Snyder PJ, Atkinson LE. Testosterone transdermal delivery system. In: Bhasin S, Gabelnick HL, Spieler JM, Swerdloff RS, Wang C, Kelly C, eds. Pharmacology, Biology, and Clinical Applications of Androgen. Wiley-Liss, New York, 1996, pp. 437–447.

89. Wu FCW, Bancroft J, Davidson DW, Nicol K. The behavioural effects of testosterone undecanoate in adult men with Klinefelter's syndrome: a controlled study. Clin Endocrinol 1982;16:489–497.

90. Nielsen FH, Hunt CD, Mullen LM, Hunt JR. Effect of dietary boron on mineral, estrogen, and testosterone metabolism in postmenopausal women. FASEB J 1987;1(5):394–397.

91. Rubin RT, Poland RE, Lesser IM. Neuroendocrine aspects of primary endogenous depression VIII. Pituitary-gonadal axis activity in male patients and matched control subjects. Psychoneuroendocrinology 1989;14(3):217–229.

92. Vogel W, Klaiber EL, Broverman DM. roles of the gonadal seroid hormones in psychiatric depression in men and women. Prog Neuropsychopharmacol 1978;2:487–503.

93. Ettigi PG, Brown GM. Psychoendocrine correlates in affective disorder. In: Muller EE, Agnoli A, eds. Neuroendocrine Correlates in Neurology and Psychiatry. Elsevier, Amsterdam, 1979, pp. 225–238.

94. Mason JW, Giller EL, Kosten TR. Serum testosterone differences between patients with schizophrenia and those with affective disorder. Biol Psychiatry 1988;23:357–366.

95. Rubin RT, Poland RE. Pituitary-adrenocortical and pituitary-gonadal function in affective disorder. In Brown GM, Koslow SH, Reichlin S, eds. Neuroendocrinology and Psychiatric Disorder. Raven Press, New York, 1984, pp. 151–164.

96. Levitt AJ, Joffe RT. Total and free testosterone in depressed men. Acta Psychiatrica Scandinavica 1988;77(3):346–348.

97. Unden F, Ljunggren JG, Beck-Friis J, Kjellman BF, Wetterberg L. Hypothalamic-pituitary-gonadal axis in major depressive disorders. Acta Psychiatr Scand 1988;78:138–146.

98. Davies RH, Harris B, Thomas DR, Cook N, Read G, Riad-Fahmy D. Salivary testosterone levels and major depressive illness in men. Br J Psychiatry 1992;161:629–632.

99. Yesavage JA, Davidson J, Widrow L, Berger PA. Plasma testosterone levels, depression, sexuality, and age. Biol Psychiatry 1985;20(2):222–225.

100. Altschule MD, Tillotson KJ. The use of testosterone in the treatment of depression. New Engl J Med 1948;239:1036–1038.

101. Vogel W, Klaiber EL, Broverman DM. A comparison of the antidepressant effects of a synthetic androgen (mesterolone) and amitriptyline in depressed men. J Clin Psychiatry 1985;46:6–8.

102. Morales AJ, Nolan JJ, Nelson JC, Yen SS. Effects of replacement dose of dehydroepiandrosterone in men and women of advancing age. J Clin Endocrinol Metab 1994;78:1360–1367.

103. Snow WG, Weinstock J. Sex differences among non-brain damaged adults on the Wecshler Adult Intelligence Scales: a review of the literature. J Clin Exp Neuropsychol 1990;12:873–886.

104. Christiansen K, Knussmann R. Sex hormones and cognitive functioning in men. Neuropsychobiology 1987;18(1):27–36.

105. Hassler M, Gupta D, Wollmann H. Testosterone, estradiol, ACTH and musical, spatial and verbal performance. Int J Neurosci 1992;65(1-4):45–60.

106. Morley JE, Flood JF, Kaiser FE, Jensen JM, Farr SA. Of mice and men: evidence that testosterone is related to age-related impairment of memory. Endocrine Society 76th Annual Meeting 1994;Abst #1523:581.

107. Gouchie C, Kimura D. The relationship between testosterone levels and cognitive ability patterns. Psychoneuroendocrinology 1991;16(4):323–334.

108. Shut VJ, Pellegrino JW, Hubert L, Reynolds RW. The relationship between androgen levels and human spatial abilities. Bull Psychonom Soc 1983;21:465–468.

109. Moffat SD, Hampson E. A curvilinear relationship between testosterone and spatial cognition in humans: possible influence of hand preference. Psychoneuroendocrinology 1996;21:323–337.

110. Rich JB, Brandt J, Lesh K, Dobs AS. The effect of testosterone on cognition in hypogonadal men. 1996 ICE the endocrine society page 734 #OR58–56.

111. Janowsky JS, Oviatt SK, Orwoll ES. Testosterone influences spatial cognition in older men. Behav Neurosci 1994;108(2):325–332.

112. Luisi M, Franchi F. Double-blind group comparative study of testosterone undecanoate and mesterolone in hypogonadal male patients. J Endocrinol Invest 1980;3:305–308.

113. Skakkebaek NE, Bancroft J, Davidson DW, Warner P. Androgen replacement with oral testosterone undecanoate in hypogonadal men:a double blind controlled study. Clin Endocrinol 1981;14:49–61.

114. Cunningham GR, Hirshkowitz M, Korenman SG, Karacan I. Testosterone replacement therapy and sleep-related erections in hypogonadal men. J Clin Endocrinol Metab 1990;70:792–797.

115. Arver S, Dobs AS, Meikle AW, Allen RP, Sanders SW, Mazer NA. Improvement of sexual function in testosterone deficient men treated for 1 year with a permeation enhanced testosterone transdermal system. J Urol 1996;155:1604–1608.

18 Testosterone and the Older Man

J. Lisa Tenover, MD, PhD

Contents

INTRODUCTION

Why Consider Androgen Therapy in the Older Man?

Testosterone Levels in Older Men

Although sex hormone replacement therapy (HRT) for postmenopausal women has been a standard practice for a number of years, the idea that an older man might be sex hormone deficient and could benefit from replacement therapy has only gained significant medical interest within the past decade. Lack of data on the prevalence of "androgen deficiency" in the older man is one of the reasons that the idea of HRT for this age group has been so slow in reaching the medical research community and the clinician. Currently, there is much more media hype about the purported benefits of androgen replacement therapy in the older man than there is good scientific data to support the media claims.

That serum testosterone, but not dihydrotestosterone, levels decline with normal aging in men has been shown in a number of studies *(1)*, but the prevalence of true hypogonadism in the older male population is unclear. One of the impediments in this area is how to define "testosterone deficiency," and this is a result of several factors. First, there seems to be no straightforward target organ change, physiological finding, or symptom that can be used to define "deficiency." Second, unlike the thyroid hormone axis, where elevated thyroid stimulating hormone levels can assist in defining an older person as thyroid deficient, serum gonadotropin levels are not helpful in defining older men as "testosterone deficient." Many older men, even with quite low serum testosterone levels, will have serum gonadotropin levels within the normal range, making them relatively hypogonadotropic.

From: *Contemporary Endocrinology: Hormone Replacement Therapy*
Edited by: A. W. Meikle © Humana Press Inc., Totowa, NJ

Table 1
Prevalence Data on Testosterone "Deficiency" in Older Males

Study	Ages (yr)	Study pop	Total testosterone (ng/dL)	Percent of Population	
A	50–87	817	<300	11.4%	
B	20–100	300	<317	1%	(20–40 yr)
				7%	(40–60 yr)
				22%	(60–80 yr)
				36%	(80–100 yr)
C	60–83	379	<350	36%	
			<300	19%	
			<250	8%	

A, Lunglmayr (rural Austria); B,Vermeulen and Kaufman (Belgium); C, Tenover (Seattle WA and Atlanta GA).

Lacking a firm guideline, most investigators in the area of HRT in the aging male have used the lower range of normal for the young adult male (two standard deviations below the mean) in serum levels of total testosterone or testosterone not bound to sex hormone binding globulin (non-SHBG-bound testosterone) to define the level below which an older man might be considered "testosterone deficient." Using this type of definition, the prevalence of "testosterone deficiency" still varies greatly and depends on the characteristics of the population being assessed. For example, very healthy older men generally will have higher serum testosterone levels than older men with chronic illnesses. Similarly, most of the data on serum testosterone levels with age have come from studies of Caucasian men of Western European descent. There are no good age-related data on Asian men or men of African-American descent. Some data from ethnic groups found predominantly in eastern Europe suggest that men in certain areas do not show a decline in serum testosterone levels with age. Table 1 lists some reported estimated prevalences of testosterone deficiency in older men.

Although total testosterone, free testosterone, and non-SHBG-bound testosterone all decline with age, because of concomitant increases in SHBG with age, it is the non-SHBG-bound testosterone that declines most dramatically. Some older men will have normal serum total testosterone levels, but below-normal levels of non-SHBG-bound testosterone. However, which measurement of testosterone should be used in defining older men as testosterone deficient is unclear, because the circulating form of testosterone that is available to tissues may vary by target tissue. For example, data using the rat model suggest that non-SHBG-bound testosterone is the compartment of testosterone that is available to the brain, but there are also data to suggest that testosterone bound to SHBG may be available to the prostate (for review, see ref. 2).

Perhaps it may not be fruitful at this time to try to define if there is one serum assay measurement that can define an older man as being "testosterone deficient." Androgen target organ responses to testosterone replacement therapy in the older man may vary in their threshold response (for example, to restore libido may take a much lower serum testosterone level than improving bone density). Thus, until we learn more about target end organ responses to such replacement therapy in older men, it may be more important to select men based on those who have one or more specific androgen target organ deficiencies and who also have serum testosterone levels that are low enough that meaningful changes in testosterone can be made with physiological replacement therapy.

Testosterone levels decline in the older man for a number of reasons, including concomitant disease and medications. For example, in the Massachusetts Male Aging Study, low serum testosterone levels were seen most frequently in men with diabetes mellitus and cardiovascular disease *(3)*. Medications such as cimetidine, ketoconazole, and glucocorticoids, have all been reported to lead to a decrease in serum testosterone. The presence of sleep apnea *(4)* or severe obesity also are associated with low testosterone levels.

In healthy normal weight older men who are nonsmokers and on no medications, the mechanism of testosterone decline with age has several components. First, it is the decline in testosterone production that leads to the overall serum level decline; testosterone metabolism actually slows with normal male aging. The largest contributor to the decline in testosterone production with age is the testis itself, which shows blunted testosterone production even when maximally stimulated with luteinizing hormone (LH). The hypothalamus also plays a role in that there is an increased sensitivity to sex steroid negative feedback with age. The ratio of bioactive to immunoreactive gonadotropins made by the pituitary may also decline somewhat with age, but overall this component as a contributor to the decline in testosterone production is small.

Androgen Target Organ Changes with Normal Aging

In young adult males, androgens are known to have many important physiologic actions, including effects on muscle, bone, central nervous system (CNS), prostate, bone marrow, and sexual function. Declining lean body mass and strength, loss of stamina, declining bone mineral density, decreased libido and potency, a slight lowering of red blood cell mass, and a decline in general sense of well being often are associated with male aging.

Both cross-sectional and longitudinal studies have shown that normal male aging is accompanied by an increase in upper and central body fat, a decrease in muscle tissue mass, and a decrease in some aspects of muscle strength *(5,6)*. In healthy older people, there is a strong correlation between muscle mass and muscle strength, but the causes of the decline in muscle mass and strength with age are unknown and probably multifactorial. Androgens have long been noted for their anabolic effects, and physiological replacement of testosterone to hypogonadal young men or supraphysiological treatment of eugonadal young adult men can result in increases in lean body mass, muscle size, and strength *(7,8)*.

Osteoporosis is becoming a larger clinical problem as the average life span of men increases *(9)*. Osteoporosis is a risk factor for hip fracture in the elderly, a major cause of morbidity and mortality. After age 60 yr, hip fracture rates in men increase dramatically, doubling each decade, and by age 80 yr, proximal femur fracture rates in white men approach 1.3% per man/year. In both cross-sectional and longitudinal studies healthy men have been shown to lose bone mass with age. Typical bone loss rates for vertebral bone in men, ages 30–80 yr, have been 1.2%/yr in cross-sectional studies and just over 2%/yr in longitudinal studies. Cortical bone is loss less rapidly, with reported rates varying from 0.2–1%/yr. "Hypogonadism" is considered a cause of male osteoporosis, and elderly men who are hypogonadal are at increased risk for minimal trauma hip fracture.

Various measures of sexual function seem to change as men age, including a decline in orgasmic frequency, an increase in erectile dysfunction, and a decline in the quality and quantity of sexual thoughts and enjoyment. Data to support a relationship between andro-gen levels and the decline in many aspects of sexual function with age are scarce and difficult to obtain. Measurements of the direct effects of androgens on erectile function in humans is difficult, because of the need to separate central effects (libido) from periph-eral effects (direct action on penis, blood vessels and nerves) and because there are many etiologies for impotence. Each man might have several causes for his erectile dysfunc-tion. The role of testosterone in the maintenance of libido is more secure.

Testosterone stimulates renal production of erythropoietin and has a direct effect on erythropoietic stem cells; androgen receptors are found in cultured erythroblasts. Andro-gens are known to increase reticulocyte counts, hemoglobin levels, and bone marrow erythropoietic activity in mammals, whereas castration leads to a decline in these param-eters. Studies in which hypogonadal young men are replaced with testosterone have demonstrated an increase in blood cell mass and hemoglobin levels. Healthy older men tend to have similar or slightly lower hemoglobin and hematocrit levels compared with normal young adult men.

Benign prostatic hyperplasia (BPH) and prostate cancer are common in aging men and both are, at some time in their progress, androgen dependent. The role of androgens in the initiation of preclinical prostate cancer is not known, and there are no data to indicate whether androgens enhance the progression of preclinical to clinical cancer. The patho-genesis of BPH is still largely uncertain, but there is increasing evidence that androgens, especially dihydrotestosterone, are necessary for the benign growth. Laboratory studies have suggested that prostatic-specific antigen (PSA) expression is under direct hormonal control via the androgen receptor. Androgen deprivation can lead to a reduction in serum PSA levels, decline in prostate size, and improvement of symptoms in BPH, and an initial regression of tumor in prostate cancer.

Overview of Androgen Replacement Trials in Older Men

When considering testosterone replacement therapy in older men, it is important to know the various potential benefits, the persons for whom those benefits are most likely to occur, the various potential risks, and the relative risk/benefit ratio. Unfortunately, the data available to date are limited on the beneficial and detrimental effects of androgen replacement in older men; consequently, therapeutic decisions are by necessity being made without this information. Androgen therapy trials reported in older men often involve small numbers of participants, short terms of treatment (the longest reported is 4 yr, most are 6 mo or less), are not always placebo controlled or double-blinded, use various modes of androgen replacement therapy, and often are reported in abstract form only. Nonetheless, by looking at the various study results in terms of target organ out-comes, it is possible to at least get an idea of what types of therapy benefits and risks might be anticipated. Table 2 gives a list of the potential benefits and risks of testosterone replacement therapy in the older man.

Muscle/Strength

To date, there have been at least five trials of testosterone supplementation in older men that have evaluated body composition changes; four of these trials, along with an additional three trials, have evaluated some aspect of strength (10–16). Table 3 is a summary of the body composition changes that have occurred with such therapy in these trials. Consistently, there is some change in body composition with testosterone therapy, either a

Table 2
Potential Benefits and Risks of Testosterone Replacement Therapy in Older Men

Benefits
    Maintenance or improvement in bone density
    Improvement in body composition
        Increased muscle mass
        Decreased fat mass
    Improvement in strength and stamina
    Improvement in libido and other aspects of sexual function
    Improvement in mood
Risks
    Liver toxicity
    Fluid retention
    Gynecomastia
    Exacerbation of sleep apnea
    Elevation of red blood cell mass
    Exacerbation of benign or malignant prostate disease
    Increase in cardiovascular disease

Table 3
Testosterone Supplementation and Body Composition in Older Men

Length of treatment (mo)	Study pop	Measure modality	Body fat	Lean mass
			(trend and average percent change)	
3	13	Hydrostatic	N C	▲ (3.2%)
6	8	DEXA	▼ (6.4%)	▲ (4.9%)
9	31	Total K/CT	▼ (6.4%)	N C
18	29	Bioimped/CT	▼ (14%)	▲ (5.0%)
12	17	Bioimped	N C	—

▼, decreases; ▲, increases; N C, no change.

decline in body fat, an increase in lean body mass (mostly muscle mass), or both. In general, however, the changes seen in these studies, which involved only testosterone therapy without any other concomitant modality (such as exercise), were small. For the average older man, the overall clinical relevance of the magnitude of the changes seen is uncertain.

The studies have demonstrated consistent results in terms of changes in muscle strength with testosterone therapy in the older man. In six of the seven studies, muscle strength increased in the testosterone treated group. Four of the studies evaluated grip strength alone, while at least two of the studies looked at lower extremity strength.

Bone

There have been at least eight studies to date that have reported on the effects of testosterone therapy in older men with regard to either biochemical parameters of bone turnover or bone mineral density *(11,13,15,16)*. These studies have lasted from 3–36 mo, with the shorter term studies evaluating only bone turnover parameters. Some—but not all of the studies—enrolled older men who were obviously osteoporotic at baseline. Table 4

Table 4
Testosterone Therapy Effects on Bone in Older Men

Length of treatment (mo)	Study pop	Parameters of bone turnover		Bone density	
		Formation	Degradation	L-spine	Other
3	13	N C	▼	—	—
3	8	▲	—	—	—
12	4	—	—	▲	—
36	8	N C	N C	slowed ▼	—
18	29	▼	▼	▲	—
12	4	—	—	▲	▲
6	6	—	—	▲	—
7–14	6	▼	▼	—	—

▼, decrease; ▲, increase; N C, no change.

is a summary of those study findings. The data are somewhat variable, but overall are consistent in terms of the effect on increasing bone mineral density and slowing bone degradation. Because testosterone is converted to estradiol in vivo, and because older men who have testosterone replacement often show a proportional increase in serum estradiol levels, it is unclear if the effect of testosterone therapy on bone is a direct result of testosterone itself, or a result of the increased estradiol levels. From the point of view of the use of testosterone as a therapy for prevention or treatment of osteoporosis in the older man, however, this argument is moot. What is important is whether older men can be maintained over longer periods of time than have been studied, and what level of testosterone replacement would be optimal to achieve the maximal benefit for bone.

Energy/Fatigue

Although an individual's energy or fatigue level may be difficult to quantitate (energy level is not exactly the same as endurance), the three double-blinded placebo-controlled studies of testosterone therapy in older men, which have queried their participants with regards to energy or fatigue level, have all reported an increase in energy and/or decline in fatigue level that was significantly better in those men treated with testosterone as compared to placebo.

Sexual Function

Studies that evaluate the effects of testosterone replacement on libido and erectile function in the older man are problematic, often both in study design and outcomes; however, there are some general statements that can be made. Regarding libido, the large majority of older men probably have androgen levels that are higher than the threshold required for behavioral activation, with libido usually being restored with relatively low levels of testosterone replacement. On the other hand, there is some suggestion that the threshold for androgen activation of sexual functioning may increase with age, and some men with low libido and "low-normal" serum testosterone levels have shown an improvement in libido with testosterone supplementation.

Studies have demonstrated that testosterone "deficiency" as a contributor to erectile dysfunction in the middle-aged and older man is uncommon. There are a few men, however, for whom testosterone replacement therapy might be beneficial in improving erectile dysfunction.

Mood

Several blinded placebo-controlled testosterone replacement studies in older men have evaluated effects on sense of well being or other aspects of mood. Although the study numbers are small, they have reported uniformly that the men in the testosterone group reported an improved or higher sense of well being compared to the group receiving placebo.

RISKS OF TESTOSTERONE THERAPY IN OLDER MEN

Table 4 also lists the most significant of the potential risks of testosterone therapy in the older man. Liver toxicity is on the list because of the potential of the oral methylated agents in this regard. However, the methylated testosterones are not recommended as a form of testosterone replacement for men, and none of the actual studies involving testosterone replacement in older men have used these oral agents. No problems with liver enzyme abnormalities or other evidence of liver toxicity have been reported with testosterone replacement in older men. Fluid retention is possible with testosterone replacement, especially within the first few months of therapy. For most men, however, the small amount of fluid retention is not harmful, and no cases of exacerbation of congestive heart failure or development of peripheral edema with androgen therapy have been reported.

Tender breasts or gynecomastia do occur in a small number of older men on testosterone therapy, perhaps because of the relatively greater increase in serum estradiol levels as compared to serum testosterone levels, seen in some older men on testosterone therapy. Not only has sleep apnea been shown to contribute to low serum testosterone levels, but testosterone supplementation has also been shown to exacerbate sleep apnea *(17)*. Because sleep apnea is most prevalent in the older male, screening for this condition, at least by history prior to testosterone supplementation, should not be overlooked.

Most studies of testosterone replacement in older men have shown a significant increase in red blood cell mass, hemoglobin levels, or hematocrit with the therapy. The increases reported are much larger than those usually seen when hypogonadal young adult men are given testosterone replacement; in some cases, it has been necessary with the older men to either terminate therapy or decrease the dose of testosterone given because of the development of polycythemia. Although the coexistence of sleep apnea and elevated body mass index seemed to have played a role in the development of polycythemia in certain of the men studied, this was clearly not the case for many of the men *(18,19)*. The method of testosterone replacement may affect the magnitude of the effect on hematopoeisis (Table 5).

Prostate

There have been at least sixteen testosterone replacement trials in men aged 40–89 yr of age, in which PSA or other prostate measurements were made. A composite analysis of these studies, which represent just over 500 man/yr of total observation (with longest individual follow-up being 4 yr), reveals that 13 of 16 studies reported absolutely no change in PSA with testosterone treatment, whereas the three other studies reported small

Table 5
Reported Increases in Hemoglobin and/or
Hematocrit Levels with Testosterone Replacement Therapy in Older Men

Testosterone patch	(Scrotal or transdermal)	1–3%
Testosterone enanthate	50 mg/2 wk	No change
Testosterone enanthate	100 mg/2 wk	5–12.5%
Testosterone enanthate	200 mg/2 wk	7–17%
Testosterone enanthate	300 mg/3 wk	Up to 19.6%

but statistically significant changes in PSA with therapy. All six of the studies, which additionally measured prostate size, maximum urine flow rates, or prostate symptom scores, reported no changes in these parameters with testosterone therapy. If PSA production is viewed as a general measure of prostate "activity," these results suggest that, at least in the short term, testosterone supplementation therapy does not appear to appreciably stimulate most older men's prostates. However, because both prostate cancer and BPH are diseases with long natural histories, and the experience to date with testosterone therapy in older men is limited to just over 500 man/yr of experience, little can, as yet, be said about the longer term effects of testosterone supplementation on the prostates of these older men *(20)*.

Cardiovascular System

Compared to premenopausal women, men have a higher incidence of cardiovascular disease and mortality. Whether this sexual dichotomy is owing largely to a protective effect of estrogens in women, or whether androgens also have a detrimental impact on the cardiovascular system in men, is not yet known. Epidemiological studies have demonstrated that low—rather than high—serum testosterone levels are associated with an increased risk of cardiovascular disease, but this does not address the question of changes in an individual's cardiovascular risk with testosterone therapy. Cardiovascular risk factors that may be affected by sex steroids include serum lipoprotein levels, vascular tone, platelet and red blood cell clotting parameters and atherogenesis. There are no data as of yet on the effects of testosterone therapy in older men on most of these parameters, except for serum lipoprotein levels. In general, parenteral testosterone therapy in older men leads to a decrease in total and low-density lipoprotein (LDL) cholesterol levels with no change–or a small decrease—in high-density lipoprotein (HDL) cholesterol levels. These changes in serum cholesterol levels with testosterone therapy are generally modest and the ultimate impact on cardiovascular risk is unknown.

HOW TO DECIDE IF AN OLDER MAN IS A CANDIDATE FOR TESTOSTERONE THERAPY

Given the paucity of sound clinical data on testosterone replacement in the older man, and the large amount of lay press that has popularized "testosterone" as a potential candidate for "superhormone" therapy to prevent or reverse the aging process in men, it is likely that men will come to a physician seeking replacement therapy rather than the physician suggesting that "testosterone deficiency" may be a problem. Sometimes men present to the physician with concerns about testosterone deficiency because their wives

Table 6
Symptoms, Signs or Conditions That Might Suggest
an Evaluation for "Testosterone Deficiency" in Older Men

Decreased libido
Loss of stamina
Increased irritability
Decreased "sense of well being"
Erectile dysfunction
Bilateral small testes
Breast enlargement
Significant obesity
Osteoporosis
Other evidence of pituitary hypofunction
Chronic illnesses
    Diabetes mellitus
    Chronic renal failure
    Liver disease
Chronic use of certain medications
    Ketoconazole
    Glucocorticoids
    Cimetidine

or significant others have urged them to do so. Among the symptoms that commonly lead older men to seek evaluation for androgen therapy, decreased libido, erectile dysfunction, loss of stamina, increased irritability, and decreased sense of well being are among the most common (Table 6). Many of these symptoms are vague and could be the result of a number of medical and psychiatric problems. This requires an astute clinician to rule out other possible causes prior to evaluation for possible testosterone replacement therapy. Other symptoms or findings that may guide a physician to evaluate an older man's androgen status include evidence of other areas of pituitary deficiency, the presence of osteopenia, gynecomastia, significant obesity, or the presence of certain chronic illnesses (Table 6).

In terms of the medical and psychiatric history, it is important to gather information in those areas where androgen replacement may present a potential risk. Pre-existing sleep apnea, clinically significant symptoms of BPH, family and personal history for prostate cancer, significant cardiovascular disease history, and/or history of elevated hemoglobin levels would be important to uncover.

In additional to a good medical and psychiatric history, a complete physical examination is an important part of the evaluation of the older male for whom testosterone replacement therapy is being considered. This examination is not so much to collaborate findings suggestive of hypogonadism but to assess the man for the potential for side effects involved with testosterone therapy. In fact, except for the occasional finding of bilateral small testicles, it is often difficult to discover any other clinical findings that reliably predict just which older men will have a low serum testosterone level. Particular areas of interest in regard to potential testosterone therapy risks include the cardiac/lung exam and the digital rectal examination of the prostate.

With regard to the laboratory evaluation needed in assessing a man for potential HRT, the minimum data obtainable should begin with at least two morning serum total, or non-

SHBG-bound, testosterone levels. This can be sampled on two separate mornings, or consist of two samples drawn at least 30 min apart. Once it is determined that both serum testosterone levels are in the low-normal or below normal range for young adult men, further tests should include a serum thyroid stimulating hormone level and a prolactin level. Serum LH and FSH levels and a serum estradiol level might also be considered, depending on the patient and suspected etiology of the low serum testosterone level. If the serum testosterone levels are clearly hypogonadal (<150 ng/dL), visual field testing, and evaluation for pituitary tumor may be in order. In terms of laboratory screening for parameters related to the potential risk of testosterone therapy, it is recommended that liver function tests, hemoglobin/hematocrit, and a prostate specific antigen level be measured.

Further screening that might be considered prior to initiation of therapy would depend on the findings from the history, physical examination, and laboratory studies. Among these additional studies might be sleep studies to evaluate for sleep apnea or a transrectal ultrasound of the prostate (with biopsy) to evaluate an elevated PSA or abnormal digital rectal examination of the prostate.

TESTOSTERONE REPLACEMENT THERAPY IN OLDER MEN

The decision to actually place an older man on a trial of testosterone replacement is based on:

1. Identifying one or more possible androgen target organ symptoms or findings that are present and can be monitored for efficacy of replacement.
2. Having evaluated for minimal short-term risk those areas of potential concern regarding androgen therapy (i.e., ruling out sleep apnea, significant prostate disease, and so forth).
3. Finding the patient has a serum total or non-SHBG testosterone level that is low enough that physiological androgen replacement will make a significant change in serum levels.

Therefore, if the normal range for serum total testosterone for a young adult male is 350–1100 ng/dL, an older man with two serum testosterone levels below 400 ng/dL still could have his serum testosterone level, on the average, doubled with replacement therapy and still be well within the normal adult male physiologic range. If his serum testosterone levels were 560 ng/dL, it would be difficult to change serum levels appreciably and still remain in the physiologic range.

Therapeutic Modalities

As with other hormone replacement therapy, choosing the mode of testosterone replacement in the older man involves consideration of a number of factors. These include:

1. Sex steroid serum levels to be obtained.
2. Efficacy in management of symptoms for which the therapy is being given.
3. Ease and accessibility of the therapy.
4. Therapy acceptability.
5. Side effects of the particular forms of replacement.
6. Cost, both in time and money.

Table 7 lists the major methods of testosterone therapy currently available in the US that are considered to be generally safe. (The oral methylated testosterones are not considered in this category because of their potential for liver toxicity). Also listed are the approx cost, in May 1998 dollars, for a 1-mo treatment with each form of replacement

Table 7
Types and Relative Cost of Testosterone Delivery Forms
Available in the US for Use in Replacement Therapy in Older Men

Type	Treatment regimen	Average retail cost of medication	Cost of 1 mo of therapy[a]
Injectable Esters			
Testosterone enanthate	150 mg/2 wk		
(200 mg/cc)			
Delatestryl (BTG)		5 cc/$56.19	$35.47
Generic (Steris)		10 cc/$16.59	$14.66
Testosterone cypionate	150 mg/2 wk		
(100 mg/cc)			
DEPO-testosterone (Upjohn)		10 cc/$35.35	$18.89
(200 mg/cc)			
DEPO-testosterone (Upjohn)		10 cc/$63.43	$19.34
Virilon (Steris)		10 cc/$26.40	$15.64
Testosterone propionate	15 mg 3×/wk		
(100 mg/cc)			
Generic (Schein)		10 cc/$18.01	$40.80
Patches			
Scrotal			
Testoderm (Alza)	1 patch/d		
40 cm^2 (4 mg/d)		#30	$76.49
60 cm^2 (6 mg/d)		#30	$76.49
Transdermal	2 patches/d		
Androderm TTS (SKB)		#60	$107.89
Testoderm TTS (AL$_{3a}$)	1 patch/d	#30	$103.49
Pellets			
Pellet	225 mg/3 mo		
Testopel (Bartor)		75 mg/$15.00	$35.00

[a]Calculated monthly cost of injectable ester therapy includes $6.50 cost/visit for syringe and injection; calculated monthly cost for pellets assume $60 cost for implantation.

therapy, based on average drug retail costs. There are other forms of testosterone replacement that are available for use outside the US, including testosterone topical gel; Sustenon, a mixture of testosterone esters for injection; and the oral testosterone undecanoate.

All forms of testosterone listed are probably efficacious if adequate serum testosterone levels are achieved. Selecting the form of therapy largely depends on patient preference with regard to acceptability, dosing regimen, and cost, as well as possible side effects unique to the testosterone delivery form. For example, the two most commonly used injectable esters are the enanthate and the cypionate because they can be given every one to two weeks. The propionate form needs to administered about 3 times/wk because of its shorter half life. If the man can learn to give the intramuscular testosterone injections himself, or it can administered by a family member, the cost of this therapy is extremely reasonable. Although most men complain of no or little pain from the testosterone injections, some men do not accept the idea of injections readily. In addition, the serum levels of testosterone obtained, even from once a week dosing with the enanthate or cypionate esters, are far from physiologic. High, often supraphysiologic, serum testosterone levels can occur within the first few days after injection, with nadir serum levels often falling below the normal physiologic range. For some men, such wide variations in serum testosterone levels can be noted by mood or libido changes. If the injectable ester form of testosterone is chosen as the treatment modality, it should be remembered that older men tend to metabolize testosterone more slowly than do younger men. Therefore, treatment regimens in older men usually use lower testosterone doses. For the enanthate or cypionate esters, 150 mg/2 wk, or 75 mg/wk are often the most suitable initial dosing regimens.

The patch forms of testosterone replacement give physiologic serum testosterone levels over the dosing period but have several limitations:

1. The maximum serum testosterone levels obtainable tend to be in the low-normal range and—especially with the scrotal patch—depend heavily on patient compliance with skin preparation and application instructions.
2. For cosmetic reasons, some men do not accept the idea of wearing a patch on their scrotum and/or on their skin.
3. The incidence of skin reactions to the transdermal patch is higher in older men than it is in younger men.

The pellet form of testosterone requires someone who is able to implant the pellets. Local extrusion of the pellets and infection at the site of the pellet are possible problems.

The only side effect, other than possible effects on mood or libido, that appears to have some relationship to dosing is the effect on serum red blood cell mass (*see* Table 5). If significant increases in hemoglobin levels are experienced or anticipated in a particular individual during testosterone therapy, changing to a regimen that results is a lower peak testosterone dose might be warranted.

Monitoring Treatment and Length of Treatment

Currently, much of the androgen replacement therapy in older men is done on a trial basis; that is, the therapy is rendered for a certain period of time, and the efficacy and safety of the therapy is assessed. In general, it is recommended that, in the absence of obvious adverse effects, therapy should be continued for at least six months to a year; it often takes that long for the well known "placebo effect" of sex steroid therapy to dissipate. If treatment is felt to be beneficial (and no significant adverse effects have arisen), then therapy should be continued, but reassessed at least on a yearly basis.

In monitoring for adverse effects, the patient should be seen within the first 3–4 mo after initiation of therapy. At that point, it would be important to evaluate for weight gain, peripheral edema, gynecomastia or breast tenderness, symptoms of BPH, problems with sleep, and bothersome changes in libido. In addition, it would be important to evaluate the hemoglobin and the PSA levels, as well as the serum testosterone level. Unless problems are noted, further follow-up for adverse effects should be repeated in 6–9 mo, and yearly thereafter. If possible, it is best to evaluate serum testosterone levels obtained from the treatment regimen at a time when serum levels should be in the midrange for that dosing regimen: about 1-wk into a 2-wk regimen for the injectable ester; about 4 h after the placement of the scrotal patch; or 8–12 h after placement of the transdermal patch.

CONCLUSION

As with all hormone replacement therapy, the benefits and risks of testosterone replacement for each man need to be continually reassessed. This is especially true for testosterone replacement therapy for the older man, where the data to date on the benefits and risks are scant, but new clinical information continues to be generated.

REFERENCES

1. Vermeulen A. Clinical Review 24: Androgens in the aging male. J Clin Endocrinol Metab 1991;73:221–224.
2. Tenover JS. Androgen administration to aging men. Endocrinol Metab Clin N Amer 1994;23:877–892.
3. Gray A, Feldman HA, McKinlay JB, Longcope C. Age, disease, and changing sex hormone levels in middle-aged men: results of the Massachusetts male aging study. J Clin Endocrinol Metab 1991;73:1016–1025.
4. Santamaria JD, Prior JC, Fleetham JA. Reversible reproductive dysfunction in men with obstructive sleep apnoea. Clin Endocrinol (Oxf) 1988;28:461–470.
5. Forbes GB, Reina JC. Adult lean body mass declines with age: some longitudinal observations. Metabolism 1970;19:653–663.
6. Reed R, Pearlmutter L, Yochum K, et al. The relationship between muscle mass and muscle strength in the elderly. J Am Geriatr Soc 1991;39:555–561.
7. Bhasin S, Storer TW, Berman N, et al. Testosterone replacement increases fat-free mass and muscle size in hypogonadal men. J Clin Endocrinol Metab 1997;82:407–413.
8. Bhasin S, Storer TW, Berman N, et al. The effects of supraphysiologic doses of testosterone on muscle size and strength in normal men. N Engl J Med 1996;335:1–7.
9. Orwoll ES, Klein RF. Osteoporosis in men. Endocr Rev 1995;16:87–116.
10. Tenover JL. Effects of androgen supplementation in the aging male. In: Oddens BJ, Vermeulen A, eds. Androgens and the Aging Male. Parthenon Publishing Group, New York, 1996, pp. 191–204.
11. Morley JE, Perry HM, Kaiser FE, et al. Effects of testosterone replacement therapy in older hypogonadal males: a preliminary study. J Am Geriatr Soc 1993;41:149–152.
12. Urban RJ, Bodenburg YH, Gilkison C. et al. Testosterone administration to elderly men increases skeletal muscle strength and protein synthesis. Am J Physiol 1995;269:E820–E826.
13. Tenover JS. Effects of testosterone supplementation in the aging male. J Clin Endocrinol Metab. 1992;75:1092–1098.
14. Marin P, Holmang S, Gustafsson C, et al. Androgen treatment of abdominally obese men. Obesity Res 1993;1:245–251.
15. Katznelson L, Finkelstein JS., Schoenfeld DA, et al. Increase in bone density and lean body mass during testosterone administration in men with acquired hypogonadism. J. Clin Endocrinol Metab 1996;81:4358–4365.
16. Sih R, Morley JE, Kaiser FE, et al. Testosterone replacement in older hypogonadal men: a 12-month randomized controlled trial. J Clin Endocrinol Metab 1997;82:1661–1667.
17. Sandblom RE, Matsumoto AM, Schoene RB, et al. Obstructive sleep apnea syndrome induced by testosterone administration. N Engl J Med 1983;308:508–510.
18. Drinka PJ, Jochen AL, Cuisinier M, et al. Polycythemia as a complication of testosterone replacement therapy in nursing home men with low testosterone levels. J Am Geriatr Soc 1995;43:899–901.
19. Krauss DJ, Taub HA, Lantinga LL, et al. Risks of blood volume changes in hypogonadal men treated with testosterone enanthate for erectile impotence. J Urol 1991;146:1566–1570.
20. Douglas TH, Connely RR, McLeon DG, et al. Effect of exogenous testosterone replacement on prostate-specific antigen and prostate-specific membrane antigen levels in hypogonadal men. J Surg Oncol 1995;59:246–250.

19

Applications of Androgen Therapy for Muscle Wasting Associated with Human Immunodeficiency Virus-Infection and Other Chronic Diseases

Shalender Bhasin, MD,
and Marjan Javanbakht, MPH

CONTENTS

INTRODUCTION

In many chronic illnesses, such as those associated with the human immunodeficiency virus (HIV), end stage renal disease, chronic obstructive lung disease, and some types of cancer, we can now achieve disease stability, but not cure. In these chronic disorders, muscle wasting occurs frequently, and is associated with debility, impaired quality of life, and poor disease outcome (1–11). For instance, a substantial proportion of HIV-infected men with acquired immunodeficiency syndrome (AIDS) require assistance with

From: *Contemporary Endocrinology: Hormone Replacement Therapy*
Edited by: A. W. Meikle © Humana Press Inc., Totowa, NJ

activities of daily life after hospitalization for secondary illnesses. Therefore, strategies that can reverse muscle wasting and augment muscle function may improve quality of life and reduce utilization of health care resources.

Of the various anabolic interventions being considered for promoting restitution of body cell mass in HIV-infected men, testosterone is particularly attractive because it is safe and relatively inexpensive *(12–16)*. There is agreement that testosterone can increase fat-free mass and muscle strength under specific experimental paradigms *(17–33)*. However, we do not know whether replacement doses of testosterone can produce clinically meaningful changes in body composition and muscle function in chronic illnesses associated with muscle wasting. Additionally, the HIV, like many other chronic diseases, produces a heterogeneous, complex and multisystem syndrome; therefore, anabolic therapy should be viewed as only one component of a multipronged therapeutic strategy.

The rationale for the use of androgenic steroids in chronic illnesses is based on the following hypotheses.

1. There is a high frequency of low testosterone levels in chronic illnesses associated with wasting.
2. Low testosterone levels in chronic illnesses are associated with poor disease outcomes and impaired muscle function.
3. Testosterone replacement of healthy, hypogonadal men produces increases in fat-free mass and muscle strength.
4. Androgen replacement in chronic illnesses associated with low testosterone levels will produce improvements in muscle mass and function similar to those observed in healthy, hypogonadal men.

In this chapter, we will evaluate the data pertaining to each of these hypotheses.

HIGH FREQUENCY OF LOW TESTOSTERONE LEVELS IN CHRONIC ILLNESSES ASSOCIATED WITH MUSCLE WASTING

Because we do not have good biological markers of testosterone action, hypogonadism has been defined purely in terms of low testosterone levels. We measured serum total and free testosterone levels in 150 consecutive, HIV-infected men attending our HIV clinic. Approximately, a third of these men had serum total and free testosterone levels in the hypogonadal range (S Bhasin, I Sinha-Hikim, S Arver, G Beall, unpublished observations). Other investigators have reported similar prevalence of hypogonadism in HIV-infected men *(34–43)*. Twenty percent of HIV-infected men with low testosterone levels have elevated LH and FSH levels and thus have hypergonadotropic hypogonadism. These patients presumably have primary testicular dysfunction. The remaining 80% have either normal or low LH and FSH levels; these men with hypogonadotropic hypogonadism either have a central defect at the hypothalamic or pituitary site or a dual defect involving both the testis and the hypothalamic-pituitary centers. The pathophysiology of hypogonadism in HIV-infection is complex and involves defects at multiple levels of the hypothalamic-pituitary testicular axis.

In a recent study, a majority of men with chronic obstructive lung disease had low total and free testosterone levels *(44)*. Similarly, there is a high frequency of hypogonadism in patients with cancer, end stage renal disease on hemodialysis, and liver disease *(45)*.

The pathophysiology of hypogonadism in chronic illness is multifactorial. Malnutrition, mediators and products of the systemic inflammatory response, drugs such as ketoconazole, metabolic abnormalities produced by the systemic illness all contribute to a decline in testosterone production.

LOW TESTOSTERONE LEVELS CORRELATE WITH POOR DISEASE OUTCOME

Low testosterone levels correlate with adverse disease outcome in HIV-infected men. Serum testosterone levels are lower in HIV-infected men who have lost weight than in those who have not (42). Longitudinal follow up of HIV-infected homosexual men reveals a progressive decrease in serum testosterone levels (6); this decrease is much greater in HIV-infected men who progress to AIDS than in those who do not (6). We do not know whether decrease in testosterone levels is a consequence of weight loss or is a contributory factor that precedes muscle wasting. In a longitudinal study, Dobs et al. (8) measured serum testosterone levels in a cohort of HIV-infected men and reported that serum testosterone levels decline early in the course of events that culminate in wasting. Testosterone levels correlate with muscle mass and exercise capacity in HIV-infected men (9) leading to speculation that hypogonadism may contribute to muscle wasting and debility. Although, patients with HIV-infection may lose both fat and lean tissue, the loss of lean body mass is an important aspect of the weight loss associated with wasting. The magnitude of depletion of nonfat tissues rather than weight loss is related to the death from wasting in AIDS (2–5,7,10). There is a high prevalence of sexual dysfunction in HIV-infected men (41,46). With the increasing life expectancy of HIV-infected men, frailty and sexual dysfunction have emerged as important quality of life issues.

ANABOLIC EFFECTS OF ANDROGENS IN HEALTHY, HYPOGONADAL, AND EUGONADAL MEN

Testosterone replacement increases nitrogen retention in castrated males of several animal species (23), eunuchoidal men, boys before puberty, and in women (22). Several recent studies (24–27) have reexamined the effects of testosterone on body composition and muscle mass in hypogonadal men in more detail. We administered 100 mg testosterone enanthate weekly for 10 wk to seven hypogonadal men after a 10–12-wk washout (24). Testosterone replacement was associated with a 4.5 ± 0.6 kg ($p = 0.005$) increase in body weight and 5.0 ± 0.8 kg ($p = 0.004$) increase in fat–free mass, estimated from underwater weight; body fat did not change. Similar increases in fat–free mass were observed using the deuterium water dilution method. Arm and leg muscle cross-sectional areas, assessed by magnetic resonance imaging (MRI), increased significantly. Substantial increases in muscle strength were also noted after treatment.

Brodsky et al. (25) reported a 15% increase in fat-free mass and a 11% decrease in fat mass in hypogonadal men. The muscle mass increased by 20% and accounted for 65% of the increase in fat-free mass. The muscle accretion during testosterone treatment was associated with a 56% increase in fractional muscle protein synthesis.

A sublingual, cyclodextrin-complexed, testosterone formulation produced a modest increase in fat-free mass (+0.9 kg) and muscle strength (+8.7 kg) in hypogonadal men (26); however, the testosterone dose used in this study was smaller than the doses used in previous studies.

Percent body fat is significantly greater in hypogonadal than eugonadal men *(27)*. Testosterone replacement of androgen-deficient men is associated with a significant decrease in body fat *(27)*.

The published studies are in agreement that in hypogonadal men, replacement doses of testosterone increase fat-free mass. The effects on fat mass are more variable; two studies observed a significant decrease in fat mass and two studies did not. The reasons for this discrepancy are not apparent; differences in the pretreatment body composition of the treated men, and the methods for body composition analysis, may in part account for the differences in results.

Effect of Supraphysiologic Doses of Testosterone on Body Composition

Intense controversy persisted until recently with respect to the effects of supra-physiologic doses of androgenic steroids on body composition and muscle strength *(17–20)*. Many of the previous studies were not blinded or placebo-controlled. The doses of androgens used in most studies were relatively low and it is surprising that any effects were seen at all. In some studies, the energy and protein intake was not controlled. The exercise stimulus was not standardized so that the effects of androgen could not be evaluated independent of the effects of strength training *(18,19)*. Another confounding factor in some studies was the inclusion of competitive athletes whose desire to win might preclude compliance with standardized regimens of diet, exercise, and drug administration *(17)*. We conducted a placebo-controlled, double-blind, randomized, clinical trial to separately assess the effects of supraphysiologic doses of testosterone and resistance exercise on fat–free mass, muscle size and strength *(21)*. Healthy men, 19–40 yr of age, and within 15% of their ideal weight, were randomly assigned to one of four groups: placebo but no exercise; testosterone but no exercise; placebo plus exercise; and test-osterone plus exercise. The men received 600 mg testosterone enanthate or placebo weekly for 10 wk. To assure compliance, the nursing staff in the Clinical Study Center administered all the injections. Serum total and free testosterone levels, measured seven days after each injection, increased fivefold; these were nadir levels and serum testoster-one levels at other times must have been higher. Serum LH levels were markedly suppressed in the two testosterone-treated but not placebo-treated men providing additional evidence of compliance. Men in the exercise groups underwent weight lifting exercises three times weekly; the training stimulus was standardized based on the subjects' initial 1-repetition maximum and supervised. Fat–free mass by underwater weighing, muscle size by MRI, and muscle strength of the arms and legs in bench press and squat exercises were measured before and after 10 wk of treatment.

The men given testosterone alone had greater gains in muscle size in the arm (mean ($\pm$ SE) change in triceps area 13.2 ± 3.3 vs $-2.1 \pm 2.9\%$, $p < 0.05$) and leg (change in quadriceps area 6.5 ± 1.3 vs $-1.0 \pm 1.1\%$, $p < 0.05$), than those given placebo injections. Testosterone-treatment was also associated with greater gains in strength in the bench press (increase 10 ± 4 vs $-1 \pm 2\%$, $p < 0.05$) and squat exercise capacity (increase 19 ± 6 vs $3 \pm 1\%$, $p < 0.05$) than placebo-injections. Testosterone and exercise, given together, produced greater increase in fat–free mass ($+9.5 \pm 1.0\%$), and muscle size ($+14.7 \pm 3.1\%$ in triceps area and $+14.1 \pm 1.3\%$ in quadriceps area) than either placebo or exercise alone, and greater gains in muscle strength ($+24 \pm 3\%$ in bench press strength, and $+39 \pm 4\%$ in squat exercise capacity) than either nonexercising group. We did not observe any significant changes in red cell counts or liver enzymes in any treatment group. Serum PSA levels did not change during treatment and no abnormalities were detected in the prostate on digital rectal examination during the 10-wk treatment period. Two men in the testosterone-group and one man receiving placebo injections developed acne. These results demonstrate that supraphysiologic doses of testosterone, especially when combined with strength training, increase fat–free mass, muscle size and strength in normal men.

Griggs et al. *(30)* administered testosterone enanthate at a dose of 3 mg/kg/wk to healthy men, 19–40 yr of age. This was an open-label study that was not placebo-controlled. Muscle mass, estimated from creatinine excretion, increased by a mean of 20% and ^{40}K mass increased 12% after 12 wk of testosterone treatment. In a separate study *(31,32)*, a similar dose of testosterone enanthate given for 12 mo to men with muscular dystrophy, was associated with a 4.9 kg increase in lean body mass (approx 10%) at 3 mo; these gains were maintained for 12 mo.

Young et al. *(33)* examined fat-free mass by DXA scan in 13 nonathletic men treated with 200 mg testosterone enanthate weekly for 6 mo during the course of a male contraceptive study. This was an open-label study that included untreated men as controls. Testosterone treatment increased serum testosterone levels by 90% and was associated with 9.6% increase in fat-free mass and 16.2% decrease in fat mass. Changes in muscle strength varied across different muscle groups; most consistent changes were reported in hip abduction which increased 19.2%.

Collectively, these data *(21,29–33)* demonstrate that when dietary intake and exercise stimulus are controlled, supraphysiologic doses of testosterone produce further increases in fat-free mass and strength in eugonadal men. It is likely that strength training may augment androgen effects on the muscle.

EFFECTS OF ANDROGEN REPLACEMENT ON BODY COMPOSITION AND MUSCLE FUNCTION IN HIV-INFECTION AND OTHER CHRONIC ILLNESSES

Several different anabolic interventions have been examined in the treatment of HIV related wasting including appetite stimulants such as dronabinol *(47)* and megesterol acetate *(48)*; anabolic hormones such as human growth hormone *(49–50)*, insulin-like growth factor-1 *(50)*, and androgens *(51–59)*; and modulators of immune response such as thalidomide. Dronabinol increases appetite but has not been shown to increase lean body mass *(47)*. Similarly, megesterol acetate treatment produces a modest weight gain but no significant change in lean body mass *(48)*. This progestational agent decreases serum testosterone levels and may produce symptoms of androgen deficiency.

In the two recently published clinical trials, treatment of HIV-infected men with human growth hormone (hGH) was associated with a 1.5 kg increase in lean body mass *(49,50)*. Although greater gains in weight were recorded after 6 wk of hGH treatment, these gains were not sustained with continued treatment for 12 wk. The reasons for the failure to sustain weight gains during hGH treatment are not clear; it is conceivable that weight gain early in the course of treatment is due to water retention. Growth hormone administration is associated with a high frequency of side effects including edema, arthralgias, myalgias, and jaw pain *(49,50)*. Not surprisingly, the treatment discontinuation rates were high (21–40%) in the two hGH studies *(49,50)*. The annual cost of treating HIV-infected men with hGH is substantially greater than that of testosterone replacement therapy using any of the available androgen formulations (source: PriceProbe [1997], First Data Bank/Hearst Corporation).

Several studies on the effects of androgen supplementation in HIV-infected men have been reported (51–59). However, many of these studies were not controlled clinical trials. Most of the studies were of short duration ranging from 12–24 wk. Several androgenic steroids have been studied in a limited fashion, including nandrolone decanoate, oxandrolone, oxymetholone, stanozolol, testosterone cypionate, and testosterone enanthate.

Rabkin et al. (56) administered 400 mg of testosterone cypionate biweekly in an open-label study to 75 men with HIV infection and serum testosterone levels less than 400 ng/dL. Improvements in self reported mood, sexual behavior, energy, and appetite for food were reported. The average weight gain was 1.5 kg. The study was not placebo-controlled, nor blinded. Furthermore, supraphysiological doses of testosterone were used. In a subsequent report, the same group (57) examined the effects of testosterone on body composition. Bioimpedance analysis was conducted on 29 HIV infected men receiving 400 mg biweekly of testosterone cypionate. The increase in weight consisted of a 1.2 kg increase in fat free mass ($p < 0.005$) and a 0.2 kg decrease in body fat (not significant).

In a study by Bucher et al. (51), treatment with intramuscular injections of 100 mg/week nandrolone decanoate was associated with 1.5 kg weight gain in contrast to a mean 0.15 kg weight loss in the placebo group.

Gold et al. (52) conducted an open-label study using 100 mg IM injections of nandrolone decanoate every 2 wk with no placebo controls. The study was conducted in 24 HIV infected men who had lost 5–15% of their usual body weight. Nandrolone treatment produced a significant increase in weight (mean, 0.14 kg/wk; $p < 0.05$) and lean body mass (mean 3 kg; $p < 0.005$). Quality of life parameters, and functional capacity also improved significantly during the trial.

Berger et al. (53), examined the anabolic effects of oxandrolone in a double-blind, placebo controlled, multicenter study. Sixty-three HIV positive men with >10% weight loss were randomized to receive either a placebo, 5 mg/d oxandrolone, or 15 mg/d of oxandrolone for 16 wk. The 15 mg/d oxandrolone group demonstrated statistically significant improvement in weight (1.5 lb), with subjects reporting improvements in appetite, physical activity, and strength. Subjects in the 5 mg/d maintained their body weight, whereas those receiving placebo continued to lose weight. The study failed to demonstrate changes in muscle strength. Furthermore, body composition data were not reported in this study.

The effects of the testosterone derivative oxymetholone were examined by Hengge et al. (54). Thirty HIV positive men were randomly assigned to receive either oxymetholone monotherapy or oxymetholone in combination with ketotifen which has been shown to block TNF-alpha. The average weight gain over a 30-wk period was 8.2 kg in the oxymetholone group ($p < 0.001$) and 6.1 kg ($p < 0.005$) in the combination group, while untreated controls lost an average of 1.8 kg. Karnofsky scores also improved in both treatment groups. However, this study was neither placebo-controlled, nor blinded and body composition was not evaluated.

In a case study of three AIDS patients with HIV-1 wasting myopathy, Berger et al. (53) reported favorable response to Stanozolol as evidenced by improvements in body weight, strength, muscle bulk, and overall sense of well being.

Coodley et al. (58) examined the effects of 200 mg testosterone cypionate given every 2 wk for 3 mo to 40 HIV seropositive patients with weight loss of greater than 5% of usual body weight and CD4 cell counts of $< 2 \times 10^5/L$ in a double-blind, placebo controlled study. Among the 35 patients who completed the first 3 mo of the study, there was no significant difference between the effects of testosterone and placebo treatment on weight gain. However, testosterone supplementation improved overall sense of well being ($p = 0.03$) and an increase in muscle strength ($p = 0.08$). The investigators speculate that the level of testosterone supplementation may have been inadequate to obtain an optimal response. The body composition was not assessed.

In a placebo-controlled, double-blind, clinical trial, we examined the effects of physiological testosterone replacement by means of the non-genital patch *(59)*. Forty one HIV positive men with serum testosterone levels less than 400 ng/dL were randomly assigned to receive either two placebo patches nightly or two testosterone patches, designed to release 5 mg testosterone over 24-h period. Results indicate that physiological testosterone replacement of HIV-infected men with low testosterone levels was associated with a 1.34 kg increase in lean body mass ($p = 0.02$) as well as a significantly greater reduction in fat mass than that achieved with placebo treatment alone.

There were no significant changes in liver enzymes, plasma HIV-RNA copy number, and CD4 and CD8[+] T-cell counts. There were no significant differences in the change in muscle strength between the two treatment groups over the 12-wk treatment duration.

These preliminary data in HIV-positive men are encouraging and suggest that anabolic factors such as testosterone promote weight gain and an increase in lean body mass, as well as an overall improvement in the quality of life. However, most of these studies were of short duration and it remains to be seen whether these effects can make a difference in the clinical outcomes of patients with HIV infection. We do not know whether physiological androgen replacement can produce meaningful changes in the quality of life, utilization of health care resources, and muscle function in HIV-infected men. Emerging data indicate that testosterone does not affect HIV replication, but its effects on virus shedding in the genital tract are not known.

TESTOSTERONE SUPPLEMENTATION IN OTHER CHRONIC ILLNESSES

Patients with autoimmune disorders particularly those receiving glucocorticoids often experience muscle wasting and bone loss *(62–64)*. In a placebo-controlled study, Reid et al. *(62)* administered a replacement dose of testosterone to men receiving glucocorticoids. Testosterone replacement was associated with a greater increase in fat-free mass and bone density than placebo.

There is a high frequency of low total and free testosterone levels, sexual dysfunction, infertility, delayed puberty, and growth failure in patients with end stage renal disease *(45)*. Androgen administration does not consistently improve sexual dysfunction in these patients *(65,66)*. Similarly, the effects of androgen treatment on growth and pubertal development in children with end stage renal disease remain unclear *(67,68)*. Controlled clinical trials of nadrolone decanoate have reported increased hemoglobin levels with androgen treatment in men with end stage renal disease who are on hemodialysis *(67–72)*. Prior to the advent of erythropoeitin, testosterone was commonly used to treat anemia associated with end stage renal disease. Neff et al. *(73)* compared the effects of testosterone enanthate 4 mg/kg/wk, nandrolone decanoate 3 mg/kg/wk, oxymethalone 1 mg/kg/dy, and fluoxymesterone 0.4 mg/kg/d on hemoglobin levels. Testosterone enanthate and nandrolone decanoate at the doses used were reported to be more effective in increasing hemoglobin levels than the other two androgen regimens. Testosterone increases red cell production by stimulating erythropoieitin and by augmenting erythropoieitin action. Further studies are needed to determine whether testosterone administration can reduce blood transfusion and erythropoieitin requirements in patients with end stage renal disease on hemodialysis.

Chronic obstructive lung disease is a chronic debilitating disease for which there are few effective therapies. Muscle wasting and dysfunction are recognized as correctable causes of exercise intolerance in these patients. It has been speculated that low levels of anabolic hormones such as testosterone, growth hormone and insulin-like growth factor-1 may contribute to muscle atrophy and dysfunction (44). Human growth hormone increases nitrogen retention and lean body muscle in patients with COPD; however, the effects of hGH on respiratory muscle strength and exercise tolerance remain to be established (60,61). Schols et al. (74) examined the effects of a low dose of nandrolone or placebo in 217 men and women with chronic obstructive lung disease; these authors reported modest increases in lean body mass and respiratory muscle strength.

TESTOSTERONE EFFECTS ON FAT METABOLISM

Percent body fat is increased in hypogonadal men (27). Some studies have reported a decrease in fat mass with testosterone replacement (27,29) therapy while others find no change. Epidemiologic studies (75,76) have demonstrated that serum testosterone levels are lower in middle aged men with visceral obesity, and correlate with plasma HDL levels. Testosterone replacement of middle aged men with visceral obesity improves insulin sensitivity, decreases blood glucose and blood pressure (77). Testosterone is an important determinant of regional fat distribution and metabolism in men (78).

DOES A DEFECT IN 5-ALPHA REDUCTION CONTRIBUTE TO WASTING IN HIV-INFECTED MEN?

Although the enzyme 5-alpha-reductase is expressed at low concentrations within the muscle (79), we do not know whether conversion of testosterone to dihydrotestosterone is required for mediating the androgen effects on the muscle. The men with benign prostatic hypertrophy who are treated with the 5-alpha-reductase inhibitor, do not experience muscle loss. Similarly, individuals with congenital 5-alpha-reductase deficiency have normal muscle development at puberty. These data suggest that 5-alpha reduction of testosterone is not obligatory for mediating its effects on the muscle.

Sattler et al. (80) have reported that serum DHT levels are lower and testosterone to dihydrotestosterone levels higher in HIV-infected men than healthy men. These investigators have proposed that a defect in testosterone to dihydrotestosterone conversion may contribute to wasting in a subset of HIV-infected men. If this hypothesis were true, then it would be rational to treat such patients with dihydrotestosterone rather than testosterone. A dihydrotestosterone gel is currently under clinical investigation. However, it is worth emphasizing that unlike testosterone, dihydrotestosterone can not be aromzatized to estradiol. Therefore, there is concern that suppression of endogenous testosterone and estradiol production by exogenous dihydrotestosterone may produce osteoporosis.

MECHANISMS OF TESTOSTERONE'S
ANABOLIC EFFECTS ON THE MUSCLE

Several studies are in agreement that testosterone produces muscle hypertrophy by increasing fractional muscle protein synthesis (25,32). However, the molecular basis of this anabolic effect is not known. Urban et al. (32) have proposed that testosterone stimulates the expression of insulin-like growth factor-1 and downregulates insulin like growth factor binding protein-4 in the muscle. Reciprocal changes in IGF-1 and its binding protein thus provide a potential mechanism for amplifying the anabolic signal. It is not clear whether the anabolic effects of supraphysiologic doses of testosterone are mediated through an androgen receptor mediated mechanism. In vitro binding studies (81–83) suggest that the maximum effects of testosterone should be manifest at about 300 ng/dL, i.e., serum testosterone levels that are at the lower end of the normal male range. Therefore, it is possible that the supraphysiologic doses of androgen produce muscle hypertrophy through androgen-receptor independent mechanisms, such as through an anti-glucocorticoid effect (84–86). We can not exclude the possibility that some androgen effects may be mediated through nonclassical binding sites. Testosterone effects on the muscle are modulated by a number of other factors such as the genetic background, growth hormone secretory status (84), nutrition, exercise, cytokines, thyroid hormones, and glucocorticoids. Testosterone may also affect muscle function by its effects on neuromuscular transmission (87,88).

ANDROGEN ADMINISTRATION IN WOMEN

The ovaries and the adrenal glands collectively produce approximately three hundred ug testosterone daily in healthy, menstruating women. Serum testosterone levels are lower in older women than younger women (89). Women who have undergone hysterectomy and bilateral oophorectomy and have been treated with combined estrogen and testosterone therapy report higher rates of sexual desire, arousal and number of fantasies than those who are given either estradiol alone or left untreated (90,91). Sherwin has proposed that testosterone may be important for the maintenance of sexual function in post-menopausal women. Postmenopausal women treated with estrogen xåus }≠îhyl testosterone have lower rates of bone resorption over a three month treatment period than those treated with estrogen alone (92). Most of the published androgen studies in postmenopausal women have used relatively large doses of testosterone (90–93). It is not surprising that supraphysiologic doses of testosterone increase muscle size and strength in pre- and post-menopausal women. We do not know, however, whether addition of "physiological" replacement doses of testosterone to a regimen of estrogen replacement can augment fat-free mass, muscle strength, sexual function, and bone density in postmenopausal women. The critical question is whether these beneficial anabolic effects can be achieved by testosterone doses that do not result in virilization.

Using an improved, sensitive equilibrium dialysis method, we defined the range for total and free testosterone levels during the normal menstrual cycle and measured serum free testosterone levels in HIV-infected women (94). Serum total and free testosterone levels were lower in HIV-infected women than healthy women. Testosterone levels correlated inversely with plasma HIV-RNA copy number. Serum FSH, but not LH, levels were significantly higher in HIV-infected women than controls. Serum total and free testosterone levels are lower in HIV-infected women, and correlate inversely with plasma

HIV RNA levels. Grinspoon et al. *(95)* have also reported that free testosterone levels were significantly lower in HIV-infected women with early and late wasting. Free testosterone levels correlated with muscle mass, leading these investigators to conclude that low testosterone levels contribute to wasting. However, free testosterone levels reported in that paper were measured by a tracer analog method. The biological nature of the fraction being measured by the tracer analog method used in the previous publication remains unclear. The hypothesis that androgen deficiency contributes to wasting in HIV-infected women remains to be tested. Clinical trials to assess the effects of testosterone replacement on body composition, muscle function, and overall quality of life in HIV-infected women with weight loss are in progress.

REFERENCES

1. Hellerstein MK, Kahn J, Mundi H, Viteri F. Current approach to treatment of human immunodeficiency virus associated with weight loss, pathophysiologic considerations and emerging -strategies. Sem Oncol 1990;17:17–33.
2. Kotler DP, Tierney AR, Wang J, Pierson RN. Magnitude of body cell mass depletion and the timing of death from wasting in AIDS. Am J Clin Nutr 1989;50:444–447.
3. Grunfeld C, Feingold KR. Metabolic disturbances and wasting in the acquired immunodeficiency syndrome. N Engl J Med 1992;327:329–337.
4. Sellmeyer DE, Grunfeld C. Endocrine and metabolic disturbances in human immunodeficiency virus infection and the acquired immune deficiency syndrome. Endocr Rev 1996;17:518–532.
5. Chlebowski RT, et al. Nutritional status, gastrointestinal dysfunction and survival in patients with AIDS. Am J Gastroenterol 1989;84:1288–1293.
6. Salehian B, Jacobson D, Grafe M, McCutchan A, Swerdloff R. Pituitary-testicular axin during HIV infection: a prospective study. Presented at the 18th annual meeting of the American Society of Andrology. Abstract #9, Tampa Florida, April 15-19, 1993.
7. Nahlen BL, et al. HIV wasting syndrome in the United States. AIDS 1993;7:183–188.
8. Dobs AS, Few WL, Blackman MR, Harman SM, Hoover DR, Graham NMH. Serum hormones in men with human immunodeficiency virus-associated wasting. J Clin Endocrinol Metab 1996;81:4108–4112.
9. Grinspoon S, Corcoran C, Lee K, et al. Loss of lean body and muscle mass correlates with androgen levels in hypogondal men with acquired immunodeficiency syndrome and wasting. J Clin Endocrinol Metab 1996;81:4051–4058.
10. Linden CP, Allen S, Serufilira A, et al. Predictors of mortality among HIV-infected women in Kigali, Rwanda. Ann Intern Med 1992;116:320–325.
11. Gunter PA, Mourahainen N, Cohen GR, et al. Relationship between nutritional status. CD4 counts and survival in HIV infection. Am J Clin Nutr 1992;56:762–799.
12. Bhasin S, Bremner WJ. Emerging issues in androgen replacement therapy. J Clin Endocrinol Metab 1997;82:3–8.
13. Sokol RZ, Palacios A, Campfield LA, Saul C, Swerdloff RS. Comparison of the kinetics of injectable testosterone in eugonadal and hypogonadal men. Fertil Steril 1982;37:425–430.
14. Snyder PJ, Lawrence DA Treatment of male hypogonadism with testosterone enanthate. J Clin Endocrinal Metab 1980;51:1335–1339.
15. Matsumoto AM. Effects of chronic testosterone administration in normal men: safety and efficacy of high dose testosterone and parallel dose-dependent suppression of LH, FSH and sperm production. J Clin Endocrinol Metab 1990;70:282.
16. Meikle AW, Mazer NA, Moellmer JF, et al. Enhanced transdermal delivery of testosterone across the nonscrotal skin produces physiological concentrations of testosterone and its metabolites in hypogonadal men. J Clin Endocrinol Metab 1992;74:623–628.
17. Wilson JD. Androgen abuse by athletes. Endocr Rev 1988;9:181–200.
18. Bardin CW. The anabolic action of testosterone. N Engl J Med 1996;335:52,53.
19. Casaburi R, Storer T, Bhasin S. Androgen effects on body composition and muscle performance. In: Bhasin S, Gabelnick H, Spieler JM, Swerdloff RS, Wang C, eds. Pharmacology, Biology, and Clinical Applications of Androgens: Current Status and Future Prospects. Wiley-Liss, New York, NY, 1996, pp. 283–288.

20. Mooradian AD, Morley JE, Korenman SG. Biological actions of androgens. Endocr Rev 1987;8:1–28.
21. Bhasin S, Storer TW, Berman N, Callegari C, Clevenger BA, Phillips J, Bunnell T, Tricker R, Shirazi A, Casaburi R. The effects of supraphysiologic doses of testosterone on muscle size and strength in men. N Engl J Med 1996;335:1–7.
22. Kenyon AT, Knowlton K, Sandiford I, Kock FC, Lotwin G. A comparative study of the metabolic effects of testosterone propionate in normal men and women and in eunuchoidism. Endocrinology 1940;26:26–45.
23. Kochakian CD. Comparison of protein anabolic properties of various androgens in the castrated rat. Am J Physiol 1950;60:553–558.
24. Bhasin S, Storer TW, Berman N, Yarasheski K, Phillips J, Clevenger B, Lee WP, Casaburi R. A replacement dose of testosterone increases fat-free mass and muscle size in hypogonadal men. J Clin Endocrinol Metab 1997;82:407–413.
25. Brodsky IG, Balagopal P, Nair KS. Effects of testosterone replacement on muscle mass and muscle protein synthesis in hypogonadal men—a Clinical Research Center Study. J Clin Endocrinol Metab 1996;81:3469–3475.
26. Wang C, Eyre DR, Clark R, Kleinberg D, Newman C, Iranmanesh A, Veldhuis J, Dudley RE, Berman N, Davidson T, Barstow TJ, Sinow R, Alexander G, Swerdloff RS. Sublingual testosterone replacement improves muscle mass and strength, decreases bone resorption, and increases bone resorption markers in hypogonadal men—a Clinical Research Center Study. J Clin Endocrinol Metab 1996;81:3654–3662.
27. Katznelson L, Finkelstein JS, Schoenfeld DA, Rosenthal DI, Anderson EJ, Klibanski A. Increase in bone density and lean body mass during testosterone administration in men with acquired hypogonadism. J Clin Endocrinol Metab 1996;81:4358–4365.
28. Bhasin S, Tenover JS. Sarcopenia: issues in testosterone replacement of older men. J Clin Endocrinol Metab 1997;82:1659,1660.
29. Forbes GB, Porta CR, Herr B, Griggs RC. Sequence of changes in body composition induced by testosterone and reversal of changes after the drug is stopped. JAMA 1992;267:397–399.
30. Griggs RC, Kingston W, Josefowicz RF, Herr BE, Forbes G, Halliday D. Effect of testosterone on muscle mass and muscle protein synthesis. J Appl Physiol 1989;66:498–503.
31. Griggs RC, Pandya S, Florence JM, Brooke MH, Kingston W, Miller JP, Chutkow J, Herr BE, Moxley RT. Randomized controlled trial of testosterone in myotonic dystrophy. Neurology 1989;39:219–222.
32. Urban RJ, Bodenburg YH, Gilkison C, Foxworth J, Coggan AR, Wolfe RR, Ferrando A. Testosterone administration to elderly men increases skeletal muscle strength and protein synthesis. Am J Physiol 1995;269:E820–E826.
33. Young NR, Baker HWG, Liu G, Seeman E. Body composition and muscle strength in healthy men receiving testosterone enanthate for contraception. J Clin Endocrinol Metab 1993;77:1028–1032.
34. Dobs AS, Dempsey MA, Ladenson PW, Polk BF. Endocrine disorders in men infected with human immunodeficiency virus. Am J Med 1988;84:611–615.
35. Meremich JA, McDermott MT, Asp AA, Harrison SM, Kidd GS. Evidence of endocrine involvement early in the course of human immunodeficiency virus infection. J Clin Endocrinol Metab 1990;70:566–571.
36. Villete JM, Bourin P, Dornel C, Mansour I, Boudou P, Dreux C, Rone R, Debord M, Leu F. Circadian variations in plasma levels of hypophyseal, adrenocortical, and testicular hormones in men infected with human immunodeficiency virus. J Clin Endorinol Metab 1990;70:572–577.
37. Aron DC. Endocrine complications of the acquired immunodeficiency syndrome. Arch Intern Med 1989;149:330–333.
38. Croxon TC, Chapman WE, Miller LK, Levitt CD, Senie R, Zumoff B. Changes in the hypothalamic pituitary-gonadal axis in human immunodeficiency virus-infected hypogonadal men. J Clin Endocrinol Metab 1989;68:317–321.
39. Raffi F, Brisseau J-M, Planchon B, Remi JP, Barrier JH, Grolleau J-Y. Endocrine function in 98 HIV-infected patients: a prospective study. AIDS 1991;5:729–733.
40. DePaepe ME, Vuletin JC, Lee MH, Rojas-Corona RR, Waxman M. Testicular atrophy in homosexual AIDS patients. Hum Pathol 1989;20:572–578.
41. Meyer-Bahlburg FH et al. HIV positive gay men: sexual dysfunction. Proc VI International Conference on AIDS 1989;701.
42. Coodley GO, Loveless MO, Nelson HD, Coodley MK. Endocrine function in HIV wasting syndrome. J Acquir Immune Def Retrovirol 1994;7:46–51.
43. Laudet A, Blum L, Guechot J, et al. Changes in systematic gonadal and adrenal steroids in asymptomatic human immunodeficiency virus-infected men: relationship with CD4 counts. Euro J Endocrin 1995;133:418–424.

44. Casaburi R, Goren S, Bhasin S. Substantial prevalence of low anabolic hormone levels in COPD patients undergoing rehabilitation. Am J Resp Crit Care Med 1996;153:A128.
45. Handelsman DJ, Dong Q. Hypothalamic-pituitary gonadal axis in chronic renal failure. Endocrin Metab Clinics N Am 1993;22:145–161.
46. Rabkin JG, Rabkin R, Wagner GJ. Testosterone treatment of clinical hypogonadism in patients with HIV/AIDS. Int J STD AIDS 1997;8:537–545.
47. Beal JE, Oldson R, Laubenstein L, et al. Dronabinol as a treatment for anorexia associated with weight loss in patients with AIDS. J Pain Symptom Manage 1995;10:89–97.
48. Von Roenn JH, Armstrong D, Kotler DP, et al. Megastrol acetate in patients with AIDS-related cachexia. Ann Intern Med 1994;121:393–399.
49. Schambelan M, Mulligan K, Grunfeld C, et al. Recombinant growth horone in patients with HIV-associated wasting. Ann Intern Med 1996;125:873–882.
50. Waters D, Danska J, Hardy K, Koster F. Recombinant growth hormone, insulin-like growth factor-1, and combination therapy in AIDS-associated wasting. Ann Intern Med 1996;125:865–872.
51. Bucher G, Berger DS, Fields-Gardner C, Jones R, Reiter WM. A prospective study on the safety and effect of nandrolone decanoate in HIV positive patients [abstract #Mo.B. 423] Int Conf AIDS 1996;11:26.
52. Gold J, High HA, Li Y, Michelmore H, Bodsworth NJ, Finlayson R, Furner VL, Allen BJ, Oliver CJ. Safety and efficacy of nandrolone decanoate for treatment of wasting in patients with HIV infection. AIDS 1996;10:745–752.
53. Berger JR, Pall L, Hall CD, Simpson DM, Berry PS, Dudley R. Oxandrolone in AIDS-wasting myopathy. AIDS 1996;10:1657–1662.
54. Hengge UR, Baumann M, Maleba R, Brockmeyer NH, Goos M. Oxymetholone promotes weight gain in patients with advanced human immunodeficiency virus (HIV-1) infection. Br J Nutr 1996;75(1):129–138.
55. Berger JR, Pall L, Winfield D. Effect of anabolic steroids on HIV-related wasting myopathy. South Med J 1993;86(8):865,866.
56. Rabkin JG, Rabkin R, Wagner JG. Testosterone treatment of clinical hypogonadism in patients with HIV/AIDS. Int J STD AIDS 1997;8:537–545.
57. Engelson ES, Rabkin JG, Rabkin R, Kotler DP. Effects of testosterone upon body composition. J Acquir Immune Defic Synd 1996;11:510,511.
58. Coodley GO, Coodley MK. A trial of testosterone therapy for HIV-associated weight loss. AIDS 1997;11:1347–1352.
59. Bhasin S, Storer TW, Kilbourne A, Hays R, Arver S, Sinha-Hikim I, Shen R, Guerrero M, Beall G. Effects of physiologic testosterone replacement in human immunodeficiency virus-infected men with low testosterone levels., in press.
60. Pape GS, Friedman M, Underwood LE, Clemmons DR. The effect of growth hormone on weight gain and pulmonary function in patients with chronic obstructive lung disease. Chest 1991;99:1495–1500.
61. Pichard C, Kyle U, Chevrolet JC. Lack of effects of recombinant growth hormone on muscle function in patients requiring prolonged mechaniscal ventilation: a prospective randomized controlled study. Crit Care Med 1996;24:403–413.
62. Reid IR, Wattie DJ, Evans MC, Stapleton JP. Testosterone therapy in glucocorticoid-treated men. Arch Intern Med 1996;156:1173–1177.
63. Reid IR, Ibbertson HK, France JT, Pybus J. Plasma testosterone concentrations in asthmatic men treated with glucocorticoids. Br Med J 1985;291:574–577.
64. McAdams MR, White RH, Chipps BE. Reduction of serum testosrone levels during chronic glucocorticoid therapy. Ann Intern Med 1986;104:648–651.
65. Chopp RT, Mendez R. Sexual function and hormonal abnormalities in uremic men on chronic dialysis and after renal transplantation. Fertil Steril 1978;29:661–666.
66. Barton CH, Mirahmadi MK, Vaziri ND. Effects of long term testosterone administration on pituitary-testicular axis in end-stage renal failure. Nephron 1982;31:61–64.
67. Jones RWA, El Bishti MM, Bloom SR, et al. The effects of anabolic steroids on growth, body composition, and metabolism in boys with chronic renal failure on regular hemodialysis. J Pediatrics 1980;97:559–566.
68. Kassmann Km Rappaport R, Broyer M. The short term effect of testosterone on growth in boys on hemodialysis. Clin Nephrol 1992;37:148–154.
69. Berns JS, Rudnick MR, Cohen RM. A controlled trial of recombinant erythropoieitin and nandrolone decanoate in the treatment of anemia in patients on chronic hemodialysis. Clin Nephrol 1992;37:264–267.

70. Buchwald D, Argyres S, Easterling RE, et al. Effect of nandrolone decanoate on the anemia of chronic hemodialysis patients. Nephron 1977;18:232–238.

71. Williams JL, Stein JH, Ferris TF. Nandrolone decanoate therapy for patients receiving hemodialysis. A controlled study. Arch Intern Med 1974;134:289–292.

72. Hendler ED, Goffinet JA, Ross S, et al. Controlled study of androgen therapy in anemia of patients on maintenance hemodialysis. N Engl J Med 1974;291:1046–1051.

73. Neff MS, Goldberg J, Slifkin RF, et al. A comparison of androgens for anemia in patients on hemodialysis. N Engl J Med 1981;304:871–875.

74. Schols AMW, Soeters PB, Mostert R. Physiologic effects of nutritional support and anabolic steroids in patients with chronic obstructive pulmonary disease. Am J Resp Crit Care Med 1995;152:1268–1274.

75. Seidell J, Bjorntorp P, Sjostrom L, Kvist H, Sannerstedt R. Visceral fat accumulation in men is positively associated with insulin, glucose and C-peptide levels, but negatively with testosterone levels. Metabolism 1990;39:897–901.

76. Barrett-Connors E, Khaw K-T. Endogenous sex-hormones and cardiovascular disease in men. A prospective population-based study. Circulation 1988;78:539–545.

77. Marin P, Krotkiewski M, Bjorntorp P. Androgen treatment of middle-aged, obese men: effects on metabolism, muscle, and adipose tissues. Eur J Med 1992;1:329–336.

78. Marin P, Oden B, Bjorntorp P. Assimilation and mobilization of triglycerides in subcutaneous abdominal and femoral adipose tissue in vivo in men: effects of androgens. J Clin Endocrinol Metab 1995;80:239–243.

79. Bartsch W, Krieg M, Voigt KD. Quantitation of endogenous testosterone, 5-alpha-dihydrotestosterone and 5-alpha-androstane-3-alpha, 17-beta-diol in subcellular fractions of the prostate, bulbocavernosus/levator ani muscle, skeletal muscle, and heart muscle of the rat. J Steroid Biochem 1980;13:259–267.

80. Sattler FR, Antonipillai I, Allen J, Horton R (1996) Wasting and sex hormones: evidence for the role of dihydrotestosterone in AIDS patients with weight loss. Abstract Tu.B.2376 presented at the XI International Conference on AIDS, Vancouver, Canada.

81. Dahlberg E, Snochowski M, Gustaffsson JA Regulation of the androgen and glucocorticoid receptors in the rat and mouse muscle cytosol. Endocrinology 1981;108:1431–1436.

82. Michel G, Bauheu EE. Androgen receptor in skeletal muscle: characterization and physiologic variations. Endocrinology 1980;107:2088.

83. Saartok T, Dahlberg E, Gustaffsson JA. Relative binding affinity of anabolic-androgenic steroids, comparison of the binding to the androgen receptors in skeletal muscle and in prostate as well as sex hormone binding globulin. Endocrinology 1984;114:2100–2107.

84. Konagaya M, Max SR. A possible role for endogenous glucocorticoid in orchiectomy-induced atrophy of the rat levator ani muscle: studies with RU38486, a potent glucocorticoid antagonist. J Steroid Biochem 1986;25:305–311.

85. Mayer M, Rosen F. Interaction of anabolic steroids with glucocorticoid receptor sites in rat muscle cytosol. Am J Physiol 1975;229:1381–1386.

86. Fryburg DA, Weltman A, Jahn LA, Weltman J, Samojlik E, Hintz RL, Veldhuis JD. Short-term modulation of the androgen milieu alters pulsatile, but not exercise- or growth hormone (GH)-releasing hormone-stimulated GH secretion in healthy men: impact of gonadal steroid and GH secretory changes on metabolic outcomes. J Clin Endocrinol Metab 1997;82:3710–3719.

87. Leslie M, Forger NG, Breedlove SM. Sexual dimorphism and androgen effects on spinal motoneurons innervating the rat felxor digitorum brevis. Brain Res 1991;561:269–273.

88. Blanco CE, Popper P, Micevych P. Anabolic-androgenic steroid induced alterations in choline acetyltransferase messenger RNA levels of spinal cord motoneurons in the male rat. Neuroscience 1997;78:973–882.

89. Zumoff B, Strain GW, Miller Lk, et al. Twenty-four hour mean plasma testosterone concentrations declines with age in norma premenopausal women. J Clin Endocrinol metab 1995;80:1429–1430.

90. Sherwin B, Gelfand MM, Brender W. Androgen enhances sexual motivation in females: a prospective, crossover study of sex steroid administration in surgical menopause. Psychosom Med 1997;47:339–351.

91. Burger HG, Hailes J, Nelson J, et al. Effect of combined implants of estradiol and testosterone on libido in postmenopausal women. Br Med J 1987;294:936–937.

92. Raisz LG, Wiita B, Artis A, et al. Comparison of the effects of estrogen alone and estrogen plus androgen on biochemical markers of bone formation and resorption in postmenopausal women. J Clin Endocrinol Metab 1995;81:37–43.

93. Watts NB, Notelovitz M, Timmons MC. Comparison of oral estrogens and estrogens plus androgen on bone mineral density, menopausal symptoms and lipid-lipoprotein profile in surgical menopause. Obstet Gynecol 1995;85:529–537.
94. Sinha-Hikim I, Arver S, Beall G, et al. The use of a sensitive equilibrium dialysis method for the measurement of free testosterone levels in healthy, cycling women and in human immunodeficiency virus-infected women. J Clin Endocrinol Metab 1998;83:1312.
95. Grinspoon S, Corcoran C, Miller K, et al. Body composition and endocrine function in women with acquired immunodeficiency syndrome wasting. J Clin Endocrinol Metab 1997;82:1332–1337.

20

Hormonal Male Contraception

Christina Wang, MD, and Ronald S. Swerdloff, MD

INTRODUCTION

Currently, available female methods of contraception include the combined estrogen-progesterone oral contraceptive pill, progestagen only pills, injectables, implants, intrauterine devices, vaginal rings, female condoms, tubal ligation, menses inducers (mifepristone [RU486] and misoprostol [prostaglandin E_1]), and emergency contraception using estrogens. Other less effective methods include natural family planning, lactation amenorrhea and vaginal spermicides. Methods under development include immunocontraception using antisperm antibodies, anti-zona-pellucida antibodies, or anti-hCG vaccine; new injectable progesterone esters; and emergency contraception with levonorgestrel or mifepristone. In contrast, the currently male controlled methods are limited to coitus interruptus, male condoms, and vasectomy.

CURRENTLY AVAILABLE MALE METHODS

Coitus interruptus requires high motivation and control. Male condoms are used by about 40 to 50 million men worldwide, and they have the added advantage of protection against sexually transmitted diseases. The user failure rate of condom is as high as 12% *(1)*, which is related to compliance as well as breakage. Nonlatex condoms are developed to increase acceptability.

Vasectomy is a simple outpatient procedure. The morbidity associated with vasectomy has been dramatically reduced by the "no-scalpel technique" *(2)*. Acceptability of vasectomy as a birth control method has wide geographical variation. About 45 million men had been vasectomized worldwide. These men are from the US, the United Kingdom, Australia, the Netherlands, China, Korea, and Thailand. The contraceptive efficacy of vasectomy is very high, though azoospermia is not reached immediately because time

From: *Contemporary Endocrinology: Hormone Replacement Therapy*
Edited by: A. W. Meikle © Humana Press Inc., Totowa, NJ

is required for clearance of the sperm through the ejaculatory system. Vasectomy is considered an irreversible method. Reanastomoses when performed by skilled surgeons lead to reappearance of sperm in the ejaculate in over 90% of men but pregnancy in their partners occurs only in approx 50% of vasovasostomy. Development of antisperm antibodies is the most likely cause of infertility after reanastomoses. Newer developments in this field include percutaneous introduction of intravasal occlusive devices and percutaneous intravasal injection of cured-in-place silicone to halt sperm transport.

NONHORMONAL METHODS

Gossypol, a chemical agent derived from cotton seed oil, was studied in over 8000 men in China in the 1970s *(3)*. Gossypol acts directly on the testes affecting spermatogenesis leading to spermatogenic arrest and irreversible damage to germ cells. Because of the high incidence of irreversibility and the potential of causing hypokalemia in some men, studies on gossypol have been largely discontinued in China and most other parts of the world *(4)*.

Agents with action in the postmeiotic spermatozoa or in the epididymis may decrease the function and/or number of sperm and cause infertility. Such agents will have a quicker onset of action and will not disturb the subjects' hormonal milieu. Examples of such agents include alpha-chlorohydrin and the 6-chloro-6-deoxy sugars *(5)*. Though active in the epididymal sperm resulting in infertility, these agents were discarded as leads because of unacceptable toxicity. Other agents active in the epididymis or postmeiotic spermatogenesis include the proton-pump ATPase inhibitors and imidazoles.

In the 1980s, investigators in China noted that a multiglycoside extract of the plant Tripterygium wilfordii (used in Chinese traditional medicine for psoriasis and rheumatoid arthritis) caused decrease in sperm motility and concentrations in male patients. Studies in rats confirmed that administration of this multiglycoride results in marked reduction in sperm motility suggesting that tripterygium may have its antifertility effect on the epididymis or postmeiotic sperm *(6,7)*. One of the active principles from tripterygium wilfordii, triptolide has been purified and tested in fertility studies in rats. After dosing for 35 d there was some decrease of sperm motility. When the animals were dosed for 70 d with the pure compound triptolide, sperm motility was markedly lowered with a small decrease in sperm concentration. Studies are ongoing to determine whether triptolide has any significant effect on spermatogenesis in addition to its effect on decreasing motility of epididymal spermatozoa *(8)*.

HORMONAL METHODS

Hormonal methods are based on reversible suppression of gonadotropins, testicular steroid and sperm production (Fig. 1). Many hormonal methods have been tested in clinical trials and represent the most promising lead in a new method of contraception for men *(9–12)*.

Hormonal Regulation of Spermatogenesis

Spermatogenesis is a highly organized process involving germ cell proliferation, maturation, and death. The spermatogonia undergo multiplication (mitosis) to become spermatocytes. Two meiotic divisions occur yielding haploid spermatids. The spermatids then undergo a complex process of differentiation called spermiogenesis during

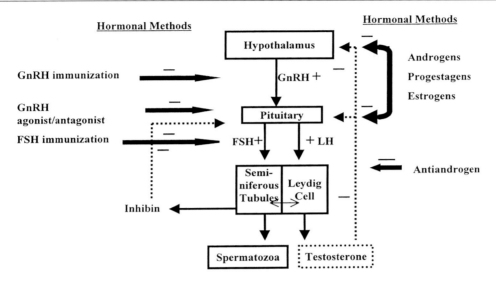

Fig. 1. Hormonal basis of male contraception.

which the acrosome and flagellum were formed. The developmental processes are arranged in defined cell association or stages of the seminiferous epithelium. These stages follow one another in a regular fashion giving rise to a wave of germ cell maturation and differentiation. In the human, the average length of the seminiferous epithelium cycle is about 73 d *(13)*. Throughout the process of spermatogenesis the germ cells are enveloped by the surrounding Sertoli cells. The Sertoli cells and germ cells cross communicate via hormones, many paracrine factors, and signals some of which are not clearly defined.

The mature spermatid is then released into the tubular lumen by a process called spermiation. The spermatids pass through the ductus efferentia and rete testes to the epididymis. During the transit through the epididymis the spermatozoa mature, acquiring both fertilizing capacity and motility, probably through maturational changes in the cell membrane induced by proteins and other substances. The transit of the spermatozoa from the testes through the vas deferences to the ejaculatory ducts takes about 14 d. Secretions from the prostate and seminal fluid contribute about 80% of the seminal fluid volume.

Spermatogenesis in man is regulated by testosterone produced by the Leydig cells in the interstitium and by the gonadotropin, follicle stimulating hormone (FSH). Both testosterone and FSH act on the germ cells probably indirectly via the Sertoli cells. Testosterone secretion is regulated by luteinizing hormone (LH) produced by the anterior pituitary gland. Both LH and FSH are secreted in a pulsatile fashion under the regulation of the GnRH. GnRH secretion by the hypothalamus is in turn regulated by a complicated network of neuropeptides and neurotransmitters. In man, it is generally accepted that both FSH and testosterone (LH) are required for initiation of spermatogenesis. Once initial maturation is induced, testosterone is required for the maintenance of spermatogenesis. Studies in men provided evidence that testosterone alone supports qualitatively normal sperm production, but both FSH and testosterone are required to maintain qualitatively and quantitatively normal spermatogenesis *(14,15)*. Recent studies from FSH receptor knockout mice and spontaneous FSH receptor mutations in men cast doubt on the obligatory role of FSH in regulation of spermatogenesis. In the FSH receptor deficient mice/humans, spermatogenesis proceeds normally albeit in some mice/humans, the sperm production is low or compromised *(16,17)*.

Leydig cell dysfunction results in low testosterone production and elevated LH levels because of decreased negative feedback on the hypothalamus-pituitary. Similarly, germ cell/Sertoli cell dysfunction results in low inhibin production and elevated FSH secretion because of attenuated negative feedback on the hypothalamic pituitary system. In addition to the gonadotropins, a large number of growth factors, cytokines, and other peptides are secreted by cells within the testis, e.g., Sertoli cells, Leydig cells, peritubular myoid cells, and macrophages that form a complex cross-communication system between germ cells and their somatic counterparts. The exact role of each of these factors in the regulation of spermatogenesis in vivo is not clear.

Androgens (Table 1)

In the 1970s, clinical studies on male hormonal methods of contraception began using testosterone enanthate (TE) as the hormonal prototype. Short term (4–6 mo) studies showed that TE administered at a weekly dose of 200 or 250 mg IM induced azoospermia in 40–60% of normal men. Oligozoospermia (defined as sperm concentration of less than 5×10^6/mL) was achieved in 90–95% of men *(18–22)*. If the interval between 200 mg TE injections was increased to 14 days, then only 45–65% of the men would reach oligozoospermia. In some studies, suppression of spermatogenesis was initially induced by weekly injections of TE and followed by spacing the frequency of TE injections to 2–4 wk. These regimens were unsuccessful since sperm production increased to above oligozoospermic levels when the interval between injections was increased to above 10 d *(22)*. In all these studies, upon discontinuation of treatment, gonadotropins and sperm counts returned to normal.

In 1985, based on the fundings of these early studies, the World Health Organization (WHO) started a multicenter study to determine whether testosterone induced azoospermia would provide effective contraception. TE was chosen as the prototype hormonal method because of its known efficacy, safety and reversibility in humans. The study included 271 couples in 10 centers in seven countries. During the suppression phase of up to 6 mo, 200 mg of TE was administered weekly by intramuscular injections until azoospermia was demonstrated in three consecutive semen analyses. The couple then entered the 12 mo efficacy phase during which the TE regimen was continued and no other methods of contraception was used. The study showed that at the end of 6 mo of TE administration, 64% of the men had persistent azoospermia. When these couples with azoospermic male partners entered the efficacy phase, there was only one pregnancy during 1,846 mo of coital exposure. This represented an efficacy rate (Pearl rate) of 0.8 (95% confidence interval 0.02 to 4.5) per 100 person/yr which, is equivalent or better than existing methods of reversible female or male available contraceptive methods *(23)*. A difference existed in the efficacy rate in centers with predominantly Asian compared to white subjects in that 91% of men in the three Asian centers achieved azoospermia compared to the 50–60% azoospermia in centers whose subjects were predominantly whites *(23)*. The ethnic differences in the suppression of spermatogenesis by androgens were also noted in the androgen plus progestagen combinations. It had been suggested that Asian men have lower spermatogenic potential *(24)*, increased germ cell apoptosis *(25)*, as well as an increased suppression of pulsatile LH secretion in response to exogenous testosterone administration *(26)*.

Table 1
Hormonal Methods of Contraception (Steroid Combinations)[a]

Androgens
    Injectables
        Testosterone enanthate (TE)
        19-Nortestosterone
        Testosterone buciclate (TB)
        Testosterone undecanoate (TU injection)
        Testosterone microspheres
    Implants
        Testosterone pellets
        7a-methyl-19 nortestosterone (MENT)
    Oral
        Testosterone undecanoate
    Transdermal
        Testosterone patches (scrotal and nonscrotal)
        Testosterone gels/creams
Androgens and Progestagens
    TE, T implants, T patches, TU inj, TB with
        Oral
            Levonorgestrel
            Desogestrel
        Implants
            Norplant
            Sinoplant
        Injectables
            Depo medroxyprogesterone acetable
            Norethisterone enanthate
            Levonorgestrel butanoate
Androgens and antiandrogens
    TE/TU oral and injectable with cyproterone acetate
Androgens and estrogens
    Testosterone and estradiol implants

[a]Products in development are shown in italics.

A second study was designed to determine whether men rendered severely oligo–zoospermic (defined as sperm concentration less than 3×10^6/mL) by 200 mg/wk TE administration would also be infertile. The answer to this question was considered very important because, to date, none of the hormonal methods of male contraception could completely suppress spermatogenesis (azoospermia) in all men. When sperm concentration was suppressed to less than 3×10^6/mL in three consecutive semen samples, then the couple would enter an efficacy phase of 12 mo. The testosterone induced severe oligo-zoospermia contraceptive efficacy study included 399 couples from 15 centers in nine countries (sponsored by WHO and by Contraceptive Research and Development Program in the US). Of the subjects, 98% achieved severe oligozoospermia or azoospermia after 6 mo of TE injections and entered the efficacy phase. There were four pregnancies in 49.5 person-years of exposure in men who had sperm concentration between 0.1 and 3×10^6/mL and none in the 230.4 person-years of observation in men who had persistent azoospermia. The combined contraceptive efficacy rate was 1.4 (95% confidence interval of 0.4 to 3.7) per 100 person-years. The occurrence of pregnancies was proportional to the sperm concentration in the ejaculate. Once azoospermia or severe oligozoospermia was attained, rebound of sperm concentration to above 3×10^6/mL was very uncommon (27). These two studies demonstrated for the first time that if a hormonal method of male contraception can render most of the men azoospermic and the remainder severely oligozoospermic, such a method would provide efficacious contraception in the couple. In these studies, as in the previous ones, all couples attained complete recovery of spermatogenesis after withdrawal of TE.

Administration of TE as a weekly injection is clearly not a practical method of contraceptive delivery. Moreover, the pharmacokinetic profile of TE with high initial serum testosterone levels followed by troughs is not the ideal for male fertility regulation. It is perceived that steady levels of testosterone might be associated with less side effects such as acne, oiliness of skin and weight gain.

Other androgen delivery systems are currently being tested or developed which may be more acceptable as a male contraceptive agent. Testosterone implants when inserted into normal volunteers led to suppression of spermatogenesis with similar efficacy as TE weekly injections provided that the serum testosterone levels are maintained in the high normal range with six 200 mg pellets (28). Testosterone biodegradable microspheres when administered to hypogonadal men provided steady serum levels for up to 70 d (29). These microspheres are technically more difficult to produce without batch to batch variations and leeching of testosterone from the microspheres. Testosterone buciclate is a product developed jointly of the WHO and the National Institute of Health. Studies in normal men showed that a single 600 mg injection provided testosterone levels within the physiological range for 16–20 wk (30). When a 1200 mg single injection of testosterone buciclate was administered to eight healthy men, azoospermia was achieved in only three men (31). Testosterone undecanoate as an oral pill was available for many years in Europe, Asia, and Australia as androgen replacement in hypogonadal men. Studies in China showed that when testosterone undecanoate was formulated in oil, a single injection resulted in normal serum testosterone levels for approx 4 wk (32). These injectable androgen preparations as well as transdermal delivery systems, are currently being tested in small scale contraceptive clinical trials in several countries.

The common side effects of androgen administration in normal men included weight gain, acne, gynecomastia, decreases in serum HDL-cholesterol levels and increases in hematocrit (33). Most of the effects are mild and apparently well tolerated by the subjects participating in the clinical studies. The long term effects of maintaining relatively high serum testosterone levels, in normal men are not known. Testosterone administration leads to a decrease in HDL-cholesterol levels without any effect on LDL-cholesterol levels (34,35). Lower HDL-cholesterol levels are associated with increased risk of coronary heart disease. Epidemiological studies, however, showed that lower testosterone levels in men are related to increased risk factors for cardiovascular disease (36,37). There are clearly many factors that may also be involved such as other lipoproteins, coagulation factors, fibrinolytic pathways, endothelial cell response and vascular reactivity. The other major concern with use of androgens is the induction of prostate dysfunction. There is no clear evidence that androgens will induce benign prostatic hyperplasia (BPH) or carcinoma of the prostate (CaP) (38,39). Although androgens are required in childhood and adulthood for BPH to develop, there is no evidence that administration of androgens to normal or hypogonadal men will result in BPH. When androgens are given to hypogonadal men, the prostate size and PSA levels increased to that of normal men. Prostate size and serum level PSA remained within the normal range *(40,41)*. The development of CaP and the progression from focal to metastatic disease is very complex. Factors that are involved include gene mutations, oncogenes, tumor suppression genes, growth factors, the number of trinucleotide repeats of the androgen receptor and androgens *(38,42,43)*. There is no clear evidence to demonstrate that exogenous androgens will lead to development of CaP or progression of histological to clinical disease. These concerns of long term androgen therapy can only be addressed by long term follow-up studies.

Because of these concerns, an androgen which cannot be 5a reduced but can be aromatized might attenuate the effects on the prostate. One such potential androgen is 7a methyl-19 nortestosterone (MENT) which is being developed as an implant,. This androgen is about 10 times as potent as testosterone on gonadotropin suppression but only four times as active on stimulation of prostate size in castrated rats *(44)*. With the recent advances in the understanding of the processes regulating the activation of the androgen receptor, it is foreseeable that androgen agonists and antagonists could be developed similar to the selective estrogen receptor modulators.

Androgen and Prostagen Combinations (Table 1)

Progestagens suppress the hypothalamic-pituitary axis when administered to normal men. Because of the suppression of endogenous testosterone production, progestagens are used together with androgens to prevent the manifestation of hypogonadism. Many androgen-progestagen combinations were used in single or multicenter, small, clinical trials supported by the WHO or the Population council *(20,45)*. The most promising progesterone was depo- medroxyprogesterone acetate (DMPA) in combination with TE or 19 nortestosterone. Combination of injections of DMPA and 19 nortestosterone at three weekly intervals lead to suppression of spermatogenesis to azoospermia in about 60% of normal white men *(46)*, but led to azoospermia in 97% of Indonesian men *(47)*. There were relatively few side effects; libido and erectile functions were retained. The main side effects included weight gain, gynecomastia and lowering of HDL-cholesterol levels.

Recently, the use of androgens plus progestagens was demonstrated to have significant advantage over the use of the same dose of androgen alone with studies of oral levonorgestrel and TE *(48)*. These investigators demonstrated clearly that when 500 mg/d of levonorgestrel was administered together with 100 mg/wk intramuscular injections of TE; this combination was significantly more effective and had a more rapid suppression of sperm concentration to less than 3×10^6/mL than TE alone. It is apparent that combinations of androgens and progestagen might allow lowering the doses of both androgens and progestagens to achieve equivalent goals. The combination of levonorgestrel plus TE suppressed HDL-cholesterol by 24% and total cholesterol by 6%. These and other investigators are studying lower doses of oral levonorgestrel as well as a desogestrel together with androgens. Long acting progestagens (e.g., levonorgestrel butanoate) or progestagen implants (Norplant, Sinoplant) may attain the same effect but have the added advantage of maintaining steady serum progestagen levels and obliterating the first pass effect of oral progestagens on liver lipoprotein metabolism. These androgen-progestagen combinations are being tested in the United States, Europe, and Asia.

Table 2
Hormonal Methods of Contraception
(Gonadotropin Suppressors With or Without Androgens)

GnRH Agonists (D Trp[6], Buserelin, Nafarelin)
   Low dose
   High dose
   Continuous infusion
   Hydrogel
GnRH Antagonist (Nal-Glu, Cetrorelix)
GnRH immunization
FSH immunization
FSH receptor antagonist
FSH antagonists
Inhibin

Antiandrogens and Androgens (Table 1)

Early studies of cyproterone acetate (CPA, an antiandrogen with progestational activity), showed that when CPA was given alone to normal men, suppression of spermatogenesis was incomplete and marked decrease in sexual function was associated with the administration of this antiandrogen (49). Subsequent studies in India suggested that combination of CPA and TE resulted in alleviation of symptoms of androgen insufficiency and marked suppression of sperm concentration (50). These studies were confirmed in a recent study using a combination of CPA plus TE which induced azoospermia or near azoospermia in all subjects. This combination had the advantage of no demonstratable effects on lipid profile and the possibility of lesser effects on the prostate gland (51). However, when CPA was combined with oral undecanoate, the suppression of spermatogenesis is reduced, where azoospermia was observed in two out of eight men (52).

Androgens and Estrogens

Androgens in combination with estradiol have been tested in rats and monkeys and induced suppression of spermatogenesis (53). The advantage of using estrogens would be to neutralize the effects of androgens on lipids. Estrogens have been shown to have synergestic effects with testosterone on prostate growth in dogs (39). Whether estrogens would have synergistic effects with androgens on growth of prostate is not known. A clinical study of androgen plus estrogen implants is currently in progress.

GnRH Analogs and Testosterone (Table 2)

GnRH agonists cause an initial and transient stimulation of gonadotropin secretion followed by progressive pituitary desensitization to GnRH with consequent suppression of FSH and LH secretion. The use of GnRH agonists (D-Trp[6], Buserelin, Nafarelin) together with testosterone had been studied in 12 clinical studies involving over 106 white normal men. The results of these studies were summarized recently (11). When GnRH agonist was administered with varying doses of TE, spermatogenesis was suppressed to azoospermia in only 20% of subjects; another 30% had sperm concentration reduced to less than 5×10^6/mL. To determine the role of treatment paradigms, GnRH agonists were administered by daily subcutaneous injections or continuous infusions.

The latter was not more successful in suppressing spermatogenesis *(54–56)*. Several possible mechanisms could explain the failure of GnRH agonists to completely inhibit spermatogenesis. Firstly, the highest agonist dose used in human clinical trials was 500 mg/d, (such a dose might not be optimal). Secondly, serum FSH levels were less suppressed than LH. Moreover escape of serum FSH some times occurred during GnRH agonist treatment. Thirdly, there was controversy whether androgens when administered with GnRH agonists enhanced or attenuated the spermatogenic suppression induced by GnRH agonists. There was evidence both in primates and humans to demonstrate that exogenous androgens at high doses might interfere with the spermatogenic suppression of GnRH agonists *(57,58)*. On the other hand, synergism between GnRH agonists and testosterone had also been reported to occur in rats and humans *(19,60)*.

A two-center study to examine whether higher doses (1–3 mg/d) of GnRH agonist (D-Trp[6]) together with low-dose TE will increase efficacy of suppression of spermatogenesis is in progress in the US, the data are under review. The advantages of GnRH agonists include lack of side effects of this group of agents and relative lower costs of synthesis compared with the antagonists.

In contrast to GnRH agonists, the GnRH antagonists interfere with the action of the endogenous hormone by competitive binding at the pituitary receptor sites. Through this action, pituitary FSH and LH secretion is rapidly and completely suppressed resulting in reduction of endogenous testosterone production and inhibition of spermatogenesis. These agents were also different from the agonists in that they were expensive to synthesize and frequently give rise to local reaction at the injection sites, presumably related to release of histamine from the mast cells. Three human trials studied the potential of the Nal-Glu GnRH antagonists in combination with various doses of TE as male contraceptives *(61,62)*. Azoospermia was achieved in 60–88% of men administered GnRH antagonists. The time to azoospermia appeared to occur earlier than with androgens alone. Upon withdrawal of the GnRH antagonist and TE, complete recovery of spermatogenesis occurred. The Nal-Glu GnRH antagonists induced pain, redness and weal formation at the injection sites. A new GnRH antagonist, Cetrorelix, has recently been studied in short-term clinical studies *(64,65)*. This GnRH antagonist apparently has little or no local side effects. A study recently completed showed that if azoospermia or severe oligozoospermia was induced by GnRH antagonist plus TE, the suppression of spermatogenesis could be maintained by the physiological dose of TE (100 mg/wk) alone *(66)*. The results of this study are important because this suggests that once suppression of gonadotropins occurred, continued suppression might require less amounts of hormonally based gonadotropin suppressive agents. Future studies with GnRH antagonists may be dependent upon the development of orally or long-acting, possibly nonpeptide GnRH antagonists by molecular drug modeling which might be safer, more acceptable and economical than the peptide analogs.

GnRH vaccines are also under development and have been tested only in men with prostate cancer.

Selective FSH Inhibition

Selective FSH inhibition as a method of male contraceptive is attractive because only spermatogenesis would be suppressed sparing the LH-testosterone axis. This approach has been explored in FSH immunization studies in non-human primates. The results were disappointing either because azoospermia was not attained or the suppression of spermatogenesis was not persistent *(67,68)*. Inhibin, which selectively inhibits FSH, has not been examined in humans. Other investigators are making and studying FSH-receptor antagonists. However, based on the study of men with inactivating mutations of the human FSH receptor, selective inhibition of FSH or FSH action probably would not result in marked or consistent suppression of spermatogenesis. These men with FSH-receptor mutations have varying phenotypes from infertility to proven fertility *(17)*.

FUTURE DEVELOPMENTS IN HORMONAL METHODS OF MALE CONTRACEPTION

In the past decade, significant advances in male contraception development have occurred. It has been shown that if suppression of spermatogenesis to azoospermia (or severe oligozoospermia) is achieved by exogenous administration of hormones, contraceptive efficacy can be attained with rates comparable to female reversible methods. Furthermore, addition of a gonadotropin suppressive agent to androgen will enhance the degree and rate of suppression of spermatogenesis by androgen alone suggesting that physiological doses of androgens may be used when administered in a combination regimen. New synthetic steroids with long-acting potential will become available for clinical investigation in the near future.

In the next decade there will be many new preparations and delivery systems for androgens. Selective androgen receptor modulators will be synthesized which may have strong gonadotropin suppressive activity, maintain sexual function, bone and muscle mass but will have little or no effect on serum lipid profile and the prostate gland. Orally active or long-acting non-peptide GnRH antagonists, with potent receptor blocking activity but without side effects, may become available. Various mechanisms to shorten the lag-time (10–14 wk) between the start of hormone administration and the suppression of spermatogenesis need to be investigated. Combination of an agent acting directly on the epididymis or on spermiogenesis might be used concomitantly with a hormonal method initially to accelerate the development of azoospermia. Studies need to be designed to assess which potential method or modes of administration of contraceptive agents might be acceptable to men from different cultural, ethnic and geographical backgrounds.

ACKNOWLEDGMENT

Supported by the GCRC grant, M01 RR00425 and NIH training grant, DK07571-11. We thank Sally Avancena, MA, for her assistance in the preparation of this manuscript.

REFERENCES

1. Trussel J, Kost K. Contraceptive failure in the United States: a critical review of literature. Studies Family Planning 1987;18:237–283.
2. Liu X, Li S. Vasal sterilization in China. Contraception 1993;48:255–265.
3. National Coordinating Group on Male Antifertility Agents. Gossypol: a new antifertility agent for males. Chinese Med J 1978;4:417–428.
4. Meng GD, Zhu JC, Chen ZW, Wong LT, Zhang GY, Hu YZ, Ding JH, Wang XH, Qian SZ, Wang C, Machin D, Pinol A, Waites GMH. Recovery to normal sperm production following cessation of gossypol treatment: a two center study in China. Int J Androl 1988;11:1–11.
5. Ford WCL, Waites GMH. A reversible contraceptive action of some 6–chloro–6–deoxy sugars in the male rat. J Reprod Fertil 1978;52:152–157.

6. Qian SZ. Tripterygium Wilfordii: a Chinese herb effective in male fertility regulation. Contraception 1987;36:247–263.

7. Qian SZ, Xu Y, Zhang JW. Recent progress in research on tripterygium: a male antifertility plant. Contraception 1995;51:121–129.

8. Lue YH, Sinha–Hikim AP, Wang C, Leung A, Baravarian S, Reutrakul V, Sangsawan R, Chaichang S, Swerdloff RS. Triptolide: a potential male contraceptive. J Andro 1998;in press.

9. Swerdloff RS, Wang C, Bhasin S. Male contraception: 1988 and beyond. In: Burger H, de Kretser D, eds., The Testis, 2nd ed. Raven Press, New York, 1989, pp. 547–568.

10. Waites GMH. Male fertility regulation: the challenges for the year 2000. Br Med Bulletin 1993;49:210–221.

11. Cummings DE, Bremner WJ. Prospects for new hormonal male contraceptives. Endocrinol Metabol Clinics N Am 1994;22:893–922

12. Wang C, Swerdloff RS, Waites GMH, Male contraception: 1993 and beyond. In: Van Look PFA, Perez–Palacio, eds. Contraceptive Research and Development 1984 to 1994, Oxford University Press, Delhi, 1994, pp. 121–134.

13. Clermont Y. The cycle of seminiferous epithelium in man. Am J Anat 1963;112:35–51.

14. Matsumoto AM, Paulsen CA, Bremner WJ. Stimulation of sperm production by human luteinizing hormone in gonadotropin–suppressed normal men. J Clin Endocrinol Metab 1984;59:882–885.

15. Matsumoto AM, Karpas AE, Bremner WJ. Chronic human chorionic gonadotropin administration in normal men: evidence that follicle stimulating hormone is necessary for maintenance of quantitatively normal spermatogenesis in man. J Clin Endocrinol Metab 1986;62:1184–1192.

16. Kumar TR, Wang Y, Lu N, Matzuk MM. Follicle stimulating hormone is required for ovarian follicle maturation but not male fertility. Nature Genetics 1997;15:201–204.

17. Tapanainen JA, Ailtomaki K, Min J, Vaskivuo T, Huhtaniemi IT. Men homozygous for an inactivating mutation of the follicle–stimulating hormone (FSH) receptor gene present variable suppression of spermatogenesis and fertility. Nature Genetics 1997;15:205,206.

18. Cunningham GR, Silverman VE, Kohler DO. Clinical evaluation of testosterone enanthate for induction and maintenance of reversible azoospermia in man. In: Patanelli DJ, ed. Hormonal Control of Male Fertility, DHEW Publication (NIH), Bethesda, MD, 78–1097, 1978, pp. 71–92.

19. Mauss J, Borsch G, Bormacher K, Richter E, Leyendecker G. Seminal fluid analyses, serum FSH, LH and testosterone in seven males before, during and after 250 mg testosterone enanthate weekly over 21 weeks. In: Patanelli DJ, ed. Hormonal control of male fertility, US DHEW (NIH), Bethesda, MD, 1978, pp. 93–122.

20. Paulsen CA, Bremner WJ, Leonard JM. Male Contraception: clinical trials. In: Mishell, DR Jr, ed. Raven Press, New York, 1982, pp. 157–170.

21. Swerdloff RS, Palacios A, McClure RD, Campfield LA, Brosman SA. Clinical evaluation of testosterone enanthate in the reversible suppression of spermatogenesis in the human male: efficacy, mechanism of action, and adverse effects. In: Patanelli DJ, ed. Hormonal control of male fertility, US DHEW (NIH), Bethesda, MD, 1978, pp. 41–70.

22. Patanelli DJ (ed). Hormonal control of male fertility. US DHEW Publication No. (NIH), Bethesda, MD, 1978;78–1097.

23. World Health Organization Task Force on Methods for the Regulation of Male Fertility. Contraceptive efficacy of testosterone-induced azoospermia in normal men. Lancet 1990;336:955–59.

24. Johnson L, Barnard JJ, Rodriguez L, Smith EC, Swerdloff RS, Wang XH, Wang C. Ethnic difference in testicular structure and spermatogenic potential may predispose testes of Asian men to a heightened sensitivity to steroidal contraceptives. J Androl 1998;19:348-357.

25. Sinha–Hikim A, Wang C, Lue YH, Johnson L, Wang XH, Swerdloff RS. Spontaneous germ cell apoptosis in human: evidence for ethnic differences in the susceptability of germ cells to programmed cell death. J Clin Endocrinol Metab 1998;83:152–156.

26. Wang C, Berman NG, Veldhuis JD, Der T, McDonald V, Steiner B, Swerdloff RS. Graded testosterone infusions distinguish gonadotropin negative feedback responsiveness in Asian and White men: a Clinical Research Center Study. J Clin Endocrinol Metab 1998;83:870–876.

27. World Health Organization Task Force on Methods for the Regulation of Male Fertility. Contraceptive efficacy of testosterone–induced azoospermia and oligozoospermia in normal men. Fertil Steril 1996;65:821–829.

28. Handelsman DJ, Conway AJ, Boylan LM. Suppression of human spermatogenesis by testosterone implants in man. J Clin Endocrinol Metab 1992;75:1326–1332.

29. Bhasin S, Swerdloff RS, Steiner B, Peterson MA, Meridores T, Galmirini M, Pandrian MR, Goldberg R, Berman N. A biodegradable testosterone microcapsule formulation provides uniform eugonadal levels of testosterone for 10 to 11 weeks in hypogonadal men. J Clin Endocrinol Metabol 1992;74:75–83.

30. Behre HM, Nieschlag E. Testosterone buciclate (20 Act–1) in hypogonadal men: pharmacokinetics and pharmacodynamics of the new long–acting androgen ester. J Clin Endocrinol Metab 1992;75:12.

31. Behre HM, Baus S, Kliesch S, Keck C, Simoni M, Nieschlag N. Potential of testosterone buciclate for male contraception: endocrine differences betwen responders and non-responders. J Clin Endocrinol Metab 1995;80:2394–2403.

32. Zhang GY, Gu YO, Wang XH, Cui YG, Bremner WJ. Pharmacokinetic study of injectable testosterone undecanoate in hypogonadal men. J Androl 1998;in press.

33. Wu FCW, Farley TMM, Peregoudov A, Waites GMH, World Health Organization Task Force on Methods for the Regulation of Male Fertility . Effects of testosterone enanthate in normal men: experience from a multicenter contraceptive efficacy study. Fertil Steril 1996;65:626–636.

34. Freidl KE, Jones RE, Hannan CJ, Plymate SJ. The administration of pharmacological doses of testosterone or 19–nortestosterone to normal men is not associated with increased insulin secretion or impaired glucose tolerance. J Clin Endocrinol Metab 1989;68:971.

35. Bagatell CJ, Herman JR, Matsumoto AM, Rivier JE, Bermner WJ. Metabolic and behavioral effects of high-dose, exogenous testosterone in healthy men. J Clin Endocrinol Metab. 1994;79:561–567.

36. Barrett-Connor E. Lower endogenous androgen levels and dyslipidemia in men with non–insulin dependent diabetes mellitus. Ann Int Med 1992;117:807–811.

37. Simon D, Charles M-A, Nahoul K, Orssand G, Kremski J, Hully V, Jonbert E, Papoz K, Eschwege E. Association between plasma total testosterone and cardiovascular risk factors in healthy adult men: the Telecom Study. J Clin Endocrinol Metab 1997;82:682–685.

38. Meikle AW, Smith JA. Epidemiology of prostate cancer. Urol Clin N Am 1990;17:709–718.

39. McConnell JD. Epidemiology, etiology, pathophysiology, and diagnosis of benign prostatic hyperplasia. In: Walsh K, Retik AB,Vaughan ED,Wein AJ, eds. Campbell's Urology, 7th ed. W. B. Saunders, Philadelphia, 1991, pp. 1429–1452.

40. Behre HM, Bohmeyer J, Nieschlag E. Prostate volume in testosterone-treated and untreated hypogonadal men in comparison to age-matched normal controls. Clin Endo 1994;40:341–49.

41. Meikle AW, Arver S, Dobs AS, Adolfsson J, Sanders SW, Middleton RG, Stephersen RA, Hoover DR, Rajaram L, Mazer NA. Prostate size in hypogonadal men treated with a nonscrotal permeation-enhanced testosterone transdermal system. Urology1997; 49:191–6.

42. McConnell JD. Physiologic basis of endocrine therapy for prostatic cancer. Urol Cl N Amer. 1991;19:1–13.

43. Pienta KJ. Etiology, epidemiology and prevention of carcinoma of the prostate. In: Walsh PC, Retik AB, Vaughan ED Wein AJ, eds. Campbell's Urology, 7th ed. W. B. Saunders, Philadelphia, 1997, pp. 2489–96.

44. Kumar N, Didolkar AK, Monder C, Bardin CW, Sundaran K. The biological activity of 7 a-methyl-19-nortestosterone is not amplified in male reproductive tract as is that of testosterone. Endocrinology 1992;130:3677–3683.

45. Schearer SB, Alvarez-Sanchez F, Anselmo J, Brenner P, Continlo E, Latham-Foundes A, Frick J, Heinild B, Johansson EDB. Hormonal contraception for men. Int J Andrology Suppl 1978;2:680–712.

46. Knuth UA, Nieschlag E. Endocrine approaches to male fertility control. J Clin Endocrinol Metab 1987;1:113–131.

47. World Health Organization Task Force on Methods for the Regulation of Male Fertility. Comparison of two androgens plus depo-medroxyprogesterone acetate for suppression to azoospermia in Indonesian men. Fertil Steril 1993;60:1062–68.

48. Bebb RA, Anawalt BD, Christiansen RB, Paulsen CA, Bremner WJ, Matsumoto AM. Combined administration of levonorgestrel and testosterone induces more rapid and effective suppression of spermatogenesis than testosterone alone: a promising male contraceptive approach. J Clin Endocrinol Metab 1996;81:757–62.

49. Wang C, Yeung KC. Use of low-dosage cyprosterone acetate as a male contraceptive. Contraception 1980;21:245–272.

50. Roy S. Experience in the development of hormonal contraceptive for the male. In: Asch RH, ed. Recent Advances in Human Reproduction. Fondazione per gli Studi Sulla Riproduzione Umana, Rome, 1985, pp. 95–104.

51. Meriggiola MC, Bremner WJ, Paulsen CA, Valdiserri A, Incorvaia L, Motta R, Pavani A, Capelli M, Flamigni C. A combined regimen of cyproterone acetate and testosterone enanthate as a potentially highly effective male contraceptive. J Clin Endocrinol Metab 1996;81:3018–3023.

52. Meriggiola MC, Bremner WJ, Costantino A, Pavani A, Capelli H, Flamigni C. An oral regimen of cyproterone acetate and testosterone undecanoate for spermatogenic suppression in men. Fertil Steril 1987;68:844–850.
53. Ewing L. Effects of testosterone and estradiol, silastic implants, on spermatogenesis in rats and monkeys. In: Patanelli DJ, ed. Hormonal Control of Male Fertility. US DHEW Publication No. (NIH), Bethesda, MD, 78–1097, 1978, pp. 173–194.
54. Bhasin S, Heber D, Steiner BS, Handelsman DJ, Swerdloff RS. Hormonal effects of gonadotropin-releasing hormone (GnRH) agonist and androgen. J Clin Endocrinol Metab 1985;60:998–1003.
55. Bhasin S, Steiner B, Swerdloff RS. Does constant infusion of gonadotropin-releasing hormone agonist lead to greater suppression of gonadal function in man thanits intermittent administration? Fertil Steril 1985;44:96–101.
56. Pavlou SN, Interlandi JW, Wakefield G, Rivier J, Vale W, Rabin D. Heterogeneity of sperm density profiles following 16-week therapy with continuous infusion of high-dose LHRH analog plus testosterone. J Androl 1986;7:228–233.
57. Bouchard P, Garcia E. Influence of testosterone substitution on sperm suppression by LHRH agonists. Horm Res 1987;28:175–180.
58. Behre HM, Nashan D, Hubert W, Nieschlag E. Depot gonadotropin-releasing hormone agonist blunts the androgen-induced suppression of spermatogenesis in a clinical trial of male contraception. J Clin Endocrinol Metab 1992;74:84–90.
59. Heber D, Swerdloff RS. Male contraception: synergism of gonadotropin-releasing hormone analog and testosterone in suppressing gonadotropin. Science 1980;209:936–938.
60. Bhasin S, Heber D, Steiner B, Peterson M, Blaisch B, Campfield LA, Swerdloff RS. Hormonal effects of GnRH agonist in the human male: II. Testosterone enhances gonadotrophin suppression induced by GnRH agonist. Clin Endocrinol 1984;20:119–128.
61. Pavlou SN, Wakefield GB, Island DP, Hoffman PG, LePage ME, Chan RL, Nerenberg CA, Kovacs WJ. Suppression of pituitary-gonadal function by a potent new luteinizing hormone-releasing hormone antagonist in normal men. J Clin Endocrinol Metab 1987;64:931–936.
62. Tom L, Bhasin S, Salameh W, Steiner B, Peterson M, Sokol RZ, Riveier J, Vale W, Swerdloff RS. Induction of azoospermia in normal men with combined Nal-Glu gonadotropin-releasing hormone antagonist and testosterone enanthate. J Clin Endocrinol Metab 1992;75:476–483.
63. Bagatell CJ, Matsumoto AM, Christensen RB, Rivier JE, Bremner WJ. Comparison of a gonadotropin releasing-hormone antagonist plus testosterone (T) versus T alone as potential male contraceptive regimens. J Clin Endocrinol Metab 1993;77:427–432.
64. Behre HM, Klein B, Steinmeyer E, McGregor GP, Voigt K, Nieschlag E. Effective suppression of luteinizing hormone and testosterone by single doses of the new gonadotropin-releasing hormone antagonist cetrorelix (SB-75) in normal men. J Clin Endocrinol Metab 1992;75:393–398.
65. Behre HM, Kliesch S, Puhse G, Reissmann T, Nieschlag E. High loading and low maintenance doses of a gonadotropin-releasing antagonist effectively suppress serum luteinizing hormone, follicle-stimulating hormone, and testosterone in normal men. J Clin Endocrinol Metab 1997;82:1403–1408.
66. Swerdloff RS, Bagatell CJ, Wang C, Anawalt BD, Steiner B, Berman N, Bremner WJ. Suppression of spermatogenesis in man induced by Nal-Glu gonadotropin releasing hormone antagonist and testosterone enanthate is maintained by testosterone enanthate alone. J Clin Endocrinol Metab 1998;83:2749-2757.
67. Murty GSRC, Rani CSS, Moudgal NR, Prasad MRN. Effect of passive immunization with specific antiserum to FSH on the spermatogenic process and fertility of male bonnet monkeys (macaca radiata). J Reprod Fertil (Suppl) 1979;26:147–154.
68. Nieschlag E. Reasons for abandoning immunization against FSH as an approach to fertility regulation. In: Zatuchini GI, Goldsmith A, Spieler JM, Sciana JJ, eds. Male Contraception: Advances and Future Prospects. Harper & Row, Philadelphia, 1985, pp. 395–399.

VII WOMEN

21

Primary and Secondary Hypogonadism in Women

C. Matthew Peterson, MD, FACOG, and Lawrence C. Udoff, MD, FACOG

INTRODUCTION

Hormone replacement of hypogonadal women is a highly effective preventive health care measure. Estrogen replacement results in a nearly a 50% reduction in the risks of cardiovascular disease, vertebral and hip fractures, and Alzheimer's disease. Hypogonadal symptomatology such as hot flushes, irritability, anxiety, mood disturbances, loss of libido and genitourinary atrophy are reduced and often alleviated by estrogen replacement. Numerous estrogen formulations and delivery systems are available and reviewed. Progestogens are utilized in women with a uterus to reduce the risk of endometrial hyperplasia and endometrial cancer. Available progestogen formulations are discussed. The role of androgens, phytoestrogens, and DHEA in hormone replacement therapy (HRT) are noted. Risks and complications of HRT are outlined, including the potential risk of breast cancer, reduced cardiovascular benefits after long-term use, and nuisance side effects. The future role of selective estrogen receptor modulators (SERM's) is highlighted.

HYPOGONADISM

Hypogonadism is characterized by low or undetectable circulating levels of gonadal steroids. In women, this specifically refers to lower than normal levels of estrogens, progesterone and androgens, the principal steroidal products of the ovary. Hypogonadism may be the result of a variety of different etiologic factors. In primary hypogonadism, patients never or only briefly express normal ovarian steroid synthesis. The classical presentation is gonadal dysgenesis associated with the 45, XO chromosomal

From: *Contemporary Endocrinology: Hormone Replacement Therapy*
Edited by: A. W. Meikle © Humana Press Inc., Totowa, NJ

abnormality, Turner's Syndrome. Secondary hypogonadism may be caused by several different factors, including the aging process (natural menopause), surgical castration (surgical menopause), radiation or chemotherapy (iatrogenic ovarian failure), or autoimmune or genetic factors resulting in the earlier than expected cessation of ovarian function (premature menopause). The pathophysiology and differential diagnosis of these conditions have been extensively reviewed in other texts. This chapter will primarily focus on the treatment of these conditions, which may be discussed almost irrespective of the particular diagnosis, because all these disorders share a common treatment goal: the elimination or attenuation of the complications incurred as a result of sex steroid hormone deficiency.

RATIONALE FOR TREATMENT

Prior to discussing specific hormone replacement regimens, it is important to understand clearly the goals of treatment. In general, these goals may be divided into two categories, immediate and long range. Immediate treatment goals address the present symptomatology of the hypogonadal patient, and long-range treatment goals are concerned with the prevention of long-term sequella associated with hypogonadism.

Patients with primary hypogonadism are usually referred by primary physicians for the purpose of initiating normal pubertal development, secondary sexual characteristics, and the establishment of menstrual bleeding. Patients with secondary hypogonadism, regardless of etiology, will often present with a constellation of symptoms attributed to the loss of sex steroid production. The most widely recognized of these symptoms is the hot flush, commonly referred to as "hot flash." Seventy percent of women will experience hot flushes within 3 mo of natural or surgical menopause (1). Approximately 55% of women will continue to experience these symptoms for the following 5 yr. Thirty-five percent of women will continue to have symptoms after 5 yr, through it is generally less frequent and intense. Other common complaints include irritability/anxiety, insomnia, mood disturbances and loss of libido. Physical complaints may include vaginal dryness and irritation (due to vaginal atrophy) and urinary incontinence.

Hypogonadism is also associated with an elevated risk of several serious diseases. One that is likely to have the most impact on a patient's health is the increased risk of cardiovascular disease. The evidence for this association is based mainly on epidemiological data illustrating an increased risk of cardiovascular disease with natural or surgical menopause (2) and the reduction of this risk by as much as 50% in patients receiving hormone replacement therapy (3–9). In a similar manner, hypogonadism is associated with osteoporosis and an increased fracture risk. Changes in bone metabolism that lead to osteoporosis are closely related to the decline in ovarian function. Estrogen replacement has been shown to reduce bone turnover and increase bone mineral density. Specifically, hormone replacement therapy (HRT) with estrogen reduces the risk of vertebral fractures (40%) and hip fractures (>50%) (10–14).

Alzheimer's disease has an age specific incidence that is 1.5–3 times higher in women than men (15). Recent work has demonstrated nearly a 50% reduction in the incidence of Alzheimer's Disease in estrogen users compared to nonusers (16–20). Theoretical explanations for estrogen's beneficial effects include: enhancement of growth proteins associated with axonal elongation, nerve processes and synapse formation (21); increases in choline acetyl transferase which is critical to acetylcholine production (22); and antioxidant and anti-inflammatory properties (23).

With the goals of disease prevention and the elimination of hypogonadal symptomatology in mind, the remainder of this chapter will review the numerous hormone replacement strategies available. Despite the health benefits, only 30% of patients eligible for HRT currently utilize treatment. One study documented that of women prescribed HRT, 20–30% never fill the prescription, 10% only report intermittent use and 20% discontinue treatment within 9 mo *(24)*. These statistics serve to emphasize the importance of tailoring the treatment and side effect profiles to the individual.

HORMONE REPLACEMENT STRATEGIES

Estrogens

Estrogens effects on multiple organs systems make it one of the most potent multipurpose drugs in the physician's armamentarium. Primary and secondary hypogonoadotrophic individuals utilize estrogens: for the initiation and maintenance of secondary sexual characteristics; to promote cardiovascular, bone, memory, cognitive, and genitourinary health; and, to avoid vasomotor symptoms and their related mental and emotional sequella. Numerous preparations are now available for hypoestrogenic states (Table 1). Potency of these preparations is based on molecular-binding constants, as well as activities in various bioassays, the ability to suppress gonadotropins, and/or induce hepatic synthesis (Table 2). The choice between various medications is dependent on the individual patient's particular medical situation, side effect profiles, and her particular needs and concerns *(25)*.

CLASSICAL ESTROGEN RECEPTOR CONCEPTS–ESTROGEN RECEPTOR ALPHA

Estrogen activity is dependent on binding with the estrogens receptor. This binding facilitates interaction of the DNA binding region of the receptor with cellular DNA and ultimately results in the protein product of estrogen responsive genes. The estrogen receptor is a member of the steroid receptor superfamily which contains the vitamin D, retinoic acid, and thyroid hormone receptors. These receptors conserve both the ligand and DNA binding areas. The ligand or hormone binding area is approximately 250 amino acids and is hydrophobic. Transactivating function-1 (TAF-1) site is both cell and promotor specific and has constitutive activity for the receptor. The TAF-2 site in the steroid binding domain is inducible by the ligand. The DNA binding region can fold into two dissimilar zinc fingers to interact with the estrogen responsive gene. The longer the estrogen remains bound to the complex the more potent the hormone. Proteins transcribed (estrogen responsive genes) are cell specific (i.e., hepatocytes increase protein synthesis and cervical cells produce cervical mucous) (Fig. 1) *(26)*.

CONJUGATED EQUINE ESTROGENS

The most widely utilized estrogens in hormone replacement therapy are conjugated equine estrogens (CEEs). This formulation is a combination of over ten different estrogenic compounds found in pregnant mare's urine. By US Pharmacopeia standards, the estrogenic content of CEEs are: sodium estrone sulfate 52.5–61.5%, sodium equilin sulfate 22.5–30.5%, 17 alpha-dihydroequilin sulfate 13.5–19.5%, sodium 17 alpha-estradiol sulfate 2.5%, and sodium 17 beta-dihydroequilin sulfate 0.5–4%. The major components are depicted in Fig. 2. The complexity of the receptor-ligand complexes of the various components and their metabolic derivatives renders a complete understanding of the pharamcokinetics problematic *(27)*.

Table 1
Approximate Serum Estrone and Estradiol Levels
After Various Doses and Formulations of Common Estrogens

Brand name	Estrogen	Daily dose* (mg)	Estrone (pg/mL)	Estradiol (pg/mL)
Oral				
Estrace®[a]	Micronized estradiol	1	150	40
		2	250	60
Estradiol, USP[b]		0.5	n/a	n/a
		1.0	n/a	n/a
		2.0	n/a	n/a
Ogen®[c]	Piperazine estrone sulfate (estropipate)	0.75	125	30
Ortho-Est®[d]		1.5	200	40
Estropipate, USP[e]		3.0	n/a	n/a
Menest®[f]	Esterfield estrogens	0.3	n/a	n/a
Estratab®[g]		0.625		
		1.25		
		2.5		
Estratest® H.S.[h]	Esterified estrogens plus 1.25 mg methyltestosterone	0.625	n/a	n/a
Estratest	Esterified estrogens plus 2.5 mg methyltestosterone	1.25		
Tace®[i]	Chlorotrianisene	12	n/a	n/a
Premarin®[j]	Conjugated equine estrogen	0.3	75	20
		0.625	150	40
		1.25	200	60
Vaginal creams				
Premarin®[k]	Conjugated equine estrogens	1.25	120	35
		2.5	170	65
Ogen®[l]	Piperazine estrone sulfate	1.5	n/a	n/a
Estrace®[m]	Micronized estradiol	0.1	n/a	n/a
Dienstrol®[n]	Dienstrol	0.1	n/a	n/a
Estradiol pellets				
	Estradiol pellet (not available in US)	25	n/a	60
Transdermal systems	Daily/total patch size			
Climara®[o]	Estradiol-weekly patch	0.05/3.9 mg (1.25 cm^2)	20–40	35
		0.1/7.8 mg (25 cm^2)	40–60	70
Estraderm®[p]	Estradiol-biweekly patch	0.05/4 mg (10 cm^2)	12	30
		0.1/9 mg (20 cm^2)	25	73

Table 1 (*continued*)

Brand name	Estrogen	Daily dose* (mg)	Estrone (pg/mL)	Estradiol (pg/mL)
Alora®q	Estradiol bi-weekly patch	0.05/1.5 mg	n/a	n/a
Vivelle®r	Estradiol-biweekly patch	0.0375/3.3 mg (11 cm^2)	12	30
		0.05/4.3 mg (14 cm^2)	25	50
		0.075/6.6 mg (22 cm^2)	35	75
		0.1/8.6 mg (29 cm^2)	50	90
FemPatch®s	Estradiol-weekly	0.025	10.3 mg	25
Vaginal ring system				
Estring®t	Estradiol	2–9 d	60	50

*Physicians should consult detail information supplied by the manufacturer before use.
[a]Estrace, Bristol-Myers Squibb, Princeton, NJ.
[b]Estradiol Tablets, USP, Watson, Corona, CA.
[c]Ogen Tablets, Pharmacia-Upjohn, Kalamazoo, MI.
[d]Ortho-Est Tablets, Ortho-McNeil Pharmaceuticals, Raritan, NJ.
[e]Estropipate Tablets, USP, Watson, Corona, CA.
[f]Menest Tablets, SmithKline Beecham Pharmaceuticals.
[g]Estratab Tablets, Solvay, Marietta, GA.
[h]Estratest Tablets, Solvay, Marietta, GA.
[i]Tace, Hoechst & Marion Roussel, Kansas City, MO.
[j]Premarin Tablets, Wyeth-Ayerst, Philadelphia, PA.
[k]Premarin Vaginal Cream, Wyeth-Ayerst, Philadelphia, PA.
[l]Ogen Vaginal Cream, Pharmacia-Upjohn, Kalamazoo, MI.
[m]Estrace Vaginal Cream, Bristol-Myers Squibb, Princeton, NJ.
[n]Dienstrol, Alora, Proctor & Gamble Pharmaceuticals, Cincinnati, OH.
[o]Climara Transdermal System, Berlex, Wayne, NJ.
[p]Estraderm Transdermal System, CibaGeneva, Summit, NJ.
[q]Alora, Proctor & Gamble Pharmaceuticals, Cincinnati, OH.
[r]Vivelle Transdermal System, CibaGeneva, Summit, NJ.
[s]FemPatch, Parke-Davis, Morris Plains, NJ.
[t]Estring Vaginal Ring, Pharmacia-Upjohn, Kalamazoo, MI.
Premphase, Wyeth-Ayerst, Philadelphia, PA.
Prempro, Wyeth-Ayerst, Philadelphia, PA.

Table 2
Relative Potency of Various Oral Estrogens

Estrogen	Serum FSH	Serum CBG-BC	Serum SHBG	Serum angiotensinogen
Estropipate	1.1	1.0	1.0	1.0
Micronized estradiol	1.3	1.9	1.0	0.7
Conjugated estrogens	1.4	2.5	3.2	3.5
DES	3.8	70	28	13
Ethinyl estradiol	80–200 (est)	1000 (est)	614	232

Adapted with permission from ref. *25*.

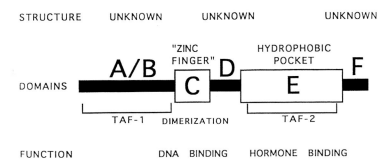

Fig. 1. Structural and functional organization of the estrogen receptor. The different domains perform different functions. The DNA binding domain (C) and the hormone binding domain (E) are the best characterized, but other important areas must be considered: TAF-1 is both cell and promoter specific and can produce constitutive activity for the receptor; the TAF-2 site, in the steroid binding domain, is inducible by the ligand. There is also a region of a few amino acids that is believed to be essential to dimerize the liganded receptor when it is located at the hormone-response element. Reprinted with permission from ref. *26*.

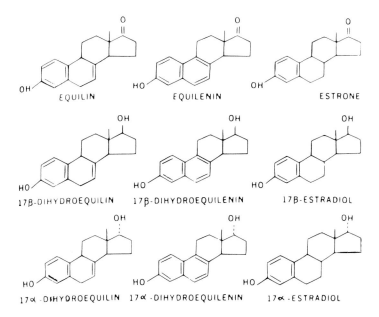

Fig. 2. The estrogenic compounds found in the urine of pregnant mares (conjugated equine estrogens). Reprinted with permission from ref. *26a*.

Once absorbed and metabolized through the liver, the estrogens circulate primarily as sulfated conjugates. These conjugated (sulfated) forms are bound primarily to albumin which significantly prolongs their half life and establishes a reservoir of estrogens. Only the hepatocyte has a membrane which is permeable to sulfated estrogens. A major portion of the activity of CEEs are attributed to the hepatic regeneration of estradiol from this conjugated estrogen reservoir. The remainder of the biologic activity of CEEs is assigned to the equine estrogens equilin and equilenin. These equine estrogens are chemically referred to as ring B unsaturated estrogens because of the additional one or two double bonds in the B ring (Fig. 2).

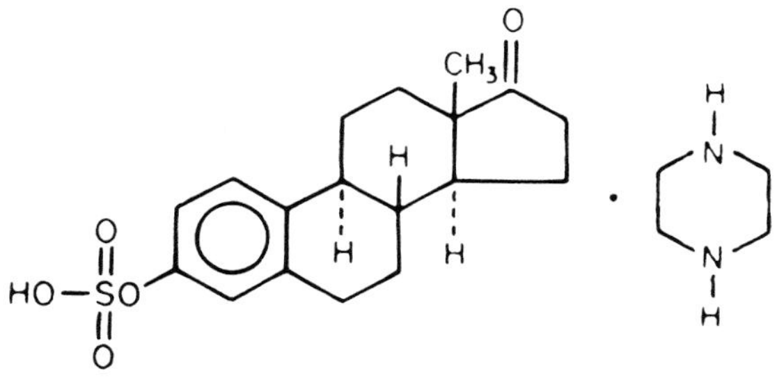

Fig. 3. Estropipate.

Equilin is known to be significantly more potent with regard to hepatic protein synthesis relative to estrone sulfate *(28)*. The pronounced hepatic protein synthesis activity of CEEs, particularly equilin, theoretically may be beneficial when considering improved lipid parameters and detrimental when considering renin substrate (angiotensinogen) *(29)*, and clotting factors *(30,31)*. With regards to the risk of deep venous thrombosis (DVT) while on hormone replacement, recent studies suggest a potentially increased risk in estrogen users which was restricted solely to the first year of use. This finding may indicate an underlying risk factor which was not controlled for such as Leiden Factor V mutation *(32)*.

Generic CEE preparations were removed from the United States market in 1991 owing to the possibility of bioinequivalence and significant differences in chemical composition *(33,34)*.

ESTERIFIED ESTROGENS

The major difference between esterified estrogens and CEEs is the percentage of estrone sulfate and equilin sulfate. Esterified estrogens have 75–85% estrone sulfate and 6–15% of sodium equilin sulfate (52.5–61.5% and 22.5–30.5% for CEE, respectively). Less than 10% are minor estrogen compounds (ring B unsaturated equine estrogens) compared to CEEs which contain up to 25% minor estrogens. Esterified estrogens are water soluble and are easily absorbed. The pharmacokinetics and hepatic metabolism resulting in the regeneration of estradiol from the conjugated (sulfated) estrone reservoir are very similar to CEEs.

ESTROPIPATE

Conjugated (sulfated) estrone is soluble and attains stability when combined with a molecule of piperazine. Estropipate is the compound piperazine estrone sulfate (Fig. 3). Piperazine is pharmacologically inert and is utilized only for its ability to stabilize the compound. Piperazine and estrone sulfate are combined in a 1:1 ratio. A dose of 0.75 mg of estropipate is equivalent to 0.625 mg of CEEs. Oral absorption is good and the drug is metabolized in the liver. Estropipate administration results in high serum concentrations of estrone sulfate, just as with CEEs. Likewise, the effects of estropipate are considered to be the result of hepatic regeneration of estradiol from the estrone sulfate reservoir.

ESTRADIOL

Natural estradiol is the common denominator of biologic activity of most of the administered estrogens (Fig. 4). It is poorly absorbed in its natural form and is

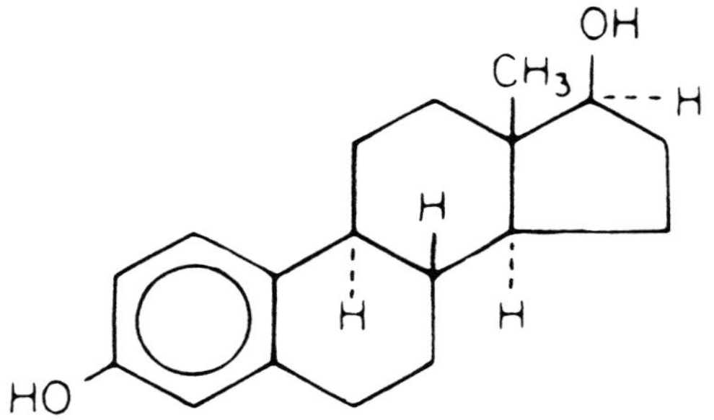

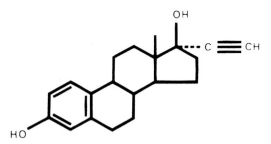

Fig. 4. Estradiol.

Fig. 5. Ethinyl Estradiol.

metabolized rapidly in a first pass effect. For this reason, micronization (micronized estradiol), or acetylation (ethinyl estradiol) are required for effective oral preparations. Micronization avoids the poor absorption through delivering the drug in particles <20 μm in diameter which allows the whole intestinal mucosa to absorb the compound *(35)*. Ethinyl estradiol is synthesized by the acetylation of estradiol with an ethinyl group at position C-17 (Fig. 5).

After absorption of any of the micronized estradiol compounds, the majority of the steroid is metabolized within the intestinal mucosa and liver to estrone sulfate (65%) and estrone (15%) *(36,37)*. As in the case of CEEs, esterified estrogens, and estropipate, the circulating reservoir of estrone sulfate and estrone created after the metabolism of absorbed micronized estradiol serves as the pool for the regeneration of estradiol *(38)*. Estrogenic induction of hepatic protein synthesis with the synthetic micronized estradiol preparations is significantly less than that found with CEEs, which may be of particular benefit when considering some relative contraindication (e.g., clotting factors in an immobilized patient, patient with personal or family history of elevated triglycerides) *(25)*.

Ethinyl estradiol is much more potent than the native steroid estradiol because it is a relatively poor substrate for the activity of 17 beta estradiol dehydrogenase which normally converts estradiol to estrone *(39)* (Table 2). Because it is spared from the rapid D ring metabolism its potency is prolonged and this effect is present regardless of oral or parenteral administration. Despite the protective C-17 acetylene group, significant metabolism by the gut and liver do occur resulting in a peripheral conversion bioavailability of somewhere between 38–59% *(40)*.

Ethinyl estradiol metabolized in the liver is converted to ethinyl estradiol-3-sulfate. This sulfated pool does not serve as a reservoir for the creation of estradiol as estrone

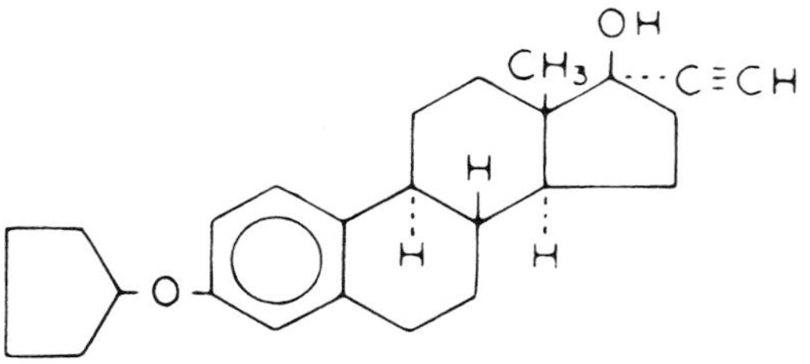

Fig. 6. Quinestrol.

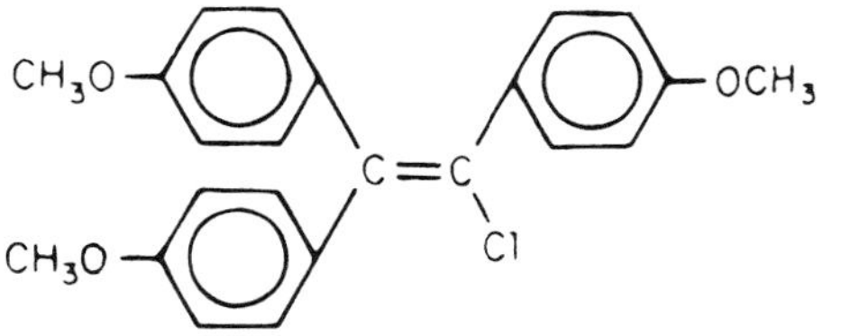

Fig. 7. Chlorotrianisene.

sulfate does for CEEs, esterified estrogens, or estropipate. Ethinyl estradiol is also a potent simulator of hepatic protein synthesis as are CEEs.

QUINESTROL

Quinestrol, the 3-cyclopentyl ether derivative of estradiol is a prodrug with no inherent estrogenic activity of its own (Fig. 6). After nearly complete absorption, intestinal and hepatic metabolism results in the formation of ethinyl estradiol and cyclopentanol. The metabolism and availability of ethinyl estradiol is as described previously.

The alkyl ether group provides resistance to hepatic metabolism, and also enhances the prodrug's lipophilicity resulting in adipose storage. This adipose storage provides a half- life of over 120 h. Thus, the alkyl ether group provides a sustained reservoir of available prodrug and allows for seven day dosing intervals. Because of these properties, quinestrol is 2–3 times more potent than ethinyl estradiol (39,42). Quinestrol is not presently marketed.

CHLOROTRIANISENE

Chlorotrianisene is a derivative of diethylstilbestrol with only 1/8 the potency of DES (Fig. 7). This drug also has extensive lipophilicity and is metabolized into other estrogenic substances after ingestion. Its potency hence is reduced if given parenterally.

Methods of Estrogen Delivery

Various preparations and their methods of administration are outlined in Table 1.

Oral administration is the most common regimen prescribed. Poor absorption of insoluble estrogens requires modification through conjugation (CEEs, esterified estrogens, estropipate) or micronization (micronized estradiol). Additionally, synthetic molecules allow oral administration (ethinyl estradiol, quinestrol, chlorotrianisene). Increased potency and prolonged half-lives make the synthetic forms less commonly utilized for hormone replacement. Oral micronized estradiol administration results in rapid conversion to estrone and estrone-3-glucuronide. Phenytoin can increase this metabolic step and reduce the desired estrogen effects. This does not occur when administered transdermally or vaginally. Transdermally administered estradiol theoretically may reduce some of the beneficial hepatic effects on lipids. Conversely, it may be the preferred method in those with a personal or family history of elevated triglycerides or who are immobilized and at risk for thromboembolic events. Transdermal delivery is particularly convenient and preferred in the postoperative state. Skin sensitivity in transdermal administration occurs in a proportion of patients and may preclude their use. Injectable estrogen administration results in higher rates of endometrial hyperplasia and addictive behavior secondary to widely fluctuating estrogen levels and other factors and is not routinely recommended *(43)*.

Vaginal preparations effectively administer estradiol and avoid hepatic effects (increased SHBG, renin substrate (angiotensinogen), and hepatic coagulation factors). Concerns over the removal of estrogen containing implants has kept this delivery system from the market in the United States.

The Breast in the Treatment of Primary Hypogonadism

Particular attention to a near–physiologic addition estrogen is required for some duration (often up to 2 yr) in order to maximize breast development in the woman with primary hypogonadism. If progestogens are added immediately with the onset of replacement therapy breast development is abnormal and often minimal. Our approach has been to initiate low dose estrogen (0.3 mg CEEs or equivalent) while monitoring breast development. Once adequate development is attained a progestogen is added. The period of isolated low dose estrogen required can be as long 1–2 yr. It is rare to induce uterine bleeding with low dose estrogen alone , but should it occur, endometrial sampling and progestogen administration is indicated.

The Future: Estrogen Receptors
Alpha and Beta and Selective Estrogen Receptor Modulators

Interactions of the estrogen receptor/ligand complexes with the DNA estrogen response element results in estrogen responsive gene transcription. In 1995, a second estrogen receptor (estrogen receptor beta) was discovered and cloned *(44,45)*. Although the two receptors appear similar physically, their distribution and subsequent gene transcriptions are very different depending on the site and substance, or ligand, binding to the receptor. Specific conformations of each of the receptor-ligand complexes are postulated to influence unique subsets of estrogen responsive genes resulting in differential modulation and hence tissue-selective outcomes. The selective estrogen receptor modulators (SERM's) have been formulated to capitalize on these differential effects. Raloxifene was recently approved for osteoporosis prevention. It apparently has no effect on the uterus or breast but may have cardioprotective effects similar to estrogen based on its interactions with estrogen receptor alpha. This generation and subsequent generations of SERM's may assist in maintaining the beneficial effects of estrogen while avoiding its adverse effects. Estrogen receptor/ligand complexes of both estrogen receptor alpha and beta will also allow further selection of effects. The isolation and enhancement of these selective activities will hopefully provide an improved safety profile for hormone replacement therapy and will be a major research and development area in the future.

Progestogens

Unopposed estrogen therapy increases the risk of endometrial cancer from five- to tenfold. The addition of a progestogen to estrogen replacement negates and may actually reduce this risk *(46,47)*. Other potential concerns with long term estrogen and estrogen/progestogen use include a potential increase in the risk of breast cancer *(48–52)*, reduced cardiovascular benefits after long-term estrogen/progestogen replacement in low risk women *(53)*, and side effects which reduce compliance (breast tenderness, PMS-like symptoms, edema, bloating, irritability and depression, and lethargy) *(24)*. Despite these concerns regarding estrogen and estrogen/progestogen regimens, present data provide little evidence of an adverse effect of the combined estrogen-progestin regimen as compared with estrogens alone on mortality *(54)*.

Thus, in postmenopausal women with and without uteri and no contraindications, presently available data indicate that the use of an estrogen/progestogen or estrogen alone regimen, respectively, of ten or more years duration is beneficial for cardiovascular, bone, memory, cognitive, and genitourinary health and to avoid vasomotor symptoms and their related mental and emotional sequella. After ten or more years use, selective estrogen receptor modulators may play an increasingly important role in maintaining the beneficial effects on the cardiovascular and bone systems without creating adverse outcomes on the breast or uterus. For women with primary hypogonadism the initiation of secondary sexual characteristics and subsequent health benefits of hormone replacement therapy appear to outweigh potential long term risks.

SYNTHETIC PROGESTOGENS

Synthetic progestogens are classified into three groups: pregnanes, estranes and gonanes *(55)* (Fig. 8). Their unique characteristics are discussed.

Pregnances. Pregnanes are derived from 17-hydroxy-progesterone. The pregnane progestogens are synthesized from natural precursor steroids (Fig. 9). The most widely used progestogen in hormone replacement therapy is the pregnane, medroxyprogesterone acetate. It is also used as a long-term injectable contraceptive (depo-medroxyprogesterone acetate given 150 mg intramuscularly for three months), and for the treatment of endometrial hyperplasia (30 mg/d). Hydroxyprogesterone caproate (250 mg intramuscularly weekly through 12 wk) is occasionally used to maintain progesterone levels in women who undergo removal of the corpus luteum during pregnancy. Megestrel is often used in cases of endometrial carcinoma.

Estranes. Estrane and gonane progestogens are derived from 19 nor-testosterone, the progestogenic parent compound used in oral contraceptives in the United States. Estranes are characterized by the presence of an ethinyl group at position 17 and by the absence of a methyl group between the A and B rings (Fig. 10). The estrane progestogens that are related structurally to norethindrone (norethynodrel, lynestrenol, norethindrone acetate, ethynodiol diacetate) are converted to this parent compound. Norethindrone is the second most commonly used progestogen in the United States for hormone replacement therapy.

Gonanes. The gonanes share the structural modifications found in the estranes and also possess an ethinyl group at position 13 and a keto group at position 3 (Fig. 11). Norgestrel was synthesized in 1963 and is a racemic mixture of dextro and levorotatory forms. The levorotatory form, levonorgestrel, provides the biologic activity. Third-gen-

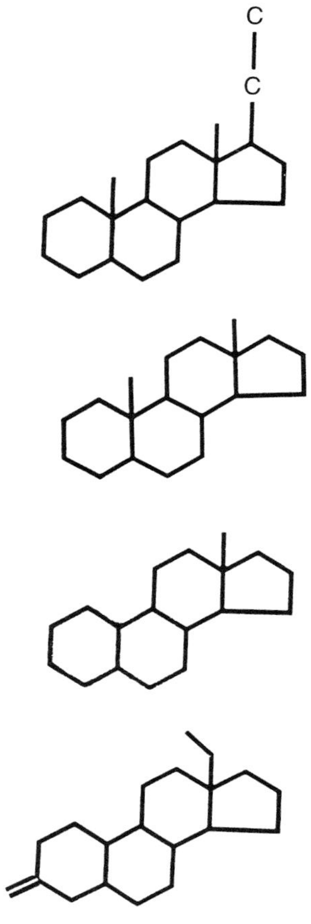

Fig. 8. Pregnane steroids have 21 carbons and include progesterone, glucocorticoids, mineralo-corticoids, and synthetic progestogens. Androstane steroids have 19 carbons and include testosterone and related steroids. Estrane steroids have an 18 carbon backbone and include estradiol and many of the 19 nortestosterone derivatives used as progestogens that have an ethinyl group at position 17 (20 carbons) and the absence of a methyl group between the A and B rings. 17-ethinyl-19 nortestosterone (norethindrone) is the estrane steroid that serves as the compound to which many estrane progestogens are metabolized. They are the second most commonly utilized progestogens in HRT. The more biologically active gonane steroids possess the structure of the estrane steroids and additionally have an ethyl group at position 13, and a keto group at position 3. The newer gonane progestogens may have reduced adverse effect (acne, hirsutism, weight gain, altered lipid, and glucose metabolism).

eration gonanes (desogestrel, gestedene, and norgestimate) have been developed to reduce unwanted side effects of progestogens such as acne, altered glucose and lipid metabolism, weight gain, and hirsutism (Fig. 12). They may be utilized in estrogen/progestogen regimens of the future.

PROGESTERONE

Progesterone preparations are synthesized from stigmasterol or diosgenin (derived from soy beans or Mexican yams, respectively) and occasionally from animal ovaries (Fig. 13).

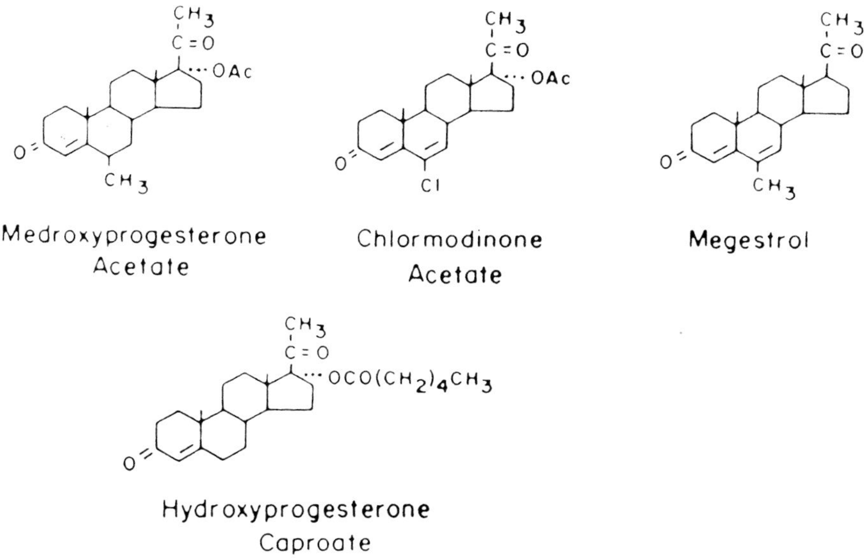

Medroxyprogesterone
Acetate

Chlormodinone
Acetate

Megestrol

Hydroxyprogesterone
Caproate

Fig. 9. The pregnane progestogens: medroxy-progesterone acetate, chlormodinone acetate, megestrol and hydroxy-progesterone caproate.

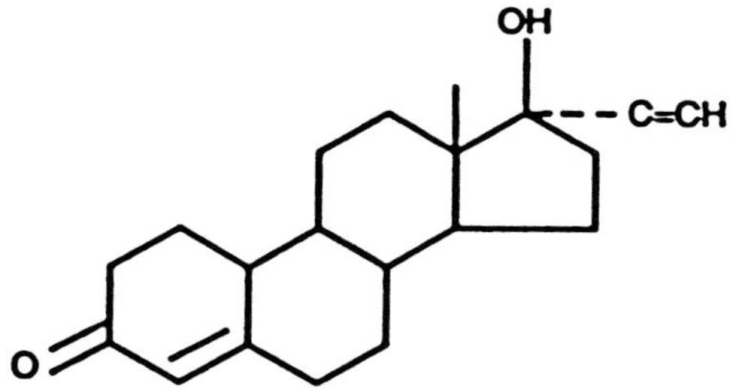

Fig. 10. The estrane progestogen norethindrone.

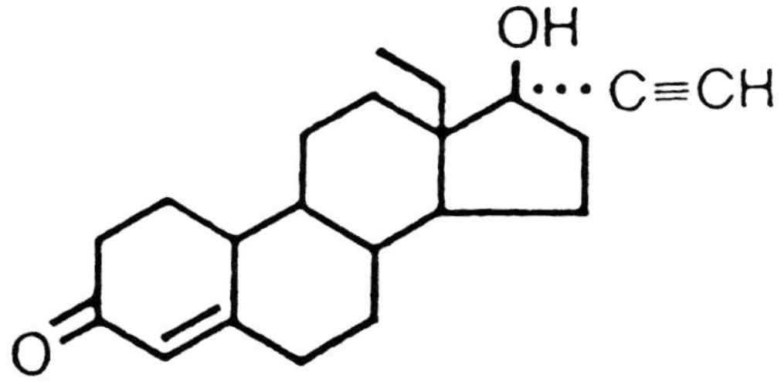

Fig. 11. The gonane progestogen levonorgestrel.

Progesterone was first synthesized for commercial uses in 1934. Its use is hampered by poor oral absorption and rapid first-pass liver metabolism. It has been used orally (micronized and unaltered), intramuscularly, rectally, and vaginally (micronized or carried in cocoa butter or polyethylene glycol vehicle in estrogen/progestogen regimens). Micronization of

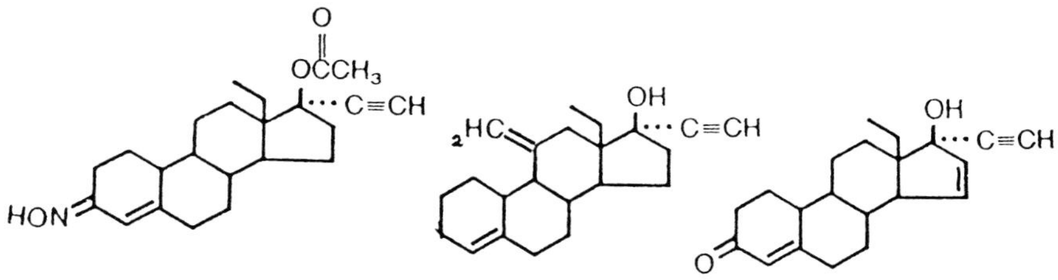

Fig. 12. Other gonane progestogens: norgestimate, desogestrel, and gestodene.

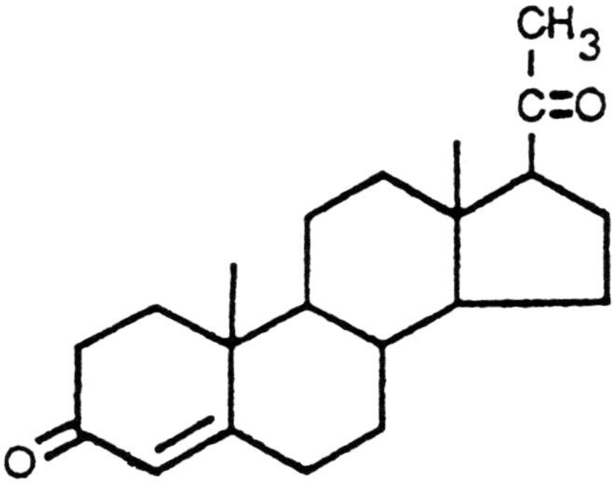

Fig. 13. Progesterone.

the progesterone in combination with lipophilic vehicles enhances oral absorption and has become increasingly popular. Orally administered micronized progesterone at a 100 mg twice to three times per day for 12 d each month in estrogen/progestogen regimens reveals rates of endometrial hyperplasia similar to that for medroxyprogesterone acetate *(56,57)*. In continuous combined regimens doses of 100 mg of oral micronized progesterone have been shown to cause an inactive endometrium and amenorrhea *(58)*.

Vaginal delivery of micronized progesterone has been shown to enhance progesterone delivery to the uterus compared to the standard intramuscular regimen and results in a synchronous secretory endometrial histologic pattern in agonadal women preparing for embryo donation *(59)*. The recommended dosage of vaginal micronized progesterone for estrogen/progestogen replacement in this setting is 800 mg/d (prior to embryo transfer in in vitro fertilization).

Only recently have studies been conducted utilizing a progesterone gel formulation. This preparation places progesterone in a 2% polycarbophil base that produces a controlled and sustained release of medication when given intravaginally. This approach takes advantage of the first uterine pass effect so that the desired endometrial impact can be obtained with lower systemic progesterone levels which could reduce progesterone related side-effects. Preliminary data has shown that in women on estrogen replacement for hypogonadism, a dose of 45–90 mg given every other day for up to 12 d induces complete secretory transition of the endometrium. Long term studies are underway to confirm the efficacy of this approach *(60)*.

Strong arguments for the use of natural progesterone as the progestogen in estrogen/ progestin replacement are being made and include the absence of adverse lipid alterations

Table 3
Common Progesterone Administration Regimens

Oral administration regimens	Estrogens	Progestogens
Cyclic sequential	1st–25th d of mo	12th–25th d of mo
Continuous sequential	Daily	1st–14th d of mo
Continuous combined	Daily	Daily
Cyclic combined	1st–25th d of mo	1st–25th d of mo
Continuous estrogen/interrupted progestin	Daily	3 d on, 3 d off

(57,61), and the absence of unwanted androgenic or estrogenic properties and their side effects *(62)*.

PROGESTOGEN REGIMENS

When progestogens are indicated (intact uterus) in hormone replacement for women the therapy is individualized to meet each woman's particular needs and desires. The most commonly used administration regimen is cyclic sequential, which has the lowest incidence of adverse effects, excluding vaginal bleeding. Cyclic sequential therapy results in withdrawal bleeding in 97% of women. After 65 yr of age, 60% continue to have bleeding on cyclic sequential delivery schedule. Continuous sequential regimens have similar rates of bleeding (Table 3).

For sequentially delivered regimens, endometrial sampling and transmission electron microscopy of ultrastructural elements have documented that the minimum progestin dose required to produce complete endometrial regression and a zero incidence of hyperplasia is 10 mg of medroxyprogesterone acetate given daily for 12 d *(63)*. A 2% incidence of hyperplasia has been reported with the use of 10 mg MPA for 10 d and a 4% incidence was noted for patient's receiving MPA for 7 d. With respect to protection against endometrial hyperplasia, based on recent clinical trials, it has been proposed that a dose of 5 mg of MPA prescribed for 14-d may be equivalent to a 10 mg dose taken over the same interval *(63)*. Clearly, one needs to consider both the dose, duration and formulation (i.e., endometrial activity) of the progestogen. Given the lack of a clearly preferred drug formulation and regimen, most practitioners will utilize progestogens in the dose range as listed in Table 2, for 12–14 d per cycle, often modified according to the patient's tolerance of progestin related side-effects. If less than customary doses are used, endometrial surveillance by endometrial biopsy is recommended.

Women routinely object to the prospect of vaginal bleeding, even if scheduled. This may be one of the reasons for the poor compliance rates seen with hormone replacement therapy. This has prompted the development of continuous combined and cyclic combined regimens aimed at inducing amenorrhea. Continuous combined regimens, such as CEE (0.625 mg/d) or micronized estradiol (1 mg/d) given with medroxyprogesterone acetate or norethindrone acetate (2.5 mg/d for both), produce spotting and bleeding in the first 3 to 6 mo but by 6 mo 60–65% are amenorrheic. Breakthrough bleeding may recur and, if persistent, a sequential (cyclic or continuous) will be required. Patient acceptance of this regimen is high *(64–66)*.

Since its introduction over a decade ago, combined continuous hormone replacement therapy has been studied in numerous clinical trials with over ten years of follow up. These studies reveal drop-out rates averaging only 20% and nearly uniform resolution of vasomotor symptoms. Approximately three quarters of the women receiving treatment for more than 6 m report no uterine bleeding. Irregular uterine bleeding during the initial months of treatment is common and may reduce patient compliance and acceptance. Endometrial atrophy is most commonly noted on endometrial biopsy. However, two symptomatic patients (return of uterine bleeding after the establishment of amenorrhea) with a history of atypical endometrial hyperplasia developed endometrial carcinoma (67).

A meta-analysis of patients on combined continuous conjugated equine estrogen and medroxyprogesterone acetate demonstrated a significant decrease in the circulating levels of total and LDL cholesterol and a significant increase in circulating HDL cholesterol post-treatment. Although such changes may be cardioprotective, no studies document decreased cardiovascular morbidity or mortality on this regimen yet. Bone density appears to be spared or increased (57).

Because of concerns regarding potential unknown risks of the continuous combined regimens, some clinicians have recommended a cyclic combined regimen. This regimen results in minimal controlled spotting for 1–3 mo followed by amenorrhea in three quarters of patients (68,69). A continuous estrogen/interrupted progestin regimen has also been developed (3 d on, 3 d off of progestin), which is theorized to reduce the metabolic effects of progestogens and also caused amenorrhea in over 75% of study participants (70). To further reduce the patient exposure to progestogens, the quarterly administration of progestogens has been investigated in limited studies. Endometrial protection was shown to be adequate, though further study is required.

Continuous combined, cyclic combined, and continuous estrogen with interrupted progestogen regimens have not demonstrated unequivocal differences in terms of the incidence of PMS-like side effects, reduction in vasomotor symptoms, improvement of lipid profile, maintenance of bone density, or patient compliance compared to cyclic sequential or continuous sequential regimens.

Progestogens presently available or soon to be released are included in Table 4.

Delivery Systems for Progestogens

Similar to estrogens, the oral route of progestin administration is the most common. Micronization has vastly improved the erratic absorption pattern seen with oral progesterone administration. The potential to reduce adverse side effects through the use of natural micronized progesterone is gaining greater appeal and vaginal delivery formulations have recently been released which, despite fluctuating serum levels, provide sustained and reliable endometrial effects. Depot medroxyprogesterone acetate is infrequently given with continuous estrogen administration as a combined continuous regimen. Injectable biopolymer delivery techniques and patch systems are under development.

HRT: Contraindications and Adverse Effects

There are several contraindications for the use of hormone replacement therapy. These include active thrombophlebitis or thromboembolic disorders, known or suspected estrogen-dependent neoplasia, and known or suspected cancer of the breast. Patients with a past history of these disorders have a relative contraindication to treatment and deserve a careful assessment of risk versus benefits prior to the institution of treatment. Other contraindications include undiagnosed abnormal genital bleeding, pregnancy and hypersensitivity to the drugs in question. Caution must be used in treating patients with impaired

Table 4
Commonly Available Progesterone

Brand name	Progestogen	mg available	Min. effective dosage*
Oral			
Provera®, generic[a]	Medroxyprogesterone acetate	2.5, 5, 10	10 mg daily
Amen®[b]	Medroxyprogesterone acetate	10	10 mg daily
Aygestin®[c]	Morethindrone acetate	5	2.5 mg daily
Megace®[d]	Megstrol acetate	20, 40	40 mg daily
Ovrette®[e]	Norgestrel	0.075	0.150 mg daily
MicicroNor®[f]	Norethindrone	0.35	1.05 mg daily
Nor-QD®[g]	Norethindrone	0.35	1.05 mg daily
Vaginal			
Progesterone®	Micronized progesterone	50, 100	800 mg in divided doses
Progesterone	Progesterone vaginal suppositories	25, 50	25 mg tx/d
Crinone®[h]	Progesterone gel 8% (90 mg)	4% (45 mg)	45–90 mg every other d
Injectable			
Depo-Provera®[i]	Medroxyprogesterone acetate	100	
Hydroxyprogesterone caproate	Hydroxyprogesterone caproate	125	
Progesterone	Progesterone	100	

*All progestogens listed have not been FDA-approved for use in HRT regimens and are not recommended for use. Physicians should consult detail information supplied by the manufacturer before use.

[a]Provera, Pharmacia-Upjohn Co., Kalamazoo, MI.
[b]Amen, Carnick Labs, Inc., Cedar Knolls, NJ.
[c]Aygestin, ESI-Lederle,Philadelphia, PA.
[d]Megace, Bristol-Myers, Syracuse, NY.
[e]Ovrette, Wyeth-Ayerst Laboratories, Philadelphia, PA.
[f]MicroNor, Ortho Pharmaceutical, Raritan, NJ.
[g]Nor-QD, G. D. Searle, Chicago, IL.
[h]Crinone, Wyeth-Ayerst Laboratories, Philadelphia, PA.
[i]Depo-Provera, Pharmacia-Upjohn, Kalamazoo, MI.

liver function owing to a concern for poor estrogen metabolism. Additionally, patients with hypertriglyceridemia (e.g., familial defects of lipoprotein metabolism) need to be carefully evaluated since they may be at risk for pancreatitis due to an estrogen associated rise in serum triglyceride levels. Other patients that warrant special consideration include those with a history of preexisting uterine fibroids which may enlarge with estrogen therapy and patients with hypercalcemia and renal insufficiency in which the prolonged use of estrogens can alter the metabolism of calcium and phosphorus.

There are numerous side-effects that may be associated with the use of HRT in menopausal women, many of which are thought to be linked to the overall poor long term compliance rates with this treatment (often reported as less than 25%). Women may experience bloating, breast tenderness, weight gain, head aches, nausea, irritability and premenstrual-like symptoms. Additionally, most women can expect uterine bleeding unless a combined continuous regimen is utilized.

Complications associated with the use of HRT are commonly attributed to the effects of estrogen on the liver. These complications include an increase, albeit small, in the incidence of venous thromboembolism, an increase in serum triglyceride levels (of possible significance to cardiac disease risk) and an increase in gallbladder disease. The effect of estrogen replacement on carbohydrate economy is unclear, but in general HRT it is not contraindicated in diabetics. HRT is not associated with detrimental effects in patients with cardivascular disease, hypertension, or with a history of cancer of the cervix, ovary, or vulva. If a progestogen is used, there is no increased risk in endometrial cancer expected, though the use of HRT in patients with a history of endometrial cancer is somewhat controversial.

One of the most publicly debated issues surrounding adverse events related to HRT is whether or not treatment is linked to an increase in the risk of breast cancer. Over 40 epidemiologic studies have been performed and the debate continues. It has been suggested that if estrogen replacement had a large impact on the risk of breast cancer, the results of the majority of these studies would be uniform. Conflicting data from large, seemingly well designed studies suggests that the epidemiological methodology employed in these studies are unable to overcome whatever recognized or unrecognized biases are present. The implication is that if a risk is present, at most the effect would be small, and is seen only after 10 yr of use. In addition, several analyses have shown that even if one assumes an increase in risk of breast cancer with the use of HRT the benefits of treatment (e.g., lower cardiovascular disease risk) outweigh the risks. Despite this line of reasoning, the fear of breast cancer remains one of the primary reasons women do not use HRT. The availability of SERM's that do not stimulate breast tissue (or that may even be protective against breast cancer) but provide some of the benefits of estrogen in other target organs such as the bone and the cardiovascular system will be an important treatment option or maintenance regimen for patients who avoid HRT because of a concern regarding breast cancer, as well as those with a history or family history of breast cancer.

Androgens

The beneficial effects from the replacement of estrogen and progesterone because of nonfunctional or absent ovarian follicles has prompted a reevaluation of ovarian androgen effects. In the United States, 130,000–195,000 women per year have their ovaries removed in conjunction with a hysterectomy.

Within the first day after total abdominal hysterectomy and bilateral salpingo-oophorectomy (TAH/BSO), plasma levels of estradiol and testosterone decrease significantly. Although estrogen levels in the premenopausal female fall from peak levels of 150–400 pg/mL to less than 20 pg/mL, testosterone levels fall in proportion to the production fraction of the premenopausal ovary, approximately 25%. In postmenopausal women, however, the fall in testosterone production may be more than the 25% total production fraction usually attributed to the premenopausal ovary *(71)*. Vermilion et al. also demonstrated the ovary to be a major contributor to the production of postmenopausal androgen levels *(72)*.

Because the number of women seeking hormone replacement therapy after oophorectomy, the rationale for the use of androgens in women should be understood. Studies of sexual behavior in bilaterally oophorectomized females reveals that estrogen replacement therapy alleviates atrophic vaginitis and dyspareunia, but does not affect motivational aspects, such as sexual desires and fantasies *(73)*.

EFFECTS OF ANDROGENS IN SURGICALLY CASTRATED ANIMALS

Animal studies have supported a role for androgens in surgically castrated primates. Testosterone propionate given to castrate rhesus monkeys increased the activity of sexually related behaviors *(74)*. Pharmacologic *(75)*, but not physiologic doses *(76)* of testosterone administered to ovariectomized female monkeys increased their sexual invitational behavior and increased lever pressing, which allowed access to a male partner *(77)*. Human studies suggest a potential benefit for sexual motivation in women, but results of such therapy in castrated females vary in the premenopausal versus postmenopausal state *(78)*.

ANDROGENS FOR WOMEN

Premenopausal Oophorectomized Women. Studies suggest that the addition of androgens to standard estrogen replacement therapy in the premenopausal woman may play a beneficial role for women who experience serious difficulty in stabilizing on standard estrogen replacement therapy and/or for those who have specific complaints regarding libido. Psychosomatic complaints are rarely improved with treatment *(79–81)*.

Postmenopausal Oophorectomized and Naturally Menopausal Women. With regard to postmenopausal oophorectomized and naturally menopausal women, the published work to date suggests that the addition of androgens to estrogen replacement regimen does not significantly enhance sexual activity or reduce depression over standard estrogen replacement alone *(82–85)*.

NEW INDICATIONS FOR ANDROGENS–OSTEOPOROSIS

Androgenic steroids are known to play a role in the maintenance of bone mass in men and women *(86,87)*. The beneficial effects of androgens, specifically dihydrotestosterone, on bone cell differentiation appears to be mediated by transforming growth factor-α, and the induction of bone cell proliferation is due to an enhanced response of osteoblastic cells to growth factors (fibroblast growth factor and insulin-like growth factor II) *(88)*.

For many years nandrolone decanoate has been shown to increase the vertebral bone mineral density (BMD) in postmenopausal women with osteoporosis *(89)*. Raisz et al. compared the effects of estrogen given alone to those of estrogen plus androgen therapy on biochemical markers of bone formation and resorption in postmenopausal women. Urinary excretion of the markers of bone resorption decreased equally in both groups. The estrogen-only group had a reduction in serum markers of bone formation; however, in women treated with the combination of estrogen and testosterone the markers of bone formation increased *(90)*.

It does appear, however, that testosterone's effects on BMD are highly dependent on the actions of estrogen in skeletal maturation and mineralization. Examples of this interaction include: the finding of severe osteoporosis in a male with normal testosterone levels but a defective estrogen receptor and an increase in BMD in postmenopausal women using combination estrogen and testosterone *(91–94)*.

It would appear that androgen replacement may potentially play a role in the treatment of women with or at high risk for osteoporosis in the future. Studies are in progress to characterize appropriate candidates and identify the potential risks (i.e., cardiovascular).

INDICATIONS/CONTRAINDICATIONS/ADVERSE EFFECTS OF METHYL TESTOSTERONE

The only Food and Drug Administration-approved combination for androgen containing hormone replacement therapy in the United States is Estratest (Solvay, Marietta, GA). Estratest is a combination of esterified estrogens (1.25 mg) and methyl testosterone (2.5 mg), whereas Estratest HS (half strength) is esterified estrogens (0.625 mg) and methyl testosterone (1.25 mg).

Androgens are responsible for the normal growth and development of male secondary sexual characteristics including growth and development of the prostate, seminal vesicles, penis, scrotum, male hair patterns (beard, chest, axillary), laryngeal enlargement, vocal cord thickening, and alterations in musculature and body fat distribution. They cause retention of nitrogen, sodium, potassium, and phosphorus and decrease urinary excretion of calcium. Protein anabolism is increased, and erythropoiesis is stimulated. Testosterone, which is metabolized by the gut, is 44% cleared by the liver on the first pass. Methyl testosterone is less extensively metabolized by the liver.

PRECAUTIONS

Patients should be observed for signs of virilization (voice deepening, hirsutism, acne, clitoromegaly). Prolonged use may result in fluid and sodium retention, and hypercalcemia may occur. Because of known hepatotoxicity of 17 alpha-alkylated androgens, liver function tests should be obtained periodically. Hemoglobin and hematocrit also should be evaluated on a periodic basis to check for polycythemia. Additionally, androgens may decrease the oral anticoagulant requirements of patients receiving such drugs, reduce insulin requirements, and lower blood glucose levels. There are rare reports of hepatocellular carcinoma in women receiving long-term high-dose therapy. Androgens decrease thyroid-binding globulin, causing lower T4 and higher T3RU.

Although the addition of androgens to postmenopausal estrogen replacement is apparently not accompanied by a significant bone-sparing effect *(95)*, further research in this area may indicate a positive effects. Parental androgen administration has been associated with hirsutism, hot flushes, decreased libido, mood changes, depression, and clitoromegaly. In some patients, testosterone levels have remained elevated with the occurrence of virilizing symptoms of 12–20 mo after an intramuscular injection *(96)*. (This parenteral [IM] product is not available in the US)

Finally, potential adverse effects on cholesterol, high density lipoprotein, high density lipoprotein 2, high density lipoprotein 3, and apolipoprotein A2 have been noted in women receiving esterified estrogens plus methyl testosterone compared to estrogen alone *(97)*.

Although these concerns are valid, retrospective and prospective studies involving the use of androgen alone and in combination with estrogens demonstrate that concerns about the adverse effects of androgen use associated with supra physiologic, self-escalated doses in men do not apply to the much lower doses combined with estrogens for hormone replacement in postmenopausal women *(98)*.

Recent clinical studies indicate that approx 5% will have a serious adverse event while taking an estrogen/androgen combination. The most commonly reported adverse events were those known to be associated with estrogen therapy (weight gain, headache, nausea, and vasodilatation) and androgen treatment (alopecia, acne, and hirsutism) *(99)*.

Summary on Androgen Use

In conclusion, androgens may be of some use in premenopausally castrated females with difficulty adjusting to estrogen replacement alone or for those with specific com-

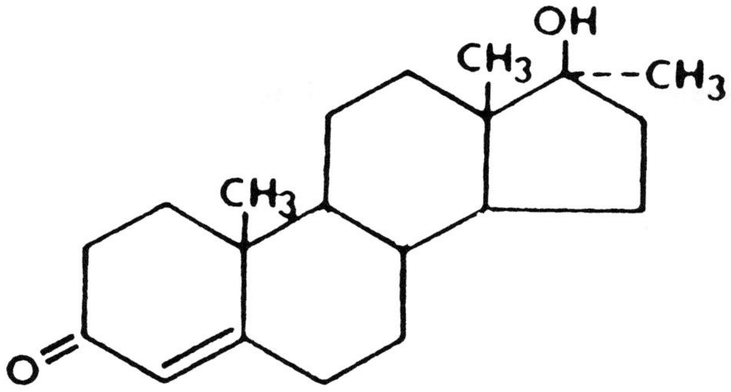

Fig. 14. Methyl testosterone.

plaints regarding decreased libido. The studies cited, and clinical experience suggests that early sexual experiences impact greatly on sexuality in later life and particular attention should be addressed to such historic factors. Interventions should address apparent causal factors. The benefit of treatment in postmenopausal females is controversial at present. Further studies to evaluate the effects on bone mineral density in this group of women may define other appropriate roles for androgens in hormone replacement regimens.

Androgen Delivery Systems

Injectable androgen administration has not been approved in the United States, thus the oral route is utilized. New transdermal delivery systems are being actively developed. The chemical structure of methyl testosterone is shown in Fig. 14.

Phytoestrogens

Despite the major health benefits derived from HRT, compliance is relatively poor. Factors associated with patient noncompliance include; concerns over an increased risk of breast cancer (RR 1.2-1.4) (24), and progestogen use with an intact uterus resulting in vaginal bleeding, PMS like symptoms, and mood swings (24).

Recent work suggests that soybean phytoestrogens may provide some of the health benefits attributed to estrogens without adverse events. Phytoestrogens are found in the legumes, particularly soy. The phytoestrogens found in soy are genistein, daidzein, and glycitein. Soybean phytoestrogens appear to be estrogen agonists for bone in experimental situations but act significantly less effectively than estrogen (CEEs) (100).

In cynomolgus monkeys, soy phytoestroogens, however, failed to maintain bone density (101). However, advantageous effects have been noted in cynomolgus monkeys in serum lipids (decreased plasma cholesterol and LDL, with increased HDL, and Apo A1) and coronary artery atherogenesis (102–105). Epidemiologic data would suggest that soy intake may reduce the risk of breast cancer (106), potentially through a reduction in circulating ovarian steroids and adrenal androgens (107). Phytoestrogens do not appear to stimulate the endometrium or genitourinary tissues (108).

The selective activities of the phytoestrogens may potentially be explained by selective estrogen receptor modulatory activities and different gene transcriptional activities of estrogen receptors alpha and beta/ligand complexes. It does appear that phytoestrogens do not increase the risks of breast and endometrial cancers and may play a supportive role in sustaining healthy bone and cardiovascular systems in women. Further research will more clearly define the potential role of the phytoestrogens in health maintenance.

DHEA

Dehydroepiandrosterone sulfate (DHEA-S) is the most abundant steroid in the body. It is primarily produced by the adrenal gland with small amounts produced by the ovary. DHEA levels vary with age. Levels are low until adrenarche and then peak at 20–30 yr, thereafter levels progressively decrease with age *(109)*.

By the seventh decade, DHEA levels are 10% of peak values. The decline in DHEAS with age results in a reduction in the formation of androgens and estrogens in peripheral target tissues.

Clinically, declining DHEA, and DHEAS levels have been associated with reduced protein synthesis, decreased body mass, and increased body fat *(110)*, cardiovascular disease in men *(111)*, various cancers *(112)*, and attenuation of the immune system *(113,114)*.

Clinical studies with appropriate controls are underway, and clear recommendations should be forthcoming. Documented side effects with use include hirsutism, decreased breast size, acne, hair loss, deepening voice, gastrointestinal discomfort, and reversible hepatitis *(115)*. Prudence suggests awaiting the results of the prospective clinical trials. For those who have self-initiated the medication, the dose should certainly be less than or equal to 50 mg. Additionally, lipids, liver function tests and testosterone levels should be monitored periodically. There is no evidence that DHEA could be used in place of estrogen replacement.

CONCLUSIONS

Regardless of the etiology of hypogonadism, treatment goals are similar. Immediate goals address the present symptomatology of the patient. This may include the treatment of hot flushes, cognitive and emotional symptoms or urogenital atrophy in patients with secondary hypogonadism or the lack of secondary sexual characteristics as in primary hypogonadal women. Treatment of primary hypogonadism attempts to mimic normal physiology (low dose isolated estrogen therapy) to allow normal breast maturation. Long-range treatment goals are concerned with the reduction of health risks such as cardiovascular disease, osteoporosis, and Alzheimer's disease which are all associated with prolonged hypogonadism. For women with a uterus, treatment utilizes an estrogen compound to directly address symptomatology and long-range concerns and a progestogen to protect against the increased risk of endometrial hyperplasia and cancer observed in women receiving unopposed estrogen therapy. In some situations, patients may benefit from an expansion of HRT to include the use of androgens and or phytoestrogens. DHEA is not considered an alternative to HRT.

Based on data currently available, there is no clear justification to recommend the use of one hormonal formulation, delivery system or treatment regimen over another. Rather, there are relative benefits that may be achieved with the various options available that are dependent on the particular characteristics of the individual patient. Medication choices will likely be even more complex in the future as the availability and activities of SERM's expands.

Many of the hormonal preparations being developed rely on transdermal delivery systems (Table 5). This expansion in technology and information will result in improved health and well-being for hypogonadal women.

Table 5
Additional Estrogen and Progestogens in Development

Product	Manufacturer
Estradiol/norethindrone acetate patches for hormone replacement	RW Johnson Pharmaceuticals, Raritan, NJ
Estradiol/progestin transdermal patches	TheraTech, Salt Lake City, Utah
17 B estradiol transdermal patches	Novo Nordic, Princeton, NJ
Norethindrone acetate and ethinyl estradiol (Fem HRT)	Warner-Lambert, Morris Plain, NJ
Conjugated estrogen and trimegesterone	Wyeth-Ayerst, Philadelphia, PA
Cyclophasic hormone replacement	RW Johnson Pharmaceuticals, Raritan, NJ
ERT/HRT transdermal patches	Wyeth-Ayerst, Philadelphia, PA
Estradiol	G. D. Searle, Skokie, IL
Beta-estradiol transdermal patches	RW Johnson Pharmaceuticals, Raritan, NJ
Estradiol/norethindrone acetate	G. D. Searle, Skokie, IL
Estradiol/norethindrone acetate transdermal patches	Cygnue, Redwood City, CA
Estradiol/progestin transdermal patches	TheraTech, Salt Lake City, UT
Estradiol/testosterone transdermal patches	TheraTech, Salt Lake City, UT
Testosterone transdermal patches	TheraTech, Salt Lake City, UT
17 Beta estradiol & norethindrone transdermal patches	Novo Nordic, Princeton, NJ
Estropipate and Medroxyprogesterone acetate	Pharmacia-Upjohn

REFERENCES

1. Hagstad A, Janson PO. The epidemiology of climacteric symptoms. Acta Obstet Gynecol Scand 1986;134:59–65.
2. Witteman JCM, Brobbee DE, Kok FJ, Hofman A, Valkenburg HA. Increased risk of atherosclerosis in women after the menopause. Br Med J 1989;298:642–644.
3. Colditz GA, Wilett WC, Stampfer MJ, Rosner B, Speizer FE, Hennekens CH. Menopause and the riskof coronary heart disease in women. N Engl J Med 1987;316:1105–1110.
4. Rosenberg L, Hennekens CH, Rosner B, Belanger C, Rothman KJ, Speizer FE. Early menopause and the risk of myocardial infarction. Am J Obstet Gynecol 1981;139:47–51.
5. Beard CM, Fuster V, Annegers FJ. Reproductive history in women with coronary heart disease: a case-control study. Am J Epidemiol 1981;120:108–114.
6. Bush, TL. Noncontraceptive estrogen use and risk of cardiovascular disease: an overview and critique of the literature. In: Kerenman, SG, eds. The menopause: Biological and Clinical Consequences of Ovarian Failure; Evolution and Management. Serono Symposia, Norwell, MA 1990, p. 211.
7. Stampfer, MJ, Colditz, GA. Estrogen replacement and coronary heart disease: a quantitative assessment of the epidemiologic evidence. Prev Med 1991;20:47–63.
8. Grady, D, Rubin, SM, Petitti, DB, et al. Hormone therapy to prevent disease and prolong life in postmenopausal women. Ann Intern Med 1992;117:1016.
9. Utian WG, Schiff I. NAMS–Gallup survey on women's knowledge, information sources and attitudes to menopause and hormone replacement therapy. Menopause 1994;1:39–48.
10. Seeman E. Osteoporosis: trials and tribulations. Am J Med 1997;18;103:74S–87S .
11. Eiken P, Kolthoff N, Nielsen SP. Effect of 10 years' hormone replacement therapy on bone mineral content in postmenopausal women. Bone 1996; 5 (Suppl):191S–193S.
12. Daly E, Roche M, Barlow D, Gray A, McPherson K, Vessey M. HRT: an analysis of benefits, risks and costs. Br Med Bull 1992;48:368–400 .
13. Van der Loos M, Paccaud F, Gutzwiller F, Chrzanowski R. Impact of hormonal prevention on fractures of the proximal femur in postmenopausal women: a simulation study. Soz Praventivmed 1988;33:162–166.

14. Speroff L, Lobo RA. Postmenopausal hormone therapy and the cardiovascular system. Heart Dis Stroke 1994;3:173–176 .

15. Jorm AF, Korten AE, Henderson AS. The prevalence of dementia: a quantitative integration of the literature. Acta Psychiatr Scand 1987; 76:465–479.

16. Paganini-Hill A, Henderson VW. Estrogen deficiency and risk of Alzheimer's disease in women. Am J Epidemiol 1994;140:256–261.

17. Paganini-Hill A, Henderson VW. Estrogen replacement therapy and risk of Alzheimer's disease. Arch Intern Med 1996;156:2213–2217.

18. Brenner De, Kukull WA, Stergachis A, et al. Postmenopausal estrogen replacement therapy and the risk of Alzheimer's disease: a population-based case-control study. Am J Epidemiol 1994;140: 262–267.

19. Mortel KF, Meyers JS. Lack of postmenopausal estrogen replacement therapy and the risk of dementia. J Neuropsychiat Clin Neurosci 1996;7:334–337.

20. Kawas C, Resnick S, Morrison A, et al. A prospective study of estrogen replacement therapy and the risk of development of Alzheimer's disease: the Baltimore Longitudinal Study of Aging. Neurology 1997;48:1517–1521.

21. Gould E, Wooley CS, Frankfurt M, McEwen BS. Gonadal steroids regulate dendritic spine density in hippocampal pyramidal cells in adulthood. J Neurosci 1990;10:1286–1291.

22. Luine VN. Estradiol increases choline acetyltransferase activity in specific basal forebrain nuclei and projection areas of female rats. Exp Neurol 1985;89:484–490.

23. Behl C, Davis JB, Lesley R, Schubert D. Hydrogen peroxide mediates amyloid beta protein toxicity. Cell 1994;77:817–827.

24. Ravnikar VA. Compliance with hormone therapy. Am J Obstet Gynecol 1987;156:1332–1334.

25. Mashchak CA, Lobo RA, Dozono-Takano R, et al. Comparison of pharmacodynamic properties of various estrogen formulations. Am J Obstet Gynecol 1982;144:511–518.

26. Jordan CV. Estrogen receptor antagonists. In: Adashi EY, Rock JA, Rosenwaks, eds. Reproductive endocrinology, surgery, and technology. Lippencott-Raven, Philadelphia, PA, 1996, p. 535.

27. Eighth Supplement to U.S.P. XXII. Easton, PA. Mack;1990;3256–3258 .

28. Lobo RL, Nguyen HN, Eggena P, Brenner PF. Biologic effects of equilin sulfate in postmenopausal women. Fertil Steril 1988;49:234–238.

29. Brosnihan KB, Weddle D, Anthony MS, Heise C, Li P, Ferrario CM. Effects of chronic hormone replacement on the renin-angiotensin system in cynomolgus monkeys. J Hypertens 1997;15:719–726.

30. Aylward M, Maddock J, Rees PL. Natural estrogen replacement therapy and blood clotting. Br Med J 1976;1:220–222.

31. Varma TR. Effect of estrogen replacement on blood coagulation factors in postmenopausal women. Int J Gynaecol Obstet 1983;21:291–296.

32. Perez-Gutthan. Hormone replacement therapy and risk of venous thromboembolism: population-based case controlled study. BMJ 1997;314:796–800.

33. Wash Drug Lett. May 13, 1991:6.

34. Bhavnani BR. Pharmacokinetics and pharmacodynamics of conjugated equine. estrogens: chemistry and metabolism. Proc Soc Exp Biol Med 1998;217:6–16 .

35. Yen SCC, Martin PL, Burnier AM, et al. Circulating estradiol, estrone, and gonadotropin levels following the administration of orally active 17 beta estradiol in post-menopausal women. J Clin Endocrinol Metab 1975;40:518–521.

36. Ryan KJ. Engel LL. Endocrinology 1953;52:287.

37. Lobo RA, Cassidenti DL. Pharmacokinetics of oral 17 beta estradiol . J Reprod Med 1992;37:77–84.

38. Kuhl H. Pharmacokinetics of oestrogens and progestogens. Maturitas 1990;12:171–197.

39. McEvoy GK, et al. eds. American Hospital Formulary Service. American Society of Hospital Pharmacists, Bethesda, MD, 1991.

40. Orme M, Back DJ, Ward S, Green S. The pharmacokinetics of ethinyl estradiol in the presence and absence of gestodene and desogestrel. Contraception 1991;43:305–316.

41. Mandel FP, Geoia Fl, Lu KH, Biologic effects of various doses of ethinyl estradiol in postmenopausal women. Obstet Gynecol 1982;59:673–679.

42. Hammond CB, Maxon WS. Estrogen replacement therapy. Clin Obstet Gynecol 1986;29:407–430.

43 Bewley S, Bewley TH. Drug dependence with estrogen replacement therapy. Lancet 1992; 339:290,291.

44. Kuiper GGJM, Enmark E, Pelto-Huikko M, Nilsson S, Gustafsson J-A.Cloning of a novel receptor expressed in rat prostate and ovary. Proc Natl Acad Sci USA 1996;93:5925–5930.

45. Mosselman S, Polman J, Dijkema R.ER beta: identification and characterization of a novel human estrogen receptor. FEBS Lett 1996;392:49–53.
46. Gambrel RD Jr. Use of progestogen therapy. Am J Obstet Gynecol 1987;156:1304–1313.
47. Persson I. Cancer risk in women receiving estrogen-progestin replacement therapy. Maturitas 1996;23:S37–S45 .
48. Persson I, Thurfjell E, Bergstrom R, Holmberg L. Hormone replacement therapy and the risk of breast cancer. Nested case-control study in a cohort of Swedish women attending mammography screening. Int J Cancer 1997;72:758–761.
49. von Schoultz B. HRT and breast cancer risk, what to advise? Eur J Obstet Gynecol Reprod Biol 1997;71:205–208.
50. Persson I, et al. Cancer incidence and mortality in women receiving estrogen and estrogen-progestin replacement therapy: long-term follow-up of a Swedish cohort. Int J Cancer 1996;67:327–332.
51. Caldas GA, Hankinson SE, Hunter DJ, Willett WC, Manson JE, Stampfer MJ, Hennekens C, Rosner B, Speizer FE. The use of estrogens and progestins and the risk of breast cancer in postmenopausal women. N Engl J Med 1995;332:1589–1593.
52. Colditz GA, Egan KM, Stampfer MJ. Hormone replacement therapy and risk of breast cancer: results from epidemiologic trials. Am J Obstet Gynecol 1993;168:1473–1480.
53. Grodstein F, Stampfer MJ, Caldas GA, Willett WC, Manson JE, Joffe M, Rosner B, Fuchs C, Hankinson SE, Hunter DJ, Hennekens CH, Speizer FE. Postmenopausal hormone therapy and mortality. N Engl J Med 1997;336:1769–1775.
54. Scarier C, Adami HO, Hoover R, Persson I. Cause-specific mortality in women receiving hormone therapy. Epidemiology 1997:1:59–65.
55. Peterson CM. Progestogens, progesterone antagonists, progesterone and androgens: Synthesis, classification, and uses. Clin Obstet Gynecol 1995;38:813–820.
56. Moyer DL, de Lignieres B, Driguez P, Pez JP. Prevention of endometrial hyperplasia by progesterone during long term estradiol replacement: influence of bleeding pattern and secretory changes. Fertil Steril 1993;59:992–997.
57. The Writing Group for the PEPI Trial. Effects of estrogen and estrogen/progestin regimens on heart disease risk factors in postmenopausal women: the postmenopausal estrogen/progestin interventions (PEPI). JAMA 1995;273:199–208.
58. Gillet JY, Andre G, Fauger B, Erny R, Buvat-Herbaut MA, et al. Induction of amenorrhea during hormone replacement therapy: optimal micronized progesterone dose. Multicenter study. Maturitas 1994;19:103–116 .
59. Miles RA, Paulson RJ, Lobo RA, Press MF, Dahmoush L, Sauer MV. Pharmacokinetics and endometrial tissue levels of progesterone after administration by intramuscular and vaginal routes: a comparative study. Fertil Steril 1994;62:485–490.
60. Casanas-Roux F, Nisolle M, Marbaix E, Smets M, Bassil S, Donnez J. Morphometric, immunohistological and three-dimensional evaluation of the endometrium of menopausal women treated by oestrogen and Crinone, a new slow-release vaginal progesterone. Hum Reprod 1996;11:357–363.
61. Jensen J, Riis BJ, Strin V, Nilas L, Christiansen C. Long term effects of percutaneous estrogens and oral progesterone on serum lipoproteins in postmenopausal women. Am J Obstet Gynecol 1987;156:66–71.
62. Shangold MM, Tomai TP, Cook JD, Jacobs SL, Zinaman MJ, Chin SY, Simon JA. Factors associated with withdrawal bleeding after administration of oral micronized progesterone in women with secondary amenorrhea. Fertil Steril 1991;56:1029–1033.
63. Whitehead MI, Hillard TC, Crook D. The role and use of progestogens. Obstet Gynecol 1990;75:559–576.
64. Woodruff JD, Pickar JH for The Menopause Study Group. Incidence of endometrial hyperplasia inpostmenopausal women taking conjugated estrogens with medroxyprogesterone acetate or conjugated estrogens alone. Am J Obstet Gynecol 1994;170:1213.
65. Ulrich LG, Barlow DH, Sturdee DW, Wells M, Campbell MJ, Nielsen B, Bragg AJ, Vessey MP. Quality of life and patient preference for sequential versus continuous combined HRT: the UK Kliofem multicenter study experience. UK Continuous Combined HRT Study Investigators. Int J Gynaecol Obstet 1997;59:S11–S17.
66. Piegsa K, Calder A, Davis JA, McKay-Hart D, Wells M, Bryden F. Endometrial status in postmenopausal women on long-term continuous combined hormone replacement therapy (Kliofem). A comparative study of endometrial biopsy, outpatient hysteroscopy and transvaginal ultrasound. Eur J Obstet Gynecol Reprod Biol 1997;72:175–180.

67. Leather AT, Savvas IA, Studd JWW. Endometrial histology and bleeding patterns after eight years of continuous combined estrogen and progestogen therapy in postmenopausal women. Obstet Gynecol 1991;78:1008–1010.

68. Darj E, Nilsson S, Axelsson O, et al. Clinical and endometrial effects of estradiol and progesterone in postmenopausal women. Maturitas 1991; 13:109–115.

69. Gambrell RD Jr. Progestogens in estrogen-replacement therapy. Clin Obstet Gynecol 1995;38:89–901.

70. Casper RF, Chapdelaine A. Estrogen and interrupted progestin: a new concept for menopausal replacement therapy. Am J Obstet Gynecol 1993;168:1188–1196.

71. Judd HL, Judd GE, Lucas WF, Yen S.C. Endocrine function of the postmenopausal ovary: concentration of androgens and estrogens in ovarian and peripheral vein blood. J Clin Endo Metab 1974;39:1020.

72. Vermilion A. The hormonal activity of the postmenopausal ovary. J Clin Endo Metab 1976;42:247–252.

73. Furuhjelm M, Karlgren E, Carstrom K. The effect of estrogen therapy on somatic and psychical symptoms in postmenopausal women. Acta Obstet Gynecol Scand 1984;63:655–661.

74. Wallem K, Goy RW. Effects of estradiol benzoate, estrone, and proprionates of testosterone or dihydrotestosterone on sexual and related behaviors of ovariectomized rhesus monkeys. Horm Behav 1977;9:228–248.

75. Michael RP, Zumpe D. Effects of androgen administration on sexual invitations by female rhesus monkeys. Anim Behav 1977;25:936–944.

76. Michael RP, Richter MC, Cain JA, et al. Artificial menstrual cycles, behavior and the role of androgens in female rhesus monkeys. Nature 1978;175:439–440.

77. Michael RP, Zumpe D, Keverne EB, et al. Neuroendocrine factors in the control of primate behavior. Rec Prog Horm Res. 1972;28:665–706.

78. Sherwin BB, Gelfand MM, Brender W. Androgen enhances sexual motivation in females: a prospective, crossover study of sex steroid administration in the surgical menopause. Psychosom Med 1985;47:339–351.

79. Sherwin BB, Gelfand MM. The role of androgen in the maintenance of sexual functioning in oophorectomized women. Psychosom Med 1987;49:397–409.

80. Sherwin BB, Gelfand MM. Differential symptoms response to parenteral estrogen and/or androgen administration in the surgical menopause. Am J Obstet Gynecol 1985, 151:153–160.

81. Young R, Wilta B, Dabbs J, et al. Comparison of estrogen plus androgen and estrogen on libido and sexual satisfaction in recently oophorectomized women. North American Menopause Society Meeting, September 17–20, 1992.

82. Dow MTG, Hart DM. Hormonal treatments of sexual unresponsiveness in postmenopausal women. Br J Obstet Gynaecol 1983;90:361–366.

83. Sherwin BB, Gelfand MM. Sex steroids and affect in "the surgical menopause: a double blind, crossover study. Psychoneuroendocrinology 1985;10:325–335.

84. Myers LS, Dixon J, Morrissette M, Carmichael M, Davidson JM. Effects of estrogen, androgen, and progestin on sexual psychophysiology and behavior in postmenopausal women. J Clin Endo Metab 1990;70:1124–1131.

85. Notelovitz M, Watts N, Timmons MC, et al. Effects of estrogen plus low dose androgen versus estrogen alone on menopausal symptoms in oophorectomized-hysterectomized women. North American Menopausal Society Meeting, September 17–20, 1992.

86. Colvard DS, Erickson, EF, Meeting PE et al, Identification of androgen receptors in normal human osteoblast-like cells. Proc Natl Acad Sci USA 1989;86:854–857.

87. Kasperk CH, Wergedeal JE, et al. Androgens directly stimulate proliferation of bone cells in vitro. Endocrinology 1989;124:1576,1577.

88. Kasperk C, Fitzsimmons R, Strong D, et al. Studies of the mechanism by which androgens enhance mitogenesis and differentiation in bone cells. J Clin Endocrinol Metab 1990;71:1322–329.

89. Need AG, Horowitz M, Bridges A, Morris H, Nordic BE. Effects of nandrolone decanoate and antiresorptive therapy on vertebral density in osteoporotic, postmenopausal women. Arch Int Med 1989;149:57–60.

90. Raisz LG, Wiita B, Artis A, et al. Comparison of the effects of estrogen alone and estrogen plus androgen on biochemical markers of bone formation and resorption in postmenopausal women. J Clin Endocrinol Metab 1995;81:37–43.

91. Smith EP, Boyd J, Frank GR, et al. Estrogen resistance caused by a mutation in the oestrogen-receptor gene in a man. N Engl J Med 1994;331:1056–1061.

92. Savvas M, Studd JWW, Fogelman I, et al. Skeletal effects of oral oestrogen compared with subcutaneous oestrogen and testosterone in postmenopausal women. Br Med J 1988;297:331–333.

93. Savvas M, Studd JWW, Norman S, et al. Increase in bone mass after one year of percutaneous oestradiol and testosterone implants in post-menopausal women who have previously received long-term oral oestrogens. Br J Obstet Gynaecol 1992; 757–760.

94. Davis SR, McCloud P, Strauss BJG, Burger HG. Testosterone enhances estradiol effects on postmenopausal bone density and sexuality. Maturitas 1995;21:227–236.

95. Garnet T, Studd, J, Watson N, Savvas M. The effects of plasma estradiol levels on increases in vertebral and femoral bone density following therapy with estradiol and estradiol with testosterone implants. Obstet Gynecol 1992;79:968–972.

96. Urman B, Pride SM, Ho Yeun BH. Elevated serum testosterone , hirsutism, and virilism associated with combined androgen-estrogen hormone replacement therapy. Obstet Gynecol. 1991;77:595–598.

97. Hickok LR, Toomey C, Speroff L. A comparison of esterified estrogens with and without methyltestosterone: effects on endometrial histology and serum lipoproteins in postmenopausal women. Obstet Gynecol 1993;82:924–927.

98. Gelfand MM, Wiita B.Int J Fertil Menopausal Stud 1996;41:412–422 .

99. Phillips E, Bauman C. Safety surveillance of esterified estrogens-methyltestosterone (Estratest and Estratest HS) replacement therapy in the United States. Clin Ther 1997;19:1070–1084 .

100. Arjmandi BH, Alkel L, Hollis BW, Amin D, Stacewicz-Sapuntzakis M, Guo P, Kukreja SC. Dietary soybean protein prevents bone loss in an ovariectomized rat model of osteoporosis.J Nutr 1996;126:161–167.

101. Jayo MJ, Anthony MS, Register TC, Rankin SE, Vest T, Clarkson TB. Dietary soy isoflavones and bone loss: a study in ovariectomized monkey. J Bone Miner Res 1996;11:S228.

102. Anthony MS, Clarkson TB, Hughes CL, Morgan TM, Burke GL. Soybean isoflavones improve cardiovascular risk factors without affecting reproductive system of peripubertal rhesus monkeys. J Nutr 1996;126:43–50.

103. Anthony MS, Burke GL, Hughes CL, Clarkson TB. Does soy supplementation improve coronary heart disease risk? Circulation 1995;91:925–929.

104. Anthony MS, Clarkson TB, Hughes CL. Plant and mammalian estrogen effects on plasma lipids of female monkeys. Circulation 1994; 90:I235.

105. Williams JK, Honore EK, Washburn SA, Clarkson TB. Effects of hormone replacement therapy on reactivity of atherosclerotic coronary arteries in cynomolgus monkeys. J Am Coll Cardiol 1994; 24:1757–1761.

106. Messina MJ, Persky V, Setchell KDR, Barnes S. Soy intake and cancer risk: a review of the in vitro and in vivo data. Nutr Cancer 1994;21:113–131.

107. Lu LJ, Anderson KE, Grady JJ, Nagamani M. Effects of soya consumption for one month on steroid hormones in premenopausal women: implications for breast cancer risk reduction. Cancer Epidemiol Biomarkers Prev 1996;5:63–70.

108. Knight DC, Eden JA. A review of the clinical effects of phytoestrogens. Obstet Gynecol 1996;87:897–904.

109. Orentreich N, Brind J, Rizer R, Vogelmen J. Age changes and sex differences in serum dehydroepiandrosterone sulfate concentration throughout adulthood. J Clin Endocrinol Metab 1984;59:551–555.

110. Nestler JE, Barlascini CO, Clore JN, Blackard WG. Dehydroepiandrosterone reduces serum low density lipoprotein levels and body fat but does not alter insulin sensitivity in normal men. J Clin Endocrinol Metab 1988;66:57–61 .

111. Barrett–Conner E, Khaw KT. Absence of an inverse relation of dehydroepiandrosterone sulfate with cardiovascular mortality in postmenopausal women. N Engl J Med 1987;317:711–715.

112. Casson PR, Buster JE. DHEA Administration to humans: panacea or palaver? Sem Repro Endo 1995;13:247–256.

113. Casson PR, Anderson RN, Herod HG. Oral dehydroepiandrosterone in physiologic doses modulates immune function in postmenopausal women. Am J Obstet Gynecol 1993; 169:1536–1539.

114. Khorran O, Vu L, Yen SCC. Activation of immune function by dehydroepiandrosterone (DHEA) in age–advanced men. J Gerontol 1997;52A M1–7.

115. Buster JE, Casson PR, Stroaughn AB, et al. Postmenopausal steroid replacement with micronized dehydroepiandrosterone: preliminary oral bioavailability and dose proportionnality studies. Am J Obstet Gynecol 1992;166:1163–1168.

22

Androgen Replacement in Women

*Susan R. Davis, MBBS, FRACP, PhD,
and Henry G. Burger, MBBS, FRACP*

CONTENTS

INTRODUCTION

There is increasing awareness of the significant and varied actions of endogenous androgens in women and acknowledgment that women may experience symptoms secondary to androgen deficiency. There is also substantial evidence that prudent testosterone replacement is effective in relieving both the physical and psychological symptoms of androgen insufficiency and is indicated for clinically affected women. Testosterone replacement for women is now available in a variety of formulations. It appears to be safe, with the caveat that doses should be restricted to the "therapeutic window" for androgen replacement in women in which the beneficial effects on well-being and quality of life can be achieved without incurring undesirable virilizing side effects.

The predominant complaint of women experiencing androgen deficiency is loss of sexual desire. Because of the complex hormonal-psychological etiology of this symptom, clinicians prescribing a hormone replacement therapy (HRT) regimen that includes an androgen component must be sensitive to the sexual and emotional needs of the affected woman and her partner, and care for the totality of the woman, not just her hormonal status. Many women who have the clinical symptoms of androgen insufficiency and low testosterone levels will respond to a replacement regimen and require no

From: *Contemporary Endocrinology: Hormone Replacement Therapy*
Edited by: A. W. Meikle © Humana Press Inc., Totowa, NJ

further intervention. However, a significant proportion of affected women have additional psycho-social issues that must be addressed, especially those who have undergone a premature menopause, or a menopause secondary to surgery or cancer therapy. Furthermore, body image issues, symptoms of post-traumatic stress, depression and other partnership problems may complicate response to hormonal therapy. Identification of such factors and appropriate professional referral will clearly optimize the overall health of such women and their response to any therapeutic intervention.

ANDROGEN PHYSIOLOGY IN THE PREMENOPAUSAL YEARS

Androgens are produced by the ovaries and the adrenals, both of which synthesize androstenedione (A), and dehydroepiandrosterone (DHEA). The ovaries are a primary site of testosterone production, however whether there is direct secretion of testosterone from the adrenals is controversial. After ovariectomy, both testosterone and A decrease by about 50% *(1)*. The adrenals also produce DHEA sulfate (DHEA-S). Conversion of the pre-androgens to testosterone peripherally accounts for at least 50% of circulating testosterone , with A being the main androgen precursor *(2)*. Androgens are produced by the ovary under the control of luteinising hormone (LH). The preovulatory phase of the menstrual cycle is associated with a rise in intrafollicular and circulating androgen levels, such that peripheral A and testosterone increase 15–20% at midcycle, followed by a secondary rise in A in the late luteal phase *(3)*. The mean daily production rate of testosterone in young healthy women is 0.43 ± 0.14 mg/d when measured in the follicular phase, with a diurnal variation, the highest rate of production occurring between 4:00 AM and midday *(4)*.

Only 1–2% of total circulating testosterone is free or biologically active; the rest is bound by sex hormone binding globulin (SHBG) and albumin. SHBG levels do not vary across the menstrual cycle, hence there is a midcycle increase in free testosterone in ovulating women *(5)*. SHBG binds, in decreasing order of affinity, DHT > testosterone >androstenediol > estradiol >estrone. In addition SHBG weakly binds DHEA, but not DHEA-S *(6)*.

Changes in SHBG levels in women can have dramatic effects on free circulating sex steroid levels. SHBG levels are suppressed by increases in circulating testosterone, glucocorticosteroids, growth hormone, and insulin (as in obesity), and increased by thyroxine and estrogens (as in pregnancy or during use of oral contraceptives).

CHANGES IN ANDROGENS WITH
THE MENOPAUSAL TRANSITION AND AGE

In contrast to estrogens, androgen levels do not fall precipitously at the menopause *(7,8)* but decline with increasing age, such that total circulating testosterone levels in women in their forties are approx 50% of those of women in their twenties *(9)*. Furthermore, as SHBG also declines with age, the ratio of testosterone to SHBG, also known as the free androgen index (FAI), does not change. However the absolute amount of circulating free testosterone in women older than 40 yr is also significantly less than women in their twenties *(9,10)*. The changes in testosterone and SHBG appear to be due partly to the decline in the adrenal production of DHEA and DHEA-S with increasing age *(11,12)*, and as one would expect the DHEA to testosterone and DHEA-S to testosterone ratios are age invariant *(9)*.

Reproductive ageing also contributes to the gradual waning of testosterone observed in the premenopausal years. The mid-cycle rise in free testosterone and A seen in younger women is absent in older reproductive aged women, in their mid forties, who continue to have regular menstrual cycles with a measurable LH surge *(5)*. In postmenopausal women total testosterone levels are positively correlated with LH, which most probably reflects ongoing stimulation of ovarian interstitial cells by LH in the postmenopausal ovary *(13)*. This is of clinical significance since the administration of exogenous estrogen, either as hormone replacement therapy or the oral contraceptive pill, may not only precipitate relative testosterone deficiency by increasing SHBG and hence lowering the absolute amount of free testosterone *(14–16)*, but also by suppressing the LH stimulus to the ovary for interstitial cell testosterone production *(16–18)*.

Indeed, clinical studies have demonstrated that following the introduction of a standard dose of 0.625 mg of conjugated equine estrogens daily, the mean testosterone to SHBG ratio, and measured free testosterone each fall by approx 30% *(14,15)*. Similarly administration of the oral contraceptive pill suppresses circulating total testosterone, with normalization of levels during the pill free menstrual phase *(16)*. The latter is less likely to be clinically manifest in younger reproductive-aged women, but on the background of declining testosterone production with age, the oral contraceptive pill may be associated with the reporting of diminished libido in women in their later reproductive years.

In evaluating women for androgen deficiency it is important to measure either SHBG in addition to total testosterone to calculate the FAI, or free testosterone directly. Because measured and estimated bioavailable testosterone are strongly correlated *(19)*, calculation of the FAI is adequate for clinical practice. The key point is that detection of a total testosterone level within the normal reproductive female range in any woman taking exogenous thyroid replacement or estrogen in any form does not exclude a physiological deficiency of bioavailable testosterone.

EVIDENCE FOR THE ROLE OF ANDROGENS IN FEMALE HEALTH AND WELL-BEING

Androgens and Female Sexuality

Satisfactory sexual function is an essential component of health and well-being, with "satisfactory" being an evaluation made by the individual in the context of her/his personal expectations and desires. Sexuality and libido are undoubtedly determined by many interacting factors. These include a person's physiological state, their physical and social environment, personal knowledge, past experiences, current expectations and of major influence, their cultural milieu. Thus, the complexity of human sexuality extends far beyond the biology of procreation.

There is a prevailing misconception that women's sexuality declines with increasing age, and that older women who continue to engage in intercourse do so to please their partner. The majority of women who undergo a natural menopause maintain their capacity for sexual desire, erotic pleasure and orgasm, although there is a general age-related decline in sexual frequency in women. However, there is a strong association between the menopause and lessening sexual and coital frequency, which is independent of age *(20)*. Some studies suggest that, compared with premenopausal women, women after their menopause report fewer sexual thoughts or fantasies, have less vaginal lubrication during sex and are less satisfied with their partners as lovers, with a low testosterone level being most closely correlated with reduced coital frequency *(21)*. However, a large community based cross-sectional study showed that 62% of a group of 45–55 yr old women reported no change in sexuality in the preceding year, although 31% reported a decrease *(22)*. The decline in sexual interest was significantly and adversely associated with menopause rather than with age. Clearly the effects of age on the health and sexual interest of men and availability of a sexual partner contribute to the observed decreases in women. Research addressing the effects on women anticipating an adverse influence of their menopause on their sexuality has shown that the correlation between anticipated changes in sexuality and what is actually experienced is weak *(23)*. The greatest predictor of a woman having a satisfying sexual relationship or experiences after her menopause is the quality of the sexual aspects of her life before the menopause, with those most content with their premenopausal sexuality least likely to report problems. Despite this general trend it is not uncommon for an individual to express frustration that she has had a very satisfying sexual relationship, but since menopause her sexuality has declined dramatically, with no other identifiable factors.

Androgens appear to play a key role in female sexuality in that diminished androgen levels in the postmenopausal years appear to contribute to the decline in sexual interest expressed by many women. Bachmann and Leiblum studied sexuality in sexagenarian women and observed that of the hormones studied, serum free testosterone was positively correlated with increased sexual desire *(24)*. Estrogen replacement will improve vasomotor symptoms, vaginal dryness and general well-being, but has little effect on libido *(25,26)*. Oral estrogen replacement therapy improves sexual satisfaction in women with atrophic vaginitis causing their dyspareunia, but women without coital discomfort appear to benefit little or not at all *(27,28)*.

Several studies have shown improvements in a number of parameters of sexuality in postmenopausal women treated with exogenous testosterone over and above the effects achieved with estrogen alone.

Estradiol and testosterone are both present in the human female brain. The highest concentrations of estradiol have been reported in the hypothalamus and the preoptic area, and of testosterone, in the substantia nigra, hypothalamus and the preoptic area *(29)*. The concentration of testosterone is several-fold higher than estradiol in each of these regions, with the highest ratio of testosterone to estradiol occurring in the hypothalamus and preoptic area which corresponds with the high aromatase activity found in these regions *(30)*. This provokes the question whether androgens act directly on the brain or only after conversion by aromatization to estrogen within the central nervous system. Support for specific direct androgen actions within the brain comes from studies of the effects of cross-sex hormone therapy in transsexuals *(31)*. Whereas the administration of androgens to female-to-male transsexuals leads to an increase in sexual motivation and arousability, the combination of anti-androgens and high dose estrogen given to male-to-female transsexuals has the opposite effect.

Androgen treatment of female-to-male transsexuals also results in improved visuospatial ability, a deterioration in verbal fluency, and increased anger readiness, whilst the reverse, including an increased tendency to indirect angry behaviour is seen in the male-to-female subjects *(31)*.

Exogenous androgen replacement in the form of testosterone, either as an injection or a subcutaneous implant enhances sexual motivation *(27,28,32–35)*. Improvements in intensity of sexual drive, arousal, frequency of sexual fantasies, satisfaction, pleasure, and relevancy have all been documented.

In contrast to the consistently observed increases in sexual motivation, improvements in coital frequency and orgasm vary considerably between studies. Certainly the failure of androgen therapy to improve coital frequency has been attributed to the relevant studies involving women with very long term relationships, such that sexual patterns are very established with a reluctance toward change. Frequency of sexual activity as a measure of efficacy of androgen therapy in women can be misleading as traditionally it is more a measure of a male partner's sexual appetite rather than the woman's. The only study in which the addition of testosterone did not show any benefit over estrogen alone was of women being treated for generalized menopausal symptoms rather than low libido *(36)*.

Testosterone replacement will be of benefit only to women who have a significant hormonal component to their sexual dysfunction. Discerning this can be quite straight-forward in many instances, for example post ovariectomy, but extremely complex in some women.

When considering whether a woman may be a candidate for androgen replacement it is essential to take a reasonably detailed, although not overly intrusive sexual history. The main feature to establish is whether there are other significant aspects of the woman's life or relationship contributing to her apparent sexual difficulties.

Androgens and Bone Function

Androgenic steroids have an important physiologic role in the development and maintenance of bone mass in women and men. Human osteoblastic cells possess androgen receptors and androgens have been shown to directly stimulate bone cell proliferation and differentiation *(37,38)*. Clinical research has demonstrated positive relationships between bone density and androgens in young, premenopausal and peri-menopausal women. Premenopausal bone loss is significantly associated with circulating testosterone levels, but not with estradiol *(39,40)*. Women who experience bone loss confined to the hip in their premenopausal years, which is not an uncommon finding, have lower total and free testosterone concentrations (by 14 and 22%, respectively) than those who do not have significant bone loss *(40)*. Consistent with these findings, hyperandrogenic women have higher bone mineral density (BMD), after correction for body mass index, than their normal female counterparts *(41)*. In the premenopausal years BMD is also strongly positively correlated with body weight *(39)*. Obesity suppresses SHBG with a resultant increase in free testosterone *(42)*. This may partially explain the relationship among obesity, free testosterone, and increased BMD, with the greater endogenous levels of biologically active free testosterone directly enhancing bone mass.

Low circulating bioavailable testosterone is significantly correlated with subsequent height loss (a surrogate measure of vertebral compression fractures) and hip fracture in postmenopausal women *(43,44)*.

Studies of both oral and parenteral estrogen and estrogen-plus-testosterone therapy in postmenopausal women have shown beneficial effects of androgens on BMD. An oral esterified estrogen-methyltestosterone combination lead to increased spinal bone mineral density over a 2-yr period, in contrast to estrogen-only therapy which prevented bone loss *(45)*. The oral estrogen-methyltestosterone combination not only suppressed several biochemical markers of bone reabsorption (as seen with estrogen alone) but was also associated with increases in the markers of bone formation *(45)*. Treatment of postmenopausal women with nandrolone decanoate has been shown to increase vertebral BMD and has been used successfully for many years to treat osteoporosis *(46)*. Combined estradiol and testosterone replacement with subcutaneous implant pellets increases bone mass in postmenopausal women *(47,48)*, with the effects in the hip and spine being greater than with estradiol implants alone *(35)*. Thus it appears that estradiol alone has an anti-reabsorptive effect on bone in postmenopausal women, whereas the addition of testoster-one, either orally or parentally results in increased bone formation.

This is further supported by studies of men, either with a mutation of the gene encoding the aromatase enzyme *(49)* or a mutation of the estrogen receptor *(50)*. These findings are encouraging, however improving BMD is only clinically important if it is associated with enhanced mechanical strength and a reduced fracture rate. To date, no studies have addressed the impact of androgens on the incidence of fracture. However, the effects of androgens on the mechanical properties of bone have been studied in feral female cyno-molgus monkeys *(51)*. Increases in intrinsic bone strength and resistance to mechanical stress were associated with increased BMD following testosterone therapy. Treatment also resulted in increased bone torsional rigidity and bending stiffness.

Androgen Replacement and Glucocorticosteroid-Related Bone Loss

Circulating DHEA and DHEA-S have been positively correlated with BMD in ageing women *(52–54)* and the progressive decline in DHEA with increasing age is believed to contribute to senile osteoporosis. It is not clear whether these adrenal pre-androgens directly influence bone metabolism or whether their effects are mediated indirectly after conversion to estradiol, A, or testosterone. Older women treated with oral DHEA have restoration of circulating A, DHT, and testosterone to premenopausal levels, as well as increases in DHEA and DHEA-S, with no changes in circulating levels of estrone or estradiol from baseline *(55)*. Furthermore, circulating DHEA-S, but not estradiol, in postmenopausal women is positively correlated with BMD *(52)*. The therapeutic admin-istration of glucocorticosteroids results in significant suppression of adrenal pre-andro-gen secretion *(56)*, which in turn may be a major factor in the development of iatrogenic osteopenia and osteoporosis with long term glucocorticosteroid use. Therefore, a pos-sible role for androgen replacement could indeed be to prevent or treat glucocorticosteroid induced bone loss in both pre and post menopausal women.

In summary, current data indicates androgen replacement, in the form of testosterone, is potentially an effective alternative to the prevention of bone loss and the treatment of osteopenia and osteoporosis. However as prospective data confirming a reduction in fracture rate with such therapy is lacking, it cannot presently be recommended for this sole indication. Further research into the biological actions of androgens in bone and clinical studies of testosterone replacement and fracture are therefore needed to define the appropriate clinical application of androgens in the prevention and treatment of bone loss.

Metabolic Effects of Androgen Therapy: Risks and Benefits

Cardiovascular Disease Risk

There are prevailing concerns regarding potential adverse metabolic effects of andro-gen replacement in women, particularly with respect to possible detrimental effects on body composition, lipid and lipoprotein metabolism and vascular function. However, available clinical data is extremely reassuring in that androgen replacement therapy in women does not appear to be associated with the undesirable metabolic consequences as seen in women with androgen excess or with an increase in cardiovascular risk.

ANDROGENS AND BODY COMPOSITION

In postmenopausal women, neither measured nor estimated bioavailable testosterone is associated with waist-to-hip ratio measurements and there does not appear to be a causal relationship between androgens and visceral adiposity in this population *(19)*. Testosterone replacement by implant is associated with a modest increase in lean body mass measured by dual photon X-ray absorptiometry, and a reduction in total body fat, with no variation in BMI *(35)*.

Testosterone levels are frequently low in human immunodeficiency virus (HIV)–positive premenopausal women *(57)* and testosterone replacement is associated with an increase in fat free mass and body cell mass in HIV-positive men *(58)*. Studies are underway to evaluate the effects of testosterone therapy on body composition parameters in HIV-positive premenopausal women, with the expectation that such therapy may result in an increase in lean body mass, and partially reverse the wasting component of this disease. It is also conceivable that testosterone replacement may be of benefit to premenopausal women suffering other illnesses associated with loss of lean body mass, such as malignant disease with cachexia.

Contrary to popular myth, neither oral nor parenteral hormone replacement therapy results in significantly increased body weight *(35,59)*. There is also no evidence that the addition of testosterone replacement leads to weight gain, although this treatment is associated with a reduction in total body fat and an increase in lean mass. With increasing age women tend to lose muscle mass and replace this with increased fat mass, with an overall tendency for weight gain in most western societies. The small increase in lean mass observed with testosterone replacement is probably of beneficial effect, which in the long term will contribute to preservation of muscle strength and skeletal stability. The only ethical issue provoked by androgen replacement therapy in older women is whether treated women who participate in competitive sport have any advantage in terms of muscle strength over their untreated counterparts.

TESTOSTERONE REPLACEMENT AND LIPIDS AND LIPOPROTEINS

Menopause, both natural and surgically induced, is associated with the development of a more adverse lipoprotein profile, however there appears to be no relationship between these observed lipid and lipoprotein changes and endogenous testosterone levels *(60)*. Postmenopausal estrogen replacement therapy results in reductions in total and low-density lipoprotein (LDL)-cholesterol and these favourable effects are not diminished with either oral or parenteral testosterone replacement *(45,46)*. Parenteral testosterone replacement does not affect high-density lipoprotein (HDL)-cholesterol *(35)*, however, HDL-cholesterol and apolipoprotein A1 decrease significantly when oral methyltestosterone is administered concurrently with oral estrogen *(45,61)*. Oral estrogen replacement is associated with increased triglyceride levels. In contrast concomitant administration of oral methyltestosterone has been associated with a reduction in triglycerides *(45)*.

The measurement of circulating lipids is an accepted surrogate for lipid metabolism. However, more direct measurement of lipid metabolism probably gives a better indication of the effects of exogenous steroid therapy on cardiovascular risk. Combined oral esterified estrogen and methyltestosterone therapy results in reduced arterial LDL degradation and cholesterol ester content in cynomolgus monkeys which does not differ from the effects observed when estrogen is given alone *(62)*. Combined estrogen and methyltestosterone therapy is also associated with reduced plasma concentrations of apoplipoprotein B, reduced LDL particle size and increased total body LDL catabolism *(62)*. Small LDL particles are more susceptible to oxidation and are hence considered to be more atherogenic. However, since estrogens appear to increase oxidative modification of LDL in the arterial wall *(62)*, the reduction in LDL particle size observed with both oral estrogen and combined therapy may not be deleterious but may merely reflect selective removal of large LDL particles from the circulation.

ANDROGEN REPLACEMENT AND VASCULAR FUNCTION

Neither circulating testosterone nor DHEA-S levels are associated with an increased risk of heart disease in postmenopausal women *(63,64)*. Intracoronary testosterone administration to anaesthetised male and female dogs induces increases in coronary artery cross-sectional area peak flow velocity and calculated volumetric blood flow which is blocked by pretreatment with an inhibitor of nitric oxide synthesis *(65)*. Furthermore, oral methyltestosterone does not diminish the beneficial effects of estrogen replacement therapy on coronary artery reactivity in cynomolgus monkeys *(66)*.

Thus, in summary, the inclusion of testosterone in a hormone replacement regimen does not appear to affect the key events in coronary artery lipid metabolism or coronary artery function. Parenteral testosterone replacement does not negate the favourable effects exerted by exogenous estrogen on lipid and lipoprotein levels, whereas oral methyltestosterone use not only opposes the HDL-cholesterol elevating effects of oral estrogen, but also reduces HDL-cholesterol levels below baseline values. Whether this effect of oral methyltestosterone in the setting of concomitant lowering of total cholesterol, LDL-cholesterol and triglyceride levels is detrimental, is not known. Certainly a high cardiac risk profile, which includes a low HDL-cholesterol level, should be considered a relative contraindication to oral testosterone replacement, but should not influence the use of parenteral testosterone replacement therapy.

ANDROGENS AND BREAST CANCER

Elevated endogenous androgen levels have been reported to be associated with breast cancer *(67,68)*. However interpretation of the available data has been limited by multiple compounding factors in these published studies. In post menopausal women with breast cancer, age-adjusted mean values of total and free testosterone have found to be higher than in controls *(69)* and intra-tumour concentrations of 5 alpha-DHT and estradiol have been reported to be greater than circulating levels of these hormones *(70)*. Androgen receptors are found in over 50% of breast tumours *(70)* and are associated with longer survival in women with operable breast cancer and a favourable response to hormone treatment in advanced disease *(71)*. As yet it is not known whether there is any relationship between exogenous androgen therapy and the occurrence of breast cancer.

VIRILIZATION WITH EXOGENOUS ANDROGEN EXCESS

Cosmetic side effects of androgen replacement are rare if supra-physiological hormone levels are avoided *(27,28,32,34,48)*, but the potential virilising effects include development of acne, hirsutism deepening of the voice and excessive libido. Women troubled by existing hirsutism or acne should not be prescribed androgen therapy. Although enhanced libido is mostly seen as a benefit of therapy, increases in sexual thoughts and fantasies may well be undesirable for some women, and this should be

Table 1
Clinical Settings in Which Androgen Replacement Therapy may be Beneficial

Premature ovarian failure, including Turner's Syndrome.
Premenopausal iatrogenic androgen deficiency states.
Symptomatic androgen deficiency due to surgical menopause, chemotherapy or irradiation.
Symptomatic androgen deficiency following natural menopause.
Potential indications:
    Glucocorticosteroid-induced bone loss.
    GNRH-analog treatment of endometriosis.
    Management of wasting syndromes.
    Premenopausal bone loss.
    Premenopausal loss of libido with diminished serum free testosterone.

clearly borne in mind if androgen replacement is being considered for the prevention or management of bone loss.

Summary

Disorders of endogenous androgen excess are clearly associated with increased cardiovascular risk, perturbations in lipid and carbohydrate metabolism, a more android weight distribution and cosmetic manifestations of virilisation. All these undesirable metabolic effects are extremely unlikely and uncommon with androgen replacement therapy with the caveat that circulating androgen levels are maintained close to, or within, the normal female reproductive range and that patients are closely clinically monitored. With respect to breast cancer risk, women who have endogenously high androgen levels do appear to be at increased risk. There is no evidence that this increase in risk can be extrapolated to so-called "physiological" exogenous androgen replacement therapy after menopause. However, until more data is available, physicians should be cognisant of the possibility that androgen replacement could influence breast cancer development and clinical vigilance must be maintained.

IDENTIFYING WOMEN MOST LIKELY TO BENEFIT FROM ANDROGEN REPLACEMENT

Although a list of potential indications for androgen therapy is provided, the decision to offer androgen replacement to a woman is based on clinical assessment, and the outcome of treatment dependent upon the subjective self-assessment of response and reporting by the patient. Biochemical measurements are of limited value, but clearly may guide the clinician away from offering androgen replacement when the free androgen index or free testosterone level is in the high normal range.

The clinical settings in which administration of androgen replacement are most likely to enhance a woman's health and well-being are listed in Table 1. Possible future indications may also include the use of androgens in wasting states, such as HIV infected individuals and malignancy-related cachexia, and to prevent or treat bone loss, particularly iatrogenic bone loss from glucocorticosteriod therapy or premenopausal bone loss.

Some women actively seek clinical assistance for loss of libido and/or inadequate restoration of well-being despite adequate estrogen/progestogen replacement. Others may volunteer such problems whilst attending their physician for another reason, however many women suffer silently, believing that this is their "lot" or are unaware of any available therapeutic options. Many women will not raise the issue of diminished libido because they find the topic awkward. Sadly, a number of young women who suffer loss of libido following cancer therapy express difficulty discussing the issue with their oncologist as they feel their problem will be seen as trivial relative to their disease recovery or remission. In many women following chemo- or radiotherapy the symptoms of the iatrogenic menopause and androgen deficiency, including fatigue, loss of well-being, depression and reduced libido, can be difficult to distinguish from the overall physical toll of their therapy and frequently their premature menopause and associated androgen insufficiency go undiagnosed and untreated. Therefore all "at risk" women should be at least directly questioned about the symptoms of androgen deficiency and made aware of the therapeutic possibilities available.

Symptoms such as fatigue and loss of well-being are extremely difficult to quantitate and similar to diminished libido, it can be very difficult for both the physician and the patient to ascertain the cause of these symptoms with certainty when the patient's circumstances are multi-factorial. The keys to dissecting out whether testosterone deficiency is a major factor and whether replacement is likely to be successful are in reality very simple and include:

1. Spending TIME talking to the patient.
2. LISTENING CAREFULLY to what the woman says, and most importantly.
3. Asking the woman WHAT SHE BELIEVES to be the fundamental problem.

In general, women are very reliable assessors of their own health and well-being and importantly are reluctant to use any therapy unless they truly believe it will result in an improvement in their health. Obviously, in assessing a woman presenting with loss of libido the physician needs to establish the individual's past sexual history, the changes that have occurred in her sexuality, the status of her current relationship, and the presence of any other extrinsic or intrinsic factors that may affect her libido, particularly stress and depression.

Premature Ovarian Failure Including Turner's Syndrome

The management of young women with premature menopause, particularly Turner's syndrome, who have never been sexually active is more difficult and perhaps controversial. Androgen replacement should be considered for such women experiencing persistent fatigue, inadequate well-being and lack of libido despite adequate estrogen and progestogen replacement. However it is obviously difficult for a woman to identify herself as having inadequate libido when she has never experienced what may be "normal." Alternatively young women who have not become sexually active should become fully informed about androgen replacement as a future option, or perhaps in some instances offered very low dose androgen replacement as a component of their HRT regimen at an earlier stage. Whether young women with premature ovarian failure should be recommended to use androgen replacement to prevent bone loss, specifically from the neck of femur, is yet to be established.

Premenopausal Iatrogenic Androgen Deficiency States

GNRH analogues are in common usage for the treatment of severe endometriosis. Clinical consequences of the use of this therapy include symptoms of estrogen deficiency, bone loss and loss of libido. Low dose testosterone replacement could possibly be used to prevent bone loss and diminish some of the symptoms which are side effects of this therapy, although this is not an established clinical indication. The use of low dose testosterone replacement to prevent or treat glucocorticosteroid-related osteopenia and osteoporosis also warrants further clinical research. The administration of androgen replacement in a setting of suppressed androgen levels with the use of the oral contraceptive pill is not currently an accepted practice. Ideally women suffering such consequences of oral contraception would be best advised to consider other forms of contraception and experience restoration of their own endogenous androgen levels following resumption of their normal ovarian function.

Androgen Replacement Following Menopause

Androgen replacement therapy has become an accepted component of hormone replacement therapy for the restoration of sexual and general well-being in women who have undergone a surgical menopause. Its use in naturally menopausal women, particularly in the perimenopausal years, remains controversial. This is because most studies published have focused on treating the surgically menopausal patient rather than the naturally menopausal woman. Most women, following natural menopause, do not experience any loss of libido. However, there is a significant sub group of women who do experience clear decline in their sexuality in association with the menopause, which anecdotally appears to be more frequent in women experiencing an earlier menopause. Androgen replacement in women who have experienced a natural menopause continues to be a neglected component of hormone replacement therapy in the management of their postmenopausal symptoms. Not only are such women usually very responsive to androgen replacement in terms of restoration of their sexuality, but they also frequently describe an increased sense of well-being and overall energy related to their androgen replacement therapy.

Whether premenopausal women who complain of loss of libido and who have low bioavailable testosterone levels should be offered androgen replacement is even more controversial. Certainly such women do appear to be at greater risk of premenopausal bone loss and it is the author's experience that some symptomatic premenopausal women with low measurable testosterone levels clinically appear to benefit from androgen therapy. At present this is a sub-group of women for whom clear recommendations cannot be made. However their symptoms should not be dismissed or too quickly attributed to other psycho-social factors, as it is possible that relative testosterone deficiency is a major contributing factor. Currently management of such women needs to be very open minded and therapy completely individualised, but we must await the results of relevant clinical studies before specific therapeutic guidelines for the premenopausal woman can be made.

Clearly androgen replacement is a far more sensitive issue for the women than HRT in general. It is essential that a physician consulting in this area is sensitive to the enormous variations in women's knowledge, expectations, sexual practices and needs and in every case tailors the therapy to the individual's circumstances.

HOW SHOULD ANDROGEN REPLACEMENT BE PRESCRIBED?

Although no form of androgen replacement is commercially available in the United States for the treatment of loss of libido in women, oral methyltestosterone can be prescribed for menopausal symptoms unresponsive to estrogen replacement alone, and tes-

Table 2
Androgen Replacement Therapy Formulations Used for Women

	Route	Frequency	Dose range
Methyltestosterone[a] (in combination with esterified estrogen).	Oral	Daily	1.25–2.5mg
Testosterone undecanoate.	Oral	Daily or	40–80 mg alternate daily
Testosterone implants.	Subcutaneous	3–6 monthly	50 mg
Nandrolone decanoate.	Intramuscular	6–12 weekly	25–50mg
Mixed testosterone esters.	Intramuscular	Monthly	50–100mg

[a]Currently available in US.

tosterone implants have been approved for replacement therapy for women in the United Kingdom. The current global therapeutic options in terms of androgen replacement therapy are listed in Table 2.

To achieve a good therapeutic response, in terms of enhanced libido, with testosterone replacement, it appears that testosterone levels often need to be restored to at least the upper end of the normal physiological range for young ovulating women. The doses of androgen replacement required to achieve such an effect usually result in an initial post administration peak testosterone level, that is supraphysiological regardless of the mode of administration.

An oral estrogen/androgen preparation is currently available in the United States in two doses, esterified estrogen 0.625 mg plus methyltestosterone 1.25 mg, or esterified estrogen 1.25 mg plus methyltestosterone 2.5 mg. Methyltestosterone is not available in any other countries because liver damage has been reported with long-term, high-dose therapy *(72)*. A more recent study has not shown any short-term (12 mo) detrimental effects of these doses of methyltestosterone combined with estrogen on hepatic enzymes or blood pressure *(72)*. Interestingly women who use esterified estrogens combined with methyltestosterone report a lower instance of nausea compared with women receiving conjugated equine estrogen alone *(72)*.

Testosterone undecanoate is an oral androgen mostly used for replacement therapy in hypogonadal men. Its clinical application in women has been little studied although in some countries its use is quite widespread. It is believed to be absorbed via the lymphatic system hence, for best effect it is recommended that testosterone undecanoate be ingested with fat, for example with a glass of milk. The clinical role for testosterone undecanoate as a replacement therapy for women at present remains unclear and further research is required before its use can be recommended.

There has now been considerable clinical experience with the administration of testosterone implants in postmenopausal women particularly in the Commonwealth countries. These implants are fused crystalline implants 4–5 mm in diameter containing testosterone BP (British Pharmacopoeia) as the active ingredient. Experience indicates that a dose of 50 mg in extremely effective and does not result in virilising side effects *(35)*. This dose is obtained by bisecting a 100-mg implant under sterile conditions. The implant is inserted, under local anaesthesia, subcutaneously, usually into the lower anterior abdominal wall using a trocar and cannula. This therapy provides a slow release of testosterone with an approximate duration of effect for a 50 mg implant of between

Table 3
Contra-indications to Testosterone Therapy

Pregnancy or lactation.
Known or suspected androgen-dependent neoplasia.
Severe acne.
Moderate–severe hirsutism.
Circumstances in which enhanced libido would be undesirable.
Androgenic alopecia.

3–6 mo. As there is significant variation in the duration of the effect, women treated with testosterone implants must be carefully monitored and serum testosterone levels measured prior to the administration of each subsequent implant. It is recommended that additional testosterone implants should not be inserted unless total testosterone is in the normal range for young women. The use of testosterone implants greater than 100mg would prudently be avoided.

The recent development of a transdermal testosterone matrix patch, intended specifically for use in women, will provide yet another therapeutic option for those requiring androgen replacement. The patch, which is now undergoing early clinical trials, is designed to deliver 150 mcg of testosterone per day over a 3–4 d period (twice-a-week application). This should raise circulating testosterone levels, on average, by approx 25 ng/dL, (about 1 nmol/L). Such a patch will have some obvious advantages over both oral and implant therapy; however, as with other hormone patches, some women may experience skin irritation or simply prefer a less conspicuous mode of therapy.

Nandrolone deconoate is approved in some countries for the treatment of postmenopausal osteoporosis. The dose, administered intramuscularly, should not exceed 50 mg and the frequency of the dose is best titrated against the patient's gross build. It is prudent that treatment is not given less than six weekly and patients should be very carefully monitored for hirsutism and voice deepening. In most women, treatment with nandronone decanoate results in cessation of bone loss over time and in some women an increase in BMD.

A final potential alternative, which is not currently generally available, is a transdermal testosterone cream or gel. Although such preparations may be regionally available on specific prescription from compounding pharmacists, there is no pharmacokinetic data available or published clinical experience pertaining to their use.

The contraindications to and side effects of testosterone replacement are listed in Tables 3 and 4. Again it is emphasised that with judicious dosing and careful patient monitoring side effects of testosterone replacement are rare. All postmenopausal women treated with testosterone replacement should be using concurrent estrogen replacement therapy. There is no clinical data available regarding the use of testosterone replacement in postmenopausal women who are not on estrogen, however one would predict that such use may well result in adverse metabolic and cosmetic side effects. The sole circumstance in which androgen therapy has been administered without concurrent estrogen use is the administration of the anabolic steroid nandrolone decanoate. Women treated with this steroid must be extremely carefully monitored for adverse effects including voice change and hirsutism which do occur when this compound is administered unopposed by estrogen.

Table 4
Side Effects from Excessive Dosage

Virilization—hirsutism, acne, temporal balding, voice deepening.
Clitoromegaly.
Fluid retention.
Hepatocellular damage—has been associated with high dose 17-a-alkylandrogens given orally.
Lipids—oral androgens may adversely affect serum levels of lipids and lipoproteins.
Drug interactions—C17 substituted derivatives of oral testosterone may decrease anticoagulant
    requirements. Androgens may elevate serum levels of oxyphenbutazone and in diabetic patients
    may rarely affect insulin requirements.

CONCLUSIONS

Testosterone, together with its metabolite, dihydrotestosterone, is the most potent physiological androgen in both men and women. Paradoxically, it is the major precursor of estrogens. Testosterone is secreted by the ovaries (and perhaps the adrenals) as well as being formed peripherally from precursors such as androstenedione. Its levels in women fall substantially during the reproductive years, with little further change at the time of spontaneous menopause. A major fall in circulating testosterone occurs following bilateral oophorectomy. The biological availability of the hormone is determined by the levels of SHBG, with factors which raise SHBG levels leading to a fall in bioavailable T. A substantial body of evidence indicates that T is an important determinant of female sexuality, and that androgen replacement enhances certain aspects of sexual function, particularly in women who have undergone oophorectomy. Physiological range androgen replacement may also have a role in the maintenance or restoration of bone mass, both following menopause and after pharmacological glucocorticoid therapy. Its role as an anabolic agent in women with wasting diseases remains to be established. At levels in or just above the physiological range, testosterone in women does not appear to have major adverse effects on cardiovascular risk factors or on vascular function. Its role, if any, in breast cancer risk remains uncertain. Androgen replacement may be particularly beneficial in women with premature ovarian failure, premenopausal iatrogenic androgen deficiency, symptomatic androgen deficiency following surgical, chemo-therapeutically-induced or radiation induced menopause and symptomatic androgen deficiency following natural menopause. Advances, particularly involving transdermal technologies, are occurring in the effort to optimise the methods of androgen replacement in women, as well as in men.

REFERENCES

1. Judd HL. Hormonal dynamics associated with the menopause. Clin Obstet Gynecol 1976;19:775–788.
2. Kirschner MAA, Bardin CW. Androgen production and metabolism in normal and virilized women. Metabolism 1972;21:667–688.
3. Judd HL, Yen, S. S. C. Serum androstenedione and testosterone levels during the menstrual cycle. J Clin Endocrinol Metab 1973;36(475):481.
4. Vierhapper H, Nowotny P, Waldhausl W. Determination of testosterone production rates in men and women using stable isotope dilution and mass spectromety. J Clin Endocrinol Metab 1997;82:1492–1496.
5. Mushayandebvu T, Castracane DV, Gimpel T, Adel T, Santoro N. Evidence for diminished midcycle ovarian androgen production in older reproductive aged women. Fertil Steril 1996;65:721–723.

6. Dunn JF, Nisula BC, Rodboard D. Transport of steroid hormones. Binding of 21 endogenous steroids to both testosterone-binding globulin and cortico-steroid-binding globulin in human plasma. J Clin Endocrinol Metab 1981;53:58–68.

7. Longcope C, Franz C, Morello C, Baker K, Johnston CC, Jr. Steroid and gonadotropin levels in women during the peri-menopausal years. Maturitas 1986;8:189–196.

8. Burger HG, Dudley EC, Hopper JL, et al. The endocrinology of the menopausal transition: a cross-sectional study of a population-based sample. J Clin Endocrinol Metab 1995;80:3537–3545.

9. Zumoff B, Strain GW, Miller LK, Rosner W. Twenty-four hour mean plasma testosterone concentration declines with age in normal premenopausal women. J Clin Endocrinol Metab 1995;80:1429–1430.

10. Rannevik G, Jeppsson S, Johnell O. A longitudinal study of the perimenopausal transition: altered profiles of steroid and pituitary hormones, SHBG and bone mineral density. Maturitas 1986;8:189–196.

11. Zumoff B, Rosenfeld RS, Strain GW. Sex differences in the 24 hour mean plasma concentrations of dehydroisoandrosterone (DHA) and dehydroisoandrosterone sulfate (DHAS) and the DHA to DHAS ratio in normal adults. J Clin Endocrinol Metab 1980;51:330–334.

12. Meldrum, Dr. Changes in circulating steroids with aging in post menopausal women. Obstet Gynecol 1997;57:624–628.

13. Bancroft J., Cawood EHH. Androgens and the menopause: a study of 40–60 year old women. Clin Endocrinol 1996;45:577–587.

14. Tazuke S, Khaw K-T, Chir MBB, and Barrett-Connor E. Exogenous estrogen and endogenous sex hormones. Medicine 1992;71:44–51.

15. Mathur RS, Landgreve SC, Moody LO, Semmens JP, Williamson HO. The effect of estrogen treatment on plasma concentrations of steroid hormones, gonadotropins, prolactin and sex hormone-binding globulin in post-menopausal women. Maturitas 1985;7:129–133.

16. Krug R, Psych D, Pietrowsky R, Fehm HL, Born J. Selective influence of menstrual cycle on perception of stimuli with reproductive significance. Psychosom Med 1994;56:410–417.

17. Ushiroyama T, Sugimoto O. Endocrine function of the peri- and postmenopausal ovary. Horm Res 1995;44:64–68.

18. Castlo-Branco C, Martinez de Osaba MJ, Fortuny A, Iglesias X, Gonzalez-Merlo J. Circulating hormone levels in menopausal women receiving different hormone replacement therapy regimens. A comparison. J Reprod Med 1995;40:556–560.

19. Goodman-Gruen D, Barrett-Connor E. Total but not bioavailable testosterone is a predictor of central adiposity in postmenopausal women. Int J Obes 1995;19:293–298.

20. Hallstrom, T. Sexuality in the climacteric. Clin Obstet Gynecol 1977;4:227–239.

21. McCoy NL, Davidson JM. A longitudinal study of the effects of menopause on sexuality. Maturitas 1985;7:203–210.

22. Dennerstein L, Smith, AMA, Morse, Burger H. Sexuality and the menopause. J Psychsom Obstet Gynecol 1994;15:56–59.

23. Frock J, Money J. Sexuality and the menopause. Psychother Psychosom 1992;57:29–33.

24. Bachmann GA. Leiblum SR. Sexuality in sexagenarian women. Maturitas 1991;13:45–50.

25. Utian WH. The true clinical features of postmenopausal oophorectomy and their response to estrogen replacement therapy. S Afr Med J 1972;46:732–737.

26. Campbell S, Whitehead,M. Oestrogen therapy and the menopausal syndrome. Clin Obstet Gynecol 1977;4:31–47.

27. Studd JWW, Chakravarti S, Oram D. The climacteric. Clin Obstet Gynecol 1977;4:3–29.

28. Sherwin BN, Gelfand MM, Brender W. Androgen enhances sexual motivation in females: a prespective, crossover study of sex steroid administration in surgical menopause. Psychosom Med 1997;47:339–351.

29. Bixo M, Backstrom T, Winblad B, Andersson A. Estradiol and testosterone in specific regions of the human female brain in different endocrine states. J Steroid Biochem Mol Biol 1995;55:297–303.

30. Roselli CE, Resko JA. Aromatase activity in the rat brain: hormone regulation and sex differences. J Steroid Biochem Mol Biol 1993;44:499–508.

31. Van Goozen, SHM, Cohen-Kettensis PT, Gooren LIG., Frijda NH, Van de Poll NE. Gender differences in behaviour: activating effects of cross-sex hormones. Psychoneuroendocrinology 1995;20:343–363.

32. Studd JWW, Colins WP, Chakravarti S. Estradiol and testosterone implants in the treatment of psycho-sexual problems in postmenopausal women. Br J Obstet Gynaecol 1977;84:314–315.

33. Burger HG, Hailes J, Menelaus M. The management of persistent symptoms with estradiol-testosterone implants: clinical, lipid and hormonal results. Maturitas 1984;6:351–358.

34. Burger HG, Hailes J, Nelson J, Menelaus M. Effect of combined implants of estradiol and testosterone on libido in postmenopausal women. Br Med J 1987;294:936–937.

35. Davis SR, McCloud PI, Strauss BJG, Burger HG. Testosterone enhances estradiol's effects on post-menopausal bone density and sexuality. Maturitas 1995;21:227–236.

36. Dow MGT, Hart DM, Forrest CA. Hormonal treatments of sexual unresponsiveness in postmenopausal women: a comparative study. Br J Obstet Gynaecol 1983;90:361–366.

37. Colvard DS, Eriksen EF, Keeting PE. Identification of androgen receptors in normal human osteoblast-like cells. Proc Natl Acad Sci USA 1989;86:854–857.

38. Kasperk CH, Wergedal JE, Farley JR, Llinkhart TA, Turner RT, Baylink DG. Androgens directly stimulate proliferation of bone cells in vitro. Endocrinology 1989;124:1576–1578.

39. Nilas L, Christiansen C. Bone mass and its relationship to age and the menopause. J Clin Endocrinol Metab 1987;65:697–699.

40. Slemenda C, Longcope C, Peacock M, Hui S, Johnston CC. Sex steroids, bone mass, and bone loss. A propspective study of pre-, peri- and postmenopausal women. J Clin Invest 1996;97:14–21.

41. Simberg N, Titinen A, Silfrast A, Viinikka L, Ylikorkala O. High bone density in hyperandrogenic women: effect of gonadotropin-releasing hormone agonist alone or in conjunction with estrogen-proges-tin replacement. J Clin Endocrinol Metab 1995;81:646–651.

42. Heiss CJ, Sanborn CF, Nichols DL. Associations of body fat distribution, circulating sex hormones and bone density in postmenopausal women. J Clin Endocrinol Metab 1995;80:1591–1596.

43. Jassal SK, Barrett-Connor E, Edelstein S. Low bioavailable testosterone levels predict future height loss in postmenopausal women. J Bone Min Res 1995;10(4):650–653.

44. Davidson BJ, Ross RK, Paganni Hill A, et al. Total free estrogens and androgens in post menopausal women with hip fractures. J Clin Endocrinol Metab 1982;54:115–120.

45. Raisz LG, Wiita B, Artis A, et al. Comparison of the effects of estrogen alone and estrogen plus androgen on biochemical markers of bone formation and resoprtion in postmenopausal women. J Clin Endocrinol Metab 1995;81:37–43.

46. Watts NB, Notelovitz M, Timmons MC. Comparison of oral estrogens and estrogens plus androgen on bone mineral density, menopausal symptoms and lipid-lipoprotein profiles in surgical menopause. Obstet Gynecol 1995;85:529–537.

47. Savvas M, Studd JWW, Fogelman I, Dooley M, Montgomery J, Murby B. Skeletal effects of oral estrogen compared with subcutaneous oestrogen and testosterone in postmenopausal women. Br Med J 1988;297:331–333.

48. Savvas M, Studd JWW, Norman S, Leather AT, Garnett, TJ. Increase in bone mass after one year of percutaneous oestradiol and testosterone implants in post menopausal women who have previously received long-term oral oestrogens. Br J Obstet Gynaecol 1992;99:757–760.

49. Morishima A, Grumbach MM, Simpson ER. Aromatase deficiency in male and female siblings caused by a novel mutuation and the physiological role of estrogens. J Clin Endocrinol Metab 1995;80:3689–3698.

50. Smith EP, Boyd J, Frank GR, et al. Estrogen resistance caused by a mutation in the oestrogen-receptor gene in a man. N Engl J Med 1994;331:1056–1061.

51. Kasra M. Grynpas MD. The effects of androgens on the mechanical properties of primate bone. Bone 1995;17:265–270.

52. Nawata H. Tariaka S. Aromatase in bone cell: association with osteoporosis in post menopausal women. J Steroid Biochem Molec Biol 1995;53:165–174.

53. Taelman P, Kayman JM, Janssens X, Vermeulen A. Persistence of increased bone resorption and possible role of dehydroepiandrosterone as a bone metabolism determinant in osteoporotic women in late menopause. Maturitas 1989;11:65–73.

54. Nordin BEC, Robertson A, Seamark RF, et al. The relation between calcium absorption serum DHEA and vertebral mineral density in postmenopausal women. J Clin Endocrinol Metab 1985;60:651–657.

55. Morales AJ, Nolan JJ, Nelson JC, Yen SSC. Effects of replacement dose of dehydroepiandrosterone in men and women of advancing age. J Clin Endocrinol Metab 1994;78:1360–1367.

56. Abraham GE. Ovarian and adrenal contribution to peripheral androgens during the menstrual cycle. J Clin Endocrinol Metab 1974;39:340–346.

57. Engelson ES, Goggin KJ, Rabkin JG, Kotler DP. Nutrition and testosterone status of HIV positive women. Proceedings of the XI Inter Conf on AIDS Vancouver 1996;332:Po.Tu.B.2382.

58. Engelson ES, Rabkin JG, Rabkin R, Kotler DP. Effects of testosterone upon body composition [Letter]. J Acquir Immune Defic Syndr Hum Retrovirol 1996;11:510–511.

59. Darling GM, Johns JA, McCloud PI, Davis SR. A comparison of combined estrogen and progestin therapy with simvastatin on serum lipids in hypercholesterolemic postmenopausal women. N Engl J Med 1997;337:595–601.
60. Wakatsuki A, Sagara Y. Lipoprotein metabolism in postmenopausal and oophorestomized women. Obstet Gynecol 1995;85:523–528.
61. Hickok LR, Toomey C, Speroff L A comparison of esterified estrogens with and without methyltestosterone: Effects on endometrial histology and serum lipoproteins in postmenopausal women. Obstet Gynecol 1993;82:919–924.
62. Wagner JD, Zhang L, Williams JK, Register TC, Ackerman DM, Wiita B, Clarkson TB, Adams MR. Esterified estrogens with and without methyltesterone decrease arterial LDL metabolism in Cynomolgus monkeys. Arterioscler Thromb Vasc Biol 1996;16:1473–1479.
63. Barrett-Connor E, Goodman-Gruen D. Prospective study of endogenous sex hormones and fatal cardiovascular disease in postmenopausal women. BMJ 1995;311:1193–1196.
64. Barrett-Connor E, Goodman-Gruen D. Dehydroepiandrosterone sulfate does not predict cardiovascular death in postmenopausal women. The Rancho Bernardo Study. Circulation 1995;91:1757–1760.
65. Chou TM, Sudhir K, Hutchison SJ, Ko E, Amidon TM, Collins P, Chatterjee K. Testosterone induces dilation of canine coronary conductance and resistance arteries in vivo. Circulation 1996;94:2614–2619.
66. Honore EK, Williams JK, Adams MR, Ackerman DM, Wagner JD. Methyltestosterone does not diminish the beneficial effects of estrogen replacement therapy on coronary arter reactivity in cynomolgus monkeys. Menopause: J North Am Menopause Soc 1996;3:20–26.
67. Secreto G, Toniolo P, Pisani P, et al. Androgens and breast cancer in premenopausal women. Cancer Res 1989;49:471–476.
68. Secreto G, Toniolo P, Berrino E, et al. Serum and urinary androgens and risk of breast cancer in postmenopausal women. Cancer Res 1991;51:2572–2576.
69. Berrino F, Muti P, Michelli A, Bolelli G, Krogh V, Sciajno R, Pisani P, Panico S, Secreto G. Serum sex hormone levels after menopause and subsequent breast cancer. J Natl Cancer Inst 1996;88:291–296.
70. Recchione C, Venturelli E, Manzari A, Cavalteri A, Martinetti A, Secreto G. Testosterone, dihydrotestosterone and oestradiol levels in postmenopausal breast cancer tissues. J Steroid Biochem Mol Biol 1995;52:541–546.
71. Bryan RM, Mercer RJ, Rennie GC, Lie TH, Morgan FJ. Androgen receptors in breast cancer. Cancer 1984;54:2436–2440.
72. Barrett-Connor E, Timmons MC, Young R, Wiita B, Estratest Working Group. Interim safety analysis of a two-year study comparing oral estrogen-androgen and conjugated estrogens in surgically menopausal women. J Women's Health 1996;5:593–602.

INDEX

DATE DUE

SEP 1 8 2000		
SEP 1 3 2000		
FEB 2 1 2003		
DEC 0 3 2003		
SEP 0 8 2011		

Demco, Inc. 38-293